PED
CLERKSHIP GUIDE

PEDIATRIC CLERKSHIP GUIDE

Second Edition

Jerold C. Woodhead, MD

Associate Professor
University of Iowa Carver College of Medicine
Director of Medical Student Education
Department of Pediatrics
University of Iowa Children's Hospital
Iowa City, Iowa

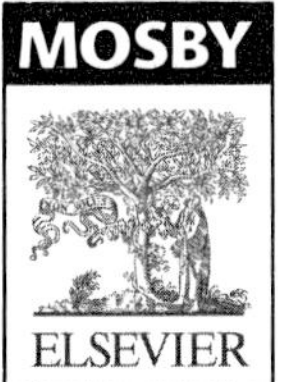

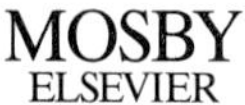

1600 John F. Kennedy Blvd.
Ste 1800
Philadelphia, PA 19103-2899

PEDIATRIC CLERKSHIP GUIDE ISBN: 978-0-323-04333-5

Notice

Knowledge and best practice in this field are constantly changing. As new research and experience broaden our knowledge, changes in practice, treatment and drug therapy may become necessary or appropriate. Readers are advised to check the most current information provided (i) on procedures featured or (ii) by the manufacturer of each product to be administered, to verify the recommended dose or formula, the method and duration of administration, and contraindications. It is the responsibility of the practitioner, relying on their own experience and knowledge of the patient, to make diagnoses, to determine dosages and the best treatment for each individual patient, and to take all appropriate safety precautions. To the fullest extent of the law, neither the Publisher nor the Editor assumes any liability for any injury and/or damage to persons or property arising out or related to any use of the material contained in this book.

The Publisher

Library of Congress Cataloging-in-Publication Data

Pediatric clerkship guide / [edited by] Jerold C. Woodhead. — 2nd ed.
p. ; cm.
Rev ed. of: Pediatric clerkship guide / [edited by] Jerold C. Woodhead. c2003.
Includes bibliographical references and index.
ISBN 978-0-323-04333-5
1. Pediatrics. 2. Clinical clerkship. I. Woodhead, Jerold C. II. Pediatric clerkship guide.
[DNLM: 1. Clinical Clerkship. 2. Pediatrics–Case Reports. 3. Pediatrics–Problems and Exercises. WS 100 P37025 2008]
RJ47.P363 2008
618.9200076—dc22

2007019389

Acquisitions Editor: James Merritt
Developmental Editor: Nicole DiCicco
Project Manager: Mary Stermel
Design Direction: Louis Forgione
Marketing Manager: Allan McKeown

Printed in the United States of America
Last digit is the print number: 9 8 7 6 5 4 3 2 1

To the memory of Steven Z. Miller and Richard Sarkin.
Their commitment to medical student education in pediatrics
and to humanism as a core professional trait
inspired all of us to be better teachers,
physicians, and human beings.
To all my family, and in memory of my parents.

Contributors

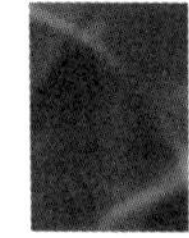

Paula Algranati, MD
Professor of Pediatrics
Director of Pediatric Medical Student Education
University of Connecticut School of Medicine
Farmington, Connecticut

Roger Berkow, MD
Professor and Vice-Chair
Department of Pediatrics
Associate Dean for Undergraduate Medical Education
University of Alabama at Birmingham School of Medicine
Pediatric Hematology/Oncology
The Children's Hospital of Alabama
University of Alabama, Birmingham
Birmingham, Alabama

Norman B. Berman, MD
Dartmouth-Hitchcock Medical Center
Lebanon, New Hampshire
Associate Professor of Pediatrics
Dartmouth Medical School
Hanover, New Hampshire

Warren P. Bishop, MD
Director, Division of Gastroenterology
Associate Professor
Department of Pediatrics
University of Iowa Children's Hospital
Iowa City, Iowa

Lavjay Butani, MD
Associate Professor and Section Chief
Pediatric Nephrology
University of California Davis Medical Center
Sacramento, California

Ken Cheyne, MD
Director of Pediatric Education
Blank Children's Hospital
Des Moines, Iowa

Cindy W. Christian, MD
Chair, Child Abuse and Neglect Prevention
The Children's Hospital of Philadelphia
Associate Professor of Pediatrics
The University of Pennsylvania School of Medicine
Philadelphia, Pennsylvania

Linda J. Cooper-Brown, PhD
Clinical Assistant Professor of Pediatrics
Division of Pediatric Psychology
University of Iowa Children's Hospital
Iowa City, Iowa

Robin R. Deterding, MD
Associate Professor and Director
Medical Student Education in Pediatrics
Department of Pediatrics
University of Colorado School of Medicine
The Children's Hospital
Denver, Colorado

Leslie H. Fall, MD
Associate Professor and Vice Chair for Education
Department of Pediatrics
Dartmouth Medical School
Children's Hospital at Dartmouth
Dartmouth-Hitchcock Medical Center
Lebanon, New Hampshire

Michael Giuliano, MD, MEd
Associate Clinical Professor of Pediatrics
Director, Cognitive Reasoning Program
State University of New York at Downstate
Brooklyn, New York
Director–NICU
Sanzari Children's Hospital
Hackensack University Medical Center
Hackensack, New Jersey

Janice L. Hanson, PhD, EdS
Assistant Professor of Medicine, Pediatrics, and Family Medicine
Uniformed Services University of the Health Sciences
Bethesda, Maryland

Adam Hartman, MD
Assistant Professor, Neurology
Pediatric Epilepsy and Child Neurology
Johns Hopkins Hospital
Baltimore, Maryland

Charles A. Jennissen, MD
Director of Pediatric Emergency Medicine
Clinical Associate Professor
Department of Emergency Medicine
University of Iowa Hospitals and Clinics
Iowa City, Iowa

Nicholas Jospe, MD
Professor of Pediatrics
Chief, Division of Pediatric Endocrinology
Golisano Children's Hospital at Strong
University of Rochester
Rochester, New York

Adam B. Kanis, MD, PhD
MAJ, US Army, MC
Chief, Medical Genetics
Tripler Army Medical Center
Department of Pediatrics
Honolulu, Hawaii

Kim M. Keppler-Noreuil, MD
Clinical Associate Professor of Pediatrics
Division of Medical Genetics
Clinical Director for Birth Defects, Iowa Registry for Congenital and Inherited Disorders
Program Director, Medical Genetics Residency Program
University of Iowa Children's Hospital
Iowa City, Iowa

Daniel P. Krowchuk, MD
Chief, General Pediatrics and Adolescent Medicine
Department of Pediatrics
Wake Forest University School of Medicine
Winston-Salem, North Carolina

Michael R. Lawless, MD
Professor
General Pediatrics and Adolescent Medicine
Wake Forest University School of Medicine
Winston-Salem, North Carolina

Anne Lyren, MD, MSc
Director, Rainbow Center for Pediatric Ethics
Rainbow Babies and Children's Hospital
Assistant Professor of Pediatrics and Bioethics
Case Western Reserve University School of Medicine
Cleveland, Ohio

Dianne M. McBrien, MD
Clinical Associate Professor of Pediatrics
Division of Developmental and Behavioral Medicine
University of Iowa Children's Hospital
Iowa City, Iowa

Stacey McConkey, MD
Clinical Assistant Professor of Pediatrics
Director, Division of Developmental and Behavioral Pediatrics
Program Director, Pediatric Residency Program
University of Iowa Children's Hospital
Iowa City, Iowa

†Steven Z. Miller, MD
A.P. Gold Associate Professor of Clinical Pediatrics
Director, Pediatric Medical Student Education
Columbia University College of Physicians and Surgeons
Director, Pediatric Emergency Medicine
Children's Hospital of New York–Presbyterian
New York, New York

Bruce Z. Morgenstern, MD
Professor of Clinical Pediatrics
University of Arizona College of Medicine
Associate Professor of Pediatrics and Adolescent Medicine
May Clinic College of Medicine
Chief, Division of Nephrology
Phoenix Children's Hospital
Phoenix, Arizona

Mary C. Ottolini, MD, MPH
Director of Pediatric Medical Student Education
Division Chief, Hospitalist Division
Professor of Pediatrics
Children's National Medical Center and
George Washington University School of Medicine
Washington, District of Columbia

Dinesh S. Pashankar, MD
Associate Professor of Pediatrics (Clinical)
Division of Pediatric Gastroenterology
Yale University School of Medicine
New Haven, Connecticut

Virginia F. Randall, MD, MPH
COL MC USA (Ret.)
Associate Professor of Pediatrics
Department of Pediatrics
Uniformed Services University of the Health Sciences
Bethesda, Maryland

†Deceased.

William V. Raszka, MD
Associate Professor of Pediatrics
Department of Pediatrics
University of Vermont College of Medicine
Given Building
Burlington, Vermont

Benjamin S. Siegel, MD
Professor of Pediatrics and Psychiatry
Director of Medical Student Education in Pediatrics
Boston University School of Medicine
Boston, Massachusetts

Timothy D. Starner, MD
Assistant Professor
Department of Pediatrics
University of Iowa Children's Hospital
Iowa City, Iowa

Jerold C. Woodhead, MD
Associate Professor
University of Iowa Carver College of Medicine
Director of Medical Student Education
Department of Pediatrics
University of Iowa Children's Hospital
Iowa City, Iowa

Preface

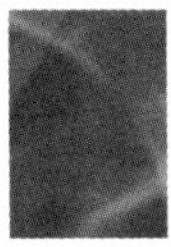

Pediatric Clerkship Guide is a resource for third-year medical students. Written by pediatric clerkship directors and other experienced pediatric educators, the guide is based on the *General Pediatric Clerkship Curriculum* developed by the Council on Medical Student Education in Pediatrics (COMSEP) and used in more than 90% of medical schools in the United States. Although specifically aimed toward medical students, the guide can assist anyone who wishes to learn the basics of health care for children.

Pediatric Clerkship Guide addresses questions that commonly arise when working with infants, children, and adolescents, whether healthy or ill. The initial section of the guide emphasizes the unique features of pediatric patients from the newborn to the adolescent. It stresses pediatric-specific clinical skills, including the interview, the physical examination, and the assessment of development. This initial section also describes key concepts, including growth, behavior, development, prevention, health promotion, interaction with patients and families, ethics, evidence-based medicine, and many other topics. The second section addresses common symptoms, physical findings, and abnormal laboratory results. The final section discusses known conditions.

Each chapter has been revised and updated. Key points focus on important concepts. Clinical cases accompany each chapter to serve as stimuli for self-directed learning; detailed explanations accompany each case. A multiple-choice practice examination based on the key concepts helps students assess mastery of the material. Explanations of the correct answers have been added as a new feature of the second edition. Updated print and electronic resources provide assistance for additional self-directed study.

Jerold C. Woodhead, MD

Acknowledgments

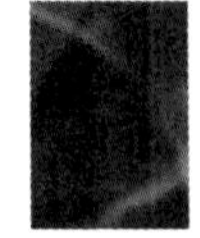

I am indebted to my patients and their families, who have taught me what it means to be a pediatrician. I especially wish to acknowledge the mentors who have guided me throughout my career, including Cathy DeAngelis, Sam Fomon, Fred Smith, and Frank Morriss. My colleagues in the Council on Medical Student Education in Pediatrics (COMSEP) deserve recognition for the innovations they have brought to the education process, their enthusiasm as teachers, and their dedication to medical students. As an organization, COMSEP has had a huge impact on pediatric medical education. The content of this book mirrors the COMSEP *General Pediatric Clerkship Curriculum,* the gold standard for education about pediatrics.

I am grateful to my co-authors for contributing to this book. Each author is an expert in her or his area, most are clerkship directors, and all are active, dedicated teachers of medical students.

Medical students also must be recognized as important contributors to this book because their needs as learners triggered its development. Over the years, students have taught me how to teach. They continue to challenge me daily to be an informed, informative teacher.

The first edition was the product of a career development award in 2001, during which I had an appointment as a scholar at the Obermann Center for Advanced Studies at the University of Iowa. Time to develop the second edition was carved out of clinical and teaching obligations. The support, encouragement, and expertise of Jim Merritt and Nicole DiCicco at Elsevier made the second edition possible.

Contents

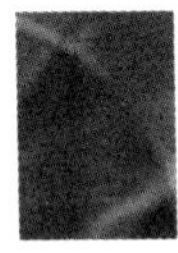

Section 1
Introduction to the Pediatric Clerkship 1

†Deceased.

†Deceased.

Section 1

Introduction to the Pediatric Clerkship

1

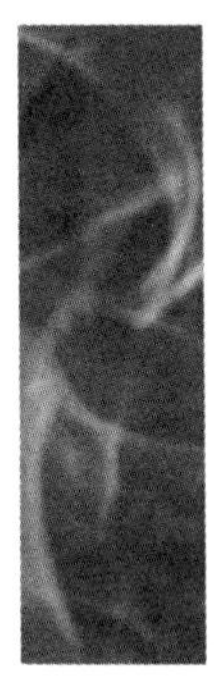

The Pediatric Clerkship

JEROLD C. WOODHEAD

What Does the Pediatric Clerkship Emphasize?

The pediatric clerkship emphasizes human growth and development, common clinical problems, uncommon but important disease processes, prevention of illness, and promotion of health. You will participate in clinical activities that take place in outpatient and inpatient services and that are supervised by both general pediatricians and subspecialists. Many clerkships also provide the opportunity to work with community-based pediatricians in practices outside the medical center. More than 90% of the pediatric clerkships in the United States are based on the Council on Medical Student Education in Pediatrics (COMSEP) *General Pediatric Clerkship Curriculum* (http://comsep.org). This book is also based on that curriculum.

How Should I Approach the Pediatric Clerkship?

Your career plans may not include a primary focus on children, but you are likely to use skills that you gain from the pediatric clerkship to interact with ill and healthy children in both your professional and personal lives. Enthusiasm, a commitment to learning, and dedication to the well-being of your patients will be crucial to your success. Time and perseverance will provide the experiences that will eventually help you achieve competency beyond your initial expectations. If you make the effort, you will develop an ability to interact successfully with infants, children, and adolescents (and their parents).

How Should I Assess My Readiness for the Clerkship?

At the start of the clerkship, take an inventory of your competency with the basic medical interview, the general physical examination, and clinical decision making, because these are the foundations for pediatric-focused skills. "Real world" experiences with healthy children, such as being a baby-sitter, lifeguard, coach, camp counselor, teacher, sibling, aunt, uncle, or parent, will give you a perspective on the patients and families with whom you will work. Clinically focused experiences with children (e.g., as an emergency medical technician or a laboratory technician) will complement the clinical skills that you will be expected to master in the clerkship. Use the clerkship objectives and a table of core clinical experiences (such as the one in Table 1-1) to make a self-assessment of your pediatric-specific knowledge and your experiences with pediatric clinical problems (e.g., none, some, a lot).

How Can I Learn Most Effectively on the Clerkship?

This text and others can assist you to expand knowledge. A list of core pediatric experiences such as the one developed by COMSEP (Table 1-1) can be used to ensure that your clinical encounters are comprehensive. Your clerkship is likely to have a specific list of core experiences in the handbook or on the Web site. The Computer-assisted Learning in Pediatrics Program (CLIPP: http://clippcases.org) is based on the COMSEP *Curriculum* and provides Web-based virtual clinical experiences to aid learning and to supplement clinical encounters.

What Clinical Skills Are the Most Difficult to Master?

To some extent, the challenges that you will face depend on your prior experiences with children and their medical care. Almost all medical students have at least some anxiety about examining children, especially newborns and toddlers. Often, students worry that they will be "exposed" as lacking in experience or ability, even if they feel quite confident about their clinical skills with adults. Many students express concern that they might frighten or hurt a young child because they lack experience with examination techniques. To adapt your skills to young patients, you may find it necessary to relearn the medical interview and the physical examination. Vital signs, laboratory tests, and imaging studies also must be interpreted taking age and development into account. Many of the reference ("normal") values for children depend on variables such as gestational age, size, muscle mass, and pubertal stage. Do not accept "normal" without checking its relevance to your specific patient.

What Resources Should I Have on Hand?

The clerkship director will likely provide suggestions for reading and also may have developed a clerkship Web site with links to good review articles and reputable print and electronic resources. Your medical library may provide access to MDConsult, Access Medicine, InformationRetriever, and a MEDLINE search engine such as Ovid, PubMed, or Grateful Med. General medical journals such as the *New England Journal of Medicine* and *JAMA* often have review articles about pediatric topics. Table 1-2 lists a sample of pediatric journals and online resources. You will benefit from access to a compendium of child-specific information, such as *The Harriet Lane Handbook* and the *Red Book* of the American Academy of Pediatrics, both of which are available in print and electronic versions. Handheld devices can provide access to many resources, including medication compendia, growth

Table 1-1

Core Pediatric Clinical Experiences

Core Experience	Site*	Patients or Examples of Symptoms, Concerns, or Diagnosis	Task†	CLIPP Cases‡
Health maintenance (well-child care)	N, O	Newborn (0–1 mo)	O P F	1
	O	Infant (1–12 mo)	O P F	2
	O	Toddler-preschool (1–5 yr)	O P F	3
	O	School-age (5–12 yr)	O P F	4
	O	Adolescent (13–19 yr)	O P F	5, 6
Growth concerns or abnormalities	I, O	Obesity, short stature, poor weight gain	P F	4, 18, 26
Nutrition concerns or abnormalities	I, O	Breast versus *formula, infant feeding, anemia, overweight*	P F	26
Development concerns or abnormalities	I, O	Language, gross motor, fine motor, or social	P F	28, 29
Behavior concerns or abnormalities	O	Sleep, colic, tantrums, toilet training, enuresis, ADHD, encopresis, school	P F	3, 4
Upper respiratory (sore throat, ear pain)	I, O	Pharyngitis, strep throat, URI, allergic rhinitis, otitis media, sinusitis, lymphadenopathy	F	11, 14
Lower respiratory (cough, wheeze)	I, O, E	Asthma, bronchiolitis, pneumonia, aspiration,	F	12, 13, 25
Gastrointestinal (nausea, vomiting, diarrhea, pain)	I, O, E	Gastroenteritis, pyloric stenosis, appendicitis, GE reflux, GERD	F	15, 16, 22, 27
Dermatology (rash, pallor)	I, O, E	Viral rash, eczema, urticaria, seborrhea, acne, anemia	P F	3, 21

(continued)

Table 1-1

Core Pediatric Clinical Experiences (Continued)

Core Experience	Site*	Patients or Examples of Symptoms, Concerns, or Diagnosis	Task†	CLIPP Cases‡
Neurologic	I, O, E	Headache, concussion, seizures, ataxia, meningitis, weakness	P F	9, 20, 24, 28, 29
Musculoskeletal (limp, pain, trauma)	I, O, E	Fracture, infection, inflammation, overuse	P F	17
Emergency	I, O, E	Respiratory distress, shock, seizures, airway obstruction, apnea, suicide, trauma, abuse	O P F	7, 23, 24, 25
Fever (with or without source)	I, O, E	Serious bacterial illness, UTI, influenza	O P F	10
Neonatal jaundice	N, I, O	Physiologic, biliary atresia, hemolysis	O P F	8
Chronic or special healthcare problems	I, O	CP, seizures, CF, asthma	O P F	8, 18, 26, 29, 30, 31

Adapted from COMSEP: http://comsep.org.

ADHD, Attention deficit hyperactivity disorder; CF, cystic fibrosis; CP, cerebral palsy; GE, gastroesophageal; GERD, gastroesophageal reflux disease; URI, upper respiratory infection; UTI, urinary tract infection.

*N, Nursery; O, outpatient; I, inpatient; E, emergency department.

†O, Observe (clinical reasoning); P, partial (history or physical examination); F, full (history, physical examination, and clinical reasoning).

‡CLIPP: http://clippcases.org.

Table 1-2

Pediatric Resources

Journals	*Ambulatory Pediatrics*
	Archives of Pediatrics and Adolescent Medicine
	Journal of Adolescent Health Care
	Journal of Pediatrics
	Pediatrics
	Pediatric Clinics of North America
	Pediatrics in Review
Online resources	CLIPP: http://clippcases.org
	GeneralPediatrics.com: www.generalpediatrics.com
	NIH Clinical Center: www.cc.nih.gov
	Normal range of resting values by age
	Pediatric blood pressure charts
	Pedicases: www.pedicases.org/
	PediatricEducation.org: www.pediatriceducation.org/
	Virtual Pediatric Hospital: www.virtualpediatrichospital.org
Information	*The Harriet Lane Handbook,* ed 17, Elsevier/Mosby, 2005
	AAP Red Book, ed 27, American Academy of Pediatrics, 2006

Table 1-3

Software for Handheld Devices

Type of Information Available	Title of Software	Web Address
General information	Pediatrics on Hand	www.pediatricsonhand.com/
Normative data	Riley Kidometer	http://kidometer.com
Drug compendia	ePocrates Rx	http://epocrates.com
	Pediatrics Lexi-Drugs	http://store.lexi.com
Growth charts	STAT Growth-BP	http://statcoder.com
Immunization schedules	Shots 2007	http://immunizationed.org

charts, immunization schedules, and many texts (Table 1-3). Numerous Web sites provide medical resources for handheld devices, both free and commercial. Some medical centers have placed formularies, laboratory data, and other resources into electronic databases that are accessible by computer or can be downloaded into handheld devices.

KEY POINTS

- Assess all of your experiences with children as you prepare for the pediatric clerkship.
- Focus your learning efforts on child development.
- Use the checklist of core pediatric clinical experiences.
- Be familiar with pediatric print and electronic resources.

2

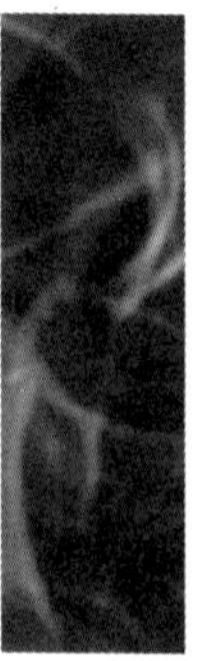

Inpatient Service

JEROLD C. WOODHEAD

What Will Help Me Be Successful on the Inpatient Service?

Your inpatient experience may be on a general pediatrics service, where patients span the age range from birth through late adolescence and manifest many different diseases and disorders. You may also spend time on a specialty service devoted to patients with specific disorders such as cardiac disease, malignancy, or gastrointestinal problems. The inpatient service occasionally may be limited to a specific age group, such as newborn infants or adolescents. In all instances, you should engage yourself with the activities of the specific service and take every opportunity to develop pediatric-specific skills in the interview and physical examination, as well as in clinical reasoning and communication. As you watch experienced clinicians work with patients and families, ask them to "think out loud" so that you may learn how they approach clinical problems and use clinical reasoning. Ask faculty and residents to observe you and give you feedback about your medical interview and physical examination skills. Request feedback about your write-ups and case presentations. Challenge yourself to make commitments about the differential diagnosis, to think critically about the evaluation process, and to develop a plan for the initial treatment of each patient. If your diagnosis, evaluation, and/or management do not match those of the resident and faculty physicians, challenge yourself to find out why. Do not expect your skills to be perfect, but strive to improve them. The list of key clinical experiences in Chapter 1 can assist you to organize your inpatient rotation.

What Is My Role on an Inpatient Service?

Your major job is to become a competent clinician. The clerkship is your opportunity to develop the basic skills that will be the foundation of your future clinical education and practice. To do this, you must be an active member of the team, not just a scribe, data collector, or "gofer." As one of a small number of students on the service, you will be highly visible, and your enthusiasm, participation, and motivation will be noted. On busy services, you will have a key role in day-to-day patient management, but if you wait to be "invited" to work up patients, you may be overlooked (or worse, viewed as uninterested). Above all, keep your eyes and ears open: You may be the only one to identify a key finding. You may be the communication link between the patient/family and the team, so talk regularly with your patients and their families, but do not attempt to give information that is beyond your level of experience and knowledge. You may be asked to discuss clinical progress with a patient and family, but a resident or staff physician will usually supervise this closely. You will often be asked to bring information from the literature to the team about specific diagnostic or management issues. The discussion on evidence-based medicine (Chapter 7) will assist with these assignments.

How Should I Present Cases?

An organized, concise presentation includes a description of the patient; a list of the relevant findings from the history, physical examination, and laboratory evaluation; and an outline of the plan for diagnosis and management. The details needed for work rounds with residents may differ importantly from those that you will provide for the attending physician. If you organize your thoughts and emphasize the key points, even the most complex case can be presented in less than 5 minutes. In almost all cases it will be acceptable to use notes when you give your presentation, but it makes sense to inquire in advance. *Practice* your case presentations before you make them. Keep flow charts of vital signs, laboratory data, and other crucial information so that the inevitable question from the attending will not require flipping through many pages of notes. Also have the immunization record and growth charts at hand so that you can refer to them if questions arise. A family pedigree often greatly aids the case presentation. Be sure to indicate who provided the information: the parent/guardian or the patient.

What Must Be Included in the Presentation?

Ask in advance about an attending's preferences for the format of patient presentations. Some physicians want details for the entire examination, whereas others want to hear only about the "important" positive and negative findings. For all case presentations in pediatrics you should include information about the patient's general appearance, age, developmental level, growth measurements, and vital signs. This allows the attending physician to develop an initial impression while you present details of the history and physical examination findings. To make the most efficient use of your time, you may decide to abbreviate information that is not immediately relevant to your case presentation; state that details are available if needed. If you decide to use terms such as "normal" or "unremarkable," be prepared to describe the physical findings that justify such a label if challenged. On many inpatient services, specific information will be needed for every patient daily; ask residents and attending physicians about the critical content for presentations.

What Clinical Notes Will I Write on Pediatric Services?

In general, the notes that you write on the pediatric services are similar to those for other services, with the addition of age-specific details such as birth history, immunization status, growth and development, and personal habits and behaviors. The Subjective, Objective, Assessment, Plan (SOAP) format is used commonly in all medical centers. You may use an electronic medical record with center-specific characteristics. Although each clerkship will have specific requirements, medical student notes generally include the following types:

- Admission note: The complete history, physical examination, problem list, differential diagnosis, and management plan.
- Progress note: A daily summary of the patient's problems and change in status, plus review of diagnostic and management issues.
- On-service note: A summary of the patient up to the time you joined the team. This note helps you learn about the patient.
- Discharge note: A summary of the hospital course, a list of final diagnoses, and the discharge plan.
- Off-service note: A summary of a patient remaining in hospital after the team changes. This note assists the next medical student.

KEY POINTS

- Participate actively.
- Read about your patient's problems.
- Practice case presentations.
- Ask for feedback about clinical notes and overall performance.

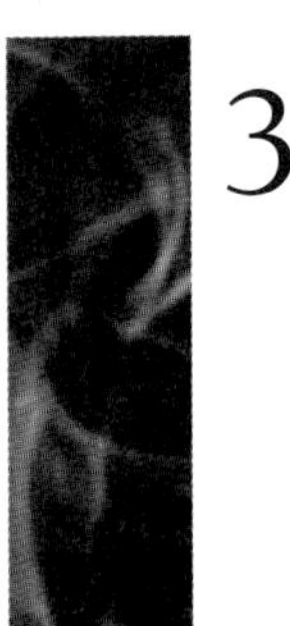

3 Outpatient Service

JEROLD C. WOODHEAD

How Should I Approach the Outpatient Service?

Your clerkship will likely have about half of its clinical activities in outpatient clinics or physician offices. Your outpatient experiences may range from general pediatrics to subspecialty services. Clinical activities may include health supervision, assessment of common pediatric illnesses, interval visits for patients with chronic conditions, management of children with special healthcare needs, and the diagnosis and management of patients with uncommon diseases and disorders. Each different clinic or outpatient activity may have its own specific approach, so you need to ask about the expectations for your participation. Be prepared, and you will find it easier to fit into the routine. At the medical center, ask a resident or faculty attending about the best way to approach patients. Each community practice will have a specific approach for patient management, so be certain to ask about expectations for your participation. Nurses and other clinic or office staff may be your best resources for practical information. Remember to seek feedback about your skills and knowledge, and then act on the recommendations. In addition, use the clinical problems presented by your patients as triggers for daily learning. The list of key clinical experiences in Chapter 1 can assist you to organize your outpatient rotation.

How Do I Manage Time in the Clinic or Office?

Time represents the most challenging aspect of outpatient rotations, especially in general pediatric clinics and pediatric office practices, because there never seems to be enough of it. Before you enter the examination room, make certain that you have a good understanding of the time allotted for your interaction with the patient. Although you may not have seen the patient before, you are likely to find documentation of the patient's previous visits to the office or clinic in the medical record. Review of the medical record will provide key information about the patient and family and may help you clarify the presenting complaint. You will need to focus your medical interview and physical examination on the specific problem because of the limited time available. When faced with multiple problems or complaints, you will find it necessary to prioritize and address only those that require immediate attention. This poses the challenge of deciding which problem is the *most* important, something that you may find difficult. Your ability to manage your time will improve with experience, just as will your ability to prioritize problems and to give efficient case presentations.

What Is a Focused Evaluation?

A focused evaluation is an assessment that emphasizes the specific concerns raised by the patient or family, with enough detail to allow identification of related problems. You will learn to interpret patient concerns, perform the relevant physical examination, and explain your findings. For example, a cough may suggest pneumonia as the only possible cause to a family. You, on the other hand, would search for many possible causes based on the cough's character, duration, triggers, and associated findings (fever, chest pain, wheeze). You would also factor in the patient's exposures, immunizations, and previous problems. Similarly, an adolescent with a chronic headache may express concern about a brain tumor, but the headache's chronicity, characteristics, and location, plus the physical examination of the head, neck, eyes, and neurologic systems, may suggest migraine or "tension" as a cause. As another example, a child with chronic diarrhea and growth below the range expected for age and family patterns may ultimately be found to have a malabsorption syndrome. The initial focused office visit will almost always require follow-up for further assessment, ongoing management, and education. You should request the opportunity to participate in the follow-up visit, if possible.

How Do I Present a Case in the Outpatient Setting?

The format and content of case presentations in the outpatient setting vary, depending on the reason for the outpatient visit. All presentations should be concise, organized, and focused on the clinical problem. Most outpatient presentations will be more concise than those on inpatient services. Always provide a brief overview of the patient's general condition, age, development, growth, and vital signs. In addition, report details of the history and physical examination so that the supervising physician will know what to look for. At the conclusion, list the clinical problem(s), commit yourself to a relevant differential diagnosis, and suggest an initial evaluation plan. Do not be afraid to "stick your neck out" if you have data to support your recommendations. Types of clinic visits and appropriate case presentations include:

- *Health supervision* (Chapter 11): This visit emphasizes the whole child, including developmental progress, nutrition, health promotion, prevention of illness and disability, and family issues. Your case presentation must address the "chief complaint of health" and contain enough information to allow the attending physician to help you provide anticipatory guidance.

- *Acute care*: This visit will likely focus on a symptom complex or problem. Your presentation will emphasize that problem and must include relevant past history, environmental exposures, family history, and the appropriate details of the focused physical examination.
- *Chronic illness or special healthcare needs* (Chapter 16): Interval visits for management of chronic illness or special needs have varying goals, depending on the nature of the patient's problem. You will need to inquire about the appropriate format for presenting case material in such settings.
- *Uncommon disorders in "diagnostic" or specialty clinics*: The patient may present a diagnostic dilemma. The evaluation will reflect the complexity of the problem, and the case presentation will resemble that for an inpatient admission. You should clarify in advance the expectations for your involvement with such patients.

What Notes Will I Write in Clinics?

Notes may be handwritten or entered into an electronic medical record. As with the inpatient service, the SOAP format is generally used. The extent of the information required will depend on the nature of the visit, as discussed previously.

KEY POINTS

- ◆ Time is often your biggest challenge, so focus on the patient's specific problems.
- ◆ Case presentations and clinical notes should be concise and include details appropriate to the type of clinic visit.
- ◆ Assign yourself a learning issue each day based on the patients that you have evaluated.

4

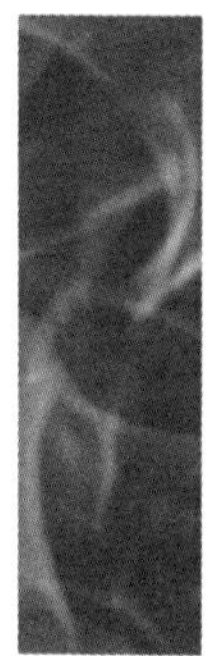

Approach to the Pediatric Patient

JEROLD C. WOODHEAD

How Do I Approach the Pediatric Patient?

Evaluation in pediatrics requires attention to development. Some patients may be unable or unwilling to cooperate, including nonverbal infants, anxious toddlers, and adolescents who are complex and protective of their privacy. The sequence, structure, and content of the interview; the optimal approach to verbal and physical interactions; and the focus of the physical examination all depend on the age and developmental stage of the patient and the reason for the evaluation. If you are aware of development, you will be able to anticipate patient responses and interpret findings. Information specific to newborn infants is found in Chapters 14 and 67; for more about adolescents, see Chapters 15, 18, and 54. Development is discussed in Chapter 9.

How Do I Begin?

Be aware of your previous experiences, current abilities, and anxieties so that you can make the best decisions during the interview and physical examination. *Ask for assistance* when performing an evaluation for the first time or whenever you have questions. *Anticipate* developmentally appropriate behaviors and reactions. *Think about your impact* on a child or adolescent: A loud voice, cold hands, and abrupt movements are likely to trigger crying and withdrawal by young patients; failure to recognize emerging independence may shut off information from an adolescent. *Watch* experienced clinicians interact with and examine patients of different ages and developmental stages. *Listen* as parents tell you about their children and adolescents. *Engage parents* as your allies to explain or interpret your questions and actions, reassure and calm children, and restrain them if necessary. Keep the parents involved when you evaluate older children and adolescents, but remember to pay attention to confidentiality, privacy, emerging maturity, and autonomy. *Ask questions directly* of children and adolescents and *listen* to what they have to say. *Be gentle, efficient,* and *persistent* during the examination, but also *be realistic*: When patients do not cooperate sufficiently to allow you to examine them, let the resident or faculty physician complete that part of the examination. On the other hand, do not "throw in the towel" too soon.

How Do I Incorporate Development into the Evaluation?

A basic understanding of development can be gained from your personal experiences and from Chapter 9. Do not make assumptions. Instead, use history, observations, and physical findings to guide your assessment of an individual's development. Careful observation of your patient will allow you to compare developmental progress with the milestones highlighted in resources such as the *Denver Developmental Assessment* (Denver II) (Figure 9-1). The *Bright Futures Pocket Guide* (www.brightfutures.org/pocket/) helps you develop a developmentally appropriate approach to patients, especially with regard to the information you provide to parents about healthy children.

How Does the Age of the Child Influence My Approach?

Understanding the dynamic process of growth, development, socialization, and maturation will allow you to plan your interview and examination. Your interactions with a child and parent will vary depending on the patient's age, the parent's experience, and the reason for the visit. As the human grows, body size increases dramatically, physiologic processes mature, cognition and behavior develop, and relationships mature and change. Parents, other family members, and the community all influence the growing child. In addition, risk factors, exposures, and disease processes change from home, to daycare, to school, and ultimately to the wider world as the adolescent gains independence and mobility. The content of health supervision visits at different ages is discussed in Chapter 11.

How Should I Approach Newborns and Young Infants?

Newborns and young infants (birth to 9 months) prefer a sleeping or quiet, alert state, so speak softly to avoid frightening an infant. The responses of the infant to your presence, to verbal interactions, and to games such as peek-a-boo can help you understand developmental progress. Before you touch the infant, wash your hands, wipe your stethoscope, and warm them both. When you do touch the infant, use gentle, gradual, rocking motions. Take advantage of the sucking reflex by using a pacifier or a gloved finger to calm an infant. Be thorough but gentle with the examination (Table 5-1). Review measurements and the pattern of growth. Listen carefully to the heart for new murmurs. Observe movements and motor skills, and assess development. Perform potentially uncomfortable maneuvers last (e.g., ear examination, Ortolani and Barlow maneuvers, Moro reflex). As discussed in Chapters 11 and 15, you must be prepared to answer many questions and provide anticipatory guidance, as parents need reassurance that they are doing the right things for their infants.

How Should I Approach Older Infants and Toddlers?

Older infants and toddlers (9 months to 3 years) usually demonstrate stranger anxiety and fear of separation from parents, beginning at about 9 months and peaking about 18 to 24 months. A calm, measured approach works best. You may need to avoid direct communication or even eye contact with a toddler until the child "warms up" to you. Sit down and speak softly to the parent, and let the child "invite" you to make direct contact. The interview must focus on the specific reasons for the visit, but health supervision (Chapter 11) will always emphasize *developmental* progress, *risks* associated with increasing mobility and independence, *exposures* to illness at home or in daycare, *immunization* status, *behaviors* such as tantrums and negativity, and *nutrition*. When you start the physical examination, look before you touch! Anything that you accomplish from a distance reduces the likelihood that an infant or toddler will "erupt," making the rest of the examination difficult if not impossible. The physical examination of a child from 15 to 36 months is usually most successful when the toddler sits on the parent's lap, with restraint provided by the parent as needed. Observe motor skills and social behaviors that signal developmental progress. Listen to language. Look for clues about illness. Most of the neurologic examination of a healthy toddler can be done by observation: language, symmetry, gait, balance, fine motor skills, and strength. Sometimes a flashlight or finger puppet can distract a child enough to allow completion of the examination. Do not hesitate to sit down on the floor with a toddler to perform parts of the examination.

How Should I Approach Young School-Age Children?

Preschool and early-school-age children (4 to 8 years) are less anxious about the doctor's office than toddlers, unless they are ill or anticipate an immunization. Children appreciate being spoken to directly and can provide information about friends, school, food, music, physical activity and sports, as well as observations and worries about illness. Parents can corroborate or correct details of the history and are generally good observers of their child's illness or developmental progress. Acknowledge a child's emerging autonomy and independence by offering options (e.g., "Which ear should I look at first?") and by asking the child to help with the examination (e.g., "Put your hands on mine so we can feel your tummy together"). Respect a child's choice about sitting with a parent or on the examination table. Some young children do not like to be undressed completely, so the examination may proceed in stages, undressing the part to be examined then putting clothes back on. But definitely examine the whole child!

How Should I Approach Older Children?

Older children (9 to 12 years) almost always cooperate with the evaluation. They generally demonstrate a concern for physical modesty and privacy. If siblings accompany a patient to the doctor's office, ask a parent to take them to the waiting room before discussing personal information or starting the physical examination. The preadolescent usually demonstrates an interest in health and the decisions that are made. Direct your questions to the child as you ask about concerns, problems, or the progress of an illness, and use language that is appropriate to the child's cognitive abilities. Listen actively to the child and respond honestly to questions. Some 10- to 12-year-olds may already have entered physical puberty but still be quite immature socially and emotionally. Use an open-ended question to start a conversation about a sensitive topic (e.g., "What have you learned in school about growing up?"). Later in the evaluation, parents can be asked to confirm details or elaborate. Observe the child before, during, and after the examination, and use these observations to aid your evaluation. Review vital signs and physical growth, including percentiles and body mass index. During the examination, draw the curtain, close the door securely, and provide a gown or drape. Explain why you are performing specific maneuvers and what you find on examination. Assess speech and language, fine motor movements, handwriting, behavior, interactions between the child and adults, and pubertal development. You must be familiar with sexual maturity rating (Figures 15-1 to 15-3).

How Should I Approach Adolescents?

Adolescents are the most adult-like patients that you will examine during the pediatric clerkship, but they are not yet adult. Adolescents challenge the inexperienced clinician because they are complex—physically, emotionally, and socially. To work successfully with adolescents, you must acquire a basic understanding of the *biopsychosocial stages of adolescence* and the *physical stages of puberty* (Chapter 15). Typically, an adolescent can interact independently and participate directly in the examination process without intervention by the parent. An adolescent may not ask about what you find but will definitely appreciate and be interested in your explanations as the examination progresses. Parents need to know that they will be asked to bring the adolescent to the office but that they will not be present in the room during the interview or examination. Adolescents need to know that their parents have a legitimate role in the healthcare process. Both need to understand that confidentiality and privacy will restrict the information that you can share unless you have permission from the patient to discuss issues with the parent and vice versa. If at all possible, these details need to be communicated in advance of the visit (see confidentiality in Chapter 6).

KEY POINTS

- Approach each patient using knowledge of development to assist your evaluation.
- You can communicate directly with patients at all ages and developmental stages.
- Parents or other caregivers are invaluable sources of information.
- Adolescents are especially sensitive to your communication style.

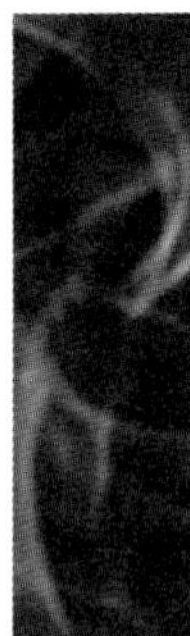

5 Physical Examination

JEROLD C. WOODHEAD and PAULA ALGRANATI

What Is Important in the Physical Examination?

The content of the physical examination depends on the patient's age, developmental stage, and the reason for the evaluation. Table 5-1 lists age-specific physical examination components. In general, a health supervision visit, a hospital admission, or the assessment of a complex complaint demands a comprehensive examination. Assessment of the daily progress of a hospitalized patient or the evaluation of a specific problem for a patient in a clinic will typically require an examination focused on the systems involved. Use of resources such as those listed in the reference section will greatly expand your knowledge of physical findings in infants, children, and adolescents.

What Can I Learn from Observation?

Observation is key to the examination at all ages, especially for infants and young children. You can learn about neurologic function and development by observing behaviors, physical abilities, and social interactions. An infant's alertness, cry, skin color, hydration status, respiratory pattern, work of breathing, and interactions with a parent all provide key information about the severity of illness. Observations of older children and adolescents should include their interactions with you and others.

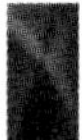

VITAL SIGNS, APPEARANCE, AND BEHAVIOR

Review vital signs and compare them with age-specific reference data (Table 5-2). "Normal" vital signs are age (and often sex and size) specific. "Normal" blood pressure (BP) is below the 90th percentile for age, sex, and height. Hypertension is defined as persistent BP readings

Table 5-1

Age and Developmental Stage–Related Focus for Physical Examination

Age	Focus
Newborn (see Chapter 14)	Assessment of gestational age Determination of appropriateness of size for gestational age Identification of birth injuries and congenital anomalies Diagnosis of acute neonatal illnesses
Infant	Assessment and monitoring of growth, development, and temperament Late manifestations of congenital anomalies or delayed sequelae of neonatal problems Tympanic membranes, emergence of teeth Signs of abuse For an *ill* infant: Observe skin color, perfusion, hydration, and oxygenation; assess respiratory effort, level of consciousness, social interaction, and quality of the cry
Toddler	Assessment and monitoring of growth and of developmental progress Observation of behavior and child-parent interactions Gait, dentition, vision, hearing (middle ear status), and blood pressure (after age 3) Signs of abuse
School-age	Assessment and monitoring of growth, including body mass index (BMI) Signs of puberty: girls after age 7 or 8 and boys after age 9 Dentition, development, behavior, blood pressure, vision, hearing, and scoliosis Focus on patient concerns Signs of abuse
Adolescent (see Chapter 15)	Assessment and monitoring of growth, including BMI, and puberty Breast self-examination for girls and testicular self-examination for boys Blood pressure, acne, dentition, signs of abuse Acute or chronic illness concerns Mental status observations

above the 95th percentile for age, sex, and height. BP is discussed in Chapter 46. Use growth charts to assess height, weight, body mass index (BMI), and head circumference. Pay attention to symmetry of growth, morphologic features, development, behavior, and the patient's interaction with parents and the examiner. Observe mental status in older children and adolescents. When evaluating an acute illness, look for disease-specific signs plus evidence of shock or toxicity, such as skin color, respiratory effort, hydration status (capillary refill), mental status,

Table 5-2

Vital Signs by Age

Age	Heart Rate* (beats per minute)	Respiratory Rate* (breaths per minute)	Blood Pressure† (mm Hg) (90th Percentile BP for 50th Percentile Height)	
			Boys	Girls
Newborn	120–170	30–80	87/68	76/68
1 year	80–160	20–40	98/53	100/58
3 years	80–120	20–30	105/61	103/62
6 years	75–115	16–22	110/70	107/69
10 years	70–110	16–20	115/75	115/74
17 years	60–110	12–20	133/83	125/80

*Adapted from Seidel H et al: *Mosby's guide to physical examination,* ed 6, St Louis, 2006, Mosby, pp 395, 444.

†"Normal" blood pressure is < 90th percentile. (Adapted from *The Harriet Lane handbook,* ed 17, Philadelphia, Mosby, 2005, pp 162–167.)

cry, and interactions. Chronic illness may result in growth abnormalities, system/organ-specific dysfunction, or other characteristic findings. A patient's appearance and physical findings may reflect a pattern of malformation that is characteristic of a syndrome or other identifiable cause of structural defects (see Chapter 62).

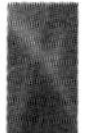

HEAD, EYES, EARS, NOSE, AND THROAT (HEENT)

HEAD

Measure head size and plot the data on the growth chart. Head circumference increases steadily from an average of 34 cm at birth to 48 cm (girls) and 49 cm (boys) by age 2; it then increases more slowly until the mean adult value of 55 cm (female) and 56 cm (male) is reached. Look at head shape and symmetry, facial features, and hair whorls. Identify the sutures and fontanels in an infant (Figure 5-1 and Chapter 14); these are usually not palpable after 15 to 18 months, occasionally earlier. The anterior fontanel is diamond shaped and at birth is approximately 2 × 2 cm (range 1 × 1 to 3 × 4 cm). The posterior fontanel is usually not palpable, even at birth, but when open it is the size of a small fingertip (< 1 × 1 cm). The superior surface of the anterior fontanel is generally level with the surface of the skull. Marked ridging or bony prominence of sutures in young infants may reflect premature fusion (synostosis). Widely separated sutures may reflect increased intracranial pressure and may be accompanied by a bulging and enlarged anterior fontanel. To determine whether the fontanel is bulging, move the infant to a sitting position, inspect the fontanel, then run your fingers across the fontanel surface. If the fontanel

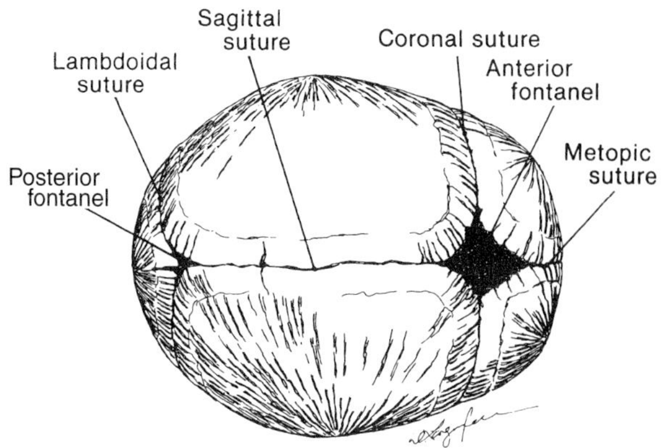

FIGURE 5-1 Cranial sutures and fontanels. (From Seidel HM et al: *Mosby's guide to physical diagnosis*, ed 6, Philadelphia, 2003, Mosby, p 258.)

protrudes convexly beyond the skull's surface, it is bulging. Dehydrated infants often display a sunken fontanel, concave with respect to the skull surface.

EYES

Identify the red reflex: Absence of the red reflex or presence of a white reflex always demands further evaluation. Assess extraocular motions and the corneal light reflection (see Eye Simulator, http://cim.ucdavis.edu/EyeRelease). Asymmetrical corneal light reflection is seen with strabismus. Young infants, especially Asian infants, commonly demonstrate pseudostrabismus, an artifact associated with prominent epicanthal folds (Figure 5-2). The corneal light reflection is symmetrical in pseudostrabismus.

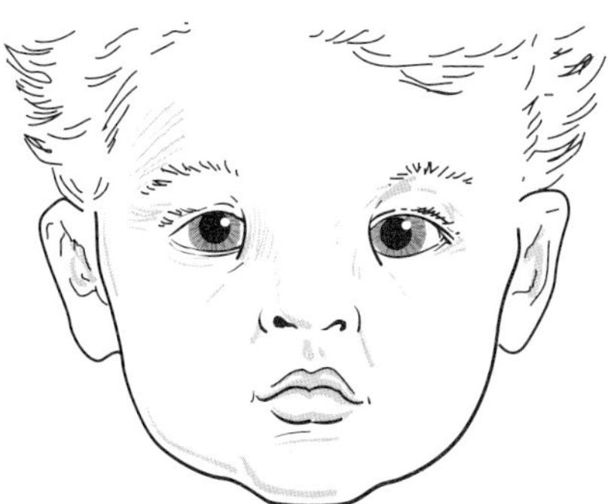

FIGURE 5-2 Child with pseudostrabismus. Note the wide nasal bridge and prominent epicanthal folds. (From Berkowitz CD: *Pediatrics: a primary care approach,* ed 2, Philadelphia, 2000, WB Saunders, p 240.)

EARS

Ask a parent to assist with the examination of the young child (see Figure 30-1). Look at the external ears to assess structure, position, and symmetry. Examine the tympanic membranes using pneumatic otoscopy. Identify the tympanic membrane's color, position, bony landmarks, light reflex, and movement to insufflation. Use a checklist as a guide (Table 30-1). Practice holding the otoscope, stabilizing the patient's head, and squeezing the bulb while examining the ear of a cooperative individual (a classmate or friend). Use the largest otoscope tip available that will fit the external canal to ensure an optimal view of the tympanic membrane. Nondisposable otoscope tips are longer and wider than the disposable tips, provide a better view of the tympanic membrane (TM), and also make a better seal for pneumatic otoscopy. Remember to clean these tips after use. If cerumen obscures the tympanic membrane, it must be removed to allow an examination. If you do not feel comfortable using a cerumen scoop, ask for assistance.

NOSE AND THROAT

Check the patency of the nasal airway. Nasal congestion may be evident from a "denasal" voice (attempts to say the letter "N" results in a sound like "D"). A cleft palate produces a "nasal" or "breathy" voice. Assess hydration and inflammation of the pharyngeal mucous membranes. When tonsils touch in the midline they are rated 4+; most young children have at least 2+ tonsils. Presence of tonsillar inflammation and exudates suggests active infection. Cleft palate is usually obvious; a submucous cleft of the palate may be identified only by a bifid or cleft uvula. Always examine the teeth and gums; distinguish between primary and permanent teeth; and identify plaque, staining, caries, gingival inflammation, and abscesses.

NECK

Cervical lymph nodes can be palpated in healthy children, but they are *not* large, immobile, tender, fluctuant, or inflamed. Figure 5-3 shows the anatomic areas drained by the cervical nodes. The thyroid gland should be small and smooth and have no nodules or tenderness. Examine the range of motion (flexion, extension, lateral bending, rotation) of the neck, and, when appropriate, test for nuchal rigidity.

CHEST

Observe the rate, pattern, and effort of breathing. Diaphragmatic breathing may be exaggerated during respiratory illness in infants and toddlers, manifested by prominent abdominal protrusion during respiration; the

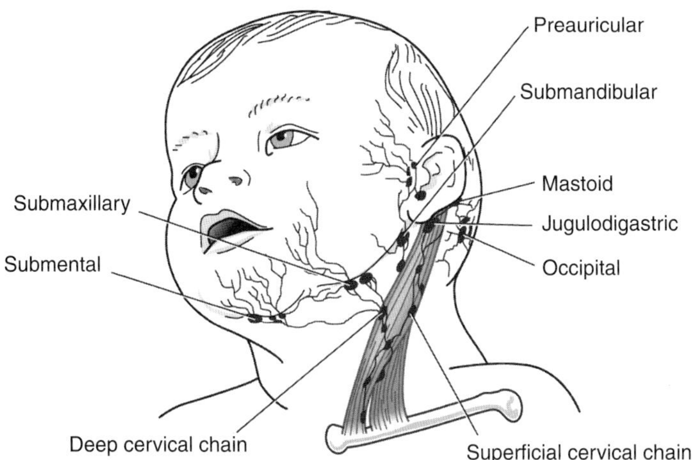

FIGURE 5-3 The lymphatic drainage and lymph nodes involved in infants and children with cervical lymphadenitis. (From Feigin RD, Cherry JD, editors: *Textbook of pediatric infectious diseases*, ed 4, Philadelphia, 1998, WB Saunders, p 171.)

cartilaginous ribs allow "collapse" of the chest during inspiration. Respiratory distress is signaled by expiratory grunting, nasal flaring, intercostal space retractions, and stridor. Wheezing, crackles, and asymmetrical breath sounds are concerning findings on auscultation. Transmitted upper airway sounds often cause confusion.

CARDIOVASCULAR

Palpate pulses in the carotid, brachial, radial, femoral, and dorsalis pedis areas. Hydration status and peripheral perfusion is best tested with capillary refill, which should be < 2 seconds. Observe and palpate precordial activity. Auscultate the heart for rhythm, rate, quality of the heart sounds, and murmurs. Young children often have prominent "sinus arrhythmia," a physiologic variation of heart rate associated with the respiratory cycle: rate increases with inspiration and decreases with expiration. You should be able to hear the physiologic splitting of the second heart sound at the second or third left intercostal space even in infants with a rapid heart rate (the splitting will be a "blurring" of the second heart sound during inspiration with return to a "crisp" sound during expiration). A venous hum is often heard when a young child is sitting and turns the head to one side; this is a continuous to-and-fro sound that disappears when supine or with head movement.

Physiologic murmurs change with position, often being more prominent when supine and diminishing when sitting. Pathologic heart murmurs are loud, often occur in diastole, and do not change with position (discussed in Chapter 48).

ABDOMEN

Examine the umbilical cord in newborns and identify the vein and the two arteries. Note the presence of granulation tissue, umbilical hernias, or a patent urachus. Observe, auscultate, and palpate the abdomen for distention, local or rebound tenderness, and masses. Palpate the liver, spleen, and kidneys. Expect the liver edge and kidneys to be palpable in a healthy newborn and young infant. Many constipated preschool children have stool in the descending colon and sigmoid that is palpable as a tubular mass in the left lower quadrant and is associated with stool in the rectal vault. If a rectal examination is necessary, you will be shown the age-appropriate technique.

GENITALIA

Before inspecting the genitalia, ask permission. This alerts parent and child or adolescent to what is coming next and also shows respect for privacy and the parent's responsibility. Explain to the child that only a doctor or a parent should look at the "private parts," "under their underwear," or "where their bathing suit covers." To observe the age-appropriate appearance of male and female genitalia, you must understand the genital changes that occur as the child grows from infancy to adolescence.

BOYS

Determine whether the penis has been circumcised. Check for phimosis in uncircumcised boys, but remember that the foreskin cannot be fully retracted until after ages 4 to 6 years in most boys. The urethral meatus should be located at the tip of the glans; if it is lower on the glans or on the shaft of the penis, hypospadias is present. Palpate the testes to ensure that both are descended into the scrotum and to identify an undescended testis (cryptorchidism), hernia, hydrocele, or testicular mass. Characterize genitalia according to sexual maturity (Tanner) stages (Chapter 15).

GIRLS

Inspect labia majora, labia minora, clitoris, urethra, vaginal orifice, and the hymen. Look for signs of virilization, imperforate hymen, labial adhesions, and injury. Characterize genitalia according to sexual maturity (Tanner) stages (Chapter 15).

 MUSCULOSKELETAL AND EXTREMITIES

The musculoskeletal examination is important at all ages. Examine the newborn's hips with Ortolani and Barlow maneuvers (Figure 5-4) to identify developmental dysplasia. The Ortolani maneuver identifies the *dislocated* hip, which will be felt to move anteriorly (reduce) into the acetabulum, with a palpable or audible "clunk." The Barlow maneuver identifies the *dislocatable* hip, which will be felt to move posteriorly (dislocate) out of the acetabulum, with a palpable or audible clunk. Use the musculoskeletal evaluation of older children and adolescents to identify restricted or excessive joint mobility, joint effusions, signs of trauma, and gait abnormalities. Figure 68-1 shows age-related variations of the legs and feet: genu varus and valgus, flexible flat feet, metarsus varus, tibial torsion, and femoral anteversion. The "2-minute musculoskeletal examination" assesses strength, symmetry, flexibility, muscle bulk, and range of motion (Figure 68-2). Common pediatric orthopedic problems are discussed in Chapter 68.

 BACK

The scapulae and iliac crests should be symmetrical in appearance, prominence, and placement. Inspect and palpate the spine along its entire length to identify curves, hair tufts, pits, dimples, or masses.

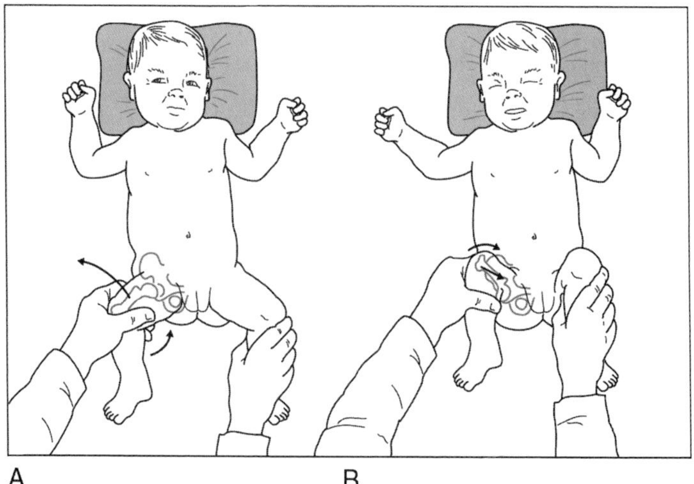

FIGURE 5-4 Ortolani (reduction) **(A)** and Barlow (dislocation) **(B)** tests. (From Berkowitz CD: *Pediatrics: a primary care approach,* ed 2, Philadelphia, 2000, WB Saunders, p 358.)

Dimples over the lower spine are common and do not need further investigation if the underlying skin is intact. If not, investigate to identify a sinus tract or underlying abnormality. A dimple in the coccygeal or gluteal cleft area is usually benign, whereas a sacral dimple may represent an occult spinal dysraphism (spina bifida occulta). Examine school-age children and adolescents for scoliosis, kyphosis, and lordosis. Figure 5-5 demonstrates the technique to identify scoliosis.

NEUROLOGIC

Observation is a key tool for the neurologic examination. Assess developmental milestones, symmetry, tone, strength, and reflexes. Primitive reflexes, including rooting, sucking, obligate grasp, Moro reflex, and tonic neck reflex, are found in healthy newborns and young infants. Persistence of primitive reflexes beyond 4 to 6 months should raise concern (Chapter 58). You should be able to demonstrate the findings that

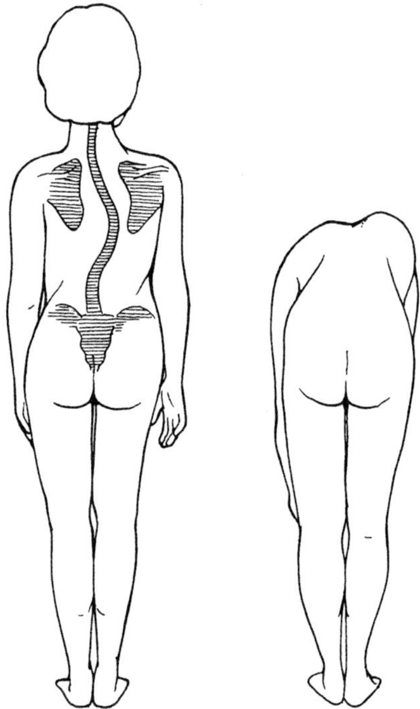

FIGURE 5-5 Examination for scoliosis: The back and spine are inspected when the patient is upright and bending forward from the waist. (From Berkowitz CD: *Pediatrics: a primary care approach,* ed 2, Philadelphia, 2000, WB Saunders, p 386.)

reflect the disappearance of primitive reflexes (e.g., the voluntary grasp of an infant older than 2 months indicates that the reflexive grasp of the newborn has disappeared).

SKIN

Observe and palpate the skin to assess color, perfusion, turgor, pigmented lesions, and rashes. Identify jaundice, petechiae, purpura, vesicles, and urticaria (Chapter 49). Examine the skin for common birthmarks and skin conditions unique to children (Chapter 57). Recognize bruises and other characteristic findings of child abuse (Chapter 24).

KEY POINTS

- History and physical examination must be based on age and developmental stage.
- Speak directly to children at all ages and use knowledge of development to assess responses.
- Observation is an important clinical skill.

BIBLIOGRAPHY

Jones KL: *Smith's recognizable patterns of human malformation,* ed 6, Philadelphia, WB Saunders, 2006.

Paller AS, Mancini AJ: *Hurwitz clinical pediatric dermatology,* Philadelphia, WB Saunders, 2006.

Robertson J, Shilkofski N: *The Harriet Lane handbook,* ed 17, Philadelphia, Mosby, 2005.

Seidel HM et al: *Mosby's guide to physical examination,* ed 6, St Louis, Mosby, 2006.

Zitelli BJ, Davis HW: *Atlas of pediatric physical diagnosis,* ed 4, Philadelphia, Mosby, 2002.

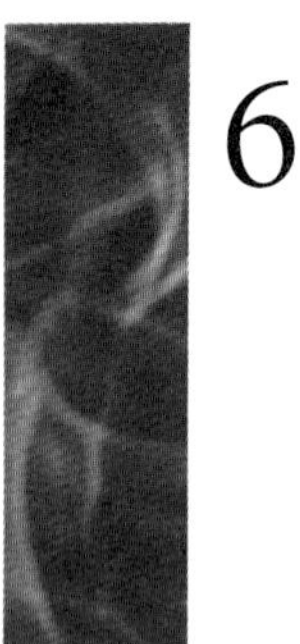

6 Ethics

ANNE LYREN and BENJAMIN S. SIEGEL

Pediatric ethics analyzes the moral aspects of decisions made in the health care of children. An ethical problem exists when there is a difference in values among the people who are involved with a medical decision. Traditional medical training emphasizes the pathophysiology of disease and answers the clinician's question, "What *can* I do?" Ethics addresses the equally important question, "What *should* I do?" Ethics is different from the law. Legal decision analysis is based on written legislation and legal precedent. The law answers the questions: "What must I do?" or "What may I do?" Ethics, on the other hand, involves breaking down a problem into its fundamental parts, examining the values and assumptions at hand, and determining the best course of action. Every decision in pediatrics has an ethical component, and attention to these issues is essential for optimal patient care.

CONSENT

Who Should Make Medical Decisions for Children?

Decision making for children is a unique and challenging process. Adult patients generally make their own medical decisions through the process of informed consent, in which a competent adult, capable of sufficient understanding, is given adequate, clear information about the proposed intervention and granted the autonomy to make choices. Most children have not reached the developmental stage at which they can ethically or legally give informed consent. To further complicate matters, many parties may be involved in the decision-making process, including the patient, parents, family members, nurses, doctors, social workers, clergy, and the courts. The ultimate goal should be to identify the child's best interest through a shared decision-making process that involves the clinician, patient, and parents. This process invokes the ethical principle of *beneficence*, which urges caregivers to identify and act according to the best interest of that particular child. The clinician provides a thorough understanding of the available medical evidence and can make recommendations based on clinical knowledge and experience. The parents bring their intimate knowledge of the child and the family. The child is represented by the parents who, as the primary caregivers, give informed consent by proxy (otherwise known as "informed permission") because they are usually best able to determine the child's best interest. Physicians have the responsibility to ensure that parental motivations are based on the child's needs rather than the parents' wishes.

All the tenets of informed consent apply to informed permission, except that parents ultimately make the decision instead of the child patient. Children gradually develop the ability to understand a diagnosis and treatment plan as they approach adolescence. Hence, the older child's ideas and opinions deserve serious consideration and can be quite enlightening in the effort to identify the child's best interest. Although older children are legally unable to give informed consent, they may still express assent and dissent that empower them to the extent of their developmental abilities. Thus the ideal decision-making scenario is a shared process: The physician provides information and recommendations, the parents give informed permission, and the child patient gives assent to interventions in his or her best interest.

CONFIDENTIALITY

What Does the Duty of Confidentiality Require in Pediatrics?

As adolescents mature from childhood to adulthood, the physician can be a unique and important advocate. As part of the process of individuation, adolescents desire more privacy in their personal lives. At the same time, they are encountering increasingly complex and challenging health issues. Physicians should respect and encourage a mature approach to health by adolescents but must be careful not to construct additional barriers for this patient population that historically has not appropriately accessed health care. Issues of confidentiality arise often within the physician/patient/parent triad, and management can be quite delicate in terms of the limits of confidentiality and the circumstances in which disclosure must occur. Although the specifics vary from state to state, the law sometimes gives an adolescent who demonstrates some degree of maturity the discretion to make healthcare decisions without the involvement of parents. This decision making relates to issues such as substance abuse, sexually transmitted diseases, pregnancy, contraception, and mental health. In some states, subgroups of adolescents, variously known as emancipated minors, mature minors, or medically emancipated minors, are considered capable of providing informed consent (based on their developmental capacity but usually 14 years or older) for all forms of care by virtue of their life experiences, which may include financial independence, being in the armed services, being declared independent by the court, pregnancy, homelessness, or marriage. Because statutes governing adolescents vary from state to state, physicians should research the laws in their practice communities. In all cases, the primary duty of the physician is to optimize the adolescent patient's care by advocating for his or her best interest.

What Are the Limits of Confidentiality in the Adolescent-Physician Relationship?

All clinical interactions are by nature confidential. Because the adolescent is the patient, in most instances he or she must give permission to share information with parents or others. Through a confidential relationship, the physician demonstrates respect for the patient's privacy while facilitating care. At the outset, the physician should establish an independent relationship with the adolescent, explaining to the patient and the parents both the breadth and the limits of confidentiality. Serious concerns that threaten the life and health of the adolescent, including suicidal ideation, significant substance use that impairs the adolescent's functioning, the potential for community violence, and sexual or physical abuse, will limit confidentiality. If the life of the patient or anyone else is in peril or the patient is being abused by parents or caretakers, the physician is mandated both ethically and legally to disclose this information to the appropriate authorities. Perhaps one of the most important roles of the physician is to facilitate communication between the adolescent and the parents, who can be important sources of support and advocacy. Under most circumstances, the adolescent should be encouraged to involve the parents in his or her health care because they ideally can provide support and help the adolescent identify his or her best interest. The physician should also encourage the parents to appreciate and embrace the adolescent's emerging maturity and independence. Confidentiality in the physician-adolescent patient relationship is key to the physician's effort to be a confidante and caregiver, ultimately acting in the best interest of the patient.

GENETIC TESTING IN CHILDREN

Under What Circumstances Should Genetic Testing of Children Be Performed?

The decision to use genetic testing for children is generally more complex than for other tests because the results have implications for family members as well as the child. Certain genetic diagnoses may subject children and their families to financial, psychological, or interpersonal prejudices that are not easily foreseeable. Genetic testing offers the possibility of great information, but it runs the risk of assuming genetic determinism—exaggerating the genetic influences on disease while devaluing the environmental ones. The decision to undertake a genetic evaluation should be based on the principle of *beneficence* with the best interest of the child as the guide.

Isn't Newborn Screening a Form of Genetic Testing? Why Is It So Widely Accepted?

Every state requires that newborn infants undergo screening to detect a number of metabolic and inherited conditions that can threaten the health and well-being of the child. The screening procedure reflects society's obligation to optimize the health of children by detecting and treating particular infant or early childhood conditions. Theoretically, each of these screening tests is carefully chosen to satisfy a number of criteria. First, the test must be highly *sensitive* so that cases are adequately identified among the masses of screened newborns. At the same time, the *specificity* should be as high as possible to avoid the anxiety that comes from a false-positive test. The screening tests must be *carried out for the entire population* of newborns to ensure detection of all cases. Effective preventive or treatment *interventions* must be available and must significantly alter the morbidity and mortality of the condition. Perhaps the most important criterion is that the test must provide a *clear benefit for the child.*

What about Screening Tests for Genetic Diseases of Adulthood?

Huntington's disease, breast cancer, and polycystic kidney disease are just a few of the adult diseases for which genetic tests are available and can be performed in childhood or even in utero. The list of diseases now known to have a genetic link is rapidly increasing in number and variety. Theoretically, identifying a predilection to such disease may lead to preemptive intervention to decrease the morbidity and mortality of the disease, but knowledge of a genetic predilection has not proved to have an impact on the future health of the patient. Physicians faced with requests for this type of testing must proceed with great caution. The psychological and social impact of this information can be much greater than anticipated and may lead to discrimination by employers, insurers, and others. Performing these tests while remaining committed to the child's best interests can be challenging. By definition, these tests detect diseases of adulthood; therefore if intervention during childhood cannot successfully and significantly alter the natural history of the disease, the testing will not be in the best interest of the child. Testing should be deferred until the child reaches late adolescence or adulthood and can make his or her own autonomous choice. Physicians faced with requests for genetic testing should keep all of these issues in mind when determining if genetic testing is in the best interest of the child.

END-OF-LIFE ISSUES

How Should Decisions Be Made for Dying Children?

Caring for dying children is one of the most challenging responsibilities in pediatrics. You will need to come to an understanding of your personal reactions to dying patients and must be sensitive to the needs of patients, family members, and the other members of the healthcare team. The emotions engendered by anticipation of a child's death have a powerful impact on families and caregivers and may be an obstacle to the appropriate care of the child. Decisions at the end of life must be guided by the child's best interest. Through a shared decision-making process, the healthcare provider should obtain informed permission from the parents as well as patient assent, when possible, to optimize these interests.

Careful, continual evaluation is critical so that when the burdens of care outweigh the benefits to the child, the treatment plan can be appropriately modified.

When Is It Appropriate to Withdraw or Withhold Support?

Healthcare providers and families often struggle when they realize that neither the current interventions nor additional ones will alter the child's progression toward death. The inevitability of death then challenges the family and the healthcare team to change the goals from cure to palliation. Parents often fear that they would be taking an active role in hastening the child's death by withholding or withdrawing support. Physicians must be prepared to help the family understand that palliation is not equivalent to giving up but instead is part of the continuum of respect and consideration for the child and his or her best interests.

What Are "Do Not Resuscitate" Orders?

"Do not resuscitate" orders are critical in end-of-life care. The physician must address this issue directly with the patient and family so that unwanted interventions do not occur at the end of a child's life. In addition, all members of the healthcare team must understand the implications of the "do not resuscitate" order. This is often a difficult issue to discuss because parents and healthcare providers may feel that withholding support is somehow preferable to withdrawing the support that is already in place. There is no ethical distinction between not initiating an intervention and removing an intervention. Viewed in light of the changing goals of treatment and the child's best interest, either treatment plan is ethically sound.

What Are Our Other Obligations to Dying Children?

As the child approaches the end of life, compassionate, developmentally appropriate communication between the healthcare provider and the family and patient remains the cornerstone of sound care. This may involve the provider in facilitating communication between the family and the patient. All questions should be answered in a clear, forthright, honest manner; misleading or overly optimistic responses do not reflect a doctor's obligation to be truthful. Physical and emotional pain should be minimized to the extent possible, even if it may hasten the dying process. Pain medication is often needed, but art, music, and child-life therapists can further enhance the quality of the child's experience. Families should continue to be intimately involved. Their well-being must be acknowledged also in an effort to optimize their experience during the progression toward the child's death and afterward. Hospice programs are expert resources. Too often, referrals to hospice care are made late or not at all, and the patient and family are not able to take full advantage of this extraordinary resource during an extremely difficult time. Encouraging the involvement of religious or spiritual supporters is always appropriate.

IMMUNIZATION AS A BENEFIT TO SOCIETY

How Should I Explain to Parents the Recommendation to Immunize Children?

Parents often question the need for immunizations. To address their concerns, you must know the risks and benefits of immunizations so that you can identify the best interest of the child. Immunizations are generally intramuscular injections and are always painful, and the current immunization schedule recommends that an infant or child receive as many as four or five injections at one visit. Each immunization has established side effects, and parents need to be aware of them. The list of available immunizations continues to change and grow and so do recent claims about vague associations between them and diseases of unclear etiology. Such claims have not been substantiated by careful medical research, yet the theories are still widely publicized and accessible. Providing parents with reliable information sources can help.

Parents may be hesitant to immunize their children against diseases such as measles and polio when the child's risk of contracting the disease is exceedingly low in the United States. These diseases are currently uncommon because of the effectiveness of immunizations. In past decades, however, these diseases affected thousands of American children and still today overwhelm many in underprivileged societies. Some countries, whose established immunization programs have been compromised by political strife, are now experiencing epidemics of diseases that were previously under control. These events reinforce the idea that widespread immunization protects the population as a whole and is likely the reason for the low prevalence of these devastating diseases in the United States.

We live in a world in which travel is fairly easy. Transient and immigrant individuals from countries with different disease risks and immunization practices enter the United States and potentially may expose others to disease. Despite this, parents may argue that immunization is not in the child's best interest because our society has a relatively low prevalence of disease. They argue that their child should not be subjected to the pain, side effects, and inconvenience of immunization to protect the society at large. Some parents may claim a religious/spiritual or philosophical exemption to immunization. Whereas all states allow certain medical exemptions approved by a physician, the laws regarding exemptions based on parental philosophical and religious/spiritual beliefs vary by state. Physicians should familiarize themselves with state laws.

The American medical profession continues to recommend routine immunization. The ethical justification for this position is based on a comprehensive view of the child's best interest that includes consideration of the principle of *justice* for all members of society. Just as there are limits to confidentiality, there are limits to pursuing the best interests of the individual. In the case of immunizations, justice imposes such a limitation. Broadly speaking, the principle of justice suggests that all members of a society must bear both the burdens and the benefits of coexistence. By refusing immunizations, parents put their own children at only a small individual risk of disease but potentially increase the risk to the entire population if the number of unimmunized children grows. Justice challenges the absolute sovereignty of the best-interest paradigm by suggesting that the best interest of the child must be balanced by the needs of society, particularly when an action, or in this case inaction, carries little risk to the child but puts the society in peril. The child has the potential to benefit directly from the immunization, which also contributes to a safer society. These benefits outweigh the individual risk to the child.

Optimal care for children goes beyond addressing the needs and interests of individual patients. Through political advocacy and increased public awareness, healthcare providers can address the welfare of all children. In a disease epidemic, the public health departments of some states have the legal power to mandate immunization administration to all susceptible children as a protection of the public health.

KEY POINTS

- Every decision in the care of children has an ethical component.
- Most pediatric patients cannot give informed consent; parents and legal guardians give informed permission.
- Children should contribute to their own medical decision making to the extent they are developmentally capable as part of the process of assent/dissent.
- Confidentiality is key to all clinical encounters, but it is especially important with adolescents.
- Genetic testing in pediatrics requires careful consideration.
- The child's best interest must guide decisions at the end of life.

Case 6-1

Grandparents bring a 6-year-old child to the office for pre-kindergarten immunizations and a routine health supervision visit. The child is staying with them while the parents are undergoing a divorce. They do not have a signed release (healthcare power of attorney) from the parents.

A. Can you examine this child and give immunizations?
B. What if this visit were for an emergent medical condition? Would you be able to manage the child?

Case 6-2

A 16-year-old adolescent requested to speak with you in private about health issues. He has a sexually transmitted disease. You discuss this health issue with him and determine that he has the developmental capacity to understand the nature of his condition, the recommended treatment, and alternatives. After the appointment, his parents demand that you tell them what you have just discussed with their son.

A. How would you reply to the parents' request?
B. Does the adolescent have a legal right to seek confidential health care?

Case 6-3

The mother of a 2-month-old infant refuses immunizations because she is afraid that immunizations will "overload" her baby's immune system.

A. Does this mother have the legal right to refuse immunizations? What is the ethical (and medical) concern?
B. What is the most reasonable approach on your part to this issue?

Case 6-4

The maternal grandmother of a 3-year-old girl was recently diagnosed with Huntington's disease. The mother of the child is currently undergoing genetic testing for this disease and would like you to test her daughter for the disease as well.

How do ethical principles guide your decision in this case?

Case 6-5

Despite intensive medical efforts, a 12-year-old boy is dying of cancer. His parents and care providers meet and determine that his goals of care should change from aggressive attempts to cure to providing palliative care. His parents state that they do not want anyone to tell the child that he is dying.

A. Is it acceptable to provide palliative care instead of cure-oriented care to this boy without his knowledge?
B. How would you manage this situation?

Case Answers

6-1 A. *Learning objective:* **Understand the legal and ethical basics of consent.** The ethical question in this case would be whether well-child care and immunizations are in the best interest of the child, which is not apparently a point of significant controversy in this situation. This case largely addresses the legal issues regarding consent to treat children. Strictly speaking, you may not even examine the child because the child's legal caregiver (the child's parent) has not given consent to your care. More importantly, you may not perform invasive procedures such as immunizations because the grandparents do not have the legal right to make the decision in place of the parents. If you can contact the parents and obtain a witnessed authorization by telephone or fax, then immunizations may be given.

6-1 B. *Learning objective:* **Recognize that in an emergency situation a physician may provide care without consent of parents or legal guardians.** Yes, in an emergency, a physician may treat a child without parental consent.

6-2 A. *Learning objective:* **Discuss the issue of confidentiality as applied to adolescents.** Inform the parents that their son is your patient and that you are guided and bound by rules of confidentiality except when the adolescent or another is at imminent risk of serious harm, such as cases of suicidality or homicidality. Encourage them to speak with their son, and encourage the boy to speak with his parents.

6-2 B. *Learning objective:* **Recognize the medical conditions for which a minor may seek confidential health care.** Yes, federal and state laws exist that offer specific provisions for adolescents seeking confidential care for some medical conditions. Sexually transmitted diseases are among the conditions for which a minor may seek confidential care. Others include substance abuse, pregnancy, contraception, and certain mental health conditions. Physicians must be aware of the confidentiality laws in the area in which they practice.

6-3 A. *Learning objective:* **Understand the conflict between personal choice and justice as applied to medical decisions.** Yes, the mother has the legal right to refuse immunizations. She puts her infant at risk and also increases the risk to society. In addition, her choice may conflict with laws regarding immunization status for children in school.

6-3 B. *Learning objective:* **Counsel families about the benefits of immunizations, both for the individual child and the larger society.** Withhold immunizations at this visit. Discuss the mother's concerns, and provide her with information from reliable sources. Continue to offer immunizations, and discuss the facts about immunizations at each visit. Also provide guidance about illness prevention for this unimmunized infant. Remind the mother that public school systems and most day-care programs require immunizations or evidence of an exemption in accordance with state laws.

6-4. *Learning objective:* **Understand the role of beneficence in making all medical decisions for children.** Beneficence instructs you to think carefully about the best interest of the child in this circumstance and not be influenced by her mother's interest. No clear evidence exists to support the assertion that the child benefits now from the knowledge that she has a disease of adult-onset for which there is currently no treatment during the latent phase. In fact, some evidence suggests that this information may make her more vulnerable to discrimination, bias, and psychological injury. Adults who are faced with the decision of whether to be tested for such diseases decide variably—some wish to have the information; others prefer not to know. Beyond satisfying her mother's desire to know, there is no reason to test the child at this time. Such testing is better left until the time at which the girl reaches the age at which she has the developmental capacity to understand the complex implications of the testing and can decide for herself whether she wants to know.

6-5 A. *Learning objective:* **Allow children to provide assent to their care and be involved to the extent that they are developmentally capable.** Although this child may not have reached an age at which he is ethically or legally able to consent to his care, his physicians have a duty to include him in discussions and decisions about his medical care to the extent he is able. Most 12-year-olds have a very good understanding of treatment goals and are able to provide meaningful assent or dissent. Not including him in this fundamental change of plans does not respect the important role he plays in his own life and risks not being truthful. Chances are this child would sense the change in plan even if no one told him. He may have worries, questions, or concerns he is reluctant to share but could be easily addressed. In addition, failing to tell him that he is dying deprives him of potential opportunities to shape the end of his life.

6-5 B. *Learning objective:* **Use multidisciplinary services at the end of life to enhance the experience of the patient and family.** Identifying the motivations for the parents' secrecy can be helpful in deciding how to approach this delicate situation. Most often, the parents are overwhelmed by sadness and do not wish to burden the child further with additional bad news. Furthermore, they may not know how to talk to their child about these issues or what hope or choices they can offer him. At these critical times, physicians must use the services of others who are specifically trained to address the needs of patients and families at the end of life. These include social workers, child-life therapists, art and music therapists, clergy, and hospice specialists.

BIBLIOGRAPHY

American Academy of Pediatrics, Committee of Bioethics: Informed consent, parental permission, and assent in pediatric practice, *Pediatrics* 95:314, 1995.

American Academy of Pediatrics, Committee on Bioethics: Responding to parental refusals of immunization of children, *Pediatrics* 115:1428, 2005.

American Academy of Pediatrics, Committee on Bioethics: Ethical issues with genetic testing in pediatrics, *Pediatrics* 107:1451, 2001.

American Academy of Pediatrics, Committee on Medical Liability: Consent by proxy for nonurgent pediatric care, *Pediatrics* 112:1185, 2003.

Himelstein BP et al: Pediatric palliative care, *N Engl J Med* 350:1752, 2004.

Society for Adolescent Medicine: Confidential health care for adolescents: position paper of the Society for Adolescent Medicine, *J Adolesc Health* 35:150, 2004.

7

Evidence-Based Medicine

LESLIE H. FALL

A 12-year-old girl in the ambulatory clinic with fever, sore throat, red tonsils, and tender cervical adenopathy has a positive rapid test for *Streptococcus*. Your attending physician quizzes you about the current evidence regarding the best treatment for this patient and asks you to look up some recent articles and present the evidence at the end of the week.

INTRODUCTION TO EVIDENCE-BASED MEDICINE (EBM)

What Do I Need to Know to Use EBM?

Using EBM requires that you understand the basic principles of epidemiology and biostatistics. In addition, you should have a working knowledge of the medical literature, including common study designs, and feel comfortable performing a basic MEDLINE search. Brief reviews are in the reference list (Gehlbach, 2002; Greenhalgh, 2006).

What Does "Evidence-Based Medicine" Mean?

EBM is the "conscientious, explicit, and judicious use of current best evidence in making decisions about the care of individual patients" (Sackett et al., 1996). EBM assumes that physicians whose practice is based on a solid understanding of the underlying evidence will provide superior patient care. EBM guides are available for interpreting most types of articles found in the medical literature. This chapter only discusses EBM for treatment questions, because these are most commonly encountered during the clerkship. Refer to the original *JAMA* series (Oxman et al., 1993) or review texts (Straus et al., 2005; Greenhalgh, 2006) for additional EBM topics.

How Does EBM Use Epidemiology and Biostatistics?

EBM asks whether valid data are clinically useful for a given patient or patient population. It brings the principles of epidemiology and biostatistics into the clinical setting, looking beyond the soundness of the study design and statistical significance. EBM may demonstrate that the results of a well-designed clinical trial do not apply to your particular patient or that the results of a relatively flawed study are still quite relevant to your patient's specific condition.

How Will I Use EBM During My Clerkship?

You will be asked often to investigate a specific clinical question in depth. EBM will help you focus the questions clearly, find relevant and quality literature, and assess its clinical usefulness. These important skills require time and practice to learn and master.

How Does EBM Relate to My Other Studies?

You will use EBM to assist with management of a specific patient or problem. The general learning during the clerkship will still come from participating directly in patient care, from reading textbooks or quality review articles, or from online resources such as the Computer-assisted Learning in Pediatrics Project (CLIPP) (http://clippcases.org).

How Do I Begin with EBM?

Before leaving the clinic or rounds, make certain that you understand the specific problem that your attending physician wants you to answer and confirm that the primary medical literature is the appropriate place to search for the answer. You should also clarify when the information is due and in what format (e.g., written or verbal presentation). Then, begin the process by focusing your questions clearly to ensure that you are addressing the specific problem and to make your literature search easier. Students commonly ask poorly formed questions, which hinders the literature search. A question such as "What is the best treatment for strep pharyngitis?" is unclear for several reasons: (1) What does "best" mean? (2) "Best" as compared to what? and (3) "Best" for whom?

How Do I Ask a Good Clinical Question?

To ensure that your question addresses the problem, consider using the PICO format: Patient, Intervention, Comparison, and Outcome. The question about appropriate treatment for streptococcal pharyngitis can be restated using the PICO format as follows: *For a 12-year-old girl with streptococcal pharyngitis* (Patient), *is a 5-day course of penicillin* (Intervention) *more efficacious than a 7-day course of penicillin* (Comparison) *for eradicating the infection* (Outcome)? Searching for the answer to this question will be easier and more rewarding than searching for the answer to the more vague question.

How Do I Use MEDLINE?

Students commonly find too many or too few articles or find articles that are not relevant. Review the basics of MEDLINE searching

(Greenhalgh 1997; Greenhalgh 2006) and ask for help from a medical librarian. The following suggestions will improve your search strategy:

1. Be sure that you understand the concepts of MeSH headings and Boolean operators ("and," "or," and "not").
2. Use the PICO format to focus the question and define search parameters.
3. Use the "age-limit" function appropriate to your patient.
   - Infant, newborn (birth to 1 month)
   - Infant (1 to 23 months)
   - Child, preschool (2 to 5 years)
   - Child (6 to 12 years)
   - Adolescent (13 to 18 years)
   - All children (all of the above)
4. Use "quality filters" to limit your search. To identify treatment articles, add "randomized controlled trial," "clinical trial," "meta-analysis," and "practice guideline" to the search strategy, or use the EBM functions of Ovid and PubMed. Ask your librarian for help.
5. Read the abstracts identified by your search and choose one to three of the best articles that are relevant to your patient. Next, read each article to gain an understanding of the study's hypothesis, methodology, and conclusions. Then, "map out" each study on paper to make the methodology and its strengths and limitations clear. This will help you determine the validity and significance of the results (Gehlbach, 2002; Greenhalgh, 2006).

How Do I Evaluate the Clinical Evidence in a Study?

Ask the following three broad questions:

1. Are the results valid?
2. What are the results?
3. Will they help me in caring for my patient?

The medical literature about treatment, diagnosis, and prognosis uses specific subsets of questions for each type of study to evaluate the data. The references (Oxman et al., 1993; Straus et al., 2005) provide guidance on how to appraise articles on topics other than treatment.

EVALUATING A THERAPEUTIC TRIAL

How Do I Begin Evaluating a Treatment Study?

Clinical trials that assess new treatments are the most common studies reported in the primary medical literature, and you should feel comfortable reading and interpreting them. Time spent to map out the study design on paper will make answering the following questions easier and will help you better describe the study design to attending physicians or residents.

How Do I Decide if the Results Are Valid?

Was the assignment of patients random?

Randomization ensures that both known and unknown determinants of outcome are evenly distributed between treatment and control groups, if the sample size is sufficiently large.

Were all patients accounted for and were patients analyzed in the groups to which they were randomized?

Every patient who entered the trial should be accounted for at its conclusion. If a substantial number of patients are reported as "lost to follow-up," the validity of the study is open to question. Patients who are "lost" often have different prognoses from those who are retained; consequently, many disappear because they have suffered adverse outcomes or because they improved before the end of the study. By preserving randomization during data analysis, all outcomes will be equally distributed in the two groups and the ultimate effect can be attributed to the treatment.

Was the study "blinded"?

The best way to avoid bias is to make the study "double-blind," so that neither investigator nor patient knows the treatment being used. For studies in which patients and treating clinicians cannot be kept blind (e.g., surgery vs. no surgery), you should note whether investigators have minimized bias by blinding those who were responsible to assess the final clinical outcomes.

Were the treatment and control groups similar?

The only important difference between groups should be whether they received the experimental therapy. Group characteristics are usually displayed in a table early in the article.

Were the groups treated equally?

Differences in care other than that under study can weaken or distort the results.

How Do I Evaluate the Results of a Therapeutic Trial?

How large was the treatment effect?

Consider a study in which death is the outcome for 20% (0.20) of patients in a control group but only 15% (0.15) of patients in a treatment group (Table 7-1). Results might be expressed in terms of absolute risk reduction or relative risk reduction.

- *Absolute risk reduction* (ARR) is the absolute difference between the proportion that died in the control group and the proportion that died in the treatment group. In this example, it would be 5%.
- *Relative risk reduction* (RRR) expresses the difference as a percentage and is more commonly used to express the impact of treatment. In this example, the new treatment reduced the risk of death by 25% relative to that occurring among control patients.

A positive RRR means that the new therapy is better than the old therapy or the control; the greater the RRR, the more effective the therapy.

Table 7-1

Evaluating the Results of a Therapeutic Trial

Measure of the Effect of Therapy	Example
Outcome without therapy (X)	20% mortality
Outcome with therapy (Y)	15% mortality
Absolute risk reduction (X – Y)	20% – 15% = 5%
Relative risk reduction: [1 – (Y/X)] × 100%	[1 – (0.15/0.2)] × 100% = 25%
Number needed to treat: 1/(X – Y)	1/0.05 = 20

RRR of zero indicates that the new therapy is no more efficacious than the old therapy or control. A negative RRR means that the new treatment is actually more harmful. If the authors do not specifically report RRR or ARR, use the data to calculate them for the outcomes that interest you. Be careful with relative reductions: You must know the absolute difference to interpret RRR. For example, ARR from 7% to 5% may not be impressive, yet it has the same RRR (25%) as ARR of 20% to 15%.

How precise was the estimate of treatment effect?
The best estimate of the true treatment effect is expressed by the confidence interval (CI), which is usually reported along with *P* values. The 95% CI includes the true RRR 95% of the time. The chance that the true RRR lies toward the extremes of this interval is low, and the chance that the true RRR lies beyond these extremes is only 5% (a property of the CI that closely relates to the "statistical significance" of $P < 0.05$). Thus if a study reports that RRR was 15% with a CI of 9% to 18%, then the treatment effect is positive. If the CI were reported as –5% to 17%, you cannot be sure of the efficacy of treatment because RRR ranges from positive (efficacious), to zero (no effect), to negative (adverse effect). In addition, the larger the sample size, the narrower the CI and the more likely the effect is real. If the CI is not reported, examine the *P* value. If the *P* value is exactly 0.05, then the lower bound of the 95% CI for the RRR lies exactly at 0 (no effect). As the *P* value decreases, the lower bound of the 95% CI for the RRR rises above 0 and an effect is more likely.

Will the New Treatment Help My Patient(s)?

Can the study results be applied to your patient?
In general, if your patient meets all of the inclusion criteria for a therapeutic trial and does not violate any of the exclusion criteria, the results of the study are applicable. If this is not the case, ask yourself whether there is some compelling reason why the results should *not* be applied to your patient. Take the patient's values into consideration.

Were all clinically important outcomes considered?
Often, researchers must substitute study endpoints that may not truly reflect the actual desired clinical endpoint. You will need to decide if these substitute outcomes are appropriate or useful.

Do benefits outweigh potential harms and costs?

Benefits are best assessed using the "number needed to treat" (NNT) (Table 7-1). The NNT is determined by the question "How many patients would need to be treated in order to prevent one adverse outcome?" In the earlier example, you would have to treat 20 patients to prevent 1 death. In addition, you need to ask whether the benefits of a given therapy outweigh its adverse effects for your patient(s). For example, treatment of mild asthmatic patients with ipratropium might result in 40 patients developing significant tachycardia for every life saved, whereas treatment of only severe asthmatics might result in 4 patients with significant tachycardia for every life saved. You need to consider your patient's asthma and clinical status before deciding to use ipratropium for the next asthma exacerbation.

PRESENTING THE EVIDENCE

What Is the Best Way to Present What I Have Learned?

Ask for recommendations about the way to present what you have learned and in what form. Written and verbal presentations should be concise, structured, and easily understood. Do not make the mistake of overly criticizing a study's methodology, results, or conclusions. Remember that most studies published in reputable journals have been peer reviewed and, although often not perfect, contain valuable data and conclusions. Although we seek black-and-white answers from the clinical literature, most medical evidence comes in shades of gray. Your job is to critically appraise the study's methodology and conclusions and to make recommendations for their application to your patient's care.

What Guidelines Should I Use for an EBM Report?

In general, a written presentation should be between one and three pages and a verbal presentation between 5 and 10 minutes. The following format, adapted from Patient-Oriented Evidence that Matters (POEMS), is appropriate for written and verbal reports (Slawson et al., 1997):

1. *Introduction*: State the clinical question, and give the references for the article(s) that you evaluated. Briefly describe your search strategy.
2. *Background*: Why did you ask this question? What population of patients are you interested in? How does the question fit into the larger context of pediatric practice?
3. *Study design*: Briefly describe the study's methodology (the "map"). Report the inclusion and exclusion criteria and whether the study results were statistically significant. Comment on the strengths and weaknesses of the study design and conclusions, but do not be overly critical.

4. *Answer the three core EBM questions:*
   - Are the results valid?
   - What are the results?
   - Will they help me in caring for my patient?
5. *Recommendations* for clinical practice: This is the most important part of the critical appraisal exercise. Make recommendations for the patient in question (and similar patients) based on what you have learned. Do not be afraid to state the conclusions from your review of the evidence, but be prepared to support them.

Are There Limits to Using EBM in Pediatrics?

Application of EBM in pediatrics is challenging because human growth and development makes longitudinal, prospective studies complicated. In contrast with the adult medical literature, there are few rigorous studies of therapeutic regimens for most of the diseases common in children. Although the U.S. Food and Drug Administration proposed regulations to require that new drugs be tested in children, this rule was rescinded and its future is in doubt.

Can I Find Online EBM Resources?

- Online tutorials teach the fundamental concepts of EBM. Look first for tutorials or links on a medical library Web site. A user-friendly online EBM tutorial co-developed by Duke University and the University of North Carolina–Chapel Hill can be found at www.hsl.unc.edu/services/tutorials/ebm/index.htm
- Collections of evidence-based reviews, meta-analyses, and practice guidelines for common clinical problems may be linked on the medical library Web site. Ask the librarian.
  - Cochrane Collaboration Child Health Field www.cochranechildhealth.ualberta.ca/reviews.html
  - American Academy of Pediatrics practice guidelines www.aappolicy.aappublications.org
  - University of Michigan Department of Pediatrics www.med.umich.edu/pediatrics/ebm/

KEY POINTS

- The question is the key element in EBM.
- Use the PICO format for your questions.
- Advance preparation will make your MEDLINE searches more efficient.
- To evaluate clinical evidence, you need to know if the study produced valid results and if the results apply to your patient.

BIBLIOGRAPHY

Gehlbach SH: *Interpreting the medical literature,* ed 4, New York, 2002, McGraw-Hill.

Greenhalgh T: The MEDLINE database, *BMJ* 315:180, 1997.

Greenhalgh T: *How to read a paper: the basics of evidence-based medicine,* ed 3, Malden, MA, 2006, Blackwell Publishing.

Oxman AD et al: Users' guides to the medical literature: I. How to get started. *JAMA* 270:2093, 1993.

Sackett DL et al: Evidence-based medicine: What it is and what it isn't. *BMJ* 312:71-72, 1996.

Slawson DC et al: Mastering medical information and the role of POEMS—patient-oriented evidence that matters. *J Family Pract* 45:195, 1997.

Straus SE, Richardson WS, Glasziou P, Haynes RB: *Evidence-based medicine: how to practice and teach EBM,* ed 3, Edinburgh, 2005, Churchill Livingstone.

8

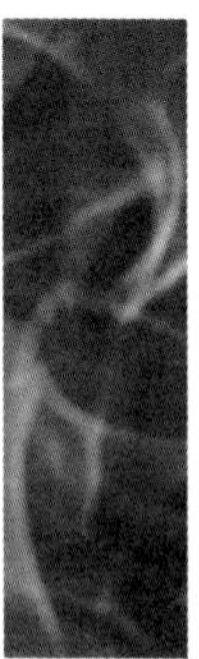

Growth

JEROLD C. WOODHEAD

What Are the Key Points I Need to Know about Growth?

The overall health of an individual affects growth and pubertal maturation through complex interactions among diseases, nutrition, and the growth process. In general, as nutrition, control of diseases, and general public health improve, populations become taller and heavier and demonstrate earlier sexual maturation. Standardized growth charts reflect the population norms and are used for ongoing surveillance. Figure 8-1 shows human growth patterns.

- *Stature and weight* change most rapidly in infancy and again during puberty. Statural growth ceases at the end of puberty, although weight may change throughout life. Weight gain is influenced by genetic, nutritional, and behavioral factors.
- *Genital growth* proceeds slowly until puberty, when it accelerates and goes through predictable stages, reflecting physiologic maturation.

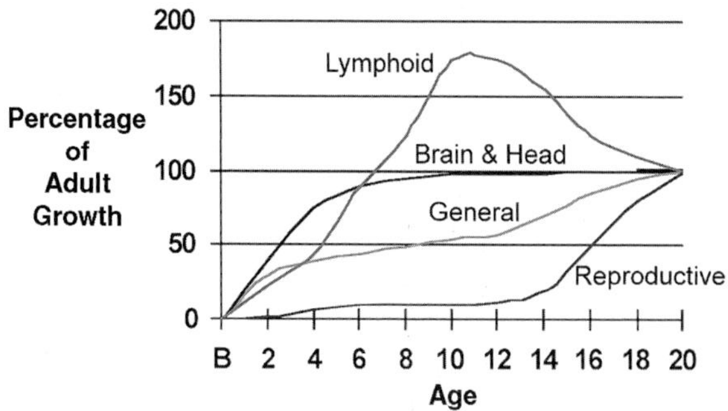

FIGURE 8-1 Human growth patterns. (Adapted from Scammon RE: The measurement of the body in childhood. In Harris JA et al, editors: *The measurement of man,* Minneapolis, 1930, University of Minnesota Press.)

- *Head circumference* (HC) increases as the brain grows rapidly in the first 2 years of life. HC growth then slows and reaches a plateau after ages 4 to 6 years.
- *Developmental and cognitive growth* continue throughout life and reflect brain and neurologic function.
- *Lymphatic* tissue has a predictable growth pattern that peaks just before puberty, reflecting exposures to infectious agents.

How Do I Measure Growth?

Most of the time, growth is measured and plotted onto growth charts by the staff of a well-functioning office or inpatient service. Deviations from expected patterns will demand interpretation and decision making. You must review growth charts for every patient, record the data in all clinical notes, and interpret the plotted points for head circumference, weight, and length or height. You will also need to consider an infant's weight-for-length and an older child's body mass index (BMI). You may be asked to make the measurements and plot the data, so observe experts taking growth measurements whenever you get the chance.

How Do I Document Growth?

Growth data are plotted on growth charts (www.cdc.gov/growthcharts/) that are gender- and age-specific. The child between 2 and 3 years of age can be plotted on either the "infant" growth chart (birth to 36 months) or the "child" growth chart (2 to 20 years). Percentiles for stature differ on the two charts because an infant is measured supine, whereas a child is measured standing. You must take the measurement technique into account when you decide which chart to use. Growth charts have also been developed for specific populations, such as those with Down syndrome, Turner syndrome, and achondroplasia. (See *The Harriet Lane Handbook,* pp 600–608.)

Do Genetic and Disease Factors Influence Growth?

The ultimate stature (height) of an individual is *genetically* determined and usually reflects the stature of the parents, if the child is healthy. Predicted stature for healthy children approximates "mean parental height":

Boy's predicted stature = [(Mother's height + k) + Father's height] ÷ 2

Girl's predicted stature = [Mother's height + (Father's height − k)] ÷ 2

where k = 5 inches in the English system and k = 13 cm in the metric system.

Growth patterns also tend to "run in families," especially if growth accelerates relatively late, as occurs with constitutional delay of growth. Parents may tell you that they were the shortest in their age group until a growth spurt occurred in high school. Key to assessment of this type of growth pattern is recognition that growth does not plateau; it follows the curve in an upward direction, even though in a percentile range lower than anticipated based on parental mean height. Genetic factors may also influence height adversely, especially when parents are both short, or in the case of disorders such as Turner and Down syndromes. Prenatal factors such as placental insufficiency and fetal alcohol syndrome cause in utero growth retardation, which may affect ultimate adult stature. Disease may adversely affect ultimate stature, as will extreme dieting during the adolescent growth spurt.

When Does Nutrition Affect Growth?

Nutrition is discussed in more detail in Chapter 10. Nutrition most strongly influences growth during infancy, especially in the first 4 months of life. The average infant gains 20 to 30 g daily between birth and 4 months, which results in a doubling of birth weight. Length also increases rapidly, with an increase of approximately 15 cm in the first 4 months. Approximately 27% of all the calories ingested in the first 4 months of life are used for synthesis and deposition of new tissue. Rapid growth demands a steady, reliable, high-quality supply of nutrients to provide approximately 100 to 110 kcal/kg/day plus adequate protein, lipid, minerals, and micronutrients. The demand placed by growth on nutritional intake falls dramatically after age 4 months. By age 1 year, growth rate has slowed and will continue to slow until puberty, when it again increases. Even during the peak of adolescent growth, the calories needed for growth do not reach the levels required at 1 year. The "energy cost of growth" is shown in Figure 8-2.

What Growth Problems Am I Likely to Encounter?

Being overweight is the most prevalent growth problem. Long-term excessive calorie intake results in excessive weight gain, and monitoring of the BMI is important during childhood to allow early intervention to prevent development of obesity. Chronic exposure to excess calories also results in acceleration of stature as weight increases, but ultimate adult height is not

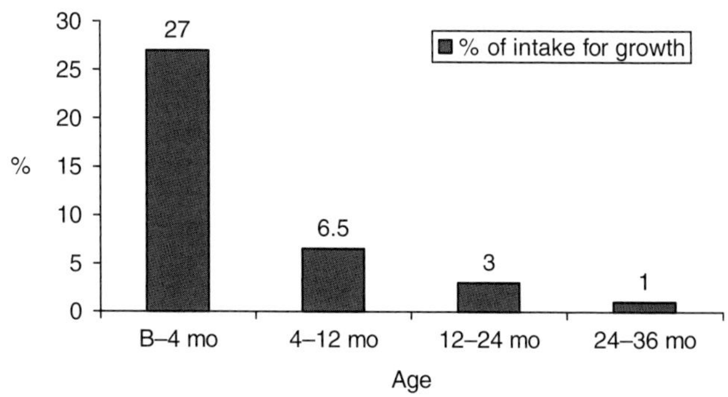

FIGURE 8-2 Energy cost of growth from birth to 3 years of age. (Adapted from Fomon SJ: *Nutrition of normal infants,* St Louis, 1993, Mosby.)

affected. In addition, physicians who care for children often are challenged by underweight, short stature, and small or large head circumference. Severe malnutrition can adversely affect ultimate stature when it occurs in childhood and during the adolescent growth spurt. Tall stature is rarely perceived as a problem by parents and patients, unless accompanied by findings associated with syndromes. Pubertal development, either early or delayed, causes concern in older children and adolescents. You must learn to assess growth in all of its dimensions if you wish to identify problems. Growth problems are discussed in Chapter 35.

KEY POINTS

- Growth is most rapid between birth and 4 months and requires a continuous supply of energy and other nutrients.
- You must learn to use and interpret growth charts.
- A child's ultimate height can be estimated if you know the heights of both biologic parents.

Case 8-1

Parents of a 2-year-old boy ask you to give them an idea about how big their son will be when he is fully grown. At present he is at the 50th percentile for length and weight. The couple also has a 6-year-old girl who is at the 75th percentile for height. They are curious about her adult stature, too.

A. How tall is this boy? How tall is the girl?
B. How can you estimate the adult stature for a child?
C. If the father is 6 feet tall and the mother is 5 feet, 6 inches tall, give estimates for both the 2-year-old boy and the 6-year-old girl.
D. If the boy has Down syndrome, what resource will you use to provide information to parents? How tall is he now? How tall will he be if he grows at the 50th percentile?

Case Answers

8-1 A. *Learning objective:* **Demonstrate the ability to measure and plot growth.** A boy at the 50th percentile is 84 cm long (34½ inches). The girl is 118 cm tall (46½ inches). Careful measurement is important, and the data must be plotted properly on growth charts. Remember that length should be measured supine up to age 2 years. After 2 years, a standing height may be obtained.

8-1 B. *Learning objective:* **Discuss the genetic influence on growth.** Information about parental stature allows you to use the equations on page 50 to estimate ultimate stature.

8-1 C. *Learning objective:* **Provide information to parents about the ultimate stature of their children.** The boy has an estimated adult stature of approximately 5 feet, 11½ inches (183 cm), the girl's estimated adult stature is 5 feet, 6½ inches (168 cm).

8-1 D. *Learning objective:* **Identify populations of children whose growth should be plotted on special growth charts.** The growth chart for individuals with Down syndrome should be used (see *The Harriet Lane Handbook,* 17 ed, pp. 600-603). Using the growth chart, you would see that a 2-year-old boy with Down syndrome at the 50th percentile for height is 80 cm tall and will have an ultimate adult stature of 145 cm if he continues to grow at the 50th percentile.

BIBLIOGRAPHY

Fiorino KN, Cox J: Nutrition and growth. In Robertson J, Shilkofski N, editors: *The Harriet Lane handbook*, ed 17, Philadelphia, 2005, Mosby, pp. 525-608.

Fomon SJ: *Nutrition of normal infants*, St Louis, 1993, Mosby.

Growth charts for healthy children: Available at www.cdc.gov/growthcharts/.

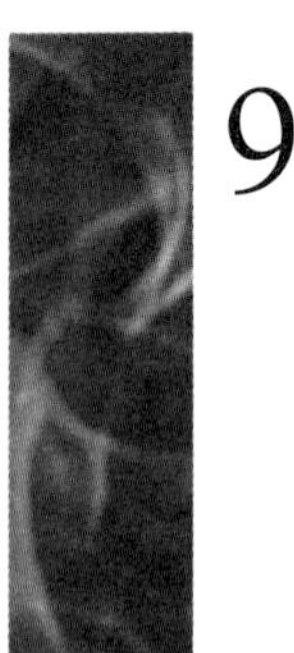

9 Developmental Assessment

JEROLD C. WOODHEAD

How Will I Learn about Development?

You will learn the *basics* of development during the clerkship, and your learning will be made easier if you make a conscious effort to *observe* infants, children, and adolescents wherever you encounter them, not just in the hospital or clinic. Ask yourself, "What does this child do that gives me clues about development?" Include observations about development at every clinical encounter, even for minor illnesses, and ask parents to tell you how they perceive their child's development compared with siblings or peers at the same age. Ask whether parents have concerns about development. *Listen* to what parents say, even if you cannot immediately provide an answer. Efforts to categorize the development of each patient will enhance your overall clinical skills and will allow you to add important information to case presentations.

What Observations Should I Make?

Watch the reaction of each patient as you enter the examination room. Observe the ways that *infants* react to parents and to the environment around them, including you. Think about how the reactions of *toddlers* provide information about their developmental progress, which will also help you gain insight about how to interact more effectively with them. Watch *children* play so that you may gain an appreciation of the progress they make physically, cognitively, socially, and emotionally. Pay attention to the ways that *children and adolescents* interact with each other, with parents, and with you. Look at physical abilities—walking, running, climbing, holding, and manipulating objects. Listen to language—content, complexity, understandability. In short, keep your eyes and ears open!

How Do I Recognize the Patterns of Developmental Progress?

Initially, identify the changes that occur with advancing age. What does a 1-month-old baby do that a newborn does not? When do you first notice that an infant can voluntarily open and close a hand? Can a 2-year-old hop on one foot? How about a 3-year-old or a 4-year-old? When can you understand most of the words and phrases spoken by a child? What behaviors do you observe in toddlers, school-age children, and adolescents? How much cooperation does a patient demonstrate during the physical examination? Soon, you will recognize that skills in a variety of areas all have predictable patterns of developmental progress and can be organized into broad categories, which will make your observations more useful. You will learn to expect certain skills and behaviors in patients at a given age. You may even begin to predict the age of a child based on developmental achievements. Frequent use of a reference for expected developmental progress will let you evaluate the observations that you make and help you become conversant with the developmental sequence more rapidly: The *Denver Developmental Assessment* (Denver II) is a widely used screening tool for children up to age 6, *Bright Futures* is a useful online resource for health supervision, and the *Early Language Milestones* provides a timeline of language development.

What Are the Major Areas of Development?

Development is usually divided into broad categories: motor, language, cognition, problem solving, and psychosocial. These categories facilitate ongoing surveillance. Each links to the others and is influenced by progress in the others. An individual's overall development represents the totality of the interaction. A practical approach to categorizing development can be found in the Denver II, which provides population-based norms for development in four "streams": gross motor, fine motor/adaptive, language, and personal/social (Figure 9-1). A separate stream devoted to cognition does not appear in the Denver II, but the fine motor/adaptive, language, and personal/social streams all reflect cognitive development. Other, more formal developmental assessment tools use more complex categorization schemes, but for your purposes during the clerkship, simple schemes suffice. The *Bright Futures Pocket Guide* provides useful lists of age-related developmental skills for day-to-day clinical evaluations.

How Do I Determine if Development Is Age-appropriate?

Most children that you encounter will have appropriate development, but some will be delayed. Your task is to understand the progress of development well enough to identify concerning patterns. The task starts with knowledge of expected development, coupled with the ability to make good observations. At some point in the clerkship, you will realize that "normal" development varies among healthy children of the same age. Some children follow the averages, whereas others "specialize" in a single area, such as language or motor development, and are "advanced" in that area and "average" or perhaps a bit "below average" in other areas. The differences are usually expected variations that do not signal the need for undue concern. Yet parents may voice worry that

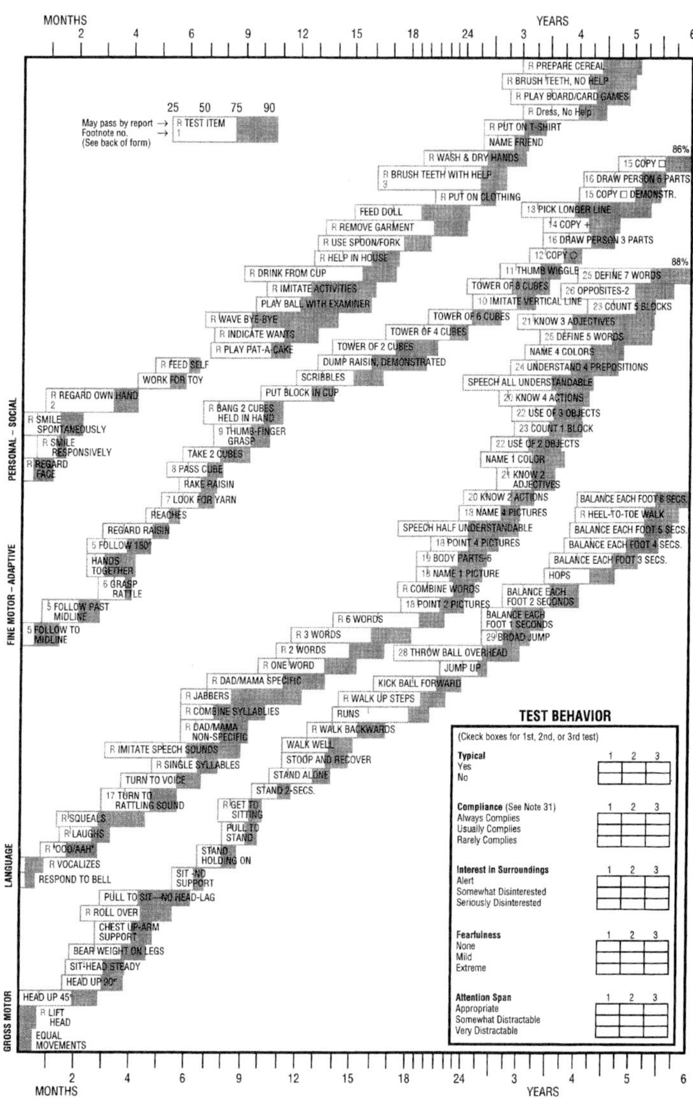

FIGURE 9-1 The Denver Developmental Assessment (Denver II). (From Frankenburg WK et al: The Denver II: A major revision and restandardization of the Denver Developmental Screening Test. *Pediatrics,* 89:91-97,1992.)

DIRECTIONS FOR ADMINISTRATION

1. Try to get child to smile by smiling, talking or waving. Do not touch him/her.
2. Child must stare at hand several seconds.
3. Parent may help guide toothbrush and put toothpaste on brush.
4. Child does not have to be able to tie shoes or button/zip in the back.
5. Move yarn slowly in an arc from one side to the other, about 8" above child's face.
6. Pass if child grasps rattle when it is touched to the backs or tips of fingers.
7. Pass if child tries to see where yarn went. Yarn should be dropped quickly from sight from tester's hand without arm movement.
8. Child must transfer cube from hand to hand without help of body, mouth, or table.
9. Pass if child picks up raisin with any part of thumb and finger.
10. Line can vary only 30 degrees or less from tester's line.
11. Make a fist with thumb pointing upward and wiggle only the thumb. Pass if child imitates and does not move any fingers other than the thumb.

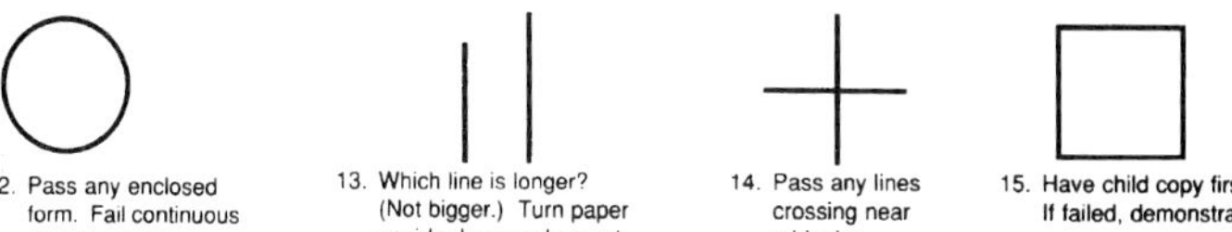

12. Pass any enclosed form. Fail continuous round motions.
13. Which line is longer? (Not bigger.) Turn paper upside down and repeat. (pass 3 of 3 or 5 of 6)
14. Pass any lines crossing near midpoint.
15. Have child copy first. If failed, demonstrate.

When giving items 12, 14, and 15, do not name the forms. Do not demonstrate 12 and 14.

16. When scoring, each pair (2 arms, 2 legs, etc.) counts as one part.
17. Place one cube in cup and shake gently near child's ear, but out of sight. Repeat for other ear.
18. Point to picture and have child name it. (No credit is given for sounds only.) If less than 4 pictures are named correctly, have child point to picture as each is named by tester.

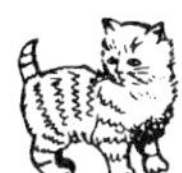 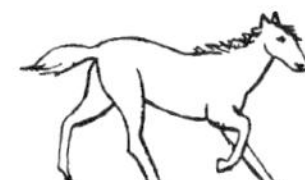 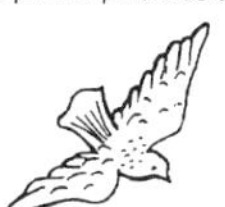 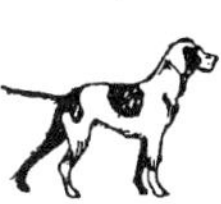 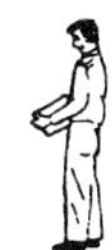

19. Using doll, tell child: Show me the nose, eyes, ears, mouth, hands, feet, tummy, hair. Pass 6 of 8.
20. Using pictures, ask child: Which one flies?... says meow?... talks?... barks?... gallops? Pass 2 of 5, 4 of 5.
21. Ask child: What do you do when you are cold?... tired?... hungry? Pass 2 of 3, 3 of 3.
22. Ask child: What do you do with a cup? What is a chair used for? What is a pencil used for? Action words must be included in answers.
23. Pass if child correctly places <u>and</u> says how many blocks are on paper. (1, 5).
24. Tell child: Put block **on** table; **under** table; **in front of** me, **behind** me. Pass 4 of 4. (Do not help child by pointing, moving head or eyes.)
25. Ask child: What is a ball?... lake?... desk?... house?... banana?... curtain?... fence?... ceiling? Pass if defined in terms of use, shape, what it is made of, or general category (such as banana is fruit, not just yellow). Pass 5 of 8, 7 of 8.
26. Ask child: If a horse is big, a mouse is __? If fire is hot, ice is __? If the sun shines during the day, the moon shines during the __? Pass 2 of 3.
27. Child may use wall or rail only, not person. May not crawl.
28. Child must throw ball overhand 3 feet to within arm's reach of tester.
29. Child must perform standing broad jump over width of test sheet (8 1/2 inches).
30. Tell child to walk forward, heel within 1 inch of toe. Tester may demonstrate. Child must walk 4 consecutive steps.
31. In the second year, half of normal children are non-compliant.

OBSERVATIONS:

FIGURE 9-1—CONT'D

their child is not following the "prescribed" developmental pattern that they have read about in books, in magazines, or on the Web. They also may be worried because family and friends have commented about their child's development. These concerns deserve serious attention.

How Do I Explain Development to a Parent?

First, you must know what "normal development" means and must understand how the child's developmental variations fit within the expected progress for an individual at a given age. You must examine the child to assess development, looking especially for those delays that signal concerns. If no problems are identified, a plan for ongoing surveillance of development will generally reassure the family and reinforce the appropriateness of the child's pattern. If, on the other hand, you encounter a child who has *not* achieved expected milestones or whose pattern deviates enough from the expected course to raise concerns, you must be able to compare the child's actual abilities with expected development. Your carefully developed observational skills will help identify the problem and also reduce the likelihood that you might overlook something. Attention to communication of "bad news" will assist you to explain concerns to parents and help them understand the need for further assessment and possible referral to a developmental specialist (see Chapter 27).

What Do I Need to Know about Development at Different Ages?

Table 9-1 lists developmental milestones from birth through adolescence.

Table 9-1

Key Developmental Issues

Age	Milestone
Newborn	Symmetry of movement and muscle tone. Flexed posture. Primitive reflexes (Moro, suck, grasp, root, etc.). Vigorous cry. Focuses on human face. Responds to voice.
Birth–6 months	Social smile by 2 months. Gradual disappearance of primitive reflexes and appearance of voluntary, symmetrical motor skills. Reaches for, holds, and then transfers object by 5–6 months. Rolling, sitting, and crawling between 4 and 6 months. Increase in social responsiveness. Vocalization with laughing, babbling and progressively complex sound production.
6–12 months	Progression of motor skills from sitting, to standing with support, to standing unsupported, to "cruising." Independent walking may not appear until later. Pincer grasp used to pick up objects by 9–10 months. Responds to name, uses single words, plays interactive games, hunts for a hidden object, feeds self with fingers. Stranger anxiety develops.
1–2 years	Walks well by 15 months and walks backward by 18 months. Language progresses from 2–4 words at age 1 year to more complex language with words and short phrases at age 2—but only ~50% understood by a stranger. Follows directions by ~18 months. Imitates words and behaviors. Drinks from a cup at 1 year and uses a spoon by 18 months. Stranger anxiety peaks.
2–4 years	Climbs stairs by 2 years, hops on both feet at age 3 years, hops on one foot at 4 years. Language increasingly complex: ~75% understandable at 3 years, essentially 100% at age 4. Knows name, age, sex. Sings.
School age	Learns address, phone number, letters, and numbers. Follows rules by 5 years. Progress in classroom activities provides good screen of development. Increasing independence in activities of daily living (dressing, eating, play, etc.).
Adolescence	Social, emotional, and personal interactions increasingly complex. Rapid changes in physical appearance and personality. School provides important clues. Increasing attention to peers and influences outside of the family. Sexuality. Habits including use of alcohol, tobacco, and illicit drugs may develop.

How Can I Avoid Making Mistakes?

You can avoid errors by actively assessing every patient based on a solid knowledge base and sound clinical skills. Challenge yourself always to define "normal." By doing so, you will develop the habit of looking for the characteristics that make development age appropriate. *Review* the child's developmental milestones. *Listen* to parental descriptions and concerns. *Take the time to observe. Describe* your findings to parents. *Do not make assumptions.* Physicians often assume that the healthy, "beautiful" child could not possibly have cognitive problems ("He doesn't look retarded"). Another dangerous assumption is that a delay in one area of development has no consequences ("She will grow out of it"). One common error is to focus only on the obvious, such as gross motor skills, while ignoring more subtle deficits in areas such as fine motor skills or language. Deficits in vision, hearing, and cognition can have a negative impact on the development of language, interactional, and problem-solving skills. Infants and young children will manifest sensory and cognitive problems by the ways that they respond to their environment. For example, a decline in vocalization between 3 and 6 months may indicate congenital neurosensory deafness, whereas delay in language later in the first or second year may suggest acquired conductive hearing loss. The combination of delays in language and social skills in a child whose development is otherwise on track may be the clue to autistic spectrum disorder. Remember that the social environment of the home has a huge influence on development, especially in language and personal and interactional skills. Knowledge of development gained from observation will prevent you from overlooking developmental problems, but it will also prevent you from labeling as "abnormal" developmental patterns and behaviors that are age appropriate.

KEY POINTS

- You learn the most about children by observing them.
- Do not make assumptions about development.
- *Bright Futures* and the Denver II are excellent resources.

Case 9-1

Parents of a 4-year-old boy who has recently been adopted from Eastern Europe are concerned that he is not developing appropriately. His past medical history has limited information about his birth. He was placed in an orphanage shortly after birth and, according to records, had "normal" developmental progress. Since arriving in the United States, he has shown many behavioral problems and uses very little language.

A. How can you assess his overall development?
B. What motor skills would you expect a 4-year-old boy to demonstrate?
C. How can you assess his language?

Case Answers

9-1 A. *Learning objective:* **Assess the development of a healthy child.** An initial assessment can be done first by observing the child playing with toys, playing with other children, and moving around the room. His interactions with parents, office staff, and you will also provide important information. A screening tool such as the Denver II will give objective information about his developmental progress.

9-1 B. *Learning objective:* **Know the sequence of the basic developmental milestones during childhood.** A 4-year-old child walks with a mature gait, climbs, and hops on one foot.

9-1 C. *Learning objective:* **Recognize that language requires the ability to hear, the cognitive ability to comprehend language, and the physical ability to produce sound.** Listen to his vocalizations. Assess ears and mouth for any abnormalities, including middle ear effusions, tympanic membrane perforations, and cleft palate. Make sure that he can hear. If needed, tympanometry and audiometry can be used.

BIBLIOGRAPHY

Coplan J: *The Early Language Milestone Scale*, ed 2 (ELM Scale 2), Austin, TX, 1993, PRO-ED.

Frankenburg WK et al: The Denver II: A major revision and restandardization of the Denver Developmental Screening Test. *Pediatrics*, 89:91-97,1992.

Green M, editor: *Bright futures: guidelines for health supervision of infants, children, and adolescents pocket guide*, ed 2, Arlington, VA, 2000, National Center for Education in Maternal and Child Health, 2000. See www.brightfutures.org to download a PDF file of the *Bright Futures Pocket Guide*.

Chung RW: Development and behavior. In Robertson J, Shilkofski N, editors: *The Harriet Lane handbook*, ed 17, Philadelphia, 2005, Mosby, pp. 231-252.

10

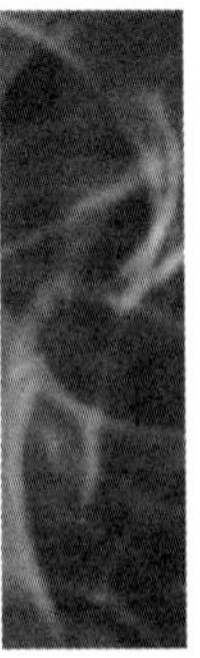

Nutrition

JEROLD C. WOODHEAD

When Should Nutrition Be Discussed?

Nutrition is one of the first topics that you will discuss with parents of newborn infants, and it will continue to be a key component of health supervision visits throughout childhood. You will need to include nutritional advice during anticipatory guidance at every health visit. Practical information can be found in *Bright Futures in Practice: Nutrition* and in the American Academy of Pediatrics' *Pediatric Nutrition Handbook*.

What Nutritional Issues Should I Discuss with Families?

Parents ask questions about breast-feeding, formula, food choices, the readiness of a child for new foods, the value of vitamin supplements, feeding behaviors, food allergy, and inadequate or excessive weight gain. To answer the questions, you need to know about the nutritional needs of human growth (see Chapter 8) and the child's developmental capabilities at different ages (see Chapter 9). Be sure to ask about nutritional beliefs that guide family eating as well as ethnic, cultural, or health-related dietary issues. Inquire about family risk factors for early cardiovascular disease and type 2 diabetes mellitus. ***Obesity** is the most prevalent nutritional disorder in the United States,* so the weight of family members, eating habits, and growth patterns (including body mass index [BMI]) will be important information. Adults who have large waist circumference are at high risk for metabolic complications associated with obesity. Recent evidence supports a similar risk for children who have a waist circumference-to-height ratio (WC:Ht) > 0.50. In other words, keeping waist circumference below half of the height is an important message. ***Poor weight gain*** occasionally causes concern for an infant or young child, and parents will need guidance to improve nutrition. ***Toddlers*** present challenges because of behavior. ***Adolescents*** need nutritional advice for topics ranging from the high-calorie needs of athletes to the severely restricted diets of individuals with eating disorders. You must be prepared to discuss the risks of obesity and of fad diets with teenagers. ***Disease*** presents nutritional challenges for acute problems, such as gastroenteritis, and chronic diseases such as diabetes mellitus, inflammatory bowel disease, cystic fibrosis, celiac disease, and chronic kidney disease. ***Unsubstantiated "nutritional" information*** from the Internet often links food with disease and vague health problems. Your best response is to provide reliable sources of information such as the Web sites of the Centers for Disease Control and Prevention (CDC) or the American Academy of Pediatrics (AAP).

Are Nutritional Deficiencies Common?

Iron and calcium deficiency affect large numbers of otherwise healthy children and adolescents in the United States, but most other nutritional deficiencies are uncommon in Western society. Nutritional deficiencies may be identified if patients or families do not eat specific foods. Iron deficiency is common among adolescent girls and may be more common in families who restrict red meat from their diets. Some ethnic groups are at high risk for calcium deficiency because they do not include dairy products in the diet, either for cultural reasons or because of the high prevalence of lactose intolerance beyond childhood. Infants nursed by women who are strict vegetarians (vegans) have high risk of B vitamin deficiency. Goat milk is deficient in folic acid and should not be the major source of nutrition for an infant or young child. Be aware that many children live in poverty and that food may not be adequate to meet their needs.

How Does Illness Affect Nutrition?

Acute illnesses such as gastroenteritis may cause inadequate intake of fluids and calories. Disease may impair nutrient absorption, as is seen with fat malabsorption in cystic fibrosis and with lactose malabsorption after prolonged diarrhea. Hereditary disaccharidase deficiency, usually lactase deficiency, typically manifests in preschool or school-age children. Disorders of lipid metabolism may require fat-restricted diets, although the restriction is usually not implemented until late childhood. Consumption of specific foods may be contraindicated in certain conditions such as celiac disease (gluten) and phenylketonuria (phenylalanine). Occasionally, foods may cause illness, as occurs with anaphylactic reactions to nuts, shellfish, and milk. Contamination of foods with bacteria, viruses, or toxins may result in diarrhea and food poisoning.

INFANTS

How Are Newborns and Young Infants Fed?

Approximately 70% of U.S. mothers begin breast-feeding at birth, but most breast-fed infants are switched to formula before 6 months. Active encouragement of breast-feeding and support from clinicians, family, and friends, plus accommodations for lactating women in the workplace, will enhance the likelihood that a mother will choose to nurse her newborn and persist with breast-feeding until the infant is at least 6 months old. Mothers who choose to formula feed or cannot breast-feed also need support, plus information about appropriate formulas. In addition, most parents begin to diversify the diets for their infants by adding "baby foods" after ages 4 to 6 months and will need advice about appropriate foods. "Whole" cow milk is not appropriate for infants younger than 12 months because it often produces occult gastrointestinal bleeding and leads to iron deficiency anemia (Chapter 63). Cow milk also has excessive protein and poorly absorbed fat and iron.

How Do Human Milk, Formulas, and Cow Milk Differ?

Table 10-1 provides a comparison of human milk, formulas, and whole cow milk. All have the same energy content, 20 kcal/oz (667 kcal/L), although human milk varies somewhat. See the nutritional formulary at your hospital or a resource such as The *Harriet Lane Handbook* for more detailed information. You can also find information about formulas designed to meet the needs of premature infants and infants with a variety of metabolic and nutritional disorders.

What Are the Benefits of Human Milk?

Human milk contains the protein, fat, carbohydrates, and essentially all other nutrients needed to promote growth from the time of full-term birth to at least 6 months of age. The volume of milk produced by the lactating mother increases in response to the infant's nursing, reaching a peak when the infant is about 4 to 6 months old. Non-nutritional components of human milk protect against infection and are especially concentrated in colostrum, the first milk produced immediately after birth. Breast-feeding promotes close contact and positive emotional and behavioral outcomes for both infant and mother. Human milk can be fortified to meet the caloric needs of premature infants.

Table 10-1

Composition of Human Milk, Standard Formulas, and Cow Milk

Nutrient	Human Milk	Cow Milk-Based Formula	Soy-Based Formula	"Whole" Cow Milk*
Energy (kcal/L)	620–700	667	667	630–680
Protein (g/L)	9	5	16.5–21	33
Fat (g/L)	32	36	36	35
Carbohydrate (g/L)	74	72	69	47
Iron (mg/L)	0.34	12	12	0.46
Vitamin D (IU/L)	50	400	400	400
Vitamin E (IU/L)	2–4	20	9.5–21	0.4–0.9
Vitamin K (IU/L)	1–4	54	100	1–4

Adapted from Fomon SJ: *Nutrition of normal infants,* St Louis, 1993, Mosby, pp 410, 427, 444.

*Vitamin D fortified.

What Is Special about the Nutrients in Human Milk?

Human milk protein is predominantly whey (60% to 70%), which is highly soluble and easily digested. Protein content decreases from 14 g/L at birth to 8 g/L at 6 months, and averages 9 g/L in mature milk. This change parallels the decrease in the infant's protein requirement. The protein content of human milk occasionally may be limiting after age 6 months for the large infant, but this is not a concern if other protein containing foods are introduced. Lipids provide about 50% of calories in human milk and the milk-fat globule contains a lipase to facilitate absorption. Human milk contains arachidonic and docosahexaenoic acids, which are essential omega-3 fatty acids not present in cow milk. Maternal dietary fat intake affects the composition of fatty acids in human milk but not the total quantity of lipid or the presence of essential fatty acids. Lactose is the principal carbohydrate source of calories in human milk; oligosaccharides provide important protection against infection. Essentially all infants digest lactose. Calcium and phosphorus are better absorbed from human milk than from formula, because they are bound to digestible proteins or are present as complexes or in ionized forms.

Which Nutrients Appear in Low Concentrations in Human Milk?

The few nutrients that have low concentrations in human milk are those that have toxic effects if taken in excess (iron, vitamin D, and fluoride) or that are synthesized by the infant after birth (vitamins D and K). The full-term infant's iron stores are adequate to maintain hemoglobin production until ages 4 to 6 months of age, after which supplementation with iron-fortified foods should be started. The infant needs 200 IU of vitamin D daily, but human milk contains $\leq$ 25 IU/L. Because most infants do not have the sun exposure needed for synthesis of vitamin D, the American Academy of Pediatrics recommends that *all breast-fed infants receive supplemental vitamin D* beginning in the first 2 months of life. Vitamin K must be administered to all newborn infants at birth to prevent vitamin K deficiency bleeding (hemorrhagic disease of the newborn). Fluoride supplementation is not necessary during infancy.

Does Human Milk Prevent Infections?

Human milk, particularly colostrum, contains secretory IgA, lysozyme, lactoferrin, cytokines, enzymes, macrophages, and other bioactive factors that protect the breast-feeding infant. Promoters of *Bifidobacterium* species in the infant's gastrointestinal tract reduce growth of pathogenic bacteria. Breast-fed infants have lower rates of otitis media, gastroenteritis, lower respiratory tract infections, and urinary tract infection. Breast-fed infants in developing countries are protected from unsanitary water that might be used to mix formula.

Does Breast-Feeding Protect against Development of Allergies?

In general, breast-fed infants have lower rates of respiratory allergies and eczema. Exclusive breast-feeding may offer protection against atopy if the mother avoids cow milk, egg, fish, peanuts, and tree nuts during lactation. Human milk contains antigens derived from the maternal diet that occasionally cause allergic reactions, including bloody diarrhea.

Is Breast-Feeding Ever *Not* Recommended?

Infants with galactosemia cannot tolerate lactose, thus must not be breast-fed. Breast-feeding is not recommended in the United States and other developed countries if the mother is infected with human immunodeficiency virus (HIV); benefits of breast-feeding by HIV-infected mothers in underdeveloped countries may outweigh the risks. In addition, women should not breast-feed if they have untreated active tuberculosis or take drugs of abuse, chemotherapeutic agents, or radioactive isotopes. Drugs such as lithium, ergotamine, and others should be discouraged if a woman is breast-feeding. Reliable information about the safety of herbal, "alternative," and "complementary" preparations is lacking. A woman who plans to breast-feed should discuss *all* medications with a physician. Drug compendia include information about use of medications during lactation.

What Should I Know about Formula?

Formulas for healthy infants are based on cow milk or soy protein isolates and have nutrient composition and energy content similar to that of human milk (Table 10-1). Lactose is the major carbohydrate in standard cow milk–based formulas. Soy protein isolate formulas are lactose free and contain glucose polymers and sucrose. Soy milk marketed to adults is *not* suitable for infants and young children. Special formulas have been developed for premature infants, infants with various metabolic diseases, and infants who must have modifications of protein, fat, or carbohydrate.

How Much Does an Infant Need to Be Fed?

The energy demands of growth are greatest in the first 4 months of life, when almost 30% of all the nutrients ingested are converted into new tissue growth (see Chapter 8). Infants need approximately 110 kcal/kg/day during the first few months of life, after which calorie need gradually declines to approximately 95 kcal/kg between ages 4 to 12 months. Healthy full-term infants voluntarily consume adequate quantities of human milk or formula and achieve appropriate growth if allowed to feed to satiety. You can reassure a breast-feeding mother that milk production is adequate if her infant is content after feeding, has at least six wet diapers each day, and follows the growth curve. You may calculate the calorie consumption of formula-fed infants by asking about the total volume fed over 24 hours because all standard formulas contain 20 kcal/oz (667 kcal/L). Formula-fed infants should *not* be encouraged to drink the last drop.

When Should Other Foods Be Added to an Infant's Diet?

In general, "solid" foods should be introduced only after 4 to 6 months of age. Before 4 months, an infant's head must be supported during feeding. After 4 months, head, neck, and trunk control allow the infant to sit with support while being fed with a spoon. In addition, by this age, maturation of the gastrointestinal tract reduces the likelihood that food proteins will enter the bloodstream unaltered and trigger adverse reactions. If foods are introduced after 4 months, cereals, fruits, vegetables, and meats may be added as the parents wish. Iron-fortified cereals and meats aid in preventing iron deficiency. The quantity of food fed at any given meal depends on appetite. Food allergy and atopy should be approached individually, based on the patient's reactions to specific foods and on a careful family history.

TODDLERS

What Nutritional Concerns Arise for Toddlers?

Parents usually have questions about the quantity and types of food that toddlers should eat. Many parents overestimate the amount of food needed, basing estimates on their own appetites. *Bright Futures in Practice: Nutrition* provides practical information to discuss with parents. The growth chart is an important tool for monitoring the consequences of adequate, inadequate, or excessive food intake. An excess of as little as 100 calories daily causes excessive weight gain. Careful attention to BMI between ages 2 and 6 years can identify the upward movement of the BMI percentile that points to calorie excess and risk for overweight. Mealtime is often a challenge for parents of toddlers who often have behavioral feeding problems related to their mastery of physical skills, emerging sense of independence, and need for attention. See Chapter 22 for a discussion of behavior problems. The toddler with a severe feeding behavior problem may fail to gain weight adequately or be at risk for child abuse (see Chapter 24).

CHILD AND ADOLESCENT

How Do I Monitor Child and Adolescent Nutrition?

Height, weight, waist circumference, and BMI of the child or adolescent serve as guides to nutritional status. As mentioned earlier, a rise in BMI between 2 and 6 years of age may be an early warning sign of calorie imbalance leading to excess weight gain. In addition, if waist circumference in children older than age 6 is greater than 50% of height (WC:Ht ratio > 0.5), the child has an increased risk for the metabolic consequences of obesity.

What Advice Should I Give about Nutrition?

You can only give advice if the patient and the family are interested in hearing it. Often, medical advice is viewed as unwanted "preaching." If you ask permission to discuss nutrition, especially the calorie imbalance that leads to overweight and obesity, you are likely to have a more receptive audience for your advice. If you also engage the patient and family in self-directed efforts to modify intake and activity, your advice may have the hoped for results. Ask about the dietary habits of the patient and the family: Who prepares meals, where does the child or adolescent eat, how often does fast food replace home-cooked meals, what is the daily consumption of carbohydrate-containing beverages such as juice and soft drinks, and what are the activity patterns of the patient and the family. *Attention to common sense makes the best advice.* Recommend a well-balanced diet that is appropriate for the energy expended by the child or adolescent and that maintains growth within the range expected for family growth patterns. Point out the high calorie content of fast foods and carbohydrate-rich drinks. Also discuss the risks of fad diets. Reinforce the benefits of regular exercise and "prescribe" a daily walk of 20 to 30 minutes duration. Use growth charts, BMI nomogram, and waist circumference (WC:Ht ratio) to demonstrate the pattern of weight gain, the goals for weight control, and as tools to monitor progress, if needed.

KEY POINTS

- Human milk is the best nutrient for newborns and young infants.
- Assist a mother who chooses not to breast-feed with selection of an iron-fortified formula.
- Iron and calcium are the most common nutritional deficiencies.
- Obesity is a major nutritional problem.

Case 10-1

The mother of a 1-week-old girl asks your advice about feeding problems. Her mother-in-law has told her that her breast milk is "thin" and that she should switch to formula to help the baby grow faster. The baby nurses every 90 minutes and wakes twice during the night to feed.

A. What information can you obtain from the history that will help you decide if the infant is receiving adequate nutrition?
B. What important facts about breast-feeding should you discuss with the mother?

Case 10-2

A 3-year-old boy has become a very picky eater over the past month. His mother says that he eats only "white" foods: milk, bread, cheese, and yogurt. He also likes sweets and juices but refuses vegetables and meat. She is worried that her son will not get adequate nutrition and is interested in a vitamin supplement for him. Over the past year, the boy's weight has increased from

50th percentile to 90th percentile and height has increased from 25th percentile to 50th percentile. BMI has increased from 75th percentile to > 95th percentile.

A. What information should you gather before you answer the mother's questions?
B. What is this boy's major nutritional problem?
C. What nutrients are likely to be missing from the diet?
D. Does he need a vitamin supplement?

Case 10-3

The mother of a 12-year-old boy is concerned because both his father and grandfather are overweight and have "heart problems." He has just started puberty but has not started his growth spurt. His weight and height are both at the 75th percentile, but the weight has increased in the past year from the 50th percentile. The physical examination shows a "spare tire" of fat around his abdomen. BMI has increased from 25th to 50th percentile last year to 75th percentile.

A. Does this boy need to go on a diet? How will you explain your decision to the mother and the boy?
B. Based on his family history, should you recommend a low-fat diet?

Case Answers

10-1 A. *Learning objective:* **Identify the infant who is not receiving adequate nutrition.** Ask about urine output: A newborn who receives adequate breast milk will have at least six wet diapers per day. Most newborns regain birth weight in the first 7 to 10 days after birth, so weigh the infant. Ask whether the mother feels breast engorgement, whether she hears the infant swallow while nursing, and whether the infant seems satisfied after a nursing session.

10-1 B. *Learning objective:* **Discuss the basics of lactation and breastfeeding.** The initial milk produced is colostrum, which provides antibodies and protective cells. Mature human milk contains protein, fat, and carbohydrate in quantities appropriate to support human growth. As growth and calorie need increase, the quantity of human milk increases to meet the need. Iron may be inadequate for an exclusively breast-fed infant older than 4 to 6 months.

10-2 A. *Learning objective:* **Identify nutritional information from the history.** Review the boy's nutritional history and growth chart. Ask about problem behaviors in addition to eating. Look at family history for growth and weight gain. If the boy has had a hematocrit done in the past, review the results.

10-2 B. *Learning objective:* **Discuss the common nutritional problems in childhood.** Obesity is the most common nutritional problem for children and adults. The number of overweight children and adolescents has tripled in the past 20 years. More than 60% of adults are overweight or obese. Most of the weight gain can be attributed to habitual overconsumption of calories: An excess of 100 calories daily for 1 year will result in weight gain of 10 to 12 pounds.

10-2 C. *Learning objective:* **Discuss the common nutritional deficiencies in childhood.** Iron deficiency is the most likely consequence of this eating pattern if it continues unchanged for months. Iron deficiency is most common between 12 and 24 months and again in adolescence. This boy's diet is not likely to be calcium deficient because of the large quantity of dairy products. Iron and calcium are the most common nutritional deficiencies among children and adolescents in the United States.

10-2 C. *Learning objective:* **Discuss the need for vitamins in childhood.** Although this boy's diet is monotonous, he most likely has adequate fat-soluble and water-soluble vitamins. Although many parents give over-the-counter vitamins to their children, a vitamin supplement is not needed. The best vitamin "supplement" is a well-balanced diet. Provide counseling to parents about ways to include a variety of foods in the diet. A dietitian has the expertise to assist with this counseling and can give practical tips for parents.

10-3 A. *Learning objective:* **Review the patterns of growth in early adolescence, especially with regard to underweight and overweight.** This boy does not need a diet, yet. His recent weight gain is a bit concerning as it suggests calorie imbalance. He does not have a past history of high BMI, at least based on last year's growth data. His BMI has increased, but it is not above the 85th percentile at which risk of overweight begins. The growth spurt begins about 2 years after the onset of pubertal changes, so you should examine him to identify his Tanner stage. Measure his waist circumference: It should be less than half of his height. Be sure to ask his permission to discuss weight at this visit and do not "preach" to him or his parents. He is likely to slim down as adolescence proceeds, but you should review his activity and eating habits with him to ensure that he knows about appropriate nutrition. Ask him to help with plans for healthy eating and activity.

10-3 B. *Learning objective:* **Discuss the nutritional approach to a family history of early cardiac disease.** You need more information about his father and grandfather before you can make any decisions. Ask about the age at which heart disease was diagnosed. Find out details about the kind of heart disease and the results of any tests and treatments. This information will help you decide on tests for the patient. A low-fat diet is not necessarily appropriate at this point; a well-balanced diet with moderation in portion size should be the major recommendation. Avoidance of excessive weight gain may be the most important "treatment."

BIBLIOGRAPHY

Work Group on Breastfeeding: Breast feeding and the use of human milk. *Pediatrics*, 115:496, 2005. See http://aappolicy.aappublications.org/cgi/content/abstract/pediatrics;115/2/496.

American Heart Association: Dietary recommendations for children and adolescents: a guide for practitioners. *Pediatrics* 117:544, 2006. See http://pediatrics.aappublications.org/cgi/content/full/pediatrics;117/2/544.

Read JS et al: Human milk, breast-feeding, and transmission of human immunodeficiency virus Type 1 in the United States. *Pediatrics* 112:1196, 2003. See http://pediatrics.aappublications.org/cgi/content/full/pediatrics;112/5/1196.

Comittee on Drugs: Transfer of drugs and other chemicals into human milk. *Pediatrics* 108:776, 2001. See www.aap.org/policy/0063.html.

Fiorino KN, Cox J: Nutrition and growth. In Robertson J, Shilkofski N, editors: *The Harriet Lane handbook*, ed 17, Philadelphia, 2005, Mosby, pp. 525-608.

Fomon SJ: *Nutrition of normal infants,* St. Louis, 1993, Mosby.

Kleinman, RE, editor: Feeding the infant. In *Pediatric nutrition handbook*, ed 5, Elk Grove Village, IL, 2004, American Academy of Pediatrics, pp. 3-22.

Story M, Holt K, Sofka D, editors: *Bright futures in practice: nutrition,* Arlington, VA, 2002, National Center for Education in Maternal and Child Health. See www.brightfutures.org/nutrition/pdf/index.html.

11

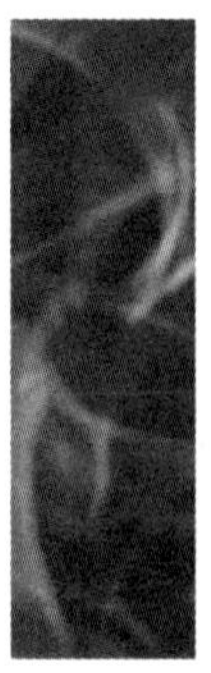

Health Supervision

JEROLD C. WOODHEAD and
MICHAEL R. LAWLESS

What Is Health Supervision?

Health supervision ("well-child check") emphasizes the health and well-being of the patient in the context of the family and the community. The health visit includes an interview, a review of developmental progress, an age-appropriate physical examination, and selected screening assessments. Personalized guidance, education of patients and families, promotion of health, and prevention of illness and injury are the goals of the visit. The *Bright Futures Pocket Guide* contains much useful information about health supervision and is available as a free download from www.brightfutures.org/pocket/index.html.

Why Emphasize Health Supervision?

Complex interactions between biologic and psychosocial factors affect the health of children and their families throughout life. A family may not be traditional, nuclear, or biologic, but it is crucial to growth and development from infancy through adolescence. Attention to families is especially important because an increasing number of children are homeless or in foster care, lack stable and effective parenting, or may be exposed to domestic violence. Chronic health conditions and special healthcare needs affect more than 25% of the patients followed in pediatric practices.

How Do I Organize the Health Supervision Visit?

The "chief complaint of health" will help you focus on the systems that contribute to the health of a child and family, just as the chief complaint of a problem helps direct your evaluation of the ill patient. The background information for the visit comes from the medical record and from the physicians, nurses, and other health professionals who have been involved in the care of the child and family. The age-appropriate assessment should be comprehensive:

- Listen to the concerns expressed by parents, children, and adolescents
- Review and update family and social history
- Review and summarize the information in the chart about illnesses and injuries
- Review previous physical findings and results of screening tests
- Review developmental progress and consider using a screening tool such as the Denver II
- Look at vital signs, growth charts, and the body mass index (BMI) nomogram
- Identify risks to the child's well-being, whether medical, social, or environmental, including the home and the community
- Determine the strengths of the child and ask about family strengths and problems
- Ask about safety, nutrition, growth, behavior, discipline, illness, and injury
- Assess immunization status at each health supervision visit; ideally, you should inquire about immunizations for all children in the family
- Observe the interactions between parent and child
- Observe the patient to assess development before you start the examination
- Base the examination on the patient's development, as discussed in Chapters 5, 8, and 9
- Select screening tests based on information from the history and examination
- Provide anticipatory guidance

What Is Anticipatory Guidance?

Anticipatory guidance provides age and developmentally focused counseling about health that is based on the concerns expressed by parents and patients. You will need the ability to answer questions and explain findings, and the knowledge to provide counseling about what can be expected during the time interval until the next visit. If at first you do not feel comfortable providing anticipatory guidance, observe an experienced pediatrician. You will be able to assume more responsibility with each subsequent patient. The focus for anticipatory guidance will be based on your interview, the physical examination, your assessment of the patient's health, and any concerns that you might have identified. Guidance must be individualized for each patient and family, although most discussions include development, behavior, education, nutrition, safety, immunizations, discipline, language, sleep, dental health, family, medical, and psychosocial topics. Anticipatory guidance can assist the family to make best use of community resources. See the *Bright Futures Pocket Guide* for age-specific suggestions.

INFANTS

What Should I Evaluate about Infant Health?

Health supervision visits are scheduled at short intervals during infancy to monitor growth and developmental progress and to initiate the primary immunization series: Hepatitis B vaccine at birth or shortly after; all other vaccines starting at age 2 months (or as soon as the infant is brought to the office to establish ongoing care—see Chapter 12). Ask about prenatal and perinatal events, the family history, and the home environment. Review developmental progress and immunization status at every visit. During the interview, observe the interaction between infant and parent and note whether the infant appears well nourished and cared for. A careful physical examination (Chapter 5) allows detection of congenital diseases and of disorders that have their roots in prenatal, intrapartum, and immediate postnatal problems but do not become apparent until after the infant is sent home from the newborn nursery. Routine hearing screen and the neonatal metabolic screen detect many congenital problems, but not all; thus, you must be attentive to the uncommon but serious disorders that occasionally appear. A screening tool such as the Denver II (see Chapter 9) can assist you to monitor development. Infant behaviors often cause concerns, sometimes because they reflect problems and other times because inexperienced parents need guidance about age-appropriate activities. Nutrition questions almost always come up, especially regarding breast-feeding (see Chapter 10). Nutritional surveillance is key early in life because rapid growth demands a high calorie intake. Screening for lead exposure should be initiated at 12 months, or even earlier in high-risk environments. When the lead level is obtained, a screen for nutritional anemia can also be done (see Chapters 13 and 50).

How Do I Assess the Family?

The adaptation of the family to the new infant gives you important insight into parenting skills and family stress. As you monitor the family, you can provide guidance for new parents and reinforcement for experienced parents. Listen actively when parents ask questions or tell about their experiences. Young parents may be unprepared for parenthood, may lack physical and financial resources, and may not have a support network of family, grandparents, neighbors, friends, and colleagues at work. Experienced parents may be concerned with older children in the family who demonstrate jealousy or show behavioral regression when a new sibling arrives. Family dysfunction may manifest during the stressful early months of new parenthood, especially with regard to crying, sleep, and financial pressures. You need to be alert to the possibility of domestic violence in any stressed family. Parental habits, such as smoking, may pose a risk for the infant. Ensure that parents pay attention to safety in the home and automobile. Inquire about family risk factors that would have an impact on immunizations or on the infant's health, such as immunocompromised relatives, or family members with active tuberculosis.

How Do I Assess the Community?

Child care is an essential community resource for mothers who must work or attend school. In some communities, child care may be lacking, which restricts parental work and education. The community itself may be unsafe, may lack public transportation, may have old housing (a risk for lead exposure), and may not have many child and family services. The "simple" becomes difficult if transportation is lacking or if medical services are located at a distance.

What Anticipatory Guidance Is Needed?

The first year of life is filled with change. Parents appreciate guidance about what to expect in the weeks or months from one health visit to the next. They benefit from practical information about feeding, sleep, behavior, developmental milestones, and common illnesses. As the infant matures, safety becomes more and more important. Information about reliable child care services can provide a valuable service to families. See the *Bright Futures Pocket Guide* for age-specific suggestions.

TODDLERS AND PRESCHOOL CHILDREN

What Problems Arise for Toddlers and Preschoolers?

Parents of toddlers and preschoolers commonly raise concerns about behavior, nutrition, language development, and intercurrent illnesses. You will need to distinguish problems that indicate health or developmental concerns from those that reflect the expected development of the child. Emerging independence makes the toddler particularly prone to confrontations with parents. Temper tantrums usually reflect the toddler's desire for attention and can trigger parental reactions that have bad consequences for the child or that reinforce the undesirable behavior. Behavior problems can also manifest at the birth of a sibling—a common occurrence in families with toddlers—with regressive behaviors, jealousy, and even aggressive outbursts occurring when the newborn is brought home. Often, behavior problems occur at bedtime or mealtime and may result in ongoing confrontation between parents and toddlers. Behavioral feeding disorders seem to peak at about age 3 years, cause much mealtime distress, and may result in either poor weight gain or excessive weight gain. Daycare or preschool exposes the child to new experiences and demands for socialization. Behavior assessment is discussed in Chapter 22. You do *not* need to do screening tests such as hematocrit, urinalysis, and tuberculin test unless the history provides a reason to do so.

What Should I Emphasize During the Evaluation?

Careful monitoring of ***growth*** measurements on growth charts and the BMI nomogram helps identify the young child at risk for failure to thrive or obesity. ***Developmental progress*** should be reviewed with parents at each visit. Observe the child's responses to environmental stimuli, both auditory and visual, and listen to the child's language. You should be able to understand approximately half of the words spoken by a 2-year-old, two-thirds to three-fourths of the words spoken by a 3-year-old, and all of the language of a 4-year-old. Delayed language may result from conductive hearing loss caused by chronic middle ear effusions or recurrent ear infections; referral to a speech and language specialist may be needed. ***Behaviors*** often trigger concerns and also prompt ineffective responses by parents. Important ***parenting skills*** should progress as the child develops. You gain important insight from observing how the parent interacts with the child for comforting, discipline, and positive reinforcement and listening to the tone of voice a parent uses to communicate with the child. Be aware of the potential for child abuse or domestic violence. Review ***immunization status***, make certain that vaccinations are up to date, and encourage yearly influenza vaccine. The ***physical examination*** may detect a congenital problem such as coarctation of the aorta or a subtle neurologic deficit that was not identified earlier. Look for physical findings that might explain any problem identified in the history. Identify early cavities and evidence of poor dental hygiene such as plaque and gingival inflammation.

How Should I Include the Family and Community?

Family issues such as finances, work, violence, and personal habits of adults (e.g., smoking, drinking) all affect the growing child. You must be aware of the possibility of child abuse in every family, especially with the toddler, whose developmentally based behaviors often challenge parental composure. Expanding family size often adds complexity to the life of the family, causing stress for both mother and father as they deal with a new infant, plus a toddler or older children. Community-related safety, resources, support, and school opportunities all must be addressed. As the child becomes older and ventures out into community-based activities, the availability of programs such as preschool and early intervention services becomes important.

What Anticipatory Guidance Is Needed?

Safety is critical. Ensure that parents and other responsible adults make the home, automobile, daycare, and other environments safe, because toddlers and preschool-age children cannot be expected to make decisions about safe behaviors. Toddlers put themselves at high risk for ingestions and choking because they explore the world by eating it. Developing motor skills and lack of experience also put toddlers at risk for falls and other trauma. The exploratory urge often induces a 3-year-old to "fly" by jumping off furniture or to pull on dangling cords attached to lamps or coffee pots. ***Entry into daycare or preschool*** exposes the child to new environments, social interactions, and educational challenges that can result in safety and behavioral concerns. Review these concerns with parents to help them make adaptations that promote safety and the child's well-being. Parents usually have many questions about recurrent infections and daycare. They also often compare the ***development*** of their child with that of others and ask about specific developmental issues such as language. ***Nutrition*** is a big concern: You will need to find out about the child's eating habits to answer the parents' questions. Ask about consumption of sweetened beverages such as juice, and the frequency of fast food meals. Provide objective data about the child's ***growth*** and nutritional status from the growth chart and BMI nomogram to assist parents to develop realistic expectations about the quantity of food needed and the up-and-down eating habits of toddlers. BMI data in particular can be used to show excessive weight gain and to plan interventions to moderate calorie intake. Tooth brushing should be encouraged as soon as teeth erupt, but it becomes especially important in the toddler years. Recommend routine dental visits. The *Bright Futures Pocket Guide* lists age-appropriate topics for anticipatory guidance.

SCHOOL-AGE CHILDREN

What Health Topics Are Important for the Older Child?

As the child enters school, motor development progresses to mastery of the complex skills associated with sports, dance, music, and other activities. New developmental challenges include formal learning and socialization, which mirror cognitive and psychosocial development. Learning and behavior in school often prompt questions about "learning disability" or "behavior problems" (see Chapters 22 and 55). This is the age group in which many life-long habits develop, so the experiences of children at home, in school, in neighborhoods, and via the media have a lasting impact. Responsibility for safety begins to be vested in the child, especially in the preadolescent. Development of decision-making skills allows choices of activities based on safety and other issues. Growth, nutrition, and illnesses remain high on the list of parental concerns.

What Should I Emphasize in the Evaluation?

Assessment of health increasingly involves the child as the historian with the parent providing details and clarifying problems. The child's responses about friends, school, food, music, physical activity, and sports assist with developmental assessment. Ask parents about school performance, physical activity, TV viewing, video games, computer use, dental care, and eating. Growth, development, behavior, nutrition, and safety continue to challenge parents. School and the expansion of the child's world beyond the family become increasingly important. Emphasize physical activities, school performance, relationships with peers and family members, personal interests, and, when applicable, pubertal progress as you assess development. Remember that physical activity and nutrition are important for this age group. Health topics become more focused on issues with lifelong consequences: blood pressure, BMI, cardiovascular risk factors, hearing, personal habits (smoking, safety), vision, and others. Approach issues such as sexuality, alcohol, drugs, and tobacco in a sensitive manner, based on the physical and emotional maturity of the child, and couch them in terms of growth and development. Immunization status should be verified yearly and attention should be paid to new vaccines or changes in recommendations, such as yearly influenza vaccine and the conjugate meningococcal vaccine. The BMI nomogram helps identify the child at risk for obesity so that intervention might mitigate weight gain and reduce the likelihood of adverse health consequences. If the waist circumference-to-height ratio (WC:Ht) is > 0.5, a child is at risk for the adverse consequences of obesity. A thorough musculoskeletal assessment by history and physical examination will ensure a child's safe participation in sports. Laboratory tests are done only if justified by history or physical examination. Tuberculosis screening should be done only for high-risk patients. This group includes immigrants and adopted children from countries where tuberculosis is endemic. If a child received Bacille Camille-Guerin (BCG) in infancy, the purified protein derivative (PPD) should still be performed (see Chapter 64).

How Do Family and Community Affect the Older Child?

Family life typically calms during school years, a lull between the storms of the toddler years and adolescence. However, problems do develop, sometimes as a result of family dysfunction, often triggered by financial stresses, and also from school-related behaviors. Occasionally a parent will request medication to "calm" a school-age child. This should trigger a careful assessment of the behavior in question. Parents sometimes need help to learn about reasonable expectations for the performance of their child—school, sports, and so forth. Discipline occasionally becomes punitive rather than instructive. Parental habits such as smoking and alcoholism have adverse consequences for children. ***The community*** has an increasingly important impact on the older child, especially related to media exposure. The physician must be aware of the availability of after-school programs, age-group sport programs, and support services for school and other problems. Big Sister or Big Brother programs help many school-age children to develop rewarding relationships with adults.

What Anticipatory Guidance Is Needed?

Guidance for school-age children tends to emphasize the upcoming year with its expected challenges in school, sports, community involvement, and family life. Guidance about safety, school, peers, and illnesses/immunizations is important. Immunizations must be updated before kindergarten and at age 11. Remember to ask about any plans by the family for travel to parts of the world where additional immunizations and preventive measures are needed. Individual attention will need to be paid to a child's personal development and health problems. The "epidemic" of obesity has its roots in childhood, so nutritional counseling is important. Encourage the child to take responsibility for personal hygiene, safety, and participation in family activities. The *Bright Futures Pocket Guide* lists age-appropriate topics for anticipatory guidance.

ADOLESCENTS

What Do Adolescents Care About?

Adolescents are not healthcare seekers by nature. The adolescent's very presence in the pediatrician's office may depend on a relationship developed during childhood, as well as on an office environment that the adolescent perceives as friendly and nonjudgmental. Adolescence is the only time in human development when an individual is aware of growth acceleration. Adolescents are very attuned to growth as it relates to anticipated physical and sexual maturity and to all-important issues of body image and appearance. This section provides a brief overview of adolescent health supervision. Chapter 15 discusses the healthy adolescent.

What Are the Key Topics for Adolescents?

Growth, development, and the major causes of morbidity are the focus for the adolescent health supervision visit. ***Growth*** rate peaks between ages 11 and 12 years in girls and between ages 13 and 14 years in boys. Peak height velocity correlates with advancing sexual maturity in boys and girls, and always precedes menarche. ***Sexual maturity*** rating should be determined at each health supervision visit. ***Nutrition*** assessment and counseling at all ages should include both the overconcern with thinness and the increasing trend toward obesity and associated type 2 diabetes mellitus. In addition, adolescents need to be reminded about the importance of balanced nutrition, the risks of "fad" diets, and the benefits of regular exercise. ***Developmental issues*** change as an individual progresses through adolescence. In ***early adolescence,*** the teenager needs guidance with the physical and emotional changes of puberty and the increasing independence from the family. In ***middle adolescence,*** pubertal growth is nearly finished so the teen's focus changes to self-identity and powerful peer alliances. As the individual reaches ***late adolescence,*** issues include the transition to more abstract thinking and more intimate relationships. Personal habits rate special attention at all stages.

What Personal Habits Should Be Discussed?

The expanded **HEADSSS** mnemonic identifies topics for discussion and evaluation of the adolescent: Home/Health, Education/Employment/Eating, Activities/Aspirations/Affiliations, Drugs, Sex, Sleep/Suicide, Shoplifting (see Chapter 15). Health habits should be discussed at each visit, including dental care, breast or testicular self-examination, management of acne, use of sunblock, and regular supervision of pigmented lesions. Major causes of adolescent mortality can be addressed by asking about use of seat belts and bike helmets, access to firearms, and exposure to violence at home, in intimate relationships, in school, or in the neighborhood. By asking about peer relations, choice of friends, and activities, you gain the opportunity to address risk-taking behaviors, such as use of alcohol, tobacco, and drugs, and you also will be able to assess signs of depression or risk for suicide. Any adolescent may temporarily have some minor areas of dysfunction in mood, family relationships, peer relationships, school performance, or unwise behavior. If you identify more than one area of dysfunction or discover severe dysfunction in any one area, the adolescent is likely to require intervention and support. Questions about menstruation, sexuality, contraception, and sexually transmitted diseases give you the opportunity to offer anticipatory guidance about these essential topics.

What Are Some Guidelines for Talking about Sensitive Topics?

Puberty, personal habits, risk-taking behaviors, and peer relations are sensitive and demand privacy if they are to be discussed in a meaningful way with the adolescent. It is easiest to introduce the topics of privacy and confidentiality as the norm for all adolescents at a visit before the onset of puberty, usually between the ages of 10 and 12 years. Parents usually accept the need for privacy during the physical examination and gradually come to recognize that privacy and confidentiality assist the adolescent to assume responsibility for personal health. *Qualified confidentiality* can be guaranteed to the adolescent and should not be violated, unless the patient poses a threat to self or others (see the discussion of confidentiality in Chapter 6).

Why Is a Complete Physical Examination Needed?

A thorough physical examination allows you to address a patient's concerns, identify physical abnormalities, and offer insight, reassurance, and guidance about physical development, a topic of great, but usually unspoken interest. The time and care spent by the examiner is interpreted by the adolescent as a sign of genuine interest. Patience, explanation, and sensitivity are particularly important when doing the first pelvic examination. Instructing a girl about breast self-examination and a boy about testicular self-examination are important cancer prevention strategies. The 2-minute musculoskeletal examination allows you to assess strength, mobility, range of motion, and coordination and to detect old injuries or other problems that make participation in contact or collision sports unwise for an individual (see Chapter 68).

Are Any Laboratory Tests Ordered Routinely?

The decision to order laboratory or other tests should be based on history and physical examination findings. Consider a hemoglobin level as a screen for anemia in boys and girls. Asymptomatic, sexually active boys should have a test of first-void urine for leukocyte esterase as a screen for the presence of unrecognized *Chlamydia* infection. A Papanicolaou smear and cervical cultures are appropriate for sexually active girls. Obtain a serum cholesterol level or lipid panel if the family history includes risk factors for cardiovascular disease or if the patient is obese or hypertensive. The intradermal PPD test for tuberculosis is done based on risk factors identified by history.

What Immunizations Should I Recommend?

Immunizations are typically given at age 11 or 12 years, just before middle school/junior high school, but older adolescents often have immunization needs, so the record should be reviewed carefully. The new tetanus-diphtheria-acellular pertussis (Tdap) vaccine should be given at age 11 years but may also be administered 5 years after the dT vaccine. Hepatitis A and conjugate-meningococcal vaccines are now both routinely recommended and should be given to any adolescent who has not yet received them. "Catch-up" vaccination for varicella, measles-mumps-rubella, and hepatitis B may be needed. Inquire about plans for foreign travel, so that appropriate immunizations and preventive measures may be provided. As adolescents prepare for college, the military, or jobs, review immunizations and remind them of the need to maintain immunizations during adult life. PPD may be needed in some situations. The vaccine to protect against human papillomavirus (HPV) was approved by the Food and Drug Administration (FDA) in June 2006 and has been recommended for routine administration to females between ages 9 and 26 years (see Chapter 12).

How Do Family and Community Affect the Adolescent?

The ***family*** affects the adolescent and is affected by the adolescent. The powerful changes occurring within the adolescent and the numerous external factors that influence behavior make family relationships pivotal. A supportive and caring family can provide guidance, understand the need for gradually increasing independence, and maintain open channels of communication. Conversely, a dysfunctional family that is consumed with domestic violence, substance abuse, or marital relationship problems may offer little support and guidance for the adolescent and can greatly magnify the stresses of adolescent adjustment. The ***community*** may support or complicate an adolescent's development and relationship with the family. A strong educational system, organized sports, and accessible recreational and entertainment activities make the community a positive force in the lives of all adolescents. Mental health and substance abuse programs that are readily available to individuals and families help the community to support those adolescents and families who need the services. Society at large influences adolescents by the standards of morality and ethics found in entertainment, government, and everyday life.

What Anticipatory Guidance Is Needed?

In many ways, anticipatory guidance is the entire focus of the adolescent health supervision visit. In addition to all of the information provided to the patient during the history and physical examination, you must remember to address nutrition, safety, and future plans. The *Bright Futures Pocket Guide* lists age-appropriate topics for anticipatory guidance.

KEY POINTS

- Health is far more than the absence of disease.
- Health supervision evaluates all components of health: personal, family, and community.
- Anticipatory guidance helps parents, older children, and adolescents understand current health status and plan for the immediate future.
- Health supervision issues are determined by age and developmental status.

Case 11-1

Prospective parents come to your office for a prenatal visit. They expect their first child in approximately 1 month. The pregnancy has been uncomplicated, and the family history is noncontributory for problems that might affect the newborn. Parents have many questions about what to expect during the first year of life.

A. How will you monitor and manage the child's health during the first year of life?
B. How will you modify your anticipatory guidance as the infant grows and develops?
C. What resources will you use to guide your health supervision program?

Case 11-2

A 13-year-old girl comes to the clinic for a health supervision visit before entry into eighth grade. Her mother expresses the concern in private that the girl has been increasingly negative and confrontational over the past several months. The girl complains that her mother will "not let me do anything fun." The girl has had appropriate growth and development and had menarche 3 months ago.

A. What issues do you need to address with the girl and her mother?
B. Where can you find more information about adolescents?

Case Answers

11-1 A. *Learning objective:* **Discuss health supervision during the first year of life.** Infants need frequent visits to the office or clinic to monitor growth, development, nutrition, and overall health. Immunizations are important during this first year. Physical examination may identify congenital or acquired problems. Family support and counseling are critical.

11-1 B. *Learning objective:* **Discuss the ways that anticipatory guidance changes as the child develops.** Growth and development change both risks and concerns. Nutrition, safety, abilities, and behaviors all change as the child grows. You must adapt advice to meet the developmental ability of the child and the experience of the parents.

11-1 C. *Learning objective:* **Identify resources for health supervision.** *Bright Futures* provides advice for this process. The Web site of the American Academy of Pediatrics also has valuable information http://aap.org.

11-2 A. *Learning objective:* **State the topics that must be addressed in an adolescent health supervision visit.** This mother and daughter need advice about communication and the process of adolescent growth and development. You must ensure that the girl does not have behaviors that pose a risk to herself or others. You also need to identify parenting abilities and responses to the girl's behaviors. Regular use of the HEADSSS mnemonic will ensure that adolescent topics are covered. Important topics include growth, sexual maturity, relationship with friends and family, educational progress, substance abuse, dietary habits, sexuality, and overall mood of the adolescent. Immunizations must be reviewed and updated. Screening tests will be done based on history.

11-2 B. *Learning objective:* **Identify sources of information about adolescents.** You can find additional information about adolescents at www.brightfutures.org/bf2/index.html and in the American Academy of Pediatrics publication, *Caring for Your Teenager.*

BIBLIOGRAPHY

Green M: *Bright futures: guidelines for health supervision,* ed 2, Arlington, VA, 2002, National Center for Education in Maternal and Child Health, www.brightfutures.org/bf2/index.html.

12

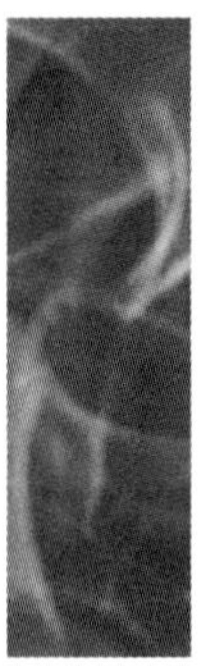

Immunization

JEROLD C. WOODHEAD

What Is Immunization?

Immunization protects against infection without the risks associated with the disease. A vaccine triggers *active immunity* by stimulating development of antibodies by a mechanism that mimics the response to infection. This process takes time, so protection does not develop immediately. The protection that results may be lifelong or may be limited in duration, necessitating booster doses of the vaccine. *Passive immunity* results when preformed antibodies are administered that provide immediate but relatively short-lived protection from infection. Examples of passive immunity include nonspecific immunoglobulin ("gamma globulin"), intravenous immune globulin (IVIG), specific immune globulin (e.g., tetanus immunoglobulin), and antitoxin (equine diphtheria antitoxin). When preformed antibodies are administered to an unimmunized individual to manage an acute exposure, subsequent administration of a vaccine is needed (if one is available) to trigger development of active immunity and provide lasting protection against disease.

What Is a Vaccine?

Vaccine is a generic term that refers to any immunobiologic agent administered as part of a program of active immunization. Most vaccines are suspensions made from attenuated (live) or killed bacteria and viruses or from specific components of those organisms. A *toxoid* is a bacterial protein (toxin) that has been rendered biologically inactive and is used as a vaccine to stimulate the active development of antibody (antitoxin). Tetanus toxoid is the major example.

What Immunizations Are Currently Recommended?

Immunization recommendations are reviewed and updated yearly, and new vaccines and combinations of vaccines are added with some regularity. Immunizations recommended in the United States are listed by the Centers for Disease Control and Prevention (www.cdc.gov/vaccines)

and the American Academy of Pediatrics (www.aap.org/healthtopics/immunizations.cfm). Table 12-1 lists currently recommended vaccines. Each state sets its own standards for *required* immunizations. Table 12-2 lists sources of reliable information.

Table 12-1

Immunizations (2007)

Vaccine		Primary Series	Booster
Hepatitis B	HepB	Birth/infancy	
Diphtheria-tetanus-acellular pertussis	DTaP	Infancy	School entry
Haemophilus influenzae type B	Hib	Infancy	N/A
Polio, trivalent inactivated	Polio	Infancy	School entry
Conjugate *Streptococcus pneumoniae*	PCV-7	Infancy	N/A
Rotavirus	RotaTeq	Infancy	N/A
Varicella*	Var	12 months	N/A
Measles-mumps-rubella*	MMR	12 months	School entry
Hepatitis A	Hep A	12 months	6 months after first dose
Human papillomavirus (HPV types 6, 11, 16, and 18)	HPV (Gardasil)	9–26 years	Second dose 2 months and third dose 6 months after first dose
Tetanus-diphtheria-acellular pertussis	Tdap	N/A	11–15 years
Conjugate meningococcal	Menactra	11–15 years	N/A
Influenza A and B	Flu	Yearly starting at 6 months (2 shots in the first year if < 9 years old)	

For specifics see www.cdc.gov/vaccines.
N/A, not applicable.
*Measles-mumps-rubella-varicella (MMRV) vaccine may be given at 12 months and at school entry.

Table 12-2

Sources for Information on Immunizations

Source	Citation or Web Site
Information for Parents	
American Academy of Pediatrics	www.aap.org/healthtopics/immunizations.cfm
CDC: "Parents: What You Need to Know"	www.cdc.gov/vaccines/spec-grps/parents.htm
Vaccine information	www.vaccineinformation.org
Healthcare Professionals	
American Academy of Pediatrics	Pickering LD, editor: *Red book: 2006 report of the Committee on Infectious Diseases,* ed 27, Elk Grove Village, IL, 2006, American Academy of Pediatrics.
CDC: Vaccine information statements	www.cdc.gov/vaccines/pubs/vis/default.htm
CDC: Immunization schedule	www.cdc.gov/vaccines/hcp.htm#sched
Immunization schedule	pda.immunizationed.org

CDC, Centers for Disease Control and Prevention.

What Affects Development of Immunity from Vaccines?

Improper storage, handling, or administration causes most immunization failures. Commonly used vaccines are 85% to 98% effective, if administered and handled properly.

Time-limited immunity develops after administration of vaccines such as diphtheria, tetanus, and pertussis; these vaccines require regular boosters to maintain immunity. Until 2005, the pertussis vaccine could not be administered to patients older than 7 years because of side effects. Inability to provide a booster dose meant that waning immunity left adolescents and adults susceptible to infection with *Bordetella pertussis*. If they developed the disease, they posed an infection risk for infants. In 2005, the acellular pertussis vaccine was approved for administration to adolescents and adults, providing the opportunity to dramatically reduce adolescent and adult disease.

Age has an important impact on vaccine success. Infants do not respond to the polysaccharide antigens of organisms such as *Haemophilus influenzae* type B and *Streptococcus pneumoniae*. Development of *conjugate vaccines* has allowed immunization of infants to these infections and has dramatically reduced infection. In addition, measles-mumps-rubella (MMR) and varicella vaccines must be administered at or after

12 months of age to trigger a reliable immune response. In an analogous fashion, the conjugate vaccine for *Neisseria meningitidis* triggers development of much longer-lived protection than did the older vaccine.

What Should I Know about Vaccine Safety?

Adverse events associated with immunization are mostly minor, such as fever or soreness at the injection site. The MMR-varicella vaccines contain live, attenuated organisms and occasionally can cause mild forms of measles and varicella approximately 1 week after immunization. Live, attenuated polio vaccine (OPV) is no longer used in the United States because of rare but clinically important reversion of the vaccine strain of virus to the wild-type with production of paralytic disease; the inactivated polio vaccine (IPV) does not pose this risk. Rare, unpredictable events have been associated with certain vaccines, including hypersensitivity reactions. Parents often ask about diseases and disorders that develop in the period following immunizations but that are not necessarily caused by the vaccination. Much publicity has been given to putative associations between vaccines and disorders such as attention deficit hyperactivity disorder, autism, multiple sclerosis, and speech and language delays. All studies to date have demonstrated convincingly that no connection exists between a vaccine and any of these conditions. To counsel parents, you must understand the evidence that has been obtained through reliable studies. The Centers for Disease Control and Prevention (CDC) and the American Academy of Pediatrics are credible sources for information about vaccine safety. The U.S. Food and Drug Administration subjects all vaccines licensed in the United States to careful scrutiny and monitors vaccine safety through the Vaccine Adverse Events Reporting System (VAERS).

KEY POINTS

- Immunization reduces morbidity and mortality of infectious disease.
- Vaccines are safe and effective.
- Reliable information is readily available in print and online sources.

Case 12-1

Parents of a newborn infant request information about the immunizations that their child will receive in the first year of life.

A. What resource will you use to provide the requested information?
B. List the diseases for which immunizations are administered in the first year of life.
C. Why are certain immunizations routinely administered only after the first year of life?

Case Answers

12-1 A. *Learning objective:* **Use current national recommendations for immunization.** Recommendations for immunizations are published annually by the Centers for Disease Control and Prevention (www.cdc.gov/vaccines).

12-1 B. *Learning objective:* **Identify the diseases for which immunizations are administered.** Immunizations routinely administered in the first year of life protect against diphtheria, tetanus, pertussis, polio, hepatitis B, *S. pneumoniae,* and *H. influenzae* type b. Hepatitis A and rotavirus were added to the recommended list in 2006.

12-1 C. *Learning objective:* **Discuss ways that the immune reaction to vaccines changes as the child ages.** The young infant does not develop reliable immunity in response to polysaccharide antigens. This led to development of conjugate vaccines against *H. influenzae* type b, and *S. pneumoniae.* Other vaccines such as MMR and varicella do not produce reliable immunity before age 12 months. Immunity to pertussis wanes ~5 years after the last dose of vaccine, which until 2005 was at school entry. Now, the acellular pertussis vaccine has been recommended for administration at age 11 years and in later adolescence and adult life.

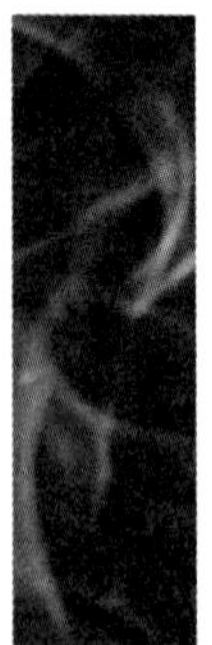

13

Lead Exposure and Poisoning

JEROLD C. WOODHEAD

ETIOLOGY

Why Is Exposure to Lead a Problem?

Lead is a neurodevelopmental toxin for the immature nervous system at even very low levels, and it has toxic effects for almost all other organ systems at higher levels. In the past, lead exposure was classified as "lead poisoning" because it was identified clinically only when high-level toxicity caused symptoms and organ failure. Now, most children identified with chronic lead exposure are asymptomatic. Adverse effects are now primarily identified in cognition, learning, and behavior among populations of affected children. Public policy in the United States and other countries has markedly reduced commercial use of lead, with a resultant reduction of environmental contamination. Public health efforts have promoted routine screening for lead exposure. The Centers for Disease Control and Prevention (CDC) has a Web site devoted to lead exposure: www.cdc.gov/lead/.

What Are the Sources of Lead?

Dust derived from deteriorating lead-based paint is currently the most important source of environmental lead in the United States. Exposure to environmental lead historically has resulted from its use in products such as paint, pottery glaze, gasoline, water pipes, inks, and pigments. Lead has even found its way into foods, such as candy in Mexico. Although lead was banned as a component of interior paint in the 1960s and from exterior house paint in 1978, lead-based paint remains on interior and exterior walls of most homes built before 1978. As this paint ages and wears, it contaminates house dust and soil, contributing to the risk of lead exposure. Renovation of old housing is a particular hazard for children because the resulting dust increases the likelihood of inhalation and ingestion of lead. Modern housing standards have replaced lead water pipes with copper and plastic, but many communities still have lead water mains. Lead was phased out as a gasoline additive starting in the late 1970s but was only completely banned in 1995. Other, less common sources of lead exposure include the following:

- Clothing worn by parents who work in lead-related industries such as battery plants, smelters, or recycling (see http://www.cdc.gov/niosh/topics/lead)
- Hobbies such as making stained glass, ammunition loading, fishing weights, jewelry making
- Imported toys and jewelry (www.cdc.gov/nceh/lead/faq/toys.htm)
- Candy imported from Mexico (see www.ocregister.com/multimedia/lead/)
- Traditional medicines and cosmetics (e.g., azarcon, greta, paylooah, surma, al kohl, ghasard, liga, bali goli)

How Is Exposure to Lead Defined and Identified?

Excessive accumulation of lead in the body is defined by an elevated blood lead level (BLL). There is no BLL threshold below which lead can be said to be safe, but BLL $\geq$ 10 μg/dl is currently used to identify a child who has excessive lead exposure. This BLL triggers environmental clean-up and close monitoring of the affected child. In the past, "lead poisoning" was a symptomatic outcome of lead toxicity. As recently as 1970, the diagnosis of excessive lead exposure required a BLL of $\geq$ 65 μg/dl. The level for diagnosis then decreased steadily as the effects of lead toxicity became better understood: $\geq$ 40 μg/dl in 1971, $\geq$ 30 μg/dl in 1975, and $\geq$ 25 μg/dl in 1985. The level was lowered to $\geq$ 10 μg/dl in 1991, because it had become apparent that adverse cognitive effects occurred at BLL between 10 and 20 μg/dl, even though no obvious "lead poisoning" symptoms could be identified. More recently, evidence of a toxic effect at even lower levels has been identified and efforts are underway to further define this risk.

How Common Are Elevated Lead Levels?

Nearly 500,000 children in the United States currently have blood lead levels $\geq$ 10 μg/dl, and more than 10 of every 100,000 employed adults have BLL $\geq$ 25 μg/dl. Although symptomatic lead poisoning has declined greatly in the United States over the past 30 years, lead exposure remains an important public health concern because the metal is still present in old housing and in many different types of work sites. Lead exposure is especially common in most of the developing world, which means that physicians who care for immigrants and adopted children must be aware of the problem.

How Does a Child Become Exposed to Lead?

Children from 6 months to 3 years of age have the highest risk for exposure to lead because their developmental progression includes crawling, exploration, and hand-to-mouth activity, all of which put them in proximity to lead in the environment. Mouthing of objects and sucking on hands introduce lead into the child's gastrointestinal tract. Pica, the consumption of nonfood items, is the behavior most associated with continuous, high-level lead ingestion. Inhalation of lead-containing dust, especially when a home is being renovated, can result in absorption across the respiratory mucosa and cause very high lead levels. Young children absorb up to 50% of lead that is either ingested or inhaled, but little is spontaneously excreted. Even low-level exposure can result in a large lead burden if it continues over many years.

EVALUATION

How Can I Detect Lead Exposure?

Detection of lead exposure and identification of elevated BLL are the responsibility of all physicians who provide health care for children. A physician must understand the epidemiology of lead exposure in a community, be able to assess risk factors from the history, and develop an active screening program to identify lead-exposed children with BLL ≥ 10 µg/dl. If the prevalence of elevated lead levels is high in a community, then *all* children should have BLL checked on a regular basis, beginning at 6 to 12 months and continuing to at least age 3 years, depending on personal risk factors identified by history. In communities where old and deteriorating housing is common, a similar approach is justified. In all communities, screening for lead exposure by history to detect risk factors is an important part of health supervision. A standardized questionnaire based on the recommendations from the Centers for Disease Control and Prevention (CDC, 1997) serves as a useful tool to identify high-risk housing, environments, and behavior (Table 13-1). Screening should be

Table 13-1

Screening Questionnaire for Detection of Lead Exposure Risk

Screening Questionnaire for Detection of Lead Exposure Risk
Basic Personal-Risk Questionnaire
Does your child live in or regularly visit a house that was built before 1950? This question could apply to a facility such as a home daycare center or the home of a babysitter or relative.
Does your child live in or regularly visit a house built before 1978 with recent or ongoing renovations or remodeling (within the last 6 months)?
Does your child have a sibling or playmate who has or did have lead poisoning?
Additional Questions for Specific Populations
Do you give your child home or folk remedies (e.g., Azarcon, paylooah, greta)?
Does your child eat candy from Mexico (e.g., picarindo, vero palerindas)?
Has your child lived in Mexico, South or Central America, Asia, or Africa, or visited longer than 2 months?
Do adults have jobs or hobbies that involve lead?

Adapted from Centers for Disease Control and Prevention: *Preventing lead poisoning in young children,* 1997.

initiated *before* the child begins to crawl and gains access to contaminated environments. Regular, repeat screening should continue throughout early childhood. Any positive response to the screening questionnaire should be followed up with a BLL determination.

How Should I React to a Patient's Blood Lead Level?

The diagnosis of ***lead exposure*** does *not* require the presence of symptoms. Most children and adults with chronic exposure to lead are asymptomatic and have BLL between 10 and 20 μg/dl. *Lead poisoning* with BLL ≥ 50 μg/dl causes problems such as anemia, abdominal colic, and seizures, but symptomatic lead poisoning is no longer common in the United States. Parents must be instructed about ways to reduce environmental lead exposure. Monitoring of BLL will be needed at intervals according to the management plan recommended by the CDC and the American Academy of Pediatrics (Table 13-2).

TREATMENT

What Is the Treatment for Lead-Exposed Children?

The best "treatment" is ***prevention***. Community action at local and statewide levels must correct the problem of deteriorating housing. ***Education*** about sources of lead in the environment, the behaviors that put young children at risk, and ways to reduce exposure is the "treatment" needed by most families. This is done optimally at regular health-supervision visits that assess risk for lead exposure, obtain testing for BLL, and communicate the importance of this effort to families. Unfortunately, families in high-risk neighborhoods often report that the risks of lead exposure, the benefits of BLL screening, and often the results of BLL tests are not communicated to them by physicians or nurses. In addition, low-income families must often travel to several different clinic sites for initial screening and subsequent BLL testing, which lowers adherence to recommended testing. ***Nutritional management*** is crucial for all children with elevated BLL, because iron and calcium deficiencies enhance the absorption of lead. Families need information about optimal iron and calcium nutrition, and iron deficiency must be treated. ***Medical treatment*** is reserved for the relatively few children with high BLL or who are symptomatic, as discussed in Table 13-2. Current treatment employs the oral chelating agent *succimer* when the BLL is ≥ 45 μg/dl. No data support succimer treatment at lower levels. Chelation should be managed at centers that specialize in the management of lead poisoning.

Table 13-2

CDC Recommendations for Management of Elevated BLL

Venous BLL (μg/dl)				
10–14	**15–19**	**20–44**	**45–69**	**≥ 70**
• Lead education Dietary Environmental • Follow-up blood lead monitoring	• Lead education Dietary Environmental • Follow-up blood lead monitoring • Proceed according to actions for 20–44 μg/dl if a follow-up BLL is in this range at least 3 months after initial venous test or BLL increases	• Lead education Dietary Environmental • Follow-up blood lead monitoring • Complete history and physical exam • Lab work: Hemoglobin or hematocrit Iron status • Environmental investigation • Lead hazard reduction • Neurodevelopmental monitoring • Abdominal x-ray (if particulate lead ingestion is suspected) with bowel decontamination if indicated	• Lead education Dietary Environmental • Follow-up blood lead monitoring • Complete history and physical exam • Complete neurologic exam • Lab work: Hemoglobin or hematocrit Iron status FEP or ZPP • Environmental investigation • Lead hazard reduction • Neurodevelopmental monitoring • Abdominal x-ray with bowel decontamination if indicated • Chelation therapy	• Hospitalize and commence chelation therapy • Proceed according to actions for 45–69 μg/dl

BLL, Blood lead level; CDC, Centers for Disease Control and Prevention; FEP, free ethrocyte protoporphyrin; ZPP, zinc protoprophyrin.
From Centers for Disease Control and Prevention: *Managing elevated blood lead levels among young children,* 2002.

KEY POINTS

- Lead is a common environmental toxin, primarily found in houses built before 1978.
- Lead exposure is defined by BLL > 10 μg/dl; symptomatic lead poisoning occurs with BLL > 50 μg/dl.
- Most lead poisoning is asymptomatic.
- The best treatment is prevention: screen at-risk patients by history and blood lead level.

Case 13-1

At a health-supervision visit, the parents of a 6-month-old girl fill out the lead screening questionnaire and indicate that their home was built before 1960 and has chipping paint. They are beginning to renovate the house and plan to scrape and sand all painted woodwork and walls. All other questions are negative. The child has just begun to crawl.

A. What are the environmental risks?
B. What developmental behaviors put the 6-month-old infant at risk? What additional behaviors will develop over the next 12 to 18 months that will increase risk?
C. What advice would you give them?
D. If the blood lead level at age 6 months is 4.0 μg/dl, are further tests necessary? If the lead level is 12 μg/dl, what further management is needed?

Case Answers

13-1 A. *Learning objective:* **Identify environmental risks that increase the likelihood of lead poisoning.** Environmental risks include lead-based paint on walls and woodwork. Dust from window ledges is likely high in lead. Dust and chipped paint may be ingested. Lead level in the soil is also likely to be high. Scraping and sanding will aerosolize lead.

13-1 B. *Learning objective:* **Discuss how developmental progress puts infants and toddlers at special risk for lead poisoning.** Current behaviors include crawling, hand-to-mouth activity, and exploration. Later, she will start walking and climbing, which increase access to contaminated areas inside and outside the house. She will have continued hand-to-mouth activity. All increase potential exposure to lead and also increase the likelihood of lead ingestion.

13-1 C. *Learning objective:* **Provide advice about prevention of lead poisoning.** When a family engages in restoration of an old house, lead-containing dust from paint and plaster cover the floor and become aerosolized. This exposes young children to markedly increased risk. The most effective way to reduce exposure is to keep the child out of the house during renovations. If the family must remain in the house during renovations, wash walls, woodwork, and window ledges daily to reduce dust. Sweep up chips. Look for chipped paint in soil around the house and remove the chips, if possible. Heavy contamination may necessitate removing soil.

13-1 D. *Learning objective:* **Interpret blood lead level test results and discuss management based on the results.** This child is at high risk largely because planned home renovations will increase environmental lead. Thus, a lead level at the 6-month visit is needed. Follow-up lead level testing will depend on the current results. If the 6-month level is 4 µg/dl, the repeat level may be done at the 12-month visit. You should stress environmental cleanliness. If the 6-month level is 12 µg/dl, then the child should be removed from the home environment and have repeat lead levels monitored over the ensuing 1 to 2 months. Subsequent tests will be based on results.

BIBLIOGRAPHY

American Academy of Pediatrics Committee on Environmental Health: Lead exposure in children: prevention, detection, and management, *Pediatrics* 116:1036, 2005. Also at http://aappolicy.aappublications.org/cgi/content/abstract /pediatrics;116/4/1036.

Centers for Disease Control and Prevention: Screening young children for lead poisoning: guidance for state and local public health officials, Atlanta, 1997, Centers for Disease Control and Prevention.

Centers for Disease Control and Prevention: Managing elevated blood lead levels among young children: recommendations from the Advisory Committee on Childhood Lead Poisoning Prevention, Atlanta, 2002.

Centers for Disease Control and Prevention: Preventing lead poisoning in young children, Atlanta, 2005, Centers for Disease Control and Prevention.

Centers for Disease Control and Prevention: Childhood lead poisoning prevention program. Available at: www.cdc.gov/nceh/lead/lead.htm.

14

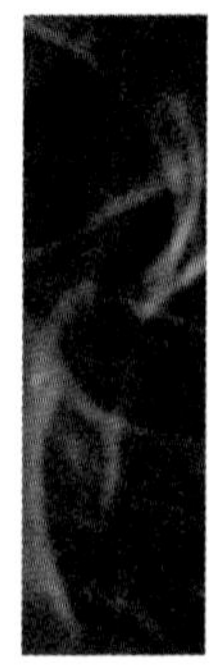

The Healthy Newborn

MICHAEL GIULIANO

What Happens at Birth?

Birth is a dramatic test of transitional physiology. The newborn must rapidly adapt cardiovascular flow and function, establish lung-based oxygenation, develop endocrine control of body metabolism, adapt neurologic responses to new stimuli, and begin to develop an immunologic defense. Unique features seen only during this transitional time can help identify many potential newborn problems. Specific problems are discussed in Chapter 67.

Where Do I Begin the History for a Newborn?

You must obtain the history of the mother, the baby, and the family. Ask about the medical, social, genetic, nutritional, drug, environmental, and infectious history. Review the mother's obstetric record, the details of labor and delivery, and the immediate postnatal events. Although much information will be in the chart, the interview offers an opportunity to build rapport and trust with the family. Open-ended questions will often bring to the surface both major and minor concerns.

What Should I Ask about the Pregnancy?

Information about previous pregnancies will often indicate potential problems for this pregnancy. Document and confirm outcomes of past pregnancies, especially complications such as prematurity, infection, preeclampsia, or major medical problems. Ask if this pregnancy was assisted with reproductive technology. Ask when prenatal care began and how the due date was determined, especially the results of any screening sonograms. Ask also about mother's overall health, including blood pressure, and whether screening tests were done for infection and gestational diabetes. Tests for genetic disorders might have included the triple screen for risk of Down syndrome, amniocentesis for chromosome analysis, or other genetic testing based on family history or ethnic background. Ask whether premature labor occurred during this pregnancy and how it was managed. Review the mother's nutrition, and ask especially if she took a daily folic acid supplement of 0.4 mg starting before conception. Some foods pose infection risks (raw meat, unpasteurized cheese, and cold cuts) while long-lived fish (shark, mackerel, etc.) may contain methyl mercury.

What Infectious Diseases Pose Risks to the Newborn?

Maternal infections may cause fetal or neonatal diseases, many of which can be treated or prevented by immunizations or prophylaxis (Table 14-1). HIV testing is now recommended for *all* pregnant women. Factors related to the risk of newborn infection include prematurity, prolonged rupture of membranes, maternal fever during labor, and chorioamnionitis. The mother's group B streptococcus (GBS) status is important: To prevent transmission of GBS from a colonized mother to the newborn, National Institutes of Health (NIH) guidelines recommend that penicillin be administered to the mother at least 4 hours before birth. It is also important to note whether the mother received any other antibiotics during labor and why. For example, antibiotic prophylaxis may be given in labor for mitral valve prolapse.

Table 14-1

Maternal Infections That Can Affect the Newborn

Organism	Key Historical Information
Varicella-zoster	Maternal and sibling history of disease or immunization. Active varicella in mother near term? Recent exposure by any nonimmune family members?
Herpes simplex I and II	Genital herpes: frequency and treatment. Active lesions at the start of labor?
Rubella, measles, mumps	Maternal immunization history or result of antibody screen
Hepatitis B	History of maternal disease and mode of disease acquisition (IV drugs, multiple sexual partners). Current status of disease (active, carrier). Family tested, immunized?
HIV	High-risk behaviors? Results of HIV testing, if done
Listeria	Consumption of cold cuts, hot dogs, or unpasteurized cheese
Tuberculosis	Immigrant from endemic country? BCG? History of contact or active disease? PPD status of mother and family members
Chlamydia	High-risk behaviors. Other STDs?
Gonococcus	High-risk behaviors. Other STDs?
Syphilis	High-risk behaviors. RPR or VDRL status? Other STDs?
Toxoplasmosis	History of exposure (cats, consumption or handling of raw meat or garden products)? Test results?
Group B streptococci	Is mother colonized? Results of screening tests? Treatment history?

BCG, Bacille Calmette-Guérin; HIV, human immunodeficiency virus; IV, intravenous; PPD, purified protein derivative; RPR, rapid plasma reagin; STD, sexually transmitted disease; VDRL, Venereal Disease Research Laboratory.

What Maternal Medical Problems Affect the Fetus?

All chronic medical problems, especially cardiac, renal, and pulmonary diseases and the drugs used to treat them, can affect the fetus and newborn. High blood pressure and diabetes during pregnancy can have profound implications for the newborn. Diseases mediated by IgG antibodies, including autoimmune thyroid disorders, myasthenia gravis, lupus, or immune thrombocytopenia, can affect the fetus and newborn. Blood transfusions or previous pregnancies, including spontaneous or elective abortions, could have led to the formation of antibodies against Rh factor, or other blood system antigens. Check the blood types of the mother and newborn because hemolysis and jaundice in the newborn could become a major issue if maternal antibodies to the fetal blood cells are present.

Are Maternal Drug or Toxin Exposures Important?

Ask about use of any prescribed or over-the-counter medication, alcohol, tobacco, and illegal drugs. Alcohol is the most common preventable cause of mental retardation, and there is no known safe amount of alcohol exposure for a fetus. Ask whether the mother had any lead exposure as a child, because lead can be mobilized during pregnancy and transferred to the fetus. Environmental lead in old housing or in the workplace can pose risks to the infant after delivery.

What Is Important in the Family History?

Begin by asking the mother about general issues, such as the ages and health status of grandparents, the baby's father, and any other children in the family. Ask whether her other children had problems in the newborn period, such as jaundice or infections. Did she breast-feed them? How have they been growing and developing? Are there any concerns about their overall health? The sudden death of a baby in the family may be your only clue to an inborn error of metabolism. Ask about major illness in the family, especially disorders with a known genetic pattern, such as cystic fibrosis, muscular dystrophy, congenital heart disease, cleft lip or palate, developmental dysplasia of the hip (DDH), hemophilia, hemoglobinopathies, and vesicoureteral reflux.

How Does the Social History Help?

The social history provides important information about the family's ability to care for the newborn, aids discharge planning, and helps plan the follow-up process. Ask whether this was a planned pregnancy and if the mother and father of the child are married, cohabiting, or no longer have a relationship. What do parents do for a living? Does the mother have the financial and health resources necessary to care for herself and her family? What social support system does the mother have? What is the location and condition of the home or apartment? Does the mother or any family member use drugs, alcohol, or tobacco products? Are any firearms present in home? Is there any indication of domestic violence?

What Happened During Labor and Delivery?

Review the labor and delivery records for evidence of fetal distress and risk factors for infection. Gestational age of the fetus and the duration of labor are important for subsequent management. If the fetal heart rate pattern was monitored during labor, did it reflect any signs of distress? If the fetus showed signs of stress, what were the results of additional testing such as a fetal scalp pH? Fetal distress might prompt emergency cesarean section, or the infant might be delivered with forceps or vacuum suction. The presence of meconium in the amniotic fluid may indicate fetal distress, as would a low Apgar score and need for resuscitation at birth.

Does the Amniotic Fluid Predict Problems?

Prenatal sonograms can identify the amount of amniotic fluid. Polyhydramnios suggests an upper gastrointestinal (GI) obstruction in the fetus. Severe oligohydramnios raises the possibility of renal abnormalities. The medical record will indicate whether meconium was present in the amniotic fluid and if special treatment was administered to the infant. Meconium-stained fluid occurs in up to 10% of term deliveries, but most infants require no intervention. A depressed newborn with meconium-stained amniotic fluid will require evaluation of the airway and possible intubation at birth.

What Is the Apgar Score?

The Apgar score assesses heart rate, respiratory rate, skin color, muscle tone, and response to stimuli at 1 minute and 5 minutes after birth, a physiologically dynamic time when the newborn must make the transition from fetal to extrauterine life (Table 14-2). Each component of the Apgar score may receive 0, 1, or 2 points. A perfectly healthy baby would have an Apgar score of 10.

Table 14-2

Apgar Scores

Score	0	1	2
Heart rate	Absent	< 100 bpm	> 100 bpm
Respiratory effort	Absent, irregular	Slow, crying	Good
Muscle tone	Limp	Some flexion of extremities	Active motion
Reflex irritability (nose suction)	No response	Grimace	Cough or sneeze
Color	Blue, pale	Acrocyanosis	Completely pink

bpm, Beats per minute.

Data from Apgar V: A proposal for new method of evaluation of the newborn infant, *Anesth Analg* 32:260, 1953.

What Transitional Issues Must I Consider?

Respiration

The newborn must make the transition from placenta-based oxygenation to lung-based ventilation at the time of delivery. The infant who makes a smooth transition will be well perfused, "pink" centrally, and have a respiratory rate between 40 and 60 breaths per minute shortly after birth. Tachypnea or prolonged need for oxygen would be an early indication that the transition has not been smooth. A newborn who did not expand the lungs and establish adequate ventilation immediately after birth would receive a low Apgar score, and resuscitation would likely have been needed in the delivery room.

Circulation

During the transition period, blood flow is "rerouted" to the lungs as pulmonary vascular resistance falls and the foramen ovale and ductus arteriosus close. Central cyanosis indicates problems such as persistence of the fetal circulatory pattern caused by elevated pulmonary vascular resistance or persistence of right-to-left shunts at the foramen ovale and ductus arteriosus. Congenital heart disease may manifest as central cyanosis that does not respond to oxygen (see Chapter 56).

Temperature control

Thermoregulation is another new demand of the transition. At birth, the newborn is suddenly thrust into a relatively cold environment and must immediately begin to generate heat. Attention is needed in the delivery room to prevent hypothermia during the transition.

Glucose control

All newborns must be monitored for signs of hypoglycemia, which include jitteriness, lethargy, poor feeding, and apnea. The fetus has a continuous supply of glucose in utero from the maternal circulation. At birth that supply suddenly stops and the newborn must generate glucose to sustain adequate blood levels. Risks for decreased glucose include maternal diabetes, birth weight that is either large or small for gestational age, and fetal stress.

Neurologic transition

Neurologic systems must make the transition from a quiet, dark environment to a loud, bright environment with multiple stimuli, such as sight, sound, and touch. Irritability, jitteriness, or lethargy could be a sign of a difficult transition to neonatal life. Rooting, sucking, swallowing, digestion, and excretion all must be mastered.

What Is Important in the Newborn's Medical History?

The baby's history after the transition period will help in determining whether this is truly a healthy newborn. Infants lose up to 10% of birth weight in the first days of life, so you must monitor for excessive weight loss. Most infants urinate and excrete meconium stool by 24 hours; if this has not occurred, you should consider the possibility of urinary tract or bowel obstruction. The initiation of feeding is crucial to monitor: How well does the infant feed, how much, and how often? If breast-feeding, is the baby latching on to the breast? Is the baby vomiting or spitting up after feeding? After the transition period, did the baby demonstrate any signs of respiratory distress, cyanosis, jaundice, temperature instability, or any unusual behaviors or neurologic findings?

What Tests Are Performed for Newborn Infants?

Most healthy newborns need few laboratory tests beyond blood glucose shortly after birth and the neonatal screen after 24 hours of age. If the baby had a screening blood glucose test, what was the result? There is still debate about the normal glucose level for a newborn, but any value below 40 mg/dl is reason for concern and intervention. Complete blood count, total and direct bilirubin levels, and serum electrolytes may be done when conditions justify. If the blood type, Coombs' test, and rapid plasma reagin (RPR) status have been assessed, they should be noted. Cultures may be done if suspicion of infection exists.

What Is Important on Physical Examination?

Good observation, gentleness, and attention to detail will ensure success. You can learn a lot about babies by just looking at them. Skin color, respiratory pattern, and position speak volumes. Some systems, such as the nervous system, are easier to evaluate in the newborn than in older children. Because newborns cannot "cooperate," do what you can before the infant begins to react to the examination. Observe first, then examine the cardiac and respiratory systems, and finally go on to the rest of the examination. The following description of the physical examination emphasizes unique newborn features. See Chapter 5 for the general physical examination.

Measurements

A baby's weight, head circumference, and length should always be plotted to determine if they are appropriate, small, or large for gestational age. Special problems can occur in each group (see Chapter 67).

Gestational age

The Ballard score is a standardized method for determining gestational age (Figure 14-1). It consists of physical and neurologic features that change in a predictable manner as the infant matures during late fetal life. These parameters should be reviewed for all newborns to assess gestational age.

Skin

The newborn is a dermatologic wonderland, with numerous skin findings at birth or shortly thereafter. Table 14-3 lists common skin findings in the newborn.

Head

The skull in a newborn is still in the process of being calcified. Fontanelles and sutures (see Chapter 5 and Figure 5-1) give the skull flexibility for the birthing process and accommodate rapid brain growth. Molding of the head into the shape of the birth canal and overriding of the sutures are common in the first few days of life and resolve

Neuromuscular maturity

Neuromuscular maturity sign	Score −1	0	1	2	3	4	5	Record score here
Posture								
Square window (wrist)	>90r	90r	60r	45r	30r	0r		
Arm recoil		180r	140–180r	110–140r	90–110r	<90r		
Popliteal angle	180r	160r	140r	120r	100r	90r	<90r	
Scarf sign								
Heel to ear								

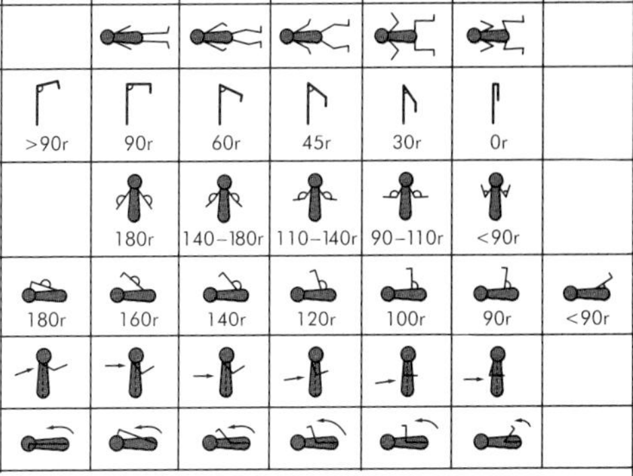

TOTAL NEUROMUSCULAR MATURITY SCORE

Physical maturity

Physical maturity sign	Score −1	0	1	2	3	4	5	Record score here
Skin	Sticky, friable, transparent	Gelatinous, red, translucent	Smooth, pink, visible veins	Superficial peeling and/or rash, few veins	Cracking, pale areas, rare veins	Parchment, deep cracking, no vessels	Leathery, cracked, wrinkled	
Lanugo	None	Sparse	Abundant	Thinning	Bald areas	Mostly bald		
Plantar surface	Heel–toe: 40–50mm: −1 <40mm: −2	>50mm, no crease	Faint red marks	Anterior transverse crease only	Creases anterior two thirds	Creases over entire sole		
Breast	Imper-ceptible	Barely perceptible	Flat areola, no bud	Stippled areola, 1–2mm bud	Raised areola, 3–4mm bud	Full areola, 5–10mm bud		
Eye/ear	Lids fused: loosely: −1 tightly: −2	Lids open, pinna flat, stays folded	Sl. curved pinna, soft, slow recoil	Well-curved pinna, soft but ready recoil	Formed and firm, instant recoil	Thick cartilage, ear stiff		
Genitals (male)	Scrotum flat, smooth	Scrotum empty, faint rugae	Testes in upper canal, rare rugae	Testes descending, few rugae	Testes down, good rugae	Testes pendulous, deep rugae		
Genitals (female)	Clitoris prominent and labia flat	Prominent clitoris and small labia minora	Prominent clitoris and enlarging minora	Majora and minora equally prominent	Majora large, minora small	Majora cover clitoris and minora		

TOTAL PHYSICAL MATURITY SCORE

Score

Neuromuscular____
Physical____
Total____

Maturity rating

Score	−10	−5	0	5	10	15	20	25	30	35	40	45	50
Weeks	20	22	24	26	28	30	32	34	36	38	40	42	44

Gestational age (weeks)

By dates____
By ultrasound____
By exam____

FIGURE 14-1 Neuromuscular and physical maturity (new Ballard score). (Adapted from Ballard JL, Khoury JC, Wedig K et al: New Ballard score, expanded to include extremely premature infants, *J Pediatr* 119:417, 1991.)

The Healthy Newborn

Table 14-3

Common Skin Findings in the Newborn

Finding	Significance
Bruising or petechiae	Birth trauma (presenting part) or nuchal cord (face). Thrombocytopenia if widely distributed
Cyanosis or mottling	Physiologic (peripheral); cardiovascular or respiratory disease (central)
Milia	Multiple small, white, keratin-filled cysts about 1 mm in diameter, most notable on the face and nose. Seen at birth
Transient neonatal pustular melanosis	Pustules that rupture shortly after birth and leave behind pigmented macules at the site of rupture. Not infectious; no treatment is needed
Sucking blisters	Clear blisters seen on fingers or wrists shortly after birth that result from vigorous in utero sucking
"Salmon patch," "angel's kiss," or "stork bite"	Flat, light red, blanching patches commonly seen on the glabella, upper eyelids, or nape of the neck. They fade with time and require no treatment
Port wine stains	Flat, intensely red-to-purple in color. Seen on the face, arms, and legs. Lesions on the eyelids, involving the distribution of the ophthalmic branch of the trigeminal nerve, can be associated with Sturge-Weber syndrome
Mongolian spots	Irregular blue-green maculae especially over the back and the buttocks. They fade with time and require no treatment. They sometimes can be confused with large bruises. Common in African American (90%) and Asian (75%) babies
Congenital melanocytic nevi	Usually small lesions varying in color from light tan to black. Rarely, they can be very large and pose a major cosmetic problem, as well as a risk for malignant melanoma
Sebaceous nevi	Yellow-orange in color, often found in the scalp. Usually oval in shape, raised, and hairless. No treatment needed
Café au lait macules	Pale tan-brown, irregular margins, from 2 mm to 2 cm in size. Presence of > 6 may be a sign of neurofibromatosis
Erythema toxicum	Erythematous macule with a small central papule, usually less than 3 cm in diameter. The cause is unknown. The rash is self-limited and requires no treatment
Jaundice	Physiologic or pathologic

spontaneously. During a normal vertex birth the presenting portion of the head receives the most trauma, which manifests as diffuse swelling or bruising of the scalp. Swelling that crosses suture lines is termed *caput succedaneum*. Caput requires no treatment because the swelling resolves in a few days. Trauma that causes bleeding into the subperiosteal space will produce a *cephalhematoma* that is limited to one cranial bone; scalp swelling will not cross suture lines. A cephalhematoma may not become evident until several hours after birth. The swelling itself does not require treatment, but the blood that is reabsorbed by the infant can contribute to elevated bilirubin levels and jaundice.

Ears
Structurally abnormal, rotated, or low-set ears may be a sign of other anomalies, especially involving the brain and urinary tract. Preauricular skin tags can be associated with renal anomalies.

Eyes
The newborn eye is difficult to examine, and you will need patience to see anything. Always evaluate the "red" reflex, which should be round and homogeneous in color. The darker the skin pigment, the less red will be the reflex; a reddish-gold color is commonly seen as the "red" reflex of a darkly pigmented infant. If there are any irregularities in the red reflex, you must rule out a congenital cataract or intraocular mass. The "white reflex" is classic for retinoblastoma. Subconjunctival hemorrhages usually reflect birth trauma, are self-limited, and require no treatment. Excessive tearing or watery discharge may indicate a blocked lacrimal duct. Conjunctival inflammation or purulent discharge may signal an infection.

Nose
The nose can be distorted or flat after vaginal delivery but recovers in a few days. Because newborns are obligatory nose-breathers, it is important to document the patency of the nares in any infant who has stridorous breathing. Choanal atresia can be a cause for respiratory distress.

Throat/Mouth
A large cleft lip and palate will be recognized immediately at delivery, but many isolated cleft palates can be missed unless the palate is carefully palpated. A bifid or notched uvula may tip you off to a submucous cleft. Occasionally, natal teeth are present. These are usually poorly formed, have poor attachments to the gum, and pose the danger of aspiration. Clear or bluish fluid-filled sacs located bilaterally on the gums are called *dental lumina cysts*. They disappear in a few weeks and require no treatment.

Chest/Lungs
The healthy newborn takes 40 to 60 breaths per minute. The diaphragm, not the chest wall, is the major respiratory muscle for the newborn. Retractions of any kind indicate increased work of breathing and call for further evaluation. Air entry should always be symmetrical; asymmetrical air entry should raise the possibility of pneumonia, pneumothorax, diaphragmatic hernia, or a congenital structural abnormality of the lungs. Coarse breath sounds heard especially right after birth usually are caused by retained lung fluid, and clear quickly. Most term infants, male and female, have breast buds at least 1 cm in diameter, from exposure to maternal hormones in utero. Galactorrhea or milky discharge from the neonatal breast occurs in up to 6% of healthy term newborns. This resolves spontaneously.

Heart
The rapid rate of the newborn heart makes examination a challenge. You must take time and will need a "fast ear" to determine whether the newborn has a cardiac abnormality. If you listen often enough and long enough, you can hear a murmur in 50% of newborn babies. Many newborn cardiac

abnormalities, such as a patent ductus arteriosus, do not require any intervention. Persistent murmurs, poor peripheral perfusion, and cyanosis are clues to cardiac problems that require investigation and intervention (see Chapter 56). Absent or weak femoral pulses may result from coarctation of the aorta. Pulse oximetry allows rapid assessment of oxygen saturation.

Abdomen

The umbilicus is the unique feature of the newborn abdomen. The umbilical cord should have two arteries and one vein. The number of vessels should be documented in the delivery room shortly after birth, because it becomes difficult to do once the cord is clamped and starts to dry out. The remnants of the umbilical cord will usually fall off by 7 to 8 days of life. Delayed separation of the cord may be an indication of a white blood cell function defect. Umbilical hernias occur commonly and result from delayed closure of the fascia through which the umbilical cord passed in utero. An umbilical hernia appears as a bulge at the umbilicus that increases with crying; the fascial defect can be palpated easily. Complications such as incarceration or strangulation of bowel occur rarely. Most umbilical hernias close spontaneously by age 4, so no treatment is recommended in the newborn period. Any palpable abdominal mass demands investigation (see Chapter 43). More than half of all newborn abdominal masses are of renal origin. Tumors are rare. An abdominal sonogram usually clarifies the nature of the mass.

Male genitalia

The newborn male has prominent scrotal rugae, which gradually disappear as maternal hormonal influence wanes. The foreskin is not retractable at birth. If newly circumcised, the exposed glans will often have a yellow exudate until it is epithelialized. Before any boy is considered for circumcision, you must first be certain that hypospadias is not present. In hypospadias, the urethral meatus is located ventral to the tip of the glans, anywhere from the lower glans all the way to the perineal area. The foreskin will be used during reconstructive surgery of hypospadias, so circumcision is contraindicated. Often, hypospadias is associated with a bifid foreskin or a chordee (ventral curvature of the penis). About 5% of full-term newborn males will have unilateral or bilateral undescended testes (cryptorchidism). The rate is much higher for premature infants. Testicular cancer and infertility are long-term complications of untreated cryptorchidism, so lack of testicular descent by ages 6 to 12 months should prompt referral to a urologist. Hydroceles occur commonly and inguinal hernias occasionally. Both result from the failure of the processus vaginalis to undergo fusion and obliteration during fetal life. Hydroceles, which are fluid-filled sacs in the scrotum, present as fixed scrotal swellings that transilluminate. Most isolated hydroceles resolve spontaneously. Inguinal hernias are 10 times more likely in males than in females. They usually are noticed as a transient bulge in the inguinal canal when the infant is straining or crying. All inguinal hernias require surgical evaluation and closure because of the risk of incarceration. Inguinal hernias can sometimes "hide" behind hydroceles and may be difficult to detect.

Female genitalia

Newborn girls have prominent labia majora and minora, which become less prominent as maternal estrogen effects diminish. A thick white vaginal discharge is often noted at birth or in the first day of life, also because of maternal estrogen effects. Newborn girls may occasionally have a small amount of vaginal bleeding in the first week of life because of estrogen withdrawal. All newborn girls should be examined for an imperforate hymen.

Ambiguous genitalia

Any newborn who is not clearly male or female requires an emergency consultation with a multidisciplinary team to determine the cause of the ambiguous genitalia. Sex assignment should be delayed until the results of the evaluation are complete.

Extremities/spine

The hip is unique in the newborn examination, although all extremities and joints need to be examined for range of motion and abnormalities. DDH occurs in as many as 1 in 1000 newborns. Mechanical, hormonal, and genetic factors can all lead to abnormal development of the femoral head and acetabular cup. This in turn causes an unstable hip joint with the femoral head either dislocated or dislocatable. DDH can lead to a lifelong disability if not recognized and treated early. The Ortolani test, the Barlow provocative test, and maneuvers to identify leg-length discrepancy, knee-height discrepancy, or asymmetrical skin folds on the legs are all used to identify a dislocated hip (see Chapter 5 and Figure 5-4).

Neurologic examination

The newborn's dominant tone is flexor, and a resting infant has flexed arms, legs, and trunk. Any asymmetry, increase, or decrease in tone may indicate significant central nervous system abnormalities. Most newborn responses are reflexive, and you should be able to elicit "primitive reflexes" including suck, root, grasp, and Moro. While observing a newborn, you will often see an isolated, rapid movement of an extremity. This is a myoclonic jerk, which can be easily extinguished by holding the extremity. Although these can be confused with seizure activity, a seizure would not be extinguished merely by holding the extremity.

What Is the Routine Care in the Nursery?

Nutritional counseling

"How are you going to feed your baby?" should be one of the first questions you ask. All mothers should be encouraged to breast-feed whenever possible. Few medications or diseases prevent a mother from breast-feeding, but you should inquire about the mother's medications and investigate whether they might have any effect on the newborn. If the mother chooses not to breast-feed, you should support this decision and discuss infant formulas. Information about human milk and formulas can be found in Chapter 10. Once the feeding method has been selected, a mother will often ask "How long should I nurse my baby?"

or "How much formula should my baby take?" Breast-fed babies generally nurse 10 minutes on each breast every 2 to 3 hours—occasionally longer and as frequently as every 90 minutes. Formula-fed babies usually take from 1 to 4 ounces every 3 to 4 hours. Feeding frequency and formula volume will change quickly over time, with each baby setting his or her own pattern of feeding. An infant who has at least six wet diapers per day and gains weight is receiving adequate amounts of breast milk or formula.

Information about weight and stools

Parents should be forewarned that newborns may lose up to 10% of birth weight before they start to grow. Initial weight loss reflects excretion of the newborn's excessive free water. Meconium stools that are passed shortly after birth are thick and blackish green in color. Stool gradually becomes soft in consistency and light yellow. Breast-fed infants have "seedy," somewhat runny stools, whereas formula-fed infants tend to have more formed stools. Most infants pass stool with each feeding, but some have a stool only once a day. Mothers should be alert to any change in the stooling pattern.

Newborn eye prophylaxis

Shortly after birth, most infants in the United States are treated with erythromycin eye ointment. Without eye prophylaxis, both *Gonococcus* and *Chlamydia* can cause neonatal conjunctivitis. In addition, chlamydial infection can spread down the respiratory tract and cause an interstitial pneumonia in the first few months of life. Eye prophylaxis dramatically decreases the risk of these problems.

Vitamin K

Infants are born vitamin K deficient and are at risk for bleeding caused by lack of this critical coagulation cofactor (see Chapter 44) This bleeding disorder can range from mild to very severe, even causing death. Breast-fed infants are at increased risk for this problem. One intramuscular dose of vitamin K (1 mg of AquaMEPHYTON) at birth has virtually eliminated vitamin K–dependent bleeding (hemorrhagic disease of the newborn).

Neonatal screening tests

All newborns are screened for inborn errors of metabolism (Chapter 62), but the disorders screened vary from state to state. The National Newborn Screening and Genetics Resource Center (http://genes-r-us.uthscsa.edu/) provides extensive information about neonatal screening, including details of state programs. The American Academy of Pediatrics has information for physicians and parents (http://aap.org/healthtopics/newbornscreening.cfm). Phenylketonuria, hypothyroidism, and galactosemia are screened by almost all states. Many states now use tandem mass spectroscopy that can screen for up to 30 inborn errors. The screening test should be done after 24 hours of age, when the infant has had several feedings. If done before 24 hours these screening tests may give false-negative results. Ensure that arrangements have been made with the follow-up health professional to repeat these tests if the infant is discharged early.

Screening for infectious diseases

Maternal infections may be transmitted to the fetus and cause disease in the newborn, so screening may be indicated based on the maternal history and results of maternal screening.

Sexually transmitted infection. Some states screen all newborns for human immunodeficiency virus (HIV) antibodies or do a nonspecific syphilis screening test (RPR). These results are needed before discharge so that appropriate evaluation and treatment can be started in a timely fashion. If a mother's HIV status is unknown, the newborn should have rapid HIV testing done immediately. Infants born to HIV-positive mothers need to be started on zidovudine shortly after birth and then must have a polymerase chain reaction test for HIV to determine if they are infected. Preventive measures, including aggressive treatment of the HIV-positive mother, cesarean section, and zidovudine treatment of the newborn, have reduced the rate of HIV transmission to as low as 1%. HIV-positive mothers cannot breast-feed their children because of the risk of transmission.

Hepatitis B. Routine immunization with hepatitis B vaccine is recommended for all newborn infants. Children born to mothers who are positive for hepatitis B surface antigen should receive hepatitis B immune globulin and hepatitis B-conjugate vaccine shortly after birth. This intervention can prevent transmission to most infants.

Varicella. Any infant born to a mother who recently developed varicella should receive a dose of varicella-zoster immune globulin (VZIG). VZIG significantly decreases the severity of neonatal varicella.

Circumcision

Circumcision remains a controversial issue. The AAP policy statement on circumcision (see *Pediatrics* 103:686, 1999) leaves the decision up to the parents. You should discuss the potential benefits (decreased urinary tract infections) and the risks (infection, bleeding, pain) of the procedure with parents and let them decide.

Hearing screening

Hearing screening is now recommended for all newborn infants (AAP policy statement: *Pediatrics* 106:798, 2000) to detect congenital hearing loss and reduce subsequent morbidity (Mehl and Thomson, 2002). Methodology varies from center to center. Inquire about the technique used in your hospital. You should find out the results of the test before your patient is discharged and whether follow-up is needed.

Jaundice

Risk factors for significant jaundice include prematurity, exclusive breast-feeding, previous siblings treated for jaundice, and East Asian race. History will identify these risks and physical examination should look for jaundice. A screening bilirubin level or transcutaneous bilirubin level should be obtained and plotted on the Bhutani curve. Close follow-up after discharge is needed for infants at high risk. If the parents notice that the infant is jaundiced they should return for evaluation. See Chapter 67 as well as the American Academy of Pediatrics Clinical Guideline for hyperbilirubinemia (see *Pediatrics* 114:297, 2004).

What Do I Need to Discuss When the Infant Is Discharged from the Nursery?

The timing of discharge for the healthy newborn has itself become controversial. The ideal length of stay for a newborn and mother is unclear. Specific criteria must be met before discharge from the newborn nursery, and it is unlikely these criteria can be met before 48 hours of life (see *Pediatrics* 113:1434, 2004). At discharge a parent should always have a clear understanding about the need for close follow-up. You must find out who will do the follow-up care of the newborn and when. Infants discharged before 48 hours of life should be seen for follow-up within 24 to 48 hours, at which time the infant can be assessed for jaundice and other problems of the immediate postnatal period and can have repeat neonatal screening done. Parents should be educated about their central role as record keepers of their child's health issues. The infant's health record card should be reviewed with the parent. It should accompany the parent and child for all medical visits.

What Safety Issues Are Important?

Car seat safety

This is a critical part of the discharge interview. Infants should ride in the back seat in safety seats that face the rear of the car. Remind parents that siblings younger than 12 years also belong in the back seat in restraints appropriate for age. They should never be seated in an air bag–equipped seat. Parents should also be reminded to use seat belts!

Sleeping position

Infants who sleep on their backs are at less risk for sudden infant death syndrome (SIDS). Parents should be instructed that infants should go to sleep only on their backs with no soft materials left in the crib.

Environmental hazards

The hazards of tobacco smoke exposure and environmental lead should be discussed at discharge and during routine health supervision. Close supervision to avoid falls or unintentional trauma from older siblings or family pets is warranted. The possibility that domestic violence exists within the family must be considered.

What Questions Might Parents Ask at Discharge?

What do I do when the baby cries?

Crying babies usually want something or need something. Most often the diaper needs changing or the baby is hungry.

When can I take my baby out?
Going out is not a concern, as long as the temperature is not too cold or hot. Clothing should be appropriate to the environmental temperature. Going into small enclosed spaces with a lot of people is a concern. Especially in the first month of life, infants should not be exposed to anyone who is sick.

What do I need to do about the umbilical cord?
Keep it dry and clean; turn the diaper edge down away from the cord. The cord will fall off in about 1 week. If you note any oozing or redness around the cord, see your doctor.

KEY POINTS

- The medical history of the newborn includes the mother's pregnancy and delivery history.
- The Apgar score provides information about the transition to extrauterine life.
- Observation is an important part of the newborn physical examination.
- Interventions and screening can prevent or minimize adverse outcomes.

Case 14-1

A newborn male infant weighs 2500 g. Apgar scores were 8 at 1 minute and 9 at 5 minutes. The mother is 16 years old and had no prenatal care. She has a history of cigarette smoking and "occasional" use of alcohol and marijuana. You are asked to examine the infant and determine gestational age

A. What findings on the physical examination would indicate that this is a full-term infant?
B. What other physical findings will you look for given the mother's history?

Case Answers

14-1 A. *Learning objective:* **Use the physical examination of the newborn to determine gestational age.** You would use the Ballard score to determine gestational age. Neurologic findings for the full-term infant include flexed body position and brisk recoil of the arm when extended from the flexed position. Prominent breast buds, creases on more than 2/3 of the soles of the feet, and a rugated scrotum are among the other important indications of physical maturity.

14-1 B. *Learning objective:* **Recognize the risk factors from the maternal history that can have an effect on fetal growth and development.** Both alcohol consumption and cigarette smoking can affect the fetus. Although signs of fetal alcohol syndrome may be subtle, you should look for the classic diagnostic findings: in utero growth retardation; a long, flat philtrum; flattened mid-face; and small head circumference. Also be aware that alcohol exposure during fetal development can cause a variety of congenital malformations, including cardiac defects, skeletal abnormalities, and eye and renal defects. Cigarette smoking causes placental insufficiency and often results in low birth weight.

BIBLIOGRAPHY

AAP, Committee on Fetus and Newborn: Hospital stay for healthy term newborns, *Pediatrics* 113:1434, 2004.

Ballard Score: www.ballardscore.com/ScoreSheet.htm

Mehl AL, Thomson V: The Colorado Newborn Hearing Screening Project, 1992–1999: on the threshold of effective population-based universal newborn hearing screening, *Pediatrics* 109:E7, 2002.

Seidel HM, Rosenstein BJ, Pathak A: *Primary care of the newborn,* ed 3, St Louis, 2001, Mosby.

15

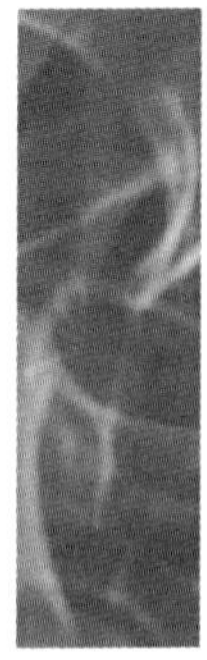

The Healthy Adolescent

KEN CHEYNE and MICHAEL R. LAWLESS

Adolescence is the period of transition between childhood and adulthood. Although often thought to be tumultuous, most adolescents navigate this transition with few difficulties. The physical changes that occur during this period are referred to as *puberty*, the psychosocial changes as *adolescence*. Special consideration must be given to ethical issues such as autonomy and confidentiality (see Chapter 6). Health supervision for the adolescent is discussed in Chapter 11.

What Is Puberty?

Puberty refers to the transition from sexual immaturity to potential fertility associated with the appearance of secondary sexual characteristics. There is a definite beginning and end.

Females go through puberty 2 years earlier than males on average. The first sign of puberty in females is breast development (thelarche). In approximately 15%, however, pubic hair (adrenarche) appears first. Unilateral onset of breast development is a normal variation, with the other breast starting to develop within six months. The usual progression of sexual maturation in females is breast budding, pubic hair growth, peak height velocity, and menarche. Most women undergo menarche within 6 months of peak height velocity. Growth usually stops 2 to 3 years after menarche.

Males have testicular enlargement (testicular length > 2.5 cm) as the first sign of puberty. The usual progression of sexual maturation in males is testicular enlargement, pubic hair growth, enlargement of the penis, and peak height velocity. Growth usually stops 2 to 3 years after peak height velocity.

What Is Sexual Maturity Rating?

Tanner published a sexual maturity rating (SMR) system for adolescent pubertal development in 1962; hence, sexual maturity ratings are also referred to as Tanner stages. In females, breast and pubic hair changes are staged. In males, genital and pubic hair growth are staged. SMR I is prepubertal. SMR V is considered adult.

SMR of breasts (Figure 15-1)

SMR I: The breasts are preadolescent. There is elevation of the papilla only.

SMR II: A small mound is formed by the elevation of the breast and papilla. The areolar diameter enlarges.

SMR III: There is further enlargement of the breast and areola with no separation of their contours.

SMR IV: There is projection of the areola and papilla to form a secondary mound above the level of the breast.

SMR V: The breasts resemble those of a mature female, as the areola has recessed to the general contour of the breast.

SMR of pubic hair (Figures 15-2 and 15-3)

SMR I: There is no pubic hair.

SMR II: There is sparse growth of long, slightly pigmented, downy hair, straight or only slightly curled, primarily at the base of the penis or along the labia.

SMR III: The hair is darker, coarser, and more curled. The hair spreads over the junction of the pubes.

SMR IV: The hair is adult in type but covers a smaller area than in the adult. It does not extend onto the thighs.

SMR V: The hair is adult in quantity and type. It extends onto the thighs.

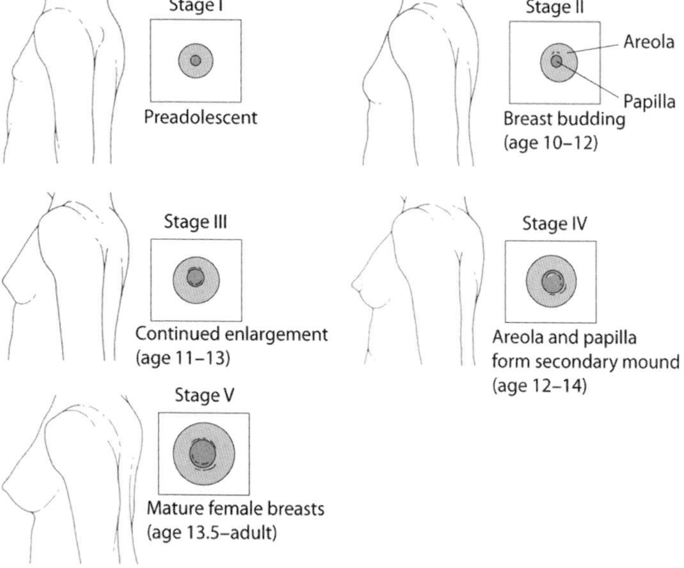

FIGURE 15-1 Sexual maturity rating (SMR) of breast development in females. (Used with permission of Ross Products Division, Abbott Laboratories Inc, Columbus, OH. From Johnson TR, Moore WM, Jefferies JE: *Children are different: development physiology,* ed 2, Columbus, OH, 1978, Ross Products Division, Abbott Laboratories Inc.)

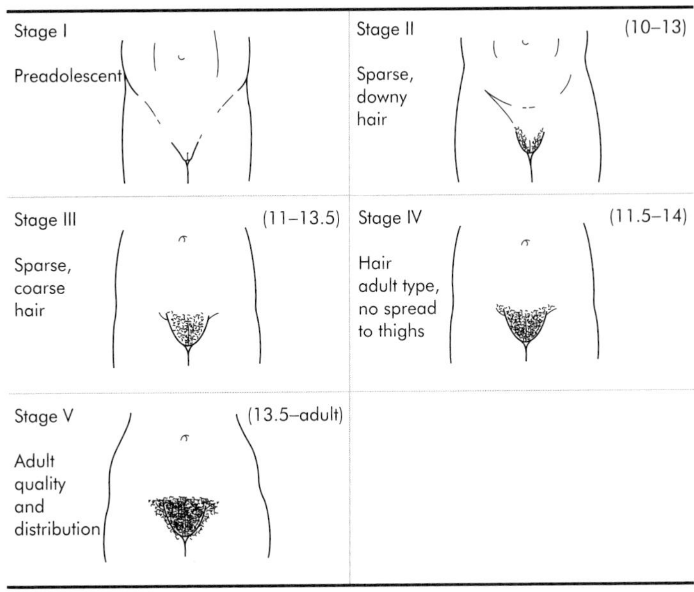

FIGURE 15-2 Sexual maturity rating (SMR) of pubic hair development in females. (Adapted from Neinstein LS: *Adolescent health care: a practical guide,* ed 2, Baltimore, 1991, Urban & Fischer Verlag.)

SMR of male genitalia (Figure 15-3)

SMR I: The penis, testes, and scrotum are of childhood size.

SMR II: Enlargement of scrotum and testes, but penis usually does not enlarge. Scrotal skin reddens.

SMR III: Further growth of testes and scrotum, with enlargement of penis, mainly in length.

SMR IV: Further growth of testes and scrotum with increased size of penis, especially in breadth.

SMR V: The genitalia are adult in size and shape.

When Is Puberty Too Early?

Female puberty is too early if there is breast development before 8 years of age or menarche before 10 years of age. Some girls may initiate breast development as early as age 6. This is more common in females of Latino or African American heritage. Although this may be normal, these girls should have regular follow-up.

Male puberty is too early if there is testicular enlargement (length > 2.5 cm) before 9 years of age.

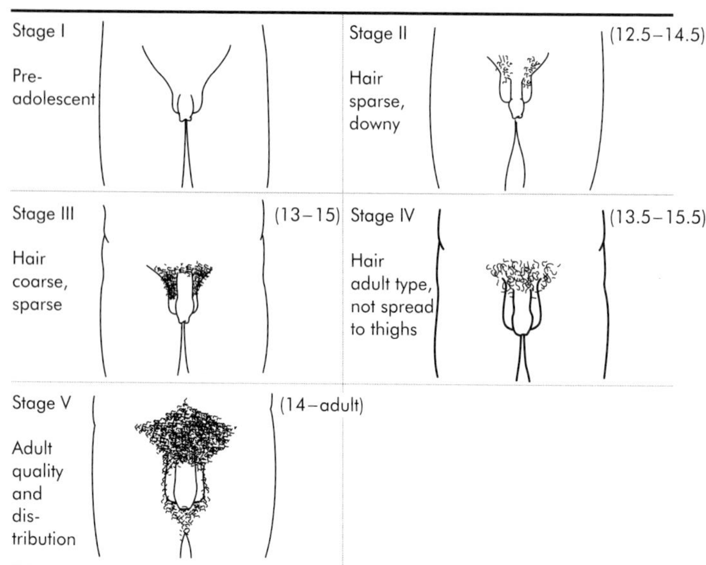

FIGURE 15-3 Sexual maturity rating (SMR) of pubic hair and genital development in males. (Adapted from Neinstein LS: *Adolescent health care: a practical guide,* ed 2, Baltimore, 1991, Urban & Fischer Verlag.)

When Is Puberty Too Late?

Females who have no breast development by 13 years of age or who have not had menarche by age 16 have delayed puberty.
Males whose testicular length has not exceeded 2.5 cm by age 14 have delayed puberty.

What Is Adolescence?

Adolescence refers to the psychosocial and developmental changes that occur as one passes from childhood to adulthood. Unlike puberty, there is not a definite beginning and end. As society becomes more complex, requiring more postsecondary training, the period of adolescence is often prolonged.

What Are the Goals of Adolescence?

There are four main goals of adolescence:

- Psychological independence or the attainment of independence from the family. Teens begin to spend more time with their friends and become increasingly less dependent on their parents. They begin to identify with other adults and often wonder why their parents can't be more like other adults they admire, such as a favorite teacher. They

begin to view their parents as having both strengths and weaknesses. Before this time, children often see their parents as infallible.
- Development of sexual identity. Adolescents come to accept the physical changes that result in an adult body and reproductive capability.
- Emergence of a stable identity. This includes choosing a career or deciding how they will support themselves in the future when they are no longer dependent on their parents.
- Development of a positive social regard or mature thought patterns.

The period of adolescence is often divided into stages labeled early, middle, and late. Although typical age ranges are associated with each stage of adolescence, each teen moves through the various stages of adolescence at his or her own unique rate to ultimately achieve a stable identity.

What Is Early Adolescence?

Early adolescence typically occurs between 11 and 14 years of age. This is a period of rapid physical growth when females are often taller than their male peers. Early adolescents ask themselves, "Am I normal?" They often compare body changes with same-sex peers. Early adolescents begin to separate from their parents as the peer group begins to have greater influence. They have intense same-sex friendships. Sexuality is undifferentiated. Early adolescent girls are often "boy crazy": Liking several boys, means that you do not have to develop a significant relationship with any one of them. Early adolescent boys often look at "girly" magazines. Thinking at this stage is concrete. If you ask young adolescents what brings them in to see you, they may respond, "My mother's car," instead of responding, "A sore throat." Early adolescents often exhibit increased self-interest and fantasy and often find themselves "on stage" in front of an "imaginary audience."

What Is Middle Adolescence?

Middle adolescence typically occurs between 15 and 17 years of age. This is a period where autonomy issues come to the forefront. Middle adolescents are often in conflict with their parents as they test limits. Peer influence is strong, as is conformity with "peer norms." They ask themselves, "Who am I?" as they focus on their personal and sexual identity. Sexual behaviors with the same and opposite sex increase. There is sexual experimentation without commitment. Middle adolescents engage in risk-taking behaviors in an ever-increasing manner. Although formal thinking is initiated at this stage, when stressed, adolescents revert to concrete thinking.

What Is Late Adolescence?

Late adolescence typically occurs between 18 and 21 years of age. Late adolescents become more concerned about the future and ask themselves, "What am I going to do with the rest of my life?" Conflict with parents decreases as peer group influence wanes. Late adolescents may be involved with numerous peer groups instead of just one as in the past. They develop close friendships, and intimacy and commitment begin to develop in their relationships. They more consistently exhibit formal thinking and conceptualize in the abstract.

What Are the Important Aspects of an Adolescent History?

A useful mnemonic for a psychosocial history in adolescents is HEADSSS:

H—*H*ome/*H*ealth

- Who lives with you?
- Have you ever lived outside of your home?

E—*E*ducation/*E*mployment/*E*ating

- Are you in any special programs in school?
- How many hours do you work per week?
- Where and with whom do you eat?
- What do you eat?

A—*A*ctivities/*A*spirations/*A*ffiliations

- What do you like to do for fun?
- In what activities do you participate in school or outside of school?
- What do you want to do when you grow up?

D—*D*rugs

- Do any of your friends smoke or use alcohol or other drugs? If the answer is yes, how do you feel about their use?
- Have you ever tried cigarettes, alcohol, marijuana, or other drugs?

S—*S*ex

- Have you and your parents talked about sex?
- Have you ever had a crush on anyone or has anyone ever had a crush on you?
- Have you ever had sex?

S—*S*leep/*S*uicide

- Do you have trouble falling asleep? On average, how many hours of sleep do you get each night?
- Have you ever thought that life isn't worth living?

S—Shoplifting (a marker for risk-taking behavior)

- Have you ever taken anything without intending to pay for it?

KEY POINTS

- Puberty refers to the time span during which secondary sexual characteristics develop. It has a definite beginning and end.
- Physical changes in puberty are classified by sexual maturity ratings.
- Adolescence has no definite beginning or end. It refers to the period between childhood and adulthood when complex biopsychosocial development occurs.
- HEADDSSS can provide important psychosocial information about an adolescent.

Case 15-1

A mother brings her 14-year-old daughter to the clinic concerned that she is "not as developed" as her friends. Most of the teen's friends have started to have their menstrual periods, but her daughter has not.

A. What additional history would be helpful?
B. What parts of the physical examination are helpful to assess pubertal development?
C. What would you tell the adolescent and her mother if the adolescent showed breast and pubic hair development? What if there is no breast development?

Case 15-2

A 16-year-old boy presents to the clinic for a health maintenance examination. His mother tells you in private that he often argues with his parents. He has had six girlfriends over the past year and was recently caught smoking a cigarette.

A. What developmental stage of adolescence does this teen demonstrate?
B. What question does this teen struggle to answer at his stage of development?
C. Describe this teen's cognitive development.

Case Answers

15-1 A. *Learning objective:* **Discuss the normal sequence of pubertal development in adolescent women.** Helpful additional historical data would be the age at the onset of breast development and whether the adolescent has gone through a growth spurt recently.

15-1 B. *Learning objective:* **Discuss use of the SMR of breasts and pubic hair to classify female pubertal development.** Although a complete physical examination is always indicated, the SMR of the adolescent's breasts and pubic hair would be most helpful. See Figures 15-1 and 15-2.

15-1 C. *Learning objective:* **Identify the normal timing of menarche in adolescent women.** If breast development is present, the adolescent and her mother could be reassured that her development is within the range of normal. Menarche typically occurs approximately 2 years after breast development appears (between 10 to 16 years of age). If there is no breast development by age 13, the girl has delayed onset of puberty.

15-2 A. *Learning objective:* **Recognize the three developmental stages of adolescence.** This teen is in middle adolescence, a time of frequent conflict and limit testing with parents. It is often a time of increasing risk-taking behavior as well.

15-2 B. *Learning objective:* **Identify the unique question that characterizes each of the three stages of adolescent development.** He is searching for his unique identity. His question is "Who am I?"

15-2 C. *Learning objective:* **Discuss the changes in cognitive functioning that occur as an adolescent matures.** Middle adolescence is the time when formal thinking (abstract thought processes) begins. When stressed, adolescents at this stage of development revert to concrete thinking, as described by Piaget.

BIBLIOGRAPHY

Elster AB, Kuznets NJ, editors: *AMA guidelines for adolescent preventive services (GAPS): recommendations and rationale*, Baltimore, 1994, Williams & Wilkins.

Goldenring JM, Rosen DS: Getting into adolescent heads: an essential update, *Contemp Pediatr* 21(1):64, 2004.

Sun SS, Schubert CM, Chumlea WC et al: National estimates of the timing of sexual maturation and racial differences among US children, *Pediatrics* 110:911, 2002.

Tanner JM: *Growth and adolescence*, ed 2, New York, 1962, Blackwell Scientific.

16

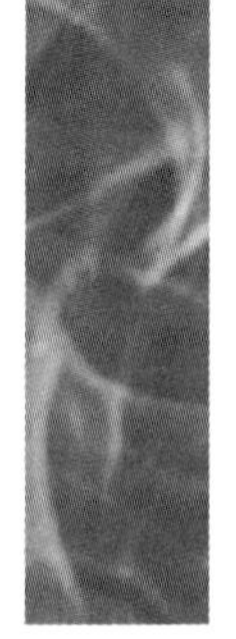

Children with Special Needs

JANICE L. HANSON and VIRGINIA F. RANDALL

What Are "Special Needs"?

In 2004, 12.8% of children younger than 18 years were found to have special healthcare needs, and 20% of households with children reported having a child with special needs. According to the U.S. Maternal and Child Health Bureau, these are children "who have or are at increased risk for a chronic physical, developmental, behavioral, or emotional condition and who also require health and related services of a type or amount beyond that required by children generally." Although some of the care these children require will be provided by pediatric subspecialists, many of their needs can be met most effectively by general pediatricians in a medical home, which is a primary care setting that is accessible, continuous, comprehensive, centered on the family, coordinated, compassionate, and culturally effective.

How Should I Approach a Child with Special Needs?

The challenges of interpersonal relationships with a child who has special needs are much like the challenges of interacting with children in general but often are intensified by the child's more complex health condition. You may find that a child's disability evokes strong emotions, just as you may find that caring for any sick child evokes thoughts, feelings, and fears surrounding your own childhood or your own children. The doctor's office is one place that the child should feel comfortable and valued. Avoid hurtful labels such as "handicapped" or "abnormal" to describe the child. Sometimes medical students and other care providers experience sadness, uneasiness, or frank anxiety as they approach these situations. These are expected reactions to suffering and it is important to acknowledge them and the experiences that led to them. Discuss your discomfort with your preceptor. As your experience grows you will find strategies to prevent these feelings from interfering with patient care or causing bias in your decisions and interactions with parents and children.

How Can I Establish Credibility?

Credibility begins by demonstrating both genuine respect for the parent and child and the desire to help with the child's health care. Understanding and acknowledging that the parents are important members of the child's healthcare team also enhances your credibility. Parents whose children have chronic medical conditions usually have learned a great deal about the conditions. They will appreciate and respect your openness to learn from them.

What Can I Do to Develop Rapport with Parents?

Call parents by their surnames, not "mom" or "dad." Assume that parents take their parenting responsibilities seriously and may be more concerned about their child's illness than a similar illness in themselves. Acknowledge and validate parents' concerns, fears, and pride: "You must have been concerned when he woke up coughing so often last night." "Sometimes nosebleeds are pretty frightening because there seems to be so much blood." "What a beautiful baby boy."

How Do I Provide Guidance for Parents?

Start by first asking an open-ended question that gives the parents an opportunity to describe their approach to parenting and the care of their child's special healthcare needs. Then, make a few suggestions or points of information based on the knowledge that you have gained from your reading. It is most helpful if these suggestions build on the parents' approach. Provide as much information about the well-child visit or the child's illness as you can. Handouts, Web sites, and peer support groups are all welcomed by parents. If parents ask a question for which you do not know the answer, admit you do not know and ask them what they think. You can help establish trust and rapport by letting the family know that you will look into the issue and discuss it with the staff. Ask about the health of parents and other members of the family. Also ask if any other family member has a chronic illness or disability. Parents appreciate your understanding the impact of a child with special needs on the whole family. Ask if parents are using any alternative medicine or home remedies to treat the child. If you are unfamiliar with the family's culture, ask parents to explain what would be done typically in their tradition to treat the child (Box 16-1). React with respect to any information.

How Should I Approach a Well-Child Visit for a Child with Special Needs?

Well-child visits and school physical examinations are part of health supervision (see Chapter 11) for all children, including those with special needs. You must pay attention to all of the typical questions that emerge as children grow and learn, but you will need to focus on the child's special needs, developmental age, and family situation. The Bright Futures Web site provides a format for health supervision,

BOX 16-1

CROSS-CULTURAL COMMUNICATION

- Learn about the cultural diversity in the population of your community.
- Read about the health practices and health beliefs you may encounter.
- Consider:
  - The appropriate distance to maintain during a conversation
  - Appropriate eye contact and touch
  - Cultural explanations of health and illness
  - Typical treatments for common childhood conditions
  - A culture's typical relationship to authority figures
- Ask the child or parent to explain some aspects of their health beliefs that may be important in the child's care. ("I'd like to better understand your thoughts on how your child became ill. Can you help me understand?")
- Avoid asking "why" questions, which may be perceived as attacking or accusing, create defensiveness, and risk shutting off communication.
- If an interpreter is needed, try to use a professional medical interpreter rather than a family member. Interpreters may be available by telephone if not available in person.
- Convey respect for the health practices and beliefs of various cultures, even when they are very different from the ones with which you are familiar.

including history, examination, anticipatory guidance, developmental surveillance, nutrition, oral health, and immunizations.

How Can I Communicate with a Child with Special Needs?

Always talk directly to a child with special needs. Use his or her first name, and use language appropriate for the age level (see Chapter 4). Touch, and if appropriate, hold the child. A child with special needs is a *child* who is usually aware of being "different" because of the chronic illness or disability. Ask parents to explain what they think you should know about the condition and its effects on their child as a unique individual. Ask parents what they think is going on and what has worked to treat their child in the past. Be aware that a child with a disability may not exhibit the same signs of an acute illness as does a child without a disability. Even the most diligent parent can miss subtle or confusing signals about an ailment. A parent may even visit the clinic to talk with you in an effort to understand confusing signals and determine whether the child has an illness needing medical attention. Ask parents if they are receiving the support and information they need. Consult with your preceptor to suggest Internet sites, national or local associations, and books.

How Can I Communicate with a Child Who Doesn't Talk?

Talk directly to the child in a soft and reassuring voice. Use the baby's or older child's name. Try to catch his or her eye and smile. Have an interesting and safe toy for children of any age to look at or reach for, such as a colorful noisemaker. Be prepared for stranger anxiety, an expected and reassuring stage of cognitive development that occurs somewhere around 9 months, although the age can vary. The child may cry the whole time you are in the room or may just stop playing and be more watchful. If you suspect stranger anxiety, ask the parent to hold the child through as much of the examination as possible. Reassure the parent that crying is typical and reflects the child's developing relationship with the parent. A young infant may tolerate being removed from a parent's arms to get a good belly and hip examination, but it will probably help if the parent stands near to reassure and amuse the child. Your ability to recognize and understand nonverbal communication from the child is important. Always show respect for the parent's estimate of the child's discomfort or degree of illness.

How Can I Communicate with a Child Who Has Begun to Talk?

Use the child's name and talk directly to the child, no matter how young. When the child is 2 or 3 years old, begin to ask questions about symptoms: "Tell me about your tummy," or "Show me where it hurts." Be ready to discuss children's books and popular TV cartoon characters seriously with the child. Washable toys (with no small parts) will help you make friends with toddlers and preschoolers and can help the small child relax and become engaged with you. Ask the parent what positions usually work best for the child during the examination. Sometimes the child is less fearful if allowed to practice first on a doll or stuffed animal with the stethoscope or flashlight. Keep up a dialogue with the child during the examination. Tell the child what you are going to do before you do it. Talk about what you are finding or seeing. The child is learning about his or her own body from you, so you can explain where the stomach is, for example, and what it does. Children are proud when they learn new things about their own bodies.

How Can I Communicate with a Child Who Uses a Communication Board or Sign Language?

Children communicate at varied levels with communication boards, other assistive devices, or sign language. Some can tell you exactly what is going on and provide reliable information during the examination. Others may be able to express themselves only in simple terms such as "yes" and "no." A nonverbal child with normal cognition will be able to communicate reliably through an interpreter. A nonverbal child with cognitive delays may have only limited ability to express concerns. Allow the child to communicate his or her needs as much as possible through the modality that works best for him or her. Sometimes, even when a device or alternative method of communication is available, a child best expresses and communicates physical and emotional states through body language and facial expressions. The parent is the best resource to help you determine how to communicate most effectively with the child. It is always important to recognize the child's ability to communicate and to express thanks for the input.

How Can I Communicate with an Adolescent Who Has Special Needs?

Adolescents with special needs have the same developmental tasks that challenge all adolescents. Be aware that each adolescent with special needs is unique. Do not underestimate their potential. Many will soon be managing their own health care, so look for ways to support their growing independence. Explain pathophysiology and give treatment options at the appropriate level. Help them learn what questions to ask healthcare providers. If contemplating a psychosocial interview, talk with the parent and adolescent together first. Explain the topics that you would like to discuss, and ask the parent and adolescent if you may have some time alone with the adolescent for the discussion. Try to "read" the relationship between each parent and adolescent, and do not assume that separating them is always best. Know the laws in your state regarding confidentiality surrounding birth control, sexually transmitted diseases, and other sensitive issues. During the physical examination, treat the adolescent as an adult and provide a gown or drape. Always have a chaperone present.

How Do I Examine a Crying or Uncooperative Child?

Acknowledge that having a child cry while at the doctor's office is often upsetting to parents. Ask parents if they know of any techniques that have helped in the past. Suggest that the child sit on the parent's lap. Proceed as gently, but quickly, as possible. For example, if the child objects to the abdominal examination, place your hand on the child's abdomen and put the child's hand on top of yours so he or she can "help" you. Have your equipment and supplies ready ahead of time so the child doesn't have to sit waiting, getting more and more apprehensive.

How Do I Perform a Painful Procedure?

Begin by realizing that what seems routine to you may be very frightening and disagreeable to a child. Explain to the parent and child what you are going to do. If it is likely to hurt, explain that, too. Telling a child, "It won't hurt," when, in fact, it will, undermines the trust that is essential for a child and parent to have in healthcare providers. If the child is on the examination table, suggest the parent stand near the child's head to talk to him or her. Ask parents (and children if appropriate) how they would like to help get the procedure done. Ask parents if they would like to hold their children on their laps and restrain them there.

What If I Inadvertently Hurt or Scare the Child?

You probably will not accidentally hurt the child, but if you do, acknowledge it immediately and apologize to the child and the parent. Tell the child, "You did a great job. You were brave!" Explain the incident thoroughly to your preceptor and document it in the chart if necessary.

What Should I Do If I Think the Child Is Very Sick?

Say in a calm voice, "I think your child needs attention right away," then leave the room and get your preceptor or another healthcare provider immediately.

What Should I Do If a Parent Does Something Not in the Best Interest of the Child?

A nonjudgmental approach seems to work the best. Nearly all parents care about their children, even parents who are doing something with which you disagree, such as smoking in the home. Find out if the parents understand the adverse effects of their behavior on the child. Help them develop a plan for altering their behavior. Talk with your preceptor about the best way to approach this circumstance.

What Are Some Safety Issues I Should Be Concerned About?

Be sure that the examination room and your personal possessions are "child proof" or out of reach. Check for small objects, accessible electrical outlets, cords on blinds, breakable objects, computer keyboards, and places from which a child could fall. A baby of any age can roll off the examination table, even a newborn. Always have your hand on the baby, if the parent does not. Remember to pay attention to standard precautions for *all* patients. Wash your hands before and after touching the child. Wear gloves when exposed to body fluids and wash your hands after removing the gloves. If a parent has to change a diaper, help with the proper disposal of the diaper, and offer facilities for the parent to wash his or her hands, too.

How Can I Advocate for Children As a Medical Student?

Ask to visit schools and the homes of children with special needs. Also take advantage of opportunities to visit homeless shelters or juvenile detention facilities. Build an understanding of the context of a child's life outside the medical-care setting because it is probably different than yours was when you were growing up. You can be a tremendous advocate by facilitating insurance paperwork, making calls to the school nurse, sending notes to the child-care center, and making copies of the day's medical visit notes for the parent.

You can also advocate for children by understanding and using care coordination, "a process that facilitates the linkage of children and their families with appropriate services and resources in a coordinated effort to achieve good health." This can be especially important for children with special healthcare needs whose care is often complicated by varied points of entry into multiple care providers and systems of care. Complex criteria often determine and limit the availability of funding among public and private payers. Primary care physicians play an important role in care coordination, along with the family, to provide a medical home for all children.

ACKNOWLEDGMENTS

We would like to thank the parent-advisors at the Uniformed Services University of the Health Sciences, particularly Kathryn Vestermark, who thoughtfully edited this chapter.

KEY POINTS

- Listen to the parents and acknowledge and validate their concerns and observations.
- Talk directly to children of all ages and abilities.
- Be sensitive to the health beliefs and practices of families.
- Keep the child's best interest as the central focus of your clinical activities.
- Be aware of your personal reactions to the challenges posed by caring for sick and healthy children.

Case 16-1

You are assigned to the office of a general pediatrician and are asked to see a 10-year-old boy with cerebral palsy for a health supervision visit. He is accompanied by his mother. The nurse's note indicates that he uses a wheelchair and a communication board. His mother told the nurse that there are no acute health problems. After you have reviewed the medical record you speak with the physician. She asks you how you will approach the visit, because this is your first experience with a child who has special needs.

A. How will you respond to the physician's question?
B. What anticipatory guidance is appropriate for this boy and his family?

Case Answers

16-1 A. *Learning Objective:* **Discuss the general approach to a child with special healthcare needs.** Early in the visit, ask the boy and his mother to show you how he uses the communication board. The child with cerebral palsy or any other special healthcare need has health supervision requirements similar to those of any other child. You will need to review immunizations, growth and development, school performance, nutrition, and all of the other areas discussed in Chapter 11. Specific information related to the boy's health problems including medications, physical or occupational therapy, and assistive devices such as orthoses will all need to be included in your assessment. Ask about family concerns and the family's adaptation to the child's condition. Listen attentively to both the mother and the child, and specifically address your questions about health, school, food preferences, and other personal topics to the boy. Speak to the boy using age-appropriate language and vocabulary, using the communication board as appropriate. Perform a careful physical examination, discuss your findings as you proceed, and answer questions. Ask the parent or your physician for guidance at any time if you have a question or feel inadequate to complete part of the evaluation. Your most important contribution may be to communicate concerns expressed by the child or his mother to the physician. You also may make key observations about physical findings that will benefit the patient.

16-1 B. *Learning Objective:* **Provide anticipatory guidance for a child with special healthcare needs.** Anticipatory guidance for this boy will include all of the topics appropriate for any 10-year-old but will be adapted to meet the special healthcare and personal needs specific to the child and family. Because children with special healthcare needs such as cerebral palsy often have multiple medical care providers in different specialties, the guidance provided at a health supervision visit must include discussion of topics relevant to care coordination. Some family topics that may come up include transportation to school, participation in camp or after-school activities, and challenges faced by the family in providing for the daily needs of the boy. Discussion of school progress may be high on the mother's list of topics. Ask whether they need any paperwork completed at this time, such as a physical form for an extracurricular activity or medication forms for school. The physician will most likely have you listen while she addresses these topics and answers the questions posed by the boy and his mother.

BIBLIOGRAPHY

American Academy of Pediatrics: The medical home. Available at: www.medicalhomeinfo.org/.

American Academy of Pediatrics Policy Statement: Care coordination in the medical home: integrated health and related systems of care for children with special health care needs, *Pediatrics* 116:1238, 2005. Also available at: http://aappolicy.aappublications.org/cgi/content/full/pediatrics;116/5/1238.

Bright Futures at Georgetown University, 2006. Available at: www.brightfutures.org/.

Jackson Allen PL: Children with special health care needs: national survey of prevalence and health care needs, *Pediatr Nurs* 30:307, 2004.

Maternal and Child Health Library: Children and adolescents with special health care needs. Available at: www.mchlibrary.info/KnowledgePaths/kp_CSHCN.html.

Newacheck PW et al: An epidemiologic profile of children with special health care needs, *Pediatrics* 102:117, 1998.

Section

2

Patients Presenting with Symptoms

17

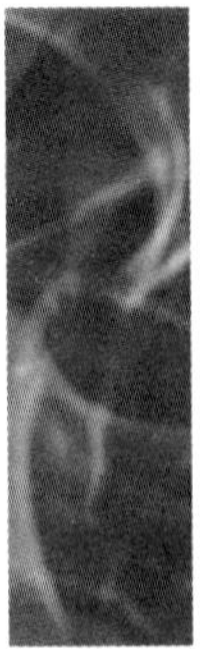

Abdominal Pain

WARREN P. BISHOP

ETIOLOGY

What Causes Abdominal Pain?

Pain identified as "abdominal" may originate from the bowel or from neighboring structures within the abdominal wall, retroperitoneum, abdomen, thorax, and pelvis. Intestinal pain is typically caused by either distention or inflammation. Distention can result from simple causes, such as constipation, or can be the consequence of obstruction or motility disturbance. Inflammation can be peptic (acid) in origin or can result from infection, allergy, injury, or autoimmunity.

How Does Age Affect the Differential Diagnosis?

Infants are more likely than older children to present with congenital lesions such as intestinal malrotation or atresia and Hirschsprung's disease. Young children are more susceptible to certain conditions, such as spontaneous intussusception. Older children are more likely than younger ones to suffer from inflammatory bowel disease. Adolescents are more likely to have sexually transmitted diseases, mittelschmerz, or ectopic pregnancy causing their distress. Some conditions can occur at any age, including urinary tract infections, trauma, pneumonia, pancreatitis, and mesenteric adenitis. Recurrent abdominal pain (RAP) occurs in 10% to 15% of children between the ages of 4 and 14 years and presents a special challenge for the pediatrician.

What Is Recurrent Abdominal Pain?

RAP may be defined as recurring attacks of abdominal pain over at least a 3-month period in children between 4 and 14 years of age. Urgent problems such as appendicitis are seldom responsible for RAP. Many children with RAP appear healthy, are growing well, have no findings on physical examination, and have no discernible abnormalities on any test or imaging study. Such children probably have functional pain and require a different management strategy than a child with a well-defined cause such as lactose intolerance or inflammatory bowel disease.

What Is Functional Pain?

Functional abdominal pain results from the motility, or function, of the intestine. Significant discomfort can result from contractions that may be excessively intense, poorly coordinated, or perceived as painful because of elevated sensitivity or anxiety. This pain is *not* "psychosomatic," in the popular sense, which implies "not real pain" or "in his head." Functional pain is typically characterized as intermittent, colicky pain not associated with meals or bowel movements. An exception is pain associated with constipation, which is often worse after eating and is relieved by defecation.

EVALUATION

How Does Pain Location Help Determine the Likely Cause?

Visceral pain tends to be poorly localized and aching or cramping in nature. In contrast, pain from somatic structures, such as the abdominal wall musculature, is easily defined as coming from a well-circumscribed area. Sometimes, as is the case with appendicitis, the discomfort begins as ill-defined visceral pain, becoming much more intense and well localized as overlying somatic structures become involved. Pain arising from the small intestine is typically periumbilical in location. Proximal gut injury (esophagus, stomach, and duodenum) tends to cause epigastric discomfort, as does inflammation of the pancreas and gallbladder. Problems arising in the colon are typically perceived directly in the same region of the abdomen.

How Do I Evaluate Acute Abdominal Pain?

Acute abdominal pain is defined as a condition of recent onset, with characteristics that indicate an urgent need for diagnosis and management. You must obtain a precise history, examine the child carefully, and, finally, order appropriate tests. Table 17-1 summarizes the information you must gather to evaluate the child with acute abdomen. Not all of the studies listed in Table 17-1 must be performed in all patients. If your history and examination lead you directly to a particular diagnosis, such as constipation, you may treat it directly.

When Should I Obtain Surgical Consultation?

Acute appendicitis should be carefully considered when evaluating any patient with acute abdominal pain. Not all patients exhibit typical features, especially if the appendix is located retrocecally or in another atypical location. Perforation of the appendix usually occurs within 24 to 48 hours of symptom onset. Therefore, you must work rapidly and enlist the help of your colleagues early in the evaluation. Surgeons should also be consulted promptly when there is evidence of obstruction, peritonitis, or mass lesion.

What Causes Recurrent Abdominal Pain?

Table 17-2 lists most of the more common causes plus features on history, physical examination, and laboratory testing that may suggest the diagnosis.

Table 17-1

Evaluation of the Child with Acute Abdominal Pain

History	
Onset	Sudden vs. gradual, preceding injury, prior episodes
Associated symptoms	Fever, nausea, dysuria, diarrhea, constipation, bloody stools or emesis, cough
Location of pain	Periumbilical, epigastric, right lower quadrant, left lower quadrant, well-localized or vague
Nature of pain	Aching, cramping, dull, sharp, burning, constant vs. colicky
Progression	Worsening, improving, changing location
Physical Examination	
General	Hydration, appearance of toxicity, growth and weight gain
Chest	Crackles, rhonchi, wheezing, tenderness of musculoskeletal structures
Abdomen	Distention, bowel sounds, tenderness (location, severity, rebound, superficial vs. deep), mass
Rectal examination	Fecal impaction, occult blood, pelvic tenderness, extrinsic mass
Laboratory/ Radiologic Evaluation	
CBC	Evidence of infection or inflammation
ESR and CRP	Evidence of inflammation or infection
Amylase, lipase	Pancreatitis
GGT	Bile duct obstruction or injury
ALT, AST	Hepatitis
Urinalysis	Urinary tract infection, hematuria (stones, obstruction)
Plain x-rays	Bowel gas pattern, evidence of obstruction, free peritoneal air, constipation, kidney stones, appendiceal fecalith
CT or ultrasound	Appendiceal abscess, intussusception, gallstones, pancreatitis, bile duct obstruction, kidney stones, renal anomalies
Barium enema	Intussusception, malrotation, less useful for appendicitis

ALT, Alanine transaminase; AST, aspartate transaminase; CBC, complete blood count; CRP, C-reactive protein; CT, computed tomography; ESR, erythrocyte sedimentation rate; GGT, gamma-glutamyltransferase.

What History Helps Evaluate RAP?

You will need to define accurately the nature and time course of the pain, determine what exacerbates and relieves it, identify associated symptoms, and decide whether or not indications of serious underlying illness are present. It is also important to assess whether genetic or environmental factors may be playing a role. It is *not* useful to approach

Table 17-2

Differential Diagnosis of Recurrent Abdominal Pain

Diagnosis	History	Examination	Laboratory
Functional pain	See text	See text	See text
Lactose intolerance	Sx worse with dairy products	Bloating, tympany	Lactose breath H_2 test
Crohn's disease	Weight loss, postprandial pain, diarrhea ± blood	Tender RLQ, Hemes + stool, perianal fissures, fistulae, growth failure	Anemia, elevated ESR, CRP
Ulcerative colitis	Bloody diarrhea, urgency, tenesmus	Heme + stool	Anemia, elevated ESR
Malrotation and obstruction	Intermittent crampy pain with bilious vomiting	Unremarkable between spells, distention, increased bowel sounds	Upper GI barium study shows malpositioned or absent ligament of Treitz
Constipation	Infrequent stools, soiling	LLQ fecal mass, impacted stool on rectal examination	Fecal mass on radiograph
Chronic pancreatitis	Epigastric pain, radiation to back, worse with food	Tender epigastrium	Elevated amylase and lipase
Gallstones	Colicky severe epigastric or RUQ pain after meals, jaundice	RUQ tenderness, jaundice	Elevated alk phos, GGT, and occasionally total and direct bilirubin; gallstones on ultrasound
Peptic ulcer disease	Burning epigastric pain	Tender epigastrium; Heme + stool	Ulcer on endoscopy
Gastroesophageal reflux	Regurgitation, heartburn	Tender epigastrium; Heme + stool	Esophagitis on endoscopy
Renal pelvic obstruction or stone	Pain radiates to flank or groin; vomiting	Enlarged kidney	Hydronephrosis on ultrasound; hematuria

alk phos, Alkaline phosphatase; CRP, C-reactive protein; ESR, erythrocyte sedimentation rate; GGT, gamma-glutamyltransferase; GI, gastrointestinal; H_2, hydrogen; LLQ, left lower quadrant; RLQ, right lower quadrant; RUQ, right upper quadrant; Sx, symptoms; +, positive; ±, variable.

the child with the attitude that the abdominal pain may not be "real." A child with pain is in need of your assistance, whether the cause is a significant underlying illness or a purely functional disorder. Table 17-3 lists questions that you should ask of every patient.

Table 17-3

Historical Data for Abdominal Pain

Onset of symptoms	***Severity of discomfort***
How long ago?	Interference with daily activities
Was there an initial illness?	Causes patient to cry or double over
What were symptoms at onset?	Pain scale rating
Location of pain	***How does pain alter lifestyle?***
Periumbilical	Missing school or other activities
Epigastric	Sleep disturbance
Upper or lower bowel quadrants	Appetite disturbance
What triggers pain?	***Associated symptoms?***
Dietary items	Fever
Activities	Diarrhea, blood in stools
Social situations (school)	Vomiting, hematemesis, bilious emesis
What alleviates pain?	Headache
Medications tried	Weight loss, poor growth
Food, rest	***Past history***
Bowel movements	Previous history of pain
Time pattern of pain	Prior surgeries
Does it awaken patient from sleep?	Travel
Is it worse in the morning?	***Family history***
Associated with meals	Inflammatory bowel disease
Investigation to date	Irritable bowel syndrome
Blood test results	Lactose intolerance, celiac disease
Radiology	Migraine headache
Stool cultures, parasitology	Biliary or pancreatic disease
Specialized testing, such as endoscopy	
Nature of pain	
Dull or aching	
Gradual or sudden onset	
Burning	
Sharp or stabbing	

What Clues Suggest the Diagnosis of Functional Pain?

Typical characteristics of functional abdominal pain are listed in Table 17-4. Often the pain results in striking limitations of activity, and missing school is common. This pattern of response to pain, such as missing school, often serves to reinforce complaints. Finally, other family members often have a history of functional abdominal pain.

Table 17-4

Typical Features of Functional Abdominal Pain

Periumbilical location	Crampy, colicky, recurrent
Pallor during attacks of pain	Missing school and other activities
Personality: often high-achiever, worrier	Danger signs absent (see Table 17-5)
Does not awaken child from sleep	Family history of abdominal pain

What Are "Danger Signs" in Recurrent Abdominal Pain?

If danger signs are present (Table 17-5), you should pursue an aggressive diagnostic course immediately. Although most of RAP is functional in nature, a small proportion of patients has serious underlying disease.

Table 17-5

Danger Signs in Recurrent Abdominal Pain

Vomiting	Fever
Pain awakens patient from sleep	Blood in emesis or stools
Weight loss	Bilious emesis
Pain *not* periumbilical in location	Abnormal screening laboratory studies

What Physical Findings Should I Look for in Recurrent Abdominal Pain?

As you conduct your physical examination, it is useful to talk to the child and parent, discussing what you are doing and what you are finding (and *not* finding!). For example, "Well, your heart and lungs check out fine. Your liver and spleen are not enlarged, and you are not very tender down here, where your appendix is." This assures the family that you are taking the child's complaint seriously and that you are conducting a thorough examination. Look at the growth chart and note whether the child is growing and gaining weight normally. Check carefully for abdominal mass lesions, including feces palpable in the left lower quadrant in the constipated child. Most children with functional pain report some degree of tenderness during abdominal palpation. Compared with appendicitis or other abscess, this tenderness is usually diffuse and unimpressive, although it might be reported as "10 out of 10." Look at the child's face—significant tenderness is usually expressed by wide-eyed, fearful anticipation of your next application of pressure. Acknowledge the reported pain, even if it does not reflect a pathologic condition. Saying, "I can tell that your tummy is a bit sore," will reassure the patient and the family that you are paying attention, while at the same time letting them know that you are not terribly concerned. If you took the opposite approach, "Your child's abdomen really isn't very tender. I tricked him by pushing with my stethoscope, and he didn't react," you will likely lose the opportunity to help the child. Don't forget to perform a rectal examination with occult blood testing.

What Initial Tests Should Be Ordered to Evaluate Recurrent Abdominal Pain?

Your goal is to rule out underlying disease without wasting healthcare resources. The initial laboratory and imaging studies in Table 17-6 should be performed for *all* patients who have RAP. Before sending the patient to the laboratory, it is useful to summarize your thoughts and plans for the family. If you say, "Your child's pain is likely cramps caused by strong intestinal muscle contractions, but I need to do additional tests to be sure I am not missing anything," you are setting yourself up for success. If you instead say, "I'm doing some tests to see what is wrong," you are in big trouble if (as you anticipate) the tests come back normal!

What Additional Tests May Be Needed?

The secondary tests listed in Table 17-6 are more invasive and more expensive and should be ordered based on the history, physical examination, and initial studies. If, for example, the child has a history of chronic bloody diarrhea and has not been thriving, a colonoscopy for suspected inflammatory bowel disease should be considered. If there is an abdominal mass without evidence of severe constipation on rectal examination, a computed tomographic (CT) scan should be ordered. A tubular, lower left-sided mass that is associated with hard stool in the rectum is likely a fecal mass caused by constipation. In this case, an enema can help you decide.

Table 17-6

Laboratory Workup in Recurrent Abdominal Pain

Initial studies—*for all patients*

- CBC, WBC, differential, ESR
- Amylase, lipase, ALT, AST, GGT, total and direct bilirubin
- Urinalysis
- Abdominal ultrasound—include liver, gallbladder, pancreas, and kidneys

Secondary studies—*select among these to investigate danger signs, abnormal physical examination findings, or lab abnormalities*

- Barium upper GI radiography with small bowel follow-through (if suspicion of inflammatory bowel disease)
- Colonoscopy (if rectal bleeding or suspicion of inflammatory bowel disease)
- CT scan (if mass lesion or abscess suspected)

ALT, Alanine transaminase; AST, aspartate transaminase; CBC, complete blood count; CT, computed tomography; ESR, erythrocyte sedimentation rate; GGT, gamma-glutamyltransferase; GI, gastrointestinal; WBC, white blood count.

TREATMENT

How Do I Treat the Patient with Recurrent Abdominal Pain?

If your workup yields a specific diagnosis, you must of course treat it. For functional pain, it is important to discuss the cause and a plan for management. As you speak to the family, you should explain that the pain is caused by vigorous intestinal motility, not by a dangerous condition. A dietary fiber supplement creates softer, bulkier stools and reduces motility-associated pain. Narcotics and antimotility agents should be avoided.

What If a Child with Recurrent Abdominal Pain Misses School Often?

When complaints of pain cause the child to stay home, the symptom becomes the focus of the family's attention, results in secondary gain for the child, and encourages a dysfunctional response to pain. It may be difficult to convince protective parents to send the child to school, but this is crucial for successful management. Once in school, the child must stay, despite attacks of pain. Most schools will allow children to rest for a short period in the nurse's office until the cramps abate. This approach nearly always results in rapid improvement.

KEY POINTS

- "Abdominal" pain may have its origin in the gastrointestinal tract, the genitourinary system, or adjacent structures and organs.
- Functional abdominal pain results from disordered bowel motility. It is not psychosomatic.
- Pain that awakens a child from sleep is a danger sign.

Case 17-1

An 11-year-old boy has been having problems with abdominal pain intermittently for several years. His mother states that when the child has pain, it usually interrupts his planned activities such as school and he stays home instead. He has seen several other doctors and has been taken to the emergency department on three occasions. Blood test results and abdominal radiographs have been normal to date, and the mother is clearly frustrated and worried. The boy indicates that his pain is periumbilical in location, is sharp and cramping in nature, does not awaken him from sleep, occurs chiefly in the morning, and is not associated with meals. He describes a constant, dull, aching sensation in addition to frequent brief attacks of more severe pain. His appetite is good, there is no vomiting or blood in the stools, and he has not lost weight.

The family has not identified triggering factors. You discover that this boy has missed 20 days of school during the first semester because of pain and has dropped out of Boy Scouts for the same reason. There is no family history of bowel disorders.

Your examination reveals diffuse complaints of pain with palpation, but no guarding, rebound tenderness, or evidence of severe discomfort. No other findings are noted on examination, including rectal examination, which revealed no evidence of tenderness or occult blood.

A. What is the most likely diagnosis, based on the history and physical examination?
B. What tests will you order? How will you explain the logic of your approach to the child and family?
C. If all laboratory test results are normal, how will you treat the patient?

Case Answers

17-1 A. *Learning objective:* **Discuss the characteristic features of the different types of abdominal pain that are detectable by history and physical examination, including "warning signs" that may point to serious disease.** History and physical examination point to functional abdominal pain for this patient. More serious causes of abdominal pain would produce clinical findings such as vomiting (especially bile stained), fever, pain that awakens the patient, and others as outlined in Table 17-5.

17-1 B. *Learning objective:* **Understand the laboratory and radiologic approach to recurrent abdominal pain, with the goal of ordering sufficient testing to rule out abnormalities, while conserving medical resources.** You should select only enough tests to reassure yourself that you are not missing a serious disorder. The standard initial tests include complete blood count and differential, tests of liver and pancreatic function, urinalysis, and abdominal ultrasound, as listed in Table 17-6. Always check stool for presence of occult blood. You need to discuss the rationale for selecting tests based on symptoms and physical findings.

17-1 C. *Learning objective:* **Interpret screening laboratory tests and understand the principles of treatment of functional abdominal pain.** Emphasize that the absence of findings on the screening laboratory tests is reassuring and confirms your impression that there is not a serious disease present. You will need to explain how each test helps with the diagnostic process. Further tests are not needed. Encourage a return to all normal activities, especially school. A fiber supplement is usually beneficial for functional pain.

BIBLIOGRAPHY

Hyams JS, Hyman E: Recurrent abdominal pain and the biopsychosocial model of medical practice, *J Pediatr* 133:473, 1998.

Irish MS: The approach to common abdominal diagnosis in infants and children, *Pediatr Clin North Am* 45:729, 1998.

Lake AM: Chronic abdominal pain in childhood: diagnosis and management, *Am Fam Physician* 59:1823, 1999.

Mason JD: The evaluation of acute abdominal pain in children, *Emerg Med Clin North Am* 14:629, 1996.

18

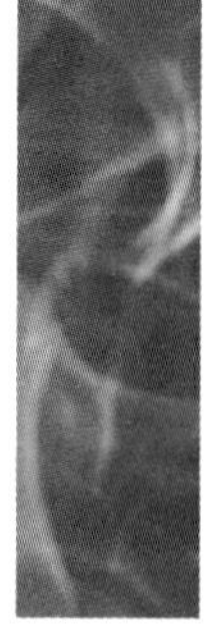

Adolescents with Health Concerns

KEN CHEYNE and MICHAEL R. LAWLESS

 DYSMENORRHEA/MENSTRUAL CRAMPS

ETIOLOGY

What Causes Dysmenorrhea?

Dysmenorrhea, or menstrual cramps, is the most common gynecologic problem experienced by adolescent women and is a leading cause of short-term school absenteeism. More than 60% of women have some degree of dysmenorrhea and most do not readily report it, so the health-care provider must routinely inquire about this symptom in the review of systems. *Primary dysmenorrhea* refers to menstrual pain for which there is no underlying pelvic pathology as a cause. It accounts for over three-fourths of the cases occurring before 25 years of age. It is caused by myometrial contraction in response to prostaglandins produced by the endometrium. Because initial menstrual periods are often anovulatory, adolescents may not complain of dysmenorrhea until several months after menarche. *Secondary dysmenorrhea* is menstrual pain associated with underlying pelvic pathology. Common causes include infection, structural abnormality of the uterus or cervix, presence of a foreign body such as an intrauterine device, a complication of pregnancy, or endometriosis.

EVALUATION

What Characterizes Dysmenorrhea?

Primary dysmenorrhea is characterized by cramping pain associated *only* with menses. No other gynecologic or systemic symptoms should be present. The adolescent who is not sexually active and who has a history consistent with primary dysmenorrhea may first be given a therapeutic trial of a prostaglandin inhibitor such as ibuprofen (see treatment section) without a pelvic examination. If primary dysmenorrhea does not respond to prostaglandin inhibitors, a pelvic examination will be needed. An adolescent who has dysmenorrhea and is sexually active or has other gynecologic symptoms must also have a pelvic examination. Other diagnostic steps in evaluating secondary dysmenorrhea include a thorough medical and psychosocial history, cultures for sexually transmitted infections (STIs), and a pregnancy test. In some cases, pelvic ultrasonography and occasionally laparoscopy are a necessary part of the diagnostic process for more complicated cases of secondary dysmenorrhea.

TREATMENT

How Do I Treat Dysmenorrhea?

Primary dysmenorrhea is treated with a prostaglandin inhibitor. A nonsteroidal antiinflammatory drug (NSAID) such as ibuprofen (400 mg every 4 to 6 hours) or naproxen (500 mg to start, then 250 mg three times daily) is a common choice. To be maximally effective, it is important that the medication be taken at the first indication that the menstrual period is beginning and continued at proper dosage for 2 or 3 days. The patient with primary dysmenorrhea who does not respond to NSAIDs, or the sexually active patient, may respond to oral contraceptives. Treatment for secondary dysmenorrhea is directed at the underlying cause, such as antibiotic therapy for an STI or hormonal suppression for endometriosis.

GYNECOMASTIA

ETIOLOGY

What Is Gynecomastia?

Gynecomastia is excessive development of the male breast. It occurs in up to two-thirds of adolescent males as a physiologic process during normal pubertal development, typically at sexual maturity rating (SMR) II and III. Enlargement of the male breast outside this peak stage of pubertal hormones may be associated with endocrine or chromosomal disorders, exogenous estrogen or androgen administered systemically or applied topically, or as a side effect of medications, including various antibiotics, cardiovascular medications, psychoactive medications, and drugs of abuse such as alcohol, marijuana, and opiates. Of particular note, gynecomastia can occur at any age as a result of anabolic steroid abuse for the purpose of enhancing athletic performance. The term *pseudo-gynecomastia* is used for apparent breast enlargement because of excessive fat tissue in overweight males.

EVALUATION

How Do I Evaluate Gynecomastia?

Physiologic gynecomastia usually has breast enlargement limited to subareolar tissue and is accompanied by mild tenderness. Often the enlargement affects only one breast, or if both breasts are affected there is some asymmetry. Noting that the affected male is in SMR II or III (see Figure 15-3) is further assurance of a physiologic basis. Development of gynecomastia in a later stage of puberty makes a pathologic cause more likely. Obtain a thorough history of medications and substances of abuse, and perform a careful physical examination looking for other evidence of abnormal hormone production or for conditions associated with gynecomastia.

TREATMENT

How Do I Treat Gynecomastia?

For most adolescent males with physiologic gynecomastia, management consists of education and reassurance that breast enlargement is a normal pubertal occurrence that is likely to resolve within 6 to 24 months. Without correct information, many boys (and their parents) worry that breast enlargement is a sign of femininity or breast cancer. If breast enlargement persists beyond 2 years, surgical reduction may be considered. Surgical reduction is reserved for the most severe cases of gynecomastia in regard to both breast size and psychological stress.

URETHRAL OR VAGINAL DISCHARGE

ETIOLOGY

What Causes Vaginal or Urethral Discharge?

A vaginal or urethral discharge should immediately raise concern about the presence of STI. About 25% of sexually active adolescents will develop an STI. Asking about sexual activity in a confidential interview is essential, with the caveat that some sexually active adolescents deny being sexually active even when the inquiry is confidential. *Chlamydia* infection and gonorrhea are the two most common bacterial causes of STI in both males and females. Nongonococcal, nonchlamydial urethritis and vaginitis are associated with *Ureaplasma urealyticum* infection and *Trichomonas*.

EVALUATION

How Do Urethral and Vaginal Discharge Present?

A male with urethral discharge often has dysuria and, less often, hematuria, scrotal pain (epididymitis), or rectal pain (proctitis). In females, leukorrhea is an asymptomatic, nonodorous, clear or white physiologic vaginal discharge that begins around menarche. Vaginal discharge caused by STI is usually malodorous, discolored, and accompanied by symptoms of itching, dysuria, and irregular menses. A malodorous vaginal discharge may occur in the absence of sexual activity if the girl has bacterial vaginosis or a vaginal foreign body. Sexually active adolescent females with abdominal pain, fever, and vomiting may have pelvic inflammatory disease.

What Findings Suggest Sexually Transmitted Infections?

In males, symptomatic *Chlamydia* infection usually presents as dysuria and urethritis with a milky white discharge 7 to 14 days after being infected. Gonorrhea in males usually presents with urethritis characterized by a yellow-green penile discharge 3 to 7 days after being infected. Women with chlamydial or gonococcal infections may present with vaginal discharge, dyspareunia, dysuria, spotting, or breakthrough bleeding while taking oral contraceptives. Both adolescent males and females may be asymptomatic with chlamydial or gonococcal infections.

How Do I Test for Gonorrhea and Chlamydia?

In males, a Gram stain of the urethral discharge can make an immediate presumptive diagnosis of gonorrhea when the characteristic gram-negative intracellular bacteria are seen. In all cases, a specimen collected by urethral swab should be tested by culture or by a nucleic acid amplification test (NAAT), which is highly sensitive and specific for chlamydial and gonorrheal infections. A urine specimen could also be used to test for gonorrhea and chlamydial infections using an NAAT.

In females, both chlamydial infection and gonorrhea are characterized by the presence of mucopus at the cervical os. A cervical specimen should be obtained using correct technique and tested by culture or NAAT for both organisms. In women, urine is also an acceptable specimen for using NAAT to test for chlamydia infection and gonorrhea.

What Other Sexually Transmitted Infections Affect Adolescent Women?

Trichomonas infection is primarily a vaginitis, although the cervix may appear friable. It is identified by wet preparation, mixing the discharge with normal saline, and finding the motile protozoan on microscopy. It can also be identified by culture or antigen detection. The vaginal pH in a woman with a *Trichomonas* infection is > 4.5.

Bacterial vaginosis causes an alteration in vaginal flora from the usually predominant lactobacilli to a predominance of *Gardnerella* and other bacteria. The resulting vaginitis has a malodorous discharge with a characteristic "fishy" odor, especially when mixed with potassium hydroxide (KOH) (the "whiff" test). The discharge also has a pH > 4.5, and on microscopy 20% or more of squamous epithelial cells have adherent bacteria (clue cells).

Yeast causes a vulvitis and vaginitis characterized by a pruritic, thick, white vaginal discharge. The discharge has a pH < 4.5, and on microscopy hyphae can be seen on KOH prep. Yeast vaginitis can occur in adolescent females who are not sexually active.

TREATMENT

Where Can I Find the Latest Information about Treatment of Sexually Transmitted Infections?

If either gonorrhea or chlamydial infection is suspected, empirical treatment should be started for *both*. Current treatment recommendations for STIs can be found on the Web site for the Centers for Disease Control and Prevention, www.cdc.gov/STD/treatment/.

KEY POINTS

- Dysmenorrhea is common but often not reported by adolescent girls. NSAIDs provide effective treatment in most cases.
- Dysmenorrhea in sexually active girls should prompt a pelvic examination.
- Gynecomastia develops in up to two-thirds of adolescent males between SMR II and III. No treatment is needed, as most cases resolve spontaneously.
- Urethral or vaginal discharge should prompt assessment for a sexually transmitted infection.

Case 18-1

Dysmenorrhea

A 14-year-old girl is concerned about cramping in her lower abdomen and back that occurs only when she menstruates. Onset of the pain was 4 months ago. Menarche was 14 months ago. Her period occurs every 4 to 5 weeks and lasts for 3 to 5 days. She is not sexually active.

A. Is the new onset of dysmenorrhea a concern?
B. Should this adolescent female have a pelvic examination?
C. If your diagnosis is primary dysmenorrhea, what is your initial treatment plan?

Case 18-2

Gynecomastia

A 14-year-old boy has had a 1-cm breast bud under his left areola for 3 months. He denies the use of any prescription or street drugs. He has not yet started his growth spurt and is otherwise healthy.

A. What is the likely diagnosis?
B. What findings on the physical examination would support your diagnosis?
C. What is this adolescent male likely concerned about?

Case 18-3

Urethral or Vaginal Discharge

A 17-year-old girl presents with a 1-week history of malodorous vaginal discharge that dries yellow on her underwear. She also complains of dysuria but denies abdominal pain, fever, or chills.

A. What additional history is important to obtain?
B. What will be your diagnostic approach to this adolescent?
C. If she were diagnosed with a sexually transmitted infection, what anticipatory guidance would you give her?

Case Answers

18-1 A. *Learning objective:* **Recognize that anovulatory menstrual periods are not associated with pain.** The initial menstrual periods are often anovulatory. Adolescent girls may not complain of dysmenorrhea until several months after menarche.

18-1 B. *Learning objective:* **List the indications for performing a pelvic examination in an adolescent with primary dysmenorrhea.** No, a pelvic examination is not indicated in a girl with primary dysmenorrhea who is not sexually active and whose pain is associated only with menses in the absence of other gynecologic symptoms.

18-1 C. *Learning objective:* **Discuss the initial treatment of primary dysmenorrhea.** Prostaglandin inhibitors such as ibuprofen and naproxen are commonly used to treat primary dysmenorrhea. They are especially useful if started just before the expected onset of the menstrual period. A calendar can assist the patient to keep track of the timing of her periods.

18-2 A. *Learning objective:* **Recognize the presenting signs and symptoms of benign adolescent gynecomastia.** The most likely diagnosis is benign adolescent gynecomastia. If the boy is obese, he probably has pseudo-gynecomastia (fat rather than breast tissue). Marijuana use can cause gynecomastia, as can exposure to estrogenic compounds.

18-2 B. *Learning objective:* **Discuss the correlation of benign adolescent gynecomastia with a typical stage of pubertal development.** Except for the palpable breast tissue, the physical examination should demonstrate SMR II or III pubertal development.

18-2 C. *Learning objective:* **Discuss the two most common concerns of an adolescent male with benign gynecomastia.** He is likely concerned that he is "turning into a girl" or that he has developed breast cancer.

18-3 A. *Learning objective:* **Recognize the risk factors for vaginitis in an adolescent.** The adolescent female should be interviewed alone to assess if she is sexually active and whether she uses condoms each time that she is sexually active. You must also ask if she has had intercourse with a new partner in the recent past. The number of sexual partners is also important information.

18-3 B. *Learning objective:* **Discuss the laboratory tests used in diagnosing vaginitis.** A pelvic examination is indicated, with appropriate testing for *Chlamydia* and gonorrhea, and a wet mount/KOH prep looking for yeast, bacterial vaginosis, or *Trichomonas.*

18-3 C. *Learning objective:* **Recognize the importance of treatment of sexual partners in the control of sexually transmitted infections.** You need to identify sexual partners, because sexually transmitted infections must be reported to the health department. You should counsel her about the importance of treatment of current and recent sexual partners. Advice about safer sex should be provided, including the use of barrier methods of contraception and responsible sexual decision making.

BIBLIOGRAPHY

Centers for Disease Control and Prevention: Sexually transmitted diseases treatment guidelines. Available at: www.cdc.gov/STD/treatment/.

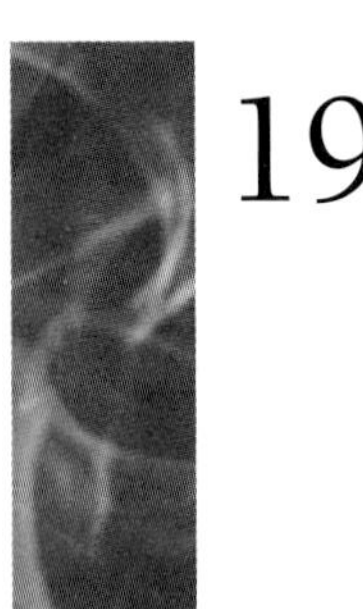

19

Allergic Symptoms

JEROLD C. WOODHEAD

ETIOLOGY

What Is Allergy?

Allergy is the term for the symptoms that develop as the result of four distinct immunopathologic mechanisms of tissue damage, classically referred to as type I to IV reactions in the Gell and Coombs classification: anaphylaxis (type I), cytotoxic (type II), immune complex (type III), and cell mediated (type IV). *Allergens* such as dust, pollen, molds, animal dander, and foods can cause allergic reactions when their antigenic properties trigger immunologic responses in susceptible individuals. Allergenic substances also include antibiotics or other medications, insect venom, and latex. The most common allergic reaction is an IgE-mediated antigen-antibody response (type I reaction) that can produce anaphylaxis, urticaria, rhinitis, asthma, and atopic dermatitis. Although characteristic of allergic responses, these reactions may also result from nonallergic mechanisms. Furthermore, a single antigen can cause any of the four types of allergic reactions. As an example, penicillin causes anaphylaxis (I), hemolysis (II), serum sickness (III), and skin sensitivity (IV). Common skin sensitizations include the rash caused by contact with poison ivy and the reaction to tuberculin in a patient who has latent tuberculosis.

How Does the Type I Reaction Cause Symptoms?

A type I allergic reaction most commonly develops when a susceptible individual becomes "sensitized" by exposure to an allergen that contacts a mucosal surface in the conjunctiva, nasal airway, pharynx, or upper or lower airway. An allergen may also be ingested or inoculated onto abraded skin. The allergen then induces B lymphocytes to secrete antigen-specific IgE, which binds to mast cells and basophils. These sensitized cells react to subsequent allergen exposure by releasing preformed mediators, primarily histamine. Other mediators that can develop during reexposure to allergens include leukotrienes, cytokines, enzymes, and chemotactic agents. The various mediators cause dilation of blood vessels, increase in vascular permeability, secretion of mucus, and contraction of smooth muscles. Symptoms such as sneezing, rhinorrhea, wheezing, and itching develop promptly after reexposure to an allergen. In addition, allergen reexposure can also trigger late activation of cell-mediated inflammation, which develops 2 to 4 hours after exposure and results in reactions lasting at least 24 hours. Late reactions promote persistent bronchodilator-resistant airway obstruction, increased airway hyperreactivity, and chronic nasal obstruction. Eosinophils are the most common cell type involved at the start of the late reaction, but any of the inflammatory leukocytes may participate.

Are Allergies Common in Childhood?

More than one-third of all children experience allergic rhinitis; up to 10% to 15% have some degree of "eczema," ranging from patches of dry skin to severe atopic dermatitis; and 5% to 10% experience asthma. Food allergies occur less frequently than respiratory allergies. They tend to be most common early in life and may persist into adulthood. Anaphylaxis, though uncommon, can be life threatening.

What Symptoms Occur in Allergy?

Allergy is often brought up as an explanation for a child's symptoms, but careful evaluation is needed to identify the true cause. Many problems that are labeled as being "allergic" often cannot be demonstrated to result from a true allergic reaction. Chronic rhinitis, for example, is often labeled as having an allergic cause, but recurrent viral infection, not allergy, probably accounts for the majority of cases. Adverse reactions to foods are also often labeled as allergic, although most are not. A specific allergic cause for most eczema cannot be identified. Asthma can have an allergic basis, but not all does. In addition to the specific manifestations caused by allergic reactions, nonallergic sequelae are common in allergic children, including otitis media, conjunctivitis, pneumonia, and skin infections. You must be prepared to evaluate and manage both the allergic and nonallergic forms of these problems.

What Is "Atopy" and How Does It Manifest?

The term *atopy* was originally coined by Coca to describe the type of abnormal hypersensitivity associated with anaphylactic-type reactions. It is currently used to label IgE-mediated allergic reactions (type I) that cause upper or lower airway disease and the syndrome of atopic dermatitis. The most common manifestations of atopy are asthma, conjunctivitis, atopic dermatitis, and rhinitis. The presence of one atopic disorder increases the likelihood that a patient will have another. For example, more than half of asthmatic children have allergic rhinitis and approximately half of children with atopic dermatitis have asthma. Interestingly, infants with asthma do not typically have allergic rhinitis. Atopy has a strong hereditary tendency: more than two-thirds of children will manifest atopic findings if both parents are atopic.

EVALUATION

How Do I Know if My Patient Has an Allergy?

History provides the key information. The patient's *symptoms* will allow you to determine whether the common target organs of allergic reactions are involved. These target organs include the nasopharyngeal and ocular mucosa, the airway and lungs, the skin, and the gastrointestinal tract. Age of the patient, exposures, seasonality, timing, and duration of symptoms all help with the diagnosis.

Do Allergic Manifestations Vary by Age?

Most allergies occur in school-age children or adolescents who have chronic or recurrent nasal congestion, runny nose, sneezing, itchy eyes, or cough and wheezing. Infants and younger children may have persistent or recurrent rash, protracted colds, or cough and wheezing. If cough and/or wheezing are prominent complaints, inquire about nighttime cough, reduced physical stamina, and a sensation of chest tightness (see Asthma in Chapter 69). Recurrent otitis media may prompt parents to raise the question of allergy, particularly if the child has chronic rhinitis; most commonly, however, the otitis is a consequence of recurrent viral infections.

What Exposures Trigger Allergic Reactions?

Onset of symptoms following specific exposures can help identify the allergen, especially if repeated events are documented. Occasionally an infant will develop bloody diarrhea, a reaction to milk protein that may have an allergic basis, although the exact mechanism is not yet known. The nutritional history and the family allergy history assume importance, but you must also ask questions about possible infection. Rarely, you will encounter a patient who has an anaphylactic reaction to a bee sting, peanuts, or another food. In this case, identification of the inciting allergen is crucial for future prevention and management. *Seasonality* or association with a *specific environmental exposure* also gives clues: symptoms may recur at a particular time of the year (e.g., ragweed allergy in late summer–early fall) or with an identifiable exposure (e.g., a pet cat). Information about the home heating system, presence of dust-trapping materials in bedrooms, and presence of pets is important. A damp basement or use of a humidifier may cause the home to have excessive humidity that promotes the growth of molds and dust mites. When a specific trigger for allergic symptoms cannot be easily identified, or when symptoms are year-round, the history must be thorough to ensure that all possibilities are considered.

How Does Family History Help with Diagnosis?

More than half of children with allergic symptoms and signs have a parent or sibling who also has allergy. Any child whose family history includes anaphylaxis or other severe allergic manifestations to specific food or environmental allergens should avoid exposure whenever possible.

How Do I Distinguish Allergy from Infection?

Duration of symptoms may give important clues to diagnosis: allergic rhinitis symptoms may persist for weeks, whereas viral upper respiratory infections typically last 5 to 7 days, although approximately 15% of children have viral symptoms that persist up to 10 to 14 days. Preschool children commonly have an average of eight upper respiratory infections per year, most in the span from November to May, so recurrent and persistent infections may confound the evaluation of chronic rhinitis. *Physical examination* should search for allergic signs that allow discrimination between allergy and infection or other causes of the findings.

What Am I Likely to Find on Head, Eyes, Ears, Nose, and Throat (HEENT) Examination?

When allergy causes nasal, pharyngeal, and ocular symptoms, the affected mucosal surfaces are typically pale and edematous, with a "cobblestone appearance" caused by lymphoid follicular hyperplasia. Mucosal inflammation is not as intense as that associated with viral or bacterial infection. Allergic rhinitis produces a watery nasal discharge, persistently obstructed nasal airway, mouth breathing, a denasal voice (loss of nasal resonance with inability to pronounce "M" and "N"), "train tracks" of thick white or yellow discharge in the posterior pharynx, and a throat-clearing sound or cough. These findings also all often accompany chronic rhinitis, of which only some is allergic. "Throat clearing" may reach such a frequency that it becomes tic-like or may develop into a "habit cough." The *allergic face* includes open mouth, dark puffy eyelids ("allergic shiners"), and nasal discharge. The nasolacrimal ducts often become obstructed in allergic rhinitis, resulting in increased lacrimation, a "tear lake," and a crusted, mucousy, and "gritty" eye discharge. This discharge is often misdiagnosed as bacterial conjunctivitis, even though conjunctival inflammation may not be a prominent finding. Secondary bacterial infection can develop with obstructed nasolacrimal ducts or with allergic conjunctivitis, but this will be marked by prominent conjunctival inflammation and usually a truly purulent discharge. An "allergic crease" on the nose reflects chronic rubbing of the nose to relieve itching or remove discharge; the "allergic salute" uses the hand to wipe the nose upward.

What Other Physical Findings Occur with Allergy?

Wheezing occurs commonly in allergic children but may be difficult to detect in infants and young children. If the history includes persistent cough, especially night cough, look carefully at the respiratory pattern: exaggerated use of abdominal accessory muscles, "squeezing" air out of the lungs in the expiratory phase, and a hyperinflated or "barrel" chest probably reflect lower airway obstruction caused by infection or asthma. Listen to the lungs with a stethoscope for prolongation of the expiratory phase or for frank wheezing (see Asthma in Chapter 69). If wheezing cannot be detected in an infant during routine auscultation, use your hands to gently squeeze the chest during the expiratory phase to generate a more forceful exhalation. This will often produce a wheeze audible by stethoscope. *Rash* may be caused by direct contact with an allergen or as a systemic allergic reaction. When caused by direct contact with an allergen such as the rhus toxin of poison ivy or poison oak, the rash will appear in the distribution of the contact on exposed areas—typically linear or perhaps even more widespread. Contact rash may also be localized to the sites of contact where a necklace touches the skin or on the feet from shoes. Skin manifestations of systemic allergy may include urticaria, erythema multiforme, and the severe findings of Stevens-Johnson syndrome. *Atopic dermatitis* ("eczema") is a complex, relatively poorly understood condition. It has been described as "an itch that rashes" and generally is signaled by severe pruritus with obvious excoriation. The rash has a wider distribution than does a contact rash, and the distribution pattern will be typical for the patient's age (see Atopic Dermatitis in Chapter 57).

Is Allergy Testing Necessary?

Most children with allergic symptoms *do not need allergy testing*. A practical initial approach to evaluate suspected allergy involves a careful history, physical examination, and selected laboratory tests to determine whether symptoms are consistent with an allergic process. Decide whether recurrent infection or a nonallergic adverse reaction can explain the symptoms. Ask about a family history of allergy. Clarify details about the environment in which symptoms develop. Look for physical findings compatible with an allergic reaction. If allergy seems a reasonable explanation for symptoms, consider a treatment trial, as outlined later. If symptoms respond to initial treatment, further evaluation may not be needed. Allergy testing may be beneficial for patients with complex allergy histories, those who do not respond to initial treatment, those whose allergies persist throughout the year, and those who have had an anaphylactic reaction.

How Is Allergy Testing Performed?

Allergy testing is most commonly performed by direct inoculation of antigen into the dermis by scratch or injection. A wheal-and-flare reaction to a "skin test" reflects an IgE response to the allergen. Both positive (histamine) and negative (sterile diluent) controls must be included in the testing. In vitro tests such as the radioallergosorbent test (RAST) also detect allergen-specific IgE.

How Is Allergy Testing Interpreted?

A physician who chooses to perform allergy testing must understand the biology and physiology of common—usually inhalant—allergens and the relationship between positive test results and actual symptoms. Allergy testing is a *bioassay for allergen-specific IgE* and does not identify clinical allergy per se. A positive test result means that IgE is detected for a specific allergen but does not mean that the patient has an allergy. The test is only valuable as a guide for treatment if symptoms correspond to the allergen that causes the positive reaction. Many asymptomatic individuals have antigen-specific IgE detectable by an allergy test but do not have allergy and do not need treatment. You must use care to select appropriate patients for testing and to avoid overinterpretation (misinterpretation) of allergy test results. Allergy skin testing can be uncomfortable for the patient and costly for the parents. Think carefully about *why* you think testing will assist management before requesting it. If allergy testing seems appropriate, you must have a plan about how the results will guide and modify your management of the patient.

What Other Tests Are Useful to Evaluate Allergy?

An elevated eosinophil count in the complete blood count (CBC) marks an inflammatory process that *may* be associated with allergy, but parasitic diseases also cause eosinophilia. Nasal swab examination for eosinophils may help in the diagnosis of chronic noninfectious rhinitis, which is often allergic. Pulmonary function testing will aid the diagnosis of asthma in older children and adolescents. Quantitative assay of serum IgE concentration does not prove useful to guide management for most allergic patients. If infection is in the differential diagnosis, cultures of the throat and of conjunctival discharge may be of value.

TREATMENT

Do Environmental Modifications Help?

Remove the offending allergen or *reduce exposure* if a specific trigger for allergic symptoms can be identified. The severity of symptoms dictates the extent to which environmental changes should be pursued. Anaphylactic shock after exposure to a food or other allergen dictates *absolute avoidance* of the exposure plus ready availability of epinephrine and supportive care. Minor symptoms, in contrast, do not justify major modifications of lifestyle. Often a family will resist removing a pet from the home, even if moderate to severe allergic symptoms develop around the pet. In that case, recommend common-sense adaptations, which might include keeping the animal outside or out of the child's bedroom and off furniture and rugs. If a pet remains in the home, frequent vacuuming and dusting may reduce ambient dander. Housecleaning should be done carefully to reduce dust exposure to the allergic child. Environmental modifications that reduce dust-trapping materials include use of allergen-proof covers on mattresses and removal of feather comforters and pillows. *Dehumidifiers* can greatly assist with mold and dust mite control. *Humidifiers have no place in the home of individuals with moderate to severe allergy* because they promote growth of molds. Reduce allergen exposure during the "allergy season" by keeping windows closed and using air conditioning. *Eliminate exposure to cigarette smoke.*

What Medications Are Useful to Treat Symptoms?

Medications directed at specific allergic symptoms are listed in Table 19-1.

How Can I Educate Patients and Families about Allergy?

The need for education is directly related to the severity of symptoms. Patients and families must be taught about risks, exposures, symptoms,

Table 19-1

Medications for Treatment of Allergy Symptoms

Class	Drug	Comments
Antihistamine		
Sedating	Chlorpheniramine maleate	OTC. Bid dosing
	Diphenhydramine HCl (Benadryl)	OTC. Weak antihistamine, short duration. Sedation common
	Hydroxyzine	Rx. Once-daily dosing often effective. Drowsiness for 4–6 hours after dose, so give at bedtime. Drowsiness diminishes after several days of treatment
Less sedating or non-sedating	Cetirizine HCl (Zyrtec)	Rx
	Fexofenadine HCl (Allegra)	Rx
	Loratadine (Claritin)	OTC
Decongestant	Pseudoephedrine HCl	Useful for nasal airway obstruction
	Oxymetazoline nasal	Nasal spray. Limit use to 3–4 days
Antiinflammatory (corticosteroid)		
Oral and systemic	Prednisone, prednisolone	Used for lower airway obstruction* or severe allergy (systemic, skin)
Inhaled, intranasal	Beclomethasone, budesonide, flunisolide, fluticasone, mometasone, triamcinolone	Topical antiinflammatory for asthma* and allergic rhinitis
Topical	Topical corticosteroid preparations (many)	Atopic and contact dermatitis†—do not use fluorinated steroids on face or diaper area
Other		
Systemic	Montelukast	Leukotriene receptor antagonist for seasonal allergies and asthma
Ocular	Olopatadine ophthalmic	Allergic conjunctivitis
	Nedocromil ophthalmic	Mast cell stabilizer for allergic conjunctivitis
Nasal	Ipratropium	Anticholinergic—nasal spray for rhinitis
Topical	Tacrolimus, picrolimus	Immune modulator for atopic dermatitis†

bid, Twice per day; OTC, over the counter; Rx, prescription.

*For specific treatment, see Asthma, Chapter 69.

†For specific treatment, see Dermatology, Chapter 57.

and management. The education needed to prevent or manage an anaphylactic reaction differs markedly from that needed to manage allergic rhinitis. If seasonal allergies are a problem, provide patients and their families with the means to make a realistic appraisal of the environment. Always discuss the benefits and side effects of treatment. Advise parents to *stop smoking*; if they cannot stop, then advise that they at least prohibit smoking around children, in the home, and in the automobile. The irritant effect of environmental tobacco smoke exacerbates the inflammation caused by allergies. Environmental exposure to tobacco smoke (second-hand smoke) greatly increases the risk of respiratory and many other problems, particularly in young children.

Can Development of Allergy Be Prevented?

Development of allergy may be prevented or delayed by avoidance of allergen exposure, especially in high-risk families. For example, exclusive breast-feeding for 6 months or more reduces exposure to allergens, promotes maturation of the infant's gastrointestinal tract, and provides secretory IgA. If there is a strong family history of allergies and atopy, some authorities recommend that a lactating mother restrict specific foods such as egg, peanuts, and milk from the diet because food allergens may be transmitted in human milk. Recent evidence, however, indicates that breast-feeding does not prevent development of eczema and atopy. Waiting to introduce "solid" foods until after 4 months of age, especially when there is a strong family history of allergy, may minimize sensitization to food allergens. Similarly, delayed introduction of foods that have a high risk of triggering allergic reactions, such as peanuts, egg, and cow's milk, may also be useful for children with allergic family histories. If family history for allergy is positive, it is far easier to tell a child that he or she cannot have a cat than to remove the cat from the home if severe allergic symptoms develop.

When Are "Allergy Shots" Useful?

Immunotherapy has been shown to be effective in reducing allergic manifestations caused by pollens, mites, insect venom, and similar environmental allergens. Mold allergies respond poorly to immunotherapy, as do food allergies. Identification of specific allergens is necessary before immunotherapy can be started, so allergy testing is mandatory. Immunotherapy consists of repeated injections of dilute allergen solutions, gradually increasing the concentration over time.

KEY POINTS

- Many symptoms attributed to "allergy" are not mediated by immune mechanisms.
- Common immune-mediated allergic reactions include rhinitis, conjunctivitis, and dermatitis.

(continued)

- Anaphylaxis is a life-threatening type I allergic reaction (IgE-mediated).
- The best "treatment" of any allergic reaction is avoidance of the allergen.
- Exposure to cigarette smoke should be prevented for all children.

Case 19-1

A 10-year-old girl has a persistent cough, nasal congestion, and "dark circles around her eyes." Symptoms have been present for several years, with worsening intensity since the family moved to your community. Her symptoms typically begin in late July and persist until the first frost. Parents bring her for evaluation in mid-August. The history indicates eczema in infancy and frequent colds year round, but especially at this time of the year. She does not wheeze and has no shortness of breath while playing soccer.

A. What additional history would assist you to determine the cause of her symptoms?
B. What physical findings would be consistent with chronic allergic rhinitis?
C. What allergens are common in your community that could account for this pattern of illness?
D. If this family lived in an area of the country that does not have freezing weather, how might allergic rhinitis manifest?

Case Answers

19-1 A. *Learning objective:* **Discuss the key historical issues that should be addressed when allergy is suspected as a cause of symptoms.** You should request details about seasonality, specific (known) triggers, episodes consistent with anaphylaxis, and family history. Information is also helpful about the environment, especially heating system, pets, tobacco smoke, and proximity to environmental allergens. Inquire about symptoms such as snoring, throat clearing, cough, hearing problems, and history of otitis media.

19-1 B. *Learning objective:* **Describe physical findings associated with allergic rhinitis.** Physical findings associated with allergic rhinitis include allergic facies: nasal crease; mouth breather; puffy, dark eyelids; pale and boggy mucosa of conjunctivae and nose; denasal voice (e.g., "m" pronounced as "eb"); and eczematoid rash.

19-1 C. *Learning objective:* **Discuss common allergens responsible for seasonal allergies.** You should know about the allergens that are common in your community. In many parts of the United States, ragweed is the primary allergen in late summer and early fall. At other seasons, grasses, molds, and tree pollens cause problems. Indoor allergens, including house dust, dust mite, and pet dander may be a year-round problem, especially if heating and air conditioning use the same ductwork.

19-1 D. *Learning objective:* **Explain how the climate of an area can affect environmental allergens and the manifestations of common allergies.** Without frost or freezing weather, allergen-producing plants may persist in the environment. This makes it more likely that symptoms will be persistent, rather than strictly seasonal, although there will still be seasonal exacerbations as plants cycle through pollen-producing times.

BIBLIOGRAPHY

Task Force on Allergic Disorders: The allergy report. American Academy of Allergy, Asthma, and Immunology (AAAAI), Milwaukee, WI, 2000.

Sears MR, Greene JM, William AR et al: Long-term relation between breastfeeding and development of atopy and asthma in children and young adults: a longitudinal study, *Lancet* 360:901, 2002.

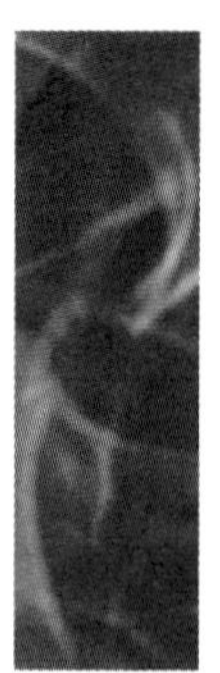

20

Arthritis and Arthralgia: Suspected Rheumatologic Disease

MARY C. OTTOLINI

ETIOLOGY

What Causes Joint Pain and Swelling?

The causes of arthritis and arthralgia in children can be grouped into three major categories: infectious, reactive, or mechanical. The differential diagnosis is based on age (Table 20-1). These clinical presentations should be distinguished from benign, self-limited "growing pains" that typically occur at night in children ages 3 to 6 years and are easily relieved by massage, nonsteroidal antiinflammatory drugs (NSAIDs), or acetaminophen.

How Do Infectious and Reactive Arthritis Differ?

Infectious arthritis results from direct infection of a bone or joint. Reactive arthritis often results from the *immune response* to infection, as in rheumatic fever. It can also reflect an *autoimmune disorder,* such as juvenile rheumatoid arthritis, or a *malignancy,* such as leukemia (Figure 20-1).

What Causes Rheumatologic Disease?

Rheumatologic diseases are autoimmune disorders in patients with the genetic predisposition to develop an exaggerated immune response to drugs, bacteria, viruses, and also to their own cells and tissues. The inciting factor is unknown for most disorders, such as systemic lupus erythematosus (SLE). The most common rheumatologic diseases in children are juvenile rheumatoid arthritis (JRA), SLE, dermatomyositis, and vasculitis (Chapter 70).

What Mechanical Problems Cause Joint Pain?

Knee and hip pain often result from mechanical or traumatic causes (see Chapter 68). Patellar-femoral syndrome and cartilage or ligament injury cause knee pain in active adolescent girls. Osgood-Schlatter disease is a common finding in physically active adolescents. Slipped capital femoral epiphysis (SCFE) occurs in obese adolescent boys,

Table 20-1

Differential Diagnosis by Age of Limp Due to Bone and Joint Pain

Newborn-4 mos	4 mos-4 yrs	5–10 yrs	11–18 yrs
	Infectious		
Osteomyelitis Arthritis *Streptococcus pyogenes* Gp A *S. pyogenes* Gp B *Staphylococcus aureus*	Osteomyelitis Discitis Arthritis *S. aureus* *S. pyogenes* Gp A *Streptococcus pneumoniae* Lyme disease Viral	Osteomyelitis Arthritis *S. aureus* *S. pyogenes* Gp A Lyme disease Viral	Osteomyelitis Arthritis *S. aureus* *S. pyogenes* Gp A *Neisseria gonorrhoeae* Lyme disease Viral
	Reactive		
Immune Response to Infection			
N/A	Lyme disease *Mycoplasma* Rheumatic fever Post *S. pyogenes* Gp A *Neisseria meningitidis* Post viral Enteritis: *Campylobacter* *Salmonella* *Shigella* *Yersinia*		
Malignancy			
N/A	Leukemia	Leukemia Osteosarcoma Ewing's sarcoma	Leukemia Osteosarcoma Osteoid osteoma
Rheumatic			
N/A	JRA	JRA Spondyloarthropathy SLE	JRA SLE Ankylosing spondylitis Spondyloarthropathy
	Mechanical		
Hip dysplasia Fracture (suspect abuse)	Toddler's fracture Salter fracture (suspect abuse)	Legg-Calvé-Perthes disease Salter fracture	Stress fracture Salter fracture Meniscus or ligament injury SCFE Osgood-Schlatter disease

JRA, Juvenile rheumatoid arthritis; N/A, not applicable; SCFE, slipped capital femoral epiphysis; SLE, systemic lupus erythematosus.

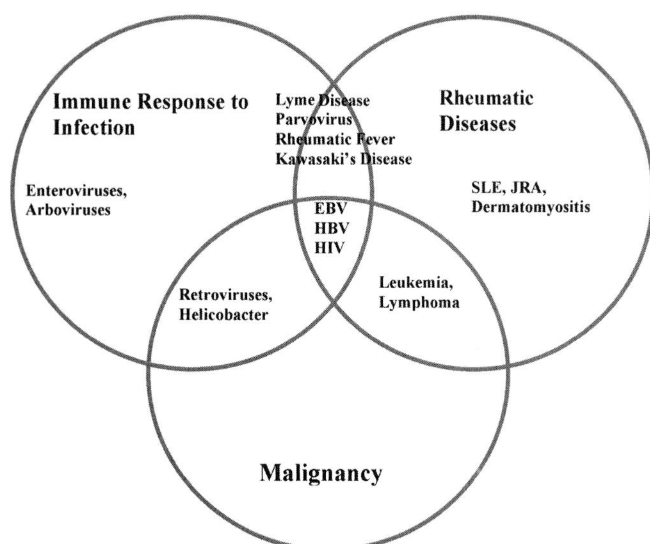

FIGURE 20-1 Differential diagnosis of reactive arthritis. EBV, Epstein Barr virus; HBV, hepatitis B virus; HIV, human immunodeficiency virus; JRA, juvenile rheumatoid arthritis; SLE, systemic lupus erythermatosis.

who present with a painful "waddling gait." Legg-Calvé-Perthes disease is seen in younger boys.

EVALUATION

What Helps Differentiate the Causes of Joint Pain?

Fever: Infection must be considered if *fever* is present because rapid diagnosis and antibiotic treatment are necessary to prevent joint destruction and sepsis. Patients with reactive arthritis may have fever, but it is uncommon in mechanical disorders. Malignancy also causes fever, arthritis, and bone or joint pain.

Pain location, quality, onset, and duration: Knee pain may be at the site of trauma or may be referred from the hip, so a careful hip examination is warranted. Patients with septic arthritis usually present with toxicity and severe pain within 24 to 48 hours of onset, whereas those with reactive arthritis or mechanical causes often have stiffness and swelling that evolves over days or weeks. Severe diffuse bone pain that is present during the day but worse at night suggests malignancy because expansion of the marrow by leukemic infiltration can cause bone pain weeks or months before blasts are seen on the peripheral smear.

History of prior infections: Many viruses and bacteria activate T cells that cross-react with joint antigens, causing a postinfectious or reactive arthritis (Table 20-1).

Underlying disease: Children with sickle cell anemia may have bone pain with a vasoocclusive crisis.

How Does Septic Arthritis Differ from Reactive Arthritis?

Children with reactive arthritis typically have low-grade fever but are not toxic-appearing. *Streptococcus, Mycoplasma,* parvovirus, and rubella can cause either direct joint infection or a reactive inflammatory response leading to arthritis. The arthritis of rheumatic fever usually involves the large joints, especially the knee; is painful out of proportion to clinical findings; and often is migratory. It responds dramatically to NSAIDs. Evaluation to exclude cardiac involvement is needed. A "toxic-appearing" febrile child with a swollen, red joint should be presumed to have a septic arthritis (see Chapter 64). Consider arthrocentesis if a limping child has a fever, especially if a septic hip is suspected. Table 20-2 lists synovial fluid findings that distinguish infectious from reactive arthritis.

How Do I Diagnose "Toxic" Synovitis?

Toxic synovitis, the most common form of reactive arthritis, occurs in boys 3 to 10 years of age who develop hip pain, limp, or refusal to bear weight 1 to 2 days after a viral upper respiratory tract infection. The hip often has limited range of motion, and pain is referred to the thigh or knee. Despite the name, these children are *not* toxic-appearing, nor do they typically have the high fever, localized tenderness, and swelling associated with bacterial infection. Radiographic or ultrasonographic examination may reveal fluid in the joint. Erythrocyte sedimentation rate (ESR) may be elevated. If arthrocentesis is performed, synovial fluid shows no infection (Table 20-2). Symptoms usually resolve in a few days with rest and NSAIDs. Persistent symptoms, especially fever and nocturnal pain, should prompt an evaluation for leukemia.

How Does Rheumatologic Disease Present in Childhood?

Rheumatologic diseases can present acutely with joint pain (arthralgia) alone, or with redness, swelling, fever, pain, and decreased range of motion (arthritis). More commonly, they have an indolent course, with progressive development of fever, stiffness, pain, or joint effusions. Unusual rashes may appear, accompanied by systemic symptoms such as weakness. Conditions that produce similar signs and symptoms

Table 20-2

Synovial Fluid Findings

	Normal	Reactive	Septic
Appearance	Clear, yellow	Turbid	Yellow-green
WBC/ml	< 200	15,000–100,000	$> 100,000$
PMN (%)	$< 30\%$	$\geq 60\%$	$\geq 90\%$
Glucose	= Serum	$\leq$ Serum	$<$ Serum
Protein (g/dl)	2.5–3.5	> 5	> 5
Culture	Negative	Negative	+ 85%–95%

PMN, Polymorphonuclear leukocytes; WBC, white blood cell; +, positive.

may have decidedly different outcomes, so your history and physical examination must be done carefully. Arthralgia is common and unless persistent does not portend a serious diagnosis. Arthritis requires a thorough evaluation.

What Laboratory Tests Should I Order?

The complete blood count (CBC) may reveal the anemia of chronic illness, especially with systemic-onset disease. Anemia may also result from gastrointestinal blood loss induced by NSAIDs and other medications. The ESR is often elevated. Decreased levels of complement (CH50, C3, and C4) and increased levels of immunoglobulins indicate activation of the inflammatory cascade. The antinuclear antibody (ANA) test is often positive at levels higher than 1:80; lower levels reflect a response to other nonspecific stimuli. ANA reactions are shown in Table 20-3.

What Imaging Studies Help in the Evaluation?

Plain films of the involved area are often nondiagnostic, especially early in the course of the disease, but may help rule out other causes. Magnetic resonance imaging reveals much more about the joint space and periarticular soft tissue. Bone scan, especially using technetium 99, can identify joint or bone inflammation.

TREATMENT

How Do I Treat Mechanical Causes of Limp and Pain?

Treatment depends on the cause and often relies on NSAIDs plus the "RICE" approach: rest, ice, compression, elevation. Early identification of Legg-Calvé-Perthes disease is crucial. Prevention of SCFE is the preferred treatment (Chapter 68).

How Do I Treat the Arthritis of Rheumatologic Diseases?

NSAIDs, such as ibuprofen and naproxen, should be the first choice for most patients. NSAIDs decrease the inflammatory response by inhibiting the production of prostaglandins through inhibition of the

Table 20-3

ANA Reactions in Rheumatologic Diseases

Antigen	Disease
Histone	Drug-induced lupus erythematosus
Ribonucleoprotein	Mixed connective tissue disease
Pm-Scl	Sclerodermatomyositis
Scl	Scleroderma
Sm	Systemic lupus erythematosus
Ro/SSA	Sjögren's syndrome, congenital heart block, annular erythema
La/SSB	Sjögren's syndrome

ANA, Antinuclear antibody; Sm, Smith antigen.

cyclooxygenase type II enzyme (COX II). Specific COX II inhibitors, such as celecoxib, are under investigation for use in children. Gastritis is the most common side effect of NSAIDs and may cause gastrointestinal blood loss and iron-deficiency anemia.

If NSAIDs Do Not Help, What Other Medications Are Useful?

Methotrexate is a second-line agent with proven efficacy for the treatment of JRA, dermatomyositis, and SLE. Effective doses are smaller than those used to treat malignancies, so side effects are minimized. The most common side effect is elevation of transaminases, but hepatic damage rarely occurs.

When Should Steroids Be Used?

Corticosteroids have both antiinflammatory and immunosuppressive effects and are crucial to controlling dermatomyositis or flare-ups of SLE. Whenever possible, prolonged, high-dose, daily steroid use should be avoided because of the adverse effects on the immune system and growth. Other side effects of steroids include psychosis, diabetes, glaucoma, Cushing's syndrome, hypertension, and osteopenia leading to pathologic fractures. Malignancy must be ruled out by a bone marrow biopsy before steroids are used for a patient with bone and joint pain or swelling.

KEY POINTS

- Infectious arthritis results from direct infection.
- Reactive arthritis occurs as an immune response to an infection, an autoimmune reaction, or from malignancy.
- Overuse and trauma are mechanical causes of arthritis.

Case 20-1

A 4-year-old boy has been limping for the past 24 hours. His mother thinks that he injured his right leg while jumping off his bed 2 days ago. He recently had a viral upper respiratory infection associated with congestion and a low-grade fever but has been well for the past week. He was active at his usual level until yesterday afternoon. When you examine him, he is afebrile and appears well, except for a pronounced limp on his right leg. He has no rash, joint swelling, or erythema. Passive movement of the right leg causes pain in the hip. Range of motion of the right hip is reduced.

A. What are possible causes of the limp?
B. What features of this child's history point to toxic synovitis?
C. What laboratory and imaging tests would assist with the evaluation of this child?

Case Answers

20-1 A. *Learning objective:* **Identify the common causes of limp in childhood.** These are trauma, toxic synovitis, Legg-Calvé-Perthes disease, and juvenile rheumatoid arthritis. Septic arthritis is not common but has serious consequences.

20-1 B. *Learning objective:* **Identify the key history to distinguish among common and serious causes of limp/joint pain.** Toxic synovitis is likely because the history includes preceding viral upper respiratory infection and absence of systemic symptoms such as high fever, rash, and morning stiffness.

20-1 C. *Learning objective:* **Identify the laboratory tests and imaging studies useful for evaluation of arthralgia and arthritis.** Given this child's specific findings, the complete blood count, differential white blood cell count, and erythrocyte sedimentation rate would be good choices for the initial workup. Plain radiograph and/or ultrasound studies of the hip would identify fluid in the joint space and deformities of the femoral head, consistent with Legg-Calvé-Perthes disease. He is not likely to need a joint aspiration for diagnosis.

BIBLIOGRAPHY

Carlson D, Hernandez J, Bloom BJ et al: Lack of *Borrelia burgdorferi* DNA in synovial samples from patients with antibiotic treatment-resistant Lyme arthritis. *Arthritis Rheum* 42:2705, 1999.

Gerber MA, Shapiro ED, Burke GS et al: Lyme disease in children in southeastern Connecticut, *N Engl J Med* 335:1270, 1996.

Kalden JR: Viral arthritis. In Klippel JH, Dieppe PA, editors: *Rheumatology*, ed 2, London, Mosby, 1998.

Nocton JJ, Miller LC, Tucker LB et al: Human parvovirus B19-asssociated arthritis in children, *J Pediatr* 122:186, 1993.

Poggio TV, Orlando N, Galanternik L et al: Microbiology of acute arthropathies among children in Argentina: Mycoplasma pneumoniae and hominis and Ureaplasma urealyticum, *Pediatr Infect Dis J* 17:304, 1998.

21

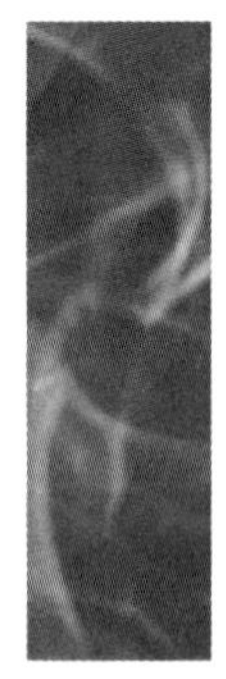

Ataxia, Dizziness, and Vertigo

ADAM HARTMAN

ETIOLOGY

What Is Ataxia?

Ataxia is the lack of control over coordinated muscular movement, including posture, eye movements, limb movements, and speech. Because of the systemic nature of most etiologies of ataxia in childhood, anatomic localization is not as useful as it is in diseases of the cerebral hemispheres. *Acute ataxia* occurs after a variety of infections, intoxications, and trauma. It can also be caused by tumors, migraines, inborn errors of metabolism, and other vascular disorders. *Chronic ataxia* is caused by tumors, hereditary conditions, congenital malformations of the posterior fossa, and inborn errors of metabolism.

What Is Dizziness?

Dizziness is a nonspecific term that usually refers to a sense of lightheadedness and unsteadiness. It is often part of the presyncopal phenomenon (see Syncope, Chapter 39) but can be caused by dehydration, hypotension, anemia, or hypoglycemia. Dizziness should be distinguished from vertigo, ataxia, and weakness. Dizziness may be seen in some dysautonomias. Cardiac causes of dizziness include arrhythmias and postural orthostatic tachycardia syndrome.

How Is Vertigo Different from Ataxia and Dizziness?

Vertigo is usually caused by a vestibular or brainstem disorder. Patients often cannot maintain a stable posture because of a sensation of motion. The differential diagnosis includes labyrinthitis, medication (e.g., aminoglycosides), migraine, seizures, motion sickness, or brainstem stroke.

EVALUATION

What History Helps in Diagnosis of Ataxia?

Most causes of ataxia can be differentiated from one another with a thorough history and physical examination. You must identify the time course (acute vs. chronic), anatomic localization (cerebellar vs. sensory), and age-related disorders. Family history is critical. It is important to distinguish age-appropriate clumsiness from pathologic ataxia. It is also important to distinguish ataxia from weakness because the causes are different.

How Does Acute Ataxia Present Most Commonly?

Acute cerebellar ataxia of childhood is the most common form of ataxia and is usually seen in toddlers and early-school-aged children. It is a diagnosis of exclusion. Viral infections such as Epstein-Barr virus, varicella, enteroviruses, and others often precede the onset of ataxia. Parents usually describe an abrupt onset: "My child was 'fine' until he woke up from a nap."

What Neurologic Findings Identify the Cause of Ataxia?

The neuroanatomy of balance requires both afferent and efferent pathways. Sensory input is crucial for feedback to motor neurons and planning centers. Diseases that affect the vestibular apparatus (e.g., labyrinthitis) can cause imbalance, as can those that affect motor planning (e.g., cerebellar tumor). When ataxia originates in the cerebellum, clinical features help localize the abnormality: Gait unsteadiness, abnormal speech, or nystagmus point to a midline lesion in the vermis. In contrast, dysmetria, demonstrated by having the child reach for a toy, or hypotonia most likely result from a lesion in the cerebellar hemispheres.

Can Physical Examination Identify the Cause of Ataxia?

Conjunctival or cutaneous telangiectasias are seen in Ataxia-Telangiectasia. Cardiac abnormalities, diabetes, and orthopedic abnormalities, including pes cavus and scoliosis, are seen in Friedreich's ataxia. Strange odors can be associated with some inborn errors of metabolism. The opsoclonus-myoclonus syndrome ("dancing eyes, dancing feet") is seen occasionally with an occult neuroblastoma. The presence or absence of reflexes can be critical in distinguishing cerebellar causes from sensory causes of ataxia.

What Workup Is Needed If a Child Has Ataxia?

In acute ataxia, consider a drug screen, sepsis/meningitis laboratory studies, and neuroimaging. The diagnosis of acute cerebellar ataxia should be made only after documentation of the infectious prodrome and the absence of other causes. Recurrent or chronic ataxia might be evaluated with neuroimaging, metabolic, or specific genetic studies, depending on clinical findings.

How Do I Evaluate the Dizzy Child?

The history and physical examination usually helps identify the most common causes. For example, dizziness in a child with gastroenteritis and fluid losses suggests dehydration. An adolescent girl with significant menstrual blood loss might be anemic. There should be no sensation of motion with simple dizziness. In most cases, no physical or neurologic abnormalities will be identified. Depending on the clinical findings, you may choose to measure orthostatic blood pressures or check electrolytes, blood glucose, or a complete blood count.

How Do I Diagnose the Cause of Vertigo?

Chronology of the event (acute, chronic), presence of cold symptoms, fever, trauma, or hearing loss, and a family history of migraine headaches or seizures usually help distinguish one cause of vertigo from the others. A history of the sensation of motion, such as that experienced while spinning around quickly, helps distinguish vertigo from other causes of unsteadiness. In older patients, the Dix-Hallpike maneuver (*www.emedicine.com/ent/topic761.htm*) can be useful to confirm vertigo.

TREATMENT

How Do I Treat the Child with Ataxia?

Acute cerebellar ataxia of childhood needs no specific therapy. Ataxia caused by a tumor is managed along with tumor treatment. Metabolic causes can be treated with specific dietary interventions and medications. Migraines are treated as outlined in Chapter 35.

How Do I Treat the Child with Dizziness?

Most transient dizziness does not require a treatment. A specific cause such as dehydration, hypotension, hypoglycemia, or anemia should be treated.

How Do I Treat the Child with Vertigo?

Migraines and seizures usually respond to standard therapies for the specific disorders. Bacterial infections are treated with antibiotics. Motion sickness can be treated with antiemetics. Vestibular damage from medications can be challenging and requires consultation with an otorhinolaryngologist. Patients with strokes should be referred to a neurologist.

KEY POINTS

- Ataxia commonly occurs after a viral infection. The ataxic child cannot control coordinated muscular movements.
- Dizziness is part of the presyncopal syndrome. It is a nonspecific term that refers to lightheadedness.
- Vertigo refers specifically to the sensation of spinning. Migraine and seizures are two causes of vertigo.

Case 21-1

A 5-year-old boy is admitted with a complicated varicella infection. He has a mild cough, has not been drinking well, but has not vomited or had diarrhea. Since waking from a nap earlier in the day, he has been unsteady on his feet and slurring his speech. He is currently taking diphenhydramine for itching and ibuprofen for fever. There is no history of trauma. He has not had any headaches. His past medical history is unremarkable. There is no family history of ataxia, seizures, migraines, or gait/balance problems. Temperature is 39° C (103.5° F). Physical examination shows multiple vesicular lesions on all skin surfaces and on the posterior pharynx. There is no nuchal rigidity, and Kernig's and Brudzinski's signs are negative. His neurologic examination is remarkable for slurred speech and abnormal finger-to-nose and heel-knee-shin tests. His gait is somewhat wide-based.

A. What is the most likely diagnosis?
B. What studies can confirm the diagnosis?
C. Is any therapy necessary?

Case Answers

21-1 A. *Learning objective:* **Using the history and physical examination, identify the likely cause of acute ataxia in a child.** This patient most likely has acute cerebellar ataxia of childhood. Onset during a viral infection, with no past history of neurologic problems, and no family history of ataxia are important clues. The absence of other neurologic findings on physical examination also points to this diagnosis.

21-1 B. *Learning objective:* **Select laboratory and imaging studies to evaluate acute ataxia.** Acute cerebellar ataxia of childhood is a diagnosis of exclusion. No specific laboratory or imaging studies are needed. A lumbar puncture can rule out meningitis, although it is not indicated in this patient. Magnetic resonance imaging, if done for other reasons (e.g., to exclude structural anomalies), might demonstrate some cerebellar enhancement on T2-weighted images.

21-1 C. *Learning objective:* **Outline treatment options for a child with acute ataxia.** No treatment is necessary for acute cerebellar ataxia. It should resolve on its own. A detailed explanation of your diagnostic findings and of the basis for your final diagnosis may well be the most important aspect of management. Follow-up to document gradual resolution of the ataxia will ensure ongoing communication with the family.

BIBLIOGRAPHY

Fenichel GM *Clinical pediatric neurology: a signs and symptoms approach,* ed 4, Philadelphia, 2005, WB Saunders.

MacGregor DL: Vertigo, *Pediatr Rev* 23:10, 2002.

22

Behavior Problems

LINDA J. COOPER-BROWN and
STACEY MCCONKEY

ETIOLOGY

How Common Are Behavior Problems?

Nearly 25% of school-age patients are evaluated by physicians for behavioral concerns ranging from minor temper tantrums to severe behaviors that cause injury to self or others. The behaviors may occur with one person or many, at home, in school, or anywhere. Severe, pervasive behavioral concerns are discussed in Chapter 55.

Why Should I Worry about a Child's Behavior?

Parents often seek assistance about behavioral problems from a child's physician. Learning about behavior will assist you to master important clinical skills that will help you address these concerns. Primary prevention of problem behavior is aided when routine care includes:

- Developmental surveillance
- Inquiry into family history and stressors
- Anticipatory guidance about age-appropriate behavioral expectations
- Coping strategies that may reduce caregiver stress
- Advice to caregivers about parenting skills
- Information about the effects of illness on behavior

How Does Behavior Relate to Child Development?

Knowledge of development helps you understand a child's behavior and identify an approach to take with the parent. Many concerns about behaviors reflect typical child development. For example, impulsivity and the inability to stay with an activity for more than a few minutes are age-appropriate for a 2-year-old but suggest the need for further evaluation of a 7-year-old. Table 22-1 lists developmental highlights that relate to behavior.

Table 22-1

Highlights of Developmental Levels

Age	Attention Span	Expressive Skills	Receptive Skills	Social Skills
12 mo	2-3 min	1 or 2 words Imitates sounds and gestures Communicates with actions and gestures	Recognizes names and words for common items	Short memory Responsive to parental and social interactions
18-24 mo	4-5 min	At least 20 words (50 @ 24 mo) 2-word phrases Uses words to make wants known	Follows simple commands Listens to simple stories, rhymes	Shows affection Imitates behavior of others Acts on impulses Limited idea of good/bad
2-3 yr	6-7 min	Sentences of 2-3 words Often asks for or directs attention to objects by naming them	Can follow a story Remembers pieces of information Follows 2-step commands	Everything happens in the world as a result of something he/she did Acts on impulses, more concerned with own needs
3-4 yr	8-9 min	Sentences of 4+ words Answers simple questions	Understands simple "who," "what," "where," "why" questions Follows 3-step command	Plays with peers Can share in small groups with supervision Reasoning is one-sided, cannot take another's perspective
4-5 yr	11-12 min	Sentences of 5+ words Communicates easily with other children, adults Talks about daily activities, experiences	Knows things used in the home Distinguishes fantasy from reality	Exploring concepts of good, bad Wants to please and be like friends

min, Minutes; mo, months.

Why Do Problem Behaviors Develop and Persist?

Behaviors persist when they are reinforced. We typically classify *reinforcers* into two categories based on the benefit to the child: *gain (positive reinforcement)* and *escape (negative reinforcement).* Problem behavior may *gain* a desired outcome, *escape* from an undesired outcome, or both. The events that initially cause a behavior problem may be completely different from the events that maintain or reinforce it. For example, a child may awaken at night crying during an acute illness and a parent may respond by comforting the child and providing medical treatment. The child's behavior and the parent's response are appropriate for the situation. Night waking and crying usually subside unless the parent continues to respond each time the child wakens or cries. The behavior may now persist because it is positively reinforced by parental attention. Or, parents may attempt a behavior management plan but give up when the child "tests the limits." Thus the child learns to persist with the problem behavior to get what he or she wants.

What Is Attention Seeking?

Attention seeking commonly occurs when children are ignored until they misbehave. Problem behavior may offer the child the only way to get what he or she wants. Children learn to gain attention through their behavior. To them, even negative attention is better than no attention.

How Does Family Stress Affect Child Behavior?

Family stressors may cause or contribute to problem behaviors. For example, a parent who has depression may be unable to engage in positive interactions or preventive measures or carry out a management plan. Domestic violence provides poor role models for anger management and communication and creates an environment with unpredictable consequences for the child's behavior.

What about Genetic, Medical, and School Influences?

Genetic or medical factors may contribute to the problem behavior. These include the child's temperament, a genetic disorder, chronic illness, and the child's cognitive skills or learning style. For example, fragile X syndrome is associated with repetitive behaviors, perseveration, and hyperactivity. *The teaching approach in the school* may trigger and reinforce problem behavior if it does not match the child's learning style. A child who learns best from visual cues may become frustrated with verbal explanations and act out in an attempt to escape demands. A child who has a learning disability may demonstrate "hyperactive" behaviors in school that only diminish after the learning disorder has been identified and an educational management program instituted (see Chapter 55).

EVALUATION

How Should I Begin an Evaluation of Behavior?

A good interview is important for gathering information.

- Be nonjudgmental.
- Be a good listener. Clarify and summarize parental concerns and key information.
- Ask about the frequency and severity of the problem.
- Determine if the behavior is appropriate for age and development.
- Identify the initial trigger and what now reinforces the behavior.
- Be certain that you have enough information and understand the concern before offering suggestions.

How Do I Determine What Reinforces a Behavior?

Table 22-2 provides examples of questions and some answers that suggest possible reinforcers.

Table 22-2

How To Identify Reinforcers of Behavior

Questions	Possible Reinforcers
1. Does the behavior happen when your attention is diverted from your child? • When you are on the phone? • When you are talking with someone? • When you are preparing meals or doing housework? **2. Do you ever scold or reason with your child about the behavior?**	**If the parent answers "yes" to question 1 or 2,** the behavior could be *reinforced by attention:* The child has learned to gain attention by exhibiting problem behavior.
3. Does the behavior happen when your child cannot have access to something? • A toy? • Food? • Going outside to play? **4. Do you ever "give in" and let your child have what he or she wants?**	**If the parent answers "yes" to question 3 or 4,** the behavior could be *reinforced by the tangible item or preferred activity:* The child has learned to gain the item or activity by exhibiting problem behavior.
5. Does the behavior happen when you ask your child to do something? • Get ready for bed? • Get dressed? • Do chores? • Do homework? **6. Do you ever "give up" and let him/her out of the task?**	**If the parent answers "yes" to question 5 or 6,** the behavior could be *reinforced by letting the child get out of undesired activities:* The child has learned to escape undesired activities by exhibiting problem behavior.

What Observations Will Help Me Assess Behavior?

Observe parent-child interactions in the clinic setting. Remember that interactions in clinic will not necessarily reflect what happens in other situations, but watch for general patterns. Observe the child's response when you use one of the positive strategies in Table 22-3. If the child responds, try instructing the parent in these alternatives. If the child is unresponsive, and especially if similar behavior occurs in other situations, referral to a psychologist may be needed for further assessment and management.

Table 22-3

Parent-Child Interaction: Potential Problems and Positive Strategies

Situation	Potential Problems	Positive Strategies
Child gets into dangerous situation (e.g., climbing)	Parent ignores or uses strategies not appropriate for development (e.g., scolding or discussion with a 2-year-old child)	Parent intervenes early and uses strategies appropriate for development (e.g., redirection with a 2-year-old child)
Child is uncooperative with exam	Parent ignores or scolds	Parent attempts to help or suggests strategies successful in other situations
Child interrupts when parent is talking with you	Parent scolds	Parent redirects (a toddler) or states when it is the child's turn to talk (a school-aged child)
Child plays well with toys or is cooperative with exam	Parent ignores	Parent provides intermittent, positive attention

What Does Physical Examination Add to the Workup?

The most important findings will be obtained from observation of unusual behaviors or parent-child interactions. You should describe and discuss them with the parent. Look for dysmorphic features that may indicate a syndrome that has an association with problem behavior, such as fragile X or fetal alcohol syndrome. Finally, because children with behavior problems are at high risk for abuse, you must perform a complete physical examination to identify bruising or unexplained injuries (see Chapter 24).

What Other Tools Can I Use?

Behavior rating scales can identify specific areas of parental or teacher concern. Developmental assessment identifies developmental levels. (Table 22-4 lists common assessment tools.) These measures do not

Table 22-4

Behavior and Developmental Assessment Tools

Behavior Rating Scales	Developmental Assessments
Connors Rating Scales	Denver Developmental Screening Test
Child Behavior Checklist	Bailey Scales of Infant Development
Pediatric Behavior Scale	Bracken Basic Concept Scale

provide information regarding the triggers and/or reinforcers of the problem behavior. This information must be obtained by asking parents and teachers to identify the situations in which problem behaviors are *likely* to occur and those in which problem behaviors are *not likely* to occur.

TREATMENT

How Should I Manage Problem Behaviors?

Although the behavior causes the concern, the *reinforcer* of the behavior must be identified to plan treatment. Table 22-5 provides examples of treatment strategies that are "matched" to the presumed reinforcers of the problem behavior.

Table 22-5

Reinforcers of Behavior Problems and Suggested Treatment Strategies

Presumed Reinforcer	Treatment Strategy
Gain (positive reinforcement) Child gets attention, tangible item, preferred activity for problem behavior	**Ignore the problem behavior** Respond only to appropriate behavior. Do not provide the attention, tangible item, or preferred activity for problem behavior. **OR** **Time out** See section dealing with "time out."
Escape (negative reinforcement) Child escapes from undesired activities for problem behavior.	**Continue the request** Do not discontinue it because of continued problem behavior. Allow the preferred activity only after he or she has complied with the request.

What Is Time-Out and Who Benefits from It?

The term *time-out* is abbreviated from "time-out from reinforcement." It is a management plan designed to *reduce* problem behavior that is reinforced by gaining attention or activities. Time-out briefly removes the child from attention or activities when he or she misbehaves. It is *not* generally used for behavior that is reinforced by escape, because removal in this case can make the problem worse. Time-out can be conducted either by sending the child to a designated area (e.g., a chair or room) or by removing attention and activities from the child (e.g., the parent walks away from the child). No attention, not even discussion, should occur when the child is in time-out, and the child should not have access to "fun" items. Time-out should end only when the child has calmed, rather than after the passage of a specific amount of time. When time-out is completed, *time-in* should begin immediately with opportunities for the child to engage in appropriate behavior and to be rewarded with attention or activities for the altered behavior. Time-in is important for *increasing* desired behaviors. Time-out/time-in is typically used with children 12 months of age and older.

How Do I Manage Behavior Triggered by Family Stress?

Identification of family stressors as a component of a child's behavior problem allows early intervention that can reduce the problem behaviors and prevent abuse and family violence. Referral should be made to a therapist who can assist with the evaluation and treatment of the stressors. You must recognize that domestic violence and child abuse occur with increased frequency in families challenged by stress. A child's behavior often reflects family stress and on occasion contributes to the increasing level of stress.

What about School Behavior Problems?

Evaluation and management of school behavior problems requires involvement of parents and school personnel. More than one treatment strategy may be needed.

- *Identify reinforcers for problem behavior.* When a teacher reports that a management program was tried and "failed," it may be that the wrong program was used. For example, if escape reinforces problem behavior, sending a child to the principal's office for misbehavior allows the child to escape tasks and reinforces behavior.
- *Match the teaching approach to the child's learning style.* A change in the teaching approach may reduce problem behavior more effectively than a behavior management program. For example, if the child has problems following three-step directions, the teacher or parent may need to break down tasks into three single-step directions.
- *Use neurocognitive testing* to look for specific learning disorders or attention deficit disorder (with or without hyperactivity) so that management may be planned (see Chapter 55).

Can Behavior Problems Be Prevented?

Problem behaviors can often be prevented by the structure of the child's environment and positive reinforcement for appropriate behavior. Some strategies may prevent behavior problems:

- *Encourage the child to use appropriate communication.* Behavior often becomes a problem because the child has learned to communicate desires through problem behavior. Caregivers can encourage the child to use more appropriate behavior to communicate wants or needs (e.g., saying "help, please" instead of having a tantrum; asking a peer to play instead of taking a toy or hitting). This provides the child with an appropriate alternative to the problem behavior.
- *Be consistent with rules and follow-through.* A child often learns that rules vary from day to day and that "pushing the right button" will make a parent eventually give in. Parents must identify acceptable and unacceptable behaviors and must determine the consequences for both. They must then apply these "rules" consistently, so that the child knows exactly what to expect for specific behaviors. Both parents should agree on the rules and strive to apply them consistently because a child quickly learns to "play" one parent against the other, exploiting even minor differences.
- *Supervise closely and intervene early.* Minor problem behaviors (e.g., teasing) may occur with increasing frequency before the appearance of more severe behaviors (e.g., pushing or hitting). If caregivers monitor possible problem situations and intervene early, the more severe problem behaviors may sometimes be prevented. Intervention might include reminding the child of the appropriate behavior or redirecting the child to alternative activities. Parents of very young children must also remember to provide close supervision to prevent injuries.
- *Provide structure and routines.* Children benefit from predictability in their environments, such as morning and bedtime routines for toothbrushing, bathing, and reading. Regularly scheduled meals, snacks, and activities should be built into the children's schedule. Chores and other less preferred tasks (e.g., homework) should be interspersed with fun activities. Activities such as television, computer time, and video games should be monitored in terms of content and amount of time permitted. Quiet time is also beneficial, especially before bed or study time.
- *"Catch" the child being good.* Parents often ignore children when they behave appropriately and provide attention only when the behavior is too severe to ignore. Instead, if parents and other caregivers regularly provide attention for appropriate behavior children will learn to display the behaviors that receive reinforcement.

KEY POINTS

- Many concerns about behaviors reflect typical child development.
- Behaviors persist when they are reinforced.
- Management is effective when parents set rules and carry them out consistently.
- Both parents should have the same approach to behaviors, as much as possible.

Case 22-1

Robert is 5 years old and refuses to eat the foods that his mother or father serve to him. He will eat only chicken nuggets from a fast-food restaurant and two or three brand-name foods. He complains that he is hungry and that his stomach hurts when parents do not give him his preferred foods at a meal. Robert's mother and father would like Robert to eat what they serve him. Physical examination is remarkable for weight at the 75th percentile, height at the 25th percentile, and body mass index (BMI) is 17.8 (95th percentile).

A. What additional information do you need?
B. How would you determine what triggers and reinforces Robert's food refusal?
C. What would you recommend?

Case 22-2

Jennifer is 4 years old and does not sit on the toilet for bowel movements. She sometimes goes days without a bowel movement and complains of abdominal pain on these occasions. She sometimes sits on the toilet to urinate but often wets her pants, especially when she has held her stool for several days. Her parents would like Jennifer to be toilet trained.

A. What additional information do you need?
B. How would you determine if there are triggers and reinforcers for the toileting problems?
C. What would you recommend?

Case Answers

22-1 A. *Learning objective:* **Discuss the approach to the evaluation of behavior problems, using the history and physical examination.** Information about growth, developmental milestones, and behavior in other settings will assist with decisions about the diagnosis and management of his dysfunctional mealtime behavior. A screening developmental assessment and observation of the child's interactions with parents and other adults can provide useful information about his general development. Perform a careful physical examination to ensure that no neurologic or other developmentally important findings are overlooked. Also notice that Robert's BMI is at the 95th percentile, which suggests that his behavior has promoted excessive weight gain and may have negative physical consequences.

22-1 B. *Learning objective:* **Identify the triggers and reinforcers for problem behaviors.** Ask his parents what they do when Robert refuses to eat and complains of being hungry. If they give him his favorite foods, it is likely that they are reinforcing his refusal and complaints by doing this. Specific observation of mealtime behaviors can assist with identification of the triggers for the behaviors.

22-1 C. *Learning objective:* **Discuss a basic approach to management of problem behaviors that have an identifiable trigger and/or reinforcer.** Behavior is likely reinforced by gaining access to favorite foods. Changing the parental response to his behaviors will likely improve his behavior. It will also affect his overall health because he is overweight and should be managed by decreasing calorie intake. Parents should be advised to offer only foods prepared for the entire family and to stop offering "fast foods" that reinforce Robert's behaviors. They can schedule occasional times when Robert is allowed to have his favorite foods, but this "reward" will only happen if he eats the meals served to him. Parents will need patience and support to carry out this management plan. They may need nutritional advice from a dietician concerning appropriate portion size and calorie needs. Regular exercise such as scheduled walks will also be beneficial for weight management. If behavior is severely disruptive to the family, referral to a child psychologist familiar with management of eating behavior will be needed.

22-2 A. *Learning objective:* **Identify possible behavioral and physical causes of problem behaviors.** Because the problem behavior relates to bowel movements, constipation, and enuresis, you should first identify any medical conditions. The history would focus on obtaining more information about bowel habits, the interventions that have been tried, presence of any illnesses or medical conditions, and family history of constipation. Find out if she was ever toilet trained for urine or stool or is in process of such training. Assess whether Jennifer shows readiness signs for toilet training, especially whether she can "bear down" to have a bowel movement. Identify any history of painful bowel movements. Ask parents if they can tell if Jennifer feels the urge for a bowel movement or urination. Ask whether she is dry when she awakens in the morning or after a nap. Ask parents if they have a toileting schedule to give Jennifer opportunities to use the toilet. A thorough physical examination (including a rectal examination) would identify anatomic or neurologic problems. Laboratory testing would identify hypothyroidism, if clinical evidence suggests this diagnosis. An abdominal radiograph may help identify the extent of stool impaction in the large bowel.

22-2 B. *Learning objective:* **Identify triggers and reinforcers for problem behavior.** If Jennifer has a past history of constipation, she may avoid sitting on the toilet because large, painful bowel movements may have caused her to "withhold" stool, worsening the constipation. Often, children engaged in play are "too busy" to sit on the toilet, which promotes constipation. Ask parents what happens if they interrupt her play to take her to the toilet to sit for a short time. Does she have tantrums? If problem behaviors occur with prompts to use the toilet, and if parents let her out of toilet sitting to avoid the tantrums, they may be reinforcing her refusal to use the toilet. This worsens constipation and leads to further stool withholding.

22-2 C. *Learning objective:* **Discuss management for problem behaviors that have identified triggers and reinforcers.** Develop a toileting schedule that includes toilet sitting at times that Jennifer may be most likely to have a bowel movement or urinate. Reinforce sitting on the toilet for brief times. Activities or highly desired items can be used to reinforce Jennifer's successful use of the toilet. Encourage a high-fiber diet, and use laxatives and enemas as needed to control constipation, if that is a component of stool withholding behavior.

23

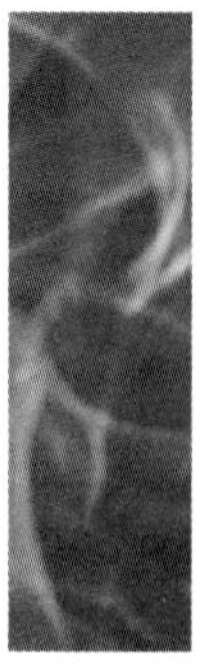

Chest Pain

NORMAN B. BERMAN

ETIOLOGY

What Are the Most Common Causes of Chest Pain?

Cardiac causes of chest pain are rare in children. Atherosclerotic coronary artery disease is essentially nonexistent in otherwise healthy children. Most chest pain in children originates in the chest wall, not in the heart. Despite this, parents often seek medical attention for a child who has chest pain because they are concerned about a "heart attack" or that the child is at risk for sudden death. These concerns are often prompted by recent events in the family or in the news.

What Are the Noncardiac Causes of Chest Pain?

Precordial catch is the term given to a chest pain that is common in adolescents. The pain is described as sharp, brief, and occurring sporadically, unassociated with exertion. One of the most characteristic features of this type of chest pain is the exacerbation by deep inspiration. *Costochondritis* is a less common chest wall pain that is due to inflammation of the costochondral joint. This pain is characterized by tenderness to palpation over the sternum and is typically much longer lasting than the precordial catch pain. Gastroesophageal reflux and other gastrointestinal causes are less common, as are pulmonary causes such as asthma or pneumothorax.

What Are the Cardiac Causes of Chest Pain?

Structural cardiac causes of chest pain

Hypertrophic cardiomyopathy and congenital coronary artery anomalies are the most common causes of sudden cardiac death in children and, as such, must always be considered in a child presenting with chest pain. Congenital heart defects are *unlikely* to cause chest pain, with the exception of severe aortic stenosis. Cardiac chest pain is uncommon but possible in children with repaired congenital heart defects.

Acquired cardiac causes of chest pain

Pericarditis is an uncommon but important cardiac cause of chest pain. Pericarditis causes a pericardial effusion to develop and thus can lead to cardiac tamponade. Pericarditis typically presents acutely with severe persistent chest pain. There is often an associated fever and respiratory symptoms.

Myocarditis is also uncommon. It often presents with signs of congestive heart failure because it impairs ventricular function. Myocarditis can cause anginal chest pain and should be considered in a patient with signs of congestive heart failure and chest pain.

Kawasaki disease is a fairly common disorder of unknown etiology. Kawasaki disease typically presents with prolonged fever (> 5 days) and other signs of vasculitis. Coronary artery aneurysms develop in up to 20% of patients with Kawasaki disease who are not treated with intravenous immunoglobulin. Aneurysms place the child at risk for myocardial ischemia and infarction, with accompanying chest pain.

Tachyarrhythmias generally do *not* cause chest pain, but some young children will describe their palpitations as chest pain.

EVALUATION

Can I Distinguish Chest Wall Pain from Cardiac Pain?

Onset. Precordial catch chest pain typically occurs sporadically, unassociated with exertion. Cardiac causes of chest pain are much more likely to be exertional.

Duration. Precordial catch chest pain is typically brief, lasting only seconds to a few minutes. Ischemic chest pain typically lasts for 10 to 15 minutes, rarely less than 1 minute.

Description. Precordial catch chest pain is typically described as sharp and is often well localized. Angina is described as a pressure or crushing sensation.

Relation to respiration. Precordial catch chest pain is classically made worse by deep inspiration. This is one of the most useful ways to distinguish it from other causes of chest pain.

Relation to exertion. Precordial catch chest pain is unrelated to exertion. Pain may occur with exercise but just as often occurs at rest. Angina occurs almost exclusively with some inciting event, usually exertion but also stress.

What Diagnostic Testing Is Needed?

A good history and physical examination are by far the most important parts of the evaluation of chest pain in children. A history consistent with chest wall pain in a child with a normal physical examination is reassuring and no further evaluation is necessary. A history of exertional chest pain that is described as pressurelike may warrant further evaluation. An electrocardiogram (ECG) is a good starting point in the diagnostic evaluation. Many cardiac causes of chest pain will present with an abnormal ECG (hypertrophic cardiomyopathy, pericarditis, myocarditis). Of course, a normal ECG cannot rule out cardiac causes of chest pain. A chest radiograph is also reasonable and can help rule out trauma and some pulmonary causes of chest pain. Referral to a pediatric cardiologist is reasonable if there remains uncertainty about the cause of the chest pain. The pediatric cardiologist may decide to order an echocardiogram to rule out hypertrophic cardiomyopathy and coronary artery anomalies. An exercise stress test may also be performed, depending on the details of the child's presentation.

TREATMENT

How Do I Treat Chest Wall Pain?

In most cases, no treatment is needed. Precordial catch chest pains are benign, do not indicate the presence of heart disease, do not place the child at any increased risk for adverse events, and are self-limited. No restrictions in activity are warranted for children with chest wall pain. *Explain* the benign nature of chest wall pain to families in a confident and reassuring manner. Make certain that the family understands why you think the chest pain is benign and why it is not cardiac in origin. In reassuring a family about an issue like chest pain, it is important to always "leave the door open," so that if the child's symptoms change the parents will feel comfortable coming back to you for reevaluation. Ibuprofen can be helpful at alleviating the pain of costochondritis.

KEY POINTS

- Cardiac causes of chest pain are rare in children and adolescents.
- Most chest pain originates in the chest wall.
- Precordial catch causes a sharp, brief pain that is aggravated by deep inspiration; it is not associated with exertion.
- The history is the most important diagnostic tool.

Case 23-1

An otherwise healthy 15-year-old boy presents with complaints of chest pains that have been occurring for the last year. The pains occur sporadically and are described as "sharp." The pains are made worse by deep inspiration and then resolve on their own in less than 1 minute.

A. What are the most common causes of chest pain in children?
B. What are the important cardiac causes of chest pain in children and how does this differ from adults?
C. What evaluation is needed for a patient who has the symptoms described?

Case Answers

23-1 A. *Learning objective:* **Discuss the common causes of chest pain in childhood.** Chest wall pain accounts for most chest pain in children. Examples include the "precordial catch syndrome" in older children and adolescents and costochondritis. Pain can also result from gastroesophageal reflux, asthma, and pneumonia.

23-1 B. *Learning objective:* **Identify the cardiac causes of chest pain in childhood, recognizing that they are uncommon and differ importantly from cardiac causes of pain in adults.** The important cardiac causes of chest pain in children and adolescents include hypertrophic cardiomyopathy, coronary artery anomalies, myocarditis, and pericarditis. The rare child with advanced Kawasaki disease and coronary artery aneurysms may have ischemic chest pain. Chest pain from coronary artery disease is otherwise extremely uncommon in children, in contrast to adult patients. Despite its uncommon occurrence, myocardial ischemia ("heart pain") is high on the list of worries expressed by patients and their parents. Your evaluation and management must address these concerns, although you do not need to do excessive testing.

23-1 C. *Learning objective:* **Discuss the management of chest wall pain.** Children and adolescents who have typical chest wall pain require no further evaluation. Electrocardiogram and chest radiograph are not necessary. An explanation of your clinical decision-making and the criteria on which it is based will ensure that patients and families understand that chest wall pain is not associated with heart disease.

24

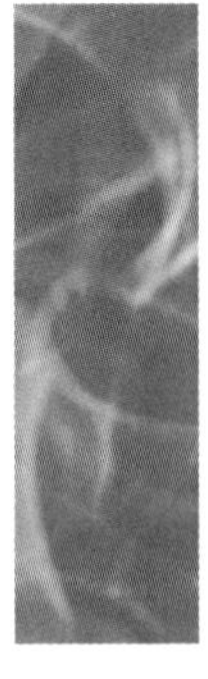

Child Abuse and Neglect

CINDY W. CHRISTIAN

ETIOLOGY

What Should I Know about Child Abuse and Neglect?

After medical school, you will be mandated by law in all 50 states and in Canada to identify and report suspected child maltreatment and to work with child protection services to protect vulnerable children. Physicians in all areas of medical practice will encounter child abuse and family violence and must identify, report, and subsequently manage the families.

How Is Child Abuse Defined?

Abuse includes all behaviors that are destructive to the normal physical or emotional development of a child. Although laws vary somewhat, only parents and guardians may be reported for physical or emotional abuse and neglect, whereas any adult may be reported for sexual abuse. Medical professionals may have cultural or religious beliefs, family upbringing, or personal experiences that influence their own perceptions of abuse, but such differences must not prevent compliance with state-specific statutes that define abuse and codify the requirements for its identification and reporting.

How Common Is Child Maltreatment?

Each year, nearly 3 million reports of suspected maltreatment are made to child protection services in the United States, and approximately 1 million of these reports are confirmed. Thousands of childhood deaths each year are attributed to abuse, primarily in children younger than 3 years. These numbers represent only official reports. The true prevalence of child abuse is unknown, because many maltreated children are not brought to the attention of public agencies. Child protection agencies are overwhelmed with referrals and can only investigate approximately 60% of reports. Furthermore, after investigation, only 55% of child victims receive services.

Does Child Abuse Have Long-Term Effects for Adults?

Recent studies in California found that more than 10% of adults suffered physical and psychological abuse as children and more than 20% reported childhood sexual abuse. Childhood exposure to socially adverse experiences such as child abuse, living with addicted parents, domestic violence, and incarcerated parents was associated with higher rates of diseases and medical problems that predict adult morbidity and early mortality.

What Factors Are Associated with Child Abuse?

Child abuse results from the complex interaction of individual, familial, and societal risk factors (Table 24-1). These are broad markers of abuse and neglect, not strong individual determinants. You must have a high index of suspicion for abuse but must not rely solely on sociodemographic variables.

Is Poverty a Risk Factor for Abuse and Neglect?

Children from families with annual incomes less than $15,000 experience some form of abuse far more often than do children from families with annual incomes more than $30,000. In particular, poor children have high rates of educational neglect, serious physical injury, and sexual abuse. Substantiation rates for abuse and neglect rise as poverty level worsens.

Are Parental Mental Health Problems Associated with Abuse and Neglect?

Substance abuse and maternal depression are strongly associated with child maltreatment. Substance abuse rates are high among abusive

Table 24-1

Risk Factors Associated with Child Abuse

Risk Factors Associated with Child Abuse
Societal Risk Factors
Poverty
Unemployment
Parental Risk Factors
Substance abuse
Maternal depression
History of childhood abuse
Domestic violence
Children of teenage mothers
Social isolation
Single-parent household
Non-related adult in the home
Child Risk Factors
Disability, including prematurity
Female gender (sexual abuse)
Male gender (emotional neglect and serious injuries)

parents, and rates of child maltreatment are high among substance abusers. Approximately 70% of families involved with the child protection system are affected by substance abuse. Depression is also a strong risk factor for physical abuse as it is highly prevalent in both the general population and among parents of abused children.

Does Abuse in Childhood Predispose a Parent to Abuse?

Intergenerational transmission of abuse is *not* inevitable. Although approximately one-third of adults who were abused in childhood later abuse or neglect their own children, the fact that an adult was abused does not in and of itself justify an investigation for possible child abuse. It *is* important, however, to assess an adult's personal history of abuse when evaluating suspected child abuse.

Does Domestic Violence Increase Risk of Child Abuse?

The concurrence of child abuse and domestic violence approaches 50% in population-based studies. In families with severe domestic violence, the child abuse rates are even greater.

Do Child Factors Contribute to Maltreatment?

Children are never blamed for their maltreatment, but a number of child factors can be identified in cases of abuse.

- Gender: *Girls* are victims of sexual abuse three times more often than boys. *Boys* sustain more serious physical injuries and more emotional neglect than girls.
- Age: The youngest children sustain the most serious injuries.
- Race: There are no significant racial differences in the incidence of abuse, but poor black children are more likely than white children to be found in the child protective service system.
- Prematurity, chronic illness, and congenital abnormalities increase risk of abuse.

EVALUATION

How Are Abused Children Identified?

The diagnosis of child abuse requires a high level of suspicion based on a detailed history, a thorough physical examination, and careful interpretation of laboratory and radiographic tests. Obvious signs of battering are not always found. In most cases, discrepancies between the history of trauma and the resulting injuries suggest the diagnosis and trigger an evaluation.

What Clinical Clues Suggest Abuse?

The history provided by the adult accompanying the child is often inaccurate or deliberately falsified. Victims of abuse are often too young, too ill, or too scared to provide a history of their assault. Abused children may manifest behavioral problems, but no single behavior is pathognomonic for abuse. Ask about family violence and sexual abuse and look for unexplained or characteristic injuries. Table 24-2 lists clinical clues that suggest abuse.

Which Bruises Should I Worry About?

Bruises are universal in healthy ambulatory children, but they are also the most common injuries identified in abused children. You must evaluate all bruises in nonambulatory infants and bruises that are patterned or in unusual distributions or locations. Mongolian spots and cultural practices such as "coining" may be mistaken for bruises caused by abuse. Illnesses that cause bruising may be mistaken for child abuse, including idiopathic thrombocytopenic purpura (ITP), hemophilia, vitamin K deficiency, Henoch-Schonlein purpura, and other coagulopathies. If a bleeding diathesis is suspected, screen with a complete blood count, platelet count, prothrombin time, partial thromboplastin time, von Willebrand panel, and an evaluation for platelet function.

Which Burns Are Suspicious for Abuse?

Inflicted burns often have patterns characteristic of the abuse mechanism and not possible with accidental injury. For example, burns caused by immersion in scalding water are found on the feet, lower legs, buttocks, and genitals and have clear lines of demarcation, sparing the areas above the water line. Burns inflicted by contact with hot solids, such as irons, radiators, stoves, or cigarettes may leave characteristic marks. Confusion occasionally occurs with toxin-mediated staphylococcal and streptococcal infections, impetigo, phytophotodermatitis, and diaper dermatitis, which can mimic abusive burns. The history and subsequent evaluation clarify the cause.

Table 24-2

Clinical Clues or "Red Flags" That Suggest Child Abuse

"Magical" injuries	Injuries without a history of trauma
History not consistent with findings	Serious injury attributed to simple household trauma or injury inflicted by a sibling
History changes over time	Varying explanations are offered as new findings emerge
History is not consonant with development	The injury is said to be self-inflicted or caused by a young sibling but is not consistent with developmental ability
Delay in seeking medical attention	Time and date of the injury must be correlated with time and date of seeking medical attention so that an explanation for the delay can be sought
Injuries diagnostic of abuse	Abused children often have multiple injuries of varying ages or patterns of injury that cannot be explained by any accidental mechanism

How Are Inflicted Fractures Identified?

No single fracture is diagnostic of child abuse. Inflicted fractures are more common in infants and young children but can be seen in all ages. Fractures in nonambulatory children should raise concern. Once children become ambulatory, accidental fractures become more common. Be suspicious of multiple or unusual fractures, and fractures of posterior ribs, metaphyses, vertebral bodies, or the scapula. Fractures of different ages raise the concern for abuse. Uncommon diseases can mimic abusive injuries, although most have other clinical manifestations that distinguish them from abuse. Children with suspicious fractures *must* be evaluated with a radiologic skeletal survey.

Is Abdominal Trauma Associated with Abuse?

Abusive abdominal injury is underrecognized and underreported because it is usually caused by blunt trauma and causes nonspecific symptoms and few external findings. Severe abdominal injury is an uncommon manifestation of abuse but can cause solid organ injury, perforation of a hollow viscus, or shearing of mesenteric vessels. Abused children tend to have multiple-organ injury, whereas accidentally injured children more commonly sustain single-organ trauma.

What Causes Death of Abused Children?

Brain injury from impact, shaking with sudden deceleration, or both is the leading cause of mortality and morbidity from physical abuse. Fathers and boyfriends most often inflict head trauma, but mothers, babysitters, and other caregivers also inflict injury. Victims of abusive head injury are generally younger than 3 years and most are infants. An infant or young child with altered mental status, unexplained lethargy, irritability, seizures, or coma *must* be evaluated for abusive head injury. History of trauma is usually minimal or lacking. Most infants with abusive head injury have retinal hemorrhages when examined by an ophthalmologist. Computed tomography (CT) scan of the head typically reveals subdural hemorrhage, often in the posterior interhemispheric fissure. Cerebral edema and subsequent infarction may not be present initially but commonly appear later. All victims of abusive head trauma require a careful physical examination and a radiologic skeletal survey to screen for other trauma. Death among victims of abusive head injury is often the result of uncontrolled intracranial pressure. Abused children with head trauma have worse outcomes than children with accidental head injury.

How Is Child Sexual Abuse Identified?

A sexually abused child is most commonly identified because the victim discloses the abuse to a parent, teacher, relative, or friend. In some cases, a child exhibits concerning behaviors and further evaluation leads to disclosure of abuse. Much less commonly, physical injury or a sexually transmitted disease leads to the diagnosis of sexual abuse.

How Common Is Genital Injury in Sexual Abuse?

Only 5% to 10% of sexually abused children have genital injuries identified at the medical evaluation. Most child sexual abuse involves activities that do not cause physical injury to a child's genitals, such as fondling, oral-genital contact, or vulvar coitus. Because children typically do not disclose the abuse in a timely way, minor injuries are likely to have healed by the time a physical examination is done. Although injury may occasionally be identified if a child is examined immediately after an abusive episode, the diagnosis of child sexual abuse does *not* require the identification of injury.

How Do I Identify Domestic Violence?

Screening for domestic violence in primary care practice may successfully uncover or prevent child abuse (Table 24-3). Talk with adolescents about abusive relationships.

TREATMENT

What Are My Responsibilities If I Identify Child Abuse?

Your chief responsibility as a medical student is to notify the supervising faculty or resident of your concerns. Laws intended to identify and protect maltreated children are specifically written to encourage early reporting of suspected abuse and do not require certainty that the child was abused. Physicians who report in good faith are protected from liability if the abuse is not confirmed, but *failing to report abuse* can result in criminal and civil penalties. All cases of sexual abuse, and many cases of physical abuse, *must* be reported to law enforcement agencies for police investigation. Although emotionally difficult and time consuming, reporting suspected maltreatment for further investigation can save or improve a child's life.

What Should I Say to the Family If I Suspect Abuse?

You should not discuss suspected abuse with a family without the direct involvement of a faculty physician. You will probably participate as a member of the team that informs the parents of an abused child about the plans for medical treatment, investigation, and follow-up. The conversation should focus on the welfare and well-being of the

Table 24-3

Some Clues to Domestic Violence
Parental alcoholism, drug abuse, or depression
History of marital turmoil
Mother is always accompanied by a controlling, domineering spouse or partner
Mother has bruises or inflicted trauma or gives a history of such trauma
Overconcern (frequent visits) for minor illnesses
Underconcern (missed appointments) for serious illnesses

child, not on apportioning blame. Displays of anger or disgust are not productive or professional.

How Do I Document Abuse?

A detailed medical history, descriptions of physical findings, results of any tests and imaging studies, and all medical diagnoses must be entered in the medical record. Include drawings and/or photographs of injuries at the time of the initial medical evaluation. This record is invaluable if physician testimony is needed for civil or criminal hearings.

Can Child Abuse Be Prevented?

Primary prevention programs, including the early nurse home visitation program for first-time young mothers that was developed more than 25 years ago by David Olds, reduce rates of abuse and neglect. Pediatricians have an important role in prevention of family violence and child maltreatment because they are trusted by families and can provide

- Anticipatory guidance regarding discipline
- Developmental information to help parents have realistic expectations
- Routine screening for domestic violence, substance abuse, and maternal depression
- Information about community resources for high-risk families

KEY POINTS

- Licensed medical professionals are mandatory reporters of abuse.
- Abuse occurs commonly but is underreported.
- Suspect inflicted trauma when injuries are not consistent with the history and/or the child's developmental stage.
- A diagnosis of sexual abuse does not require physical findings of genital trauma.

Case 24-1

A 2-month-old baby presents with lethargy and is poorly responsive. He has a small facial bruise identified on physical examination. Further evaluation reveals subdural hemorrhage and healing rib fractures.

A. Why are you concerned?
B. To whom would you report this incident?
C. What would you say to the baby's parents?

Case 24-2

A 4-month-old presents to the emergency department with inconsolable crying. The physical examination reveals tenderness and swelling of the left thigh. Radiograph reveals an acute fracture of the femur. The parents report that the baby rolled off the couch that morning.

A. How would you further assess the baby?
B. What specific issues must you address in your evaluation?
C. Should this infant be reported to child protection services?

Case 24-3

A 7-year-old girl is brought to your office after disclosing to her mother that an adult male cousin had sexually abused her over a period of many months. She tells you that her cousin put his "private" in her "butt." She has an unremarkable physical examination at your office, without evidence of genital trauma.

A. Was this child sexually abused?
B. Should this case be reported? To whom should the report be made?
C. Should this child have cultures done to identify possible sexually transmitted disease (STD)?

Case Answers

24-1 A. *Learning objective:* **Identify the child who has been subjected to intentional injury (child abuse) from history, physical examination, and imaging studies.** The infant is a victim of abusive head injury and has been repeatedly injured, as evidenced by the healing rib fractures. Lethargy and poor responsiveness indicate the need for urgent intervention and evaluation.

24-1 B. *Learning objective:* **Discuss the responsibilities of the "mandatory reporter" of abuse, and indicate to whom a report must be made.** You must report to child protective services, and because of the severity of the injuries, in this case you must also report to the police. Child protective service social workers will determine the circumstances in which the child was abused and plan for the ongoing safety of the child. They will work with families to lessen future risks for children and improve family functioning. The police investigate the possibility that a crime has been committed. In some jurisdictions, child protective services and the police work together to investigate child maltreatment. Each state has laws that define reporting methods for suspected child maltreatment. All physicians, healthcare providers, and individuals working with children are *mandated* reporters of suspected child maltreatment and should be aware of local practice for filing a report.

24-1 C. *Learning objective:* **Explain an approach to communication with a family whose child has been abused.** Conversations with parents about child abuse are among the most difficult for physicians, but they can be done professionally and in a caring manner. The task is often anxiety-provoking for the physician, but it is critical for maintenance of the patient/family/physician relationship. Although parents may be angry at the suggestion of child abuse, you will observe experienced physicians use many of the following strategies to lessen confrontation and anger: Frame the conversation around the safety and well-being of the child. Avoid being accusatory, as you are not the investigator, judge, or jury. Explain to the parents that the findings suggest (or clearly indicate) that someone has hurt the child and that the investigation of the injuries is for the child's ongoing health and safety. Ask the parents if they have been concerned about or are aware of anyone who might have hurt the child. Explain your responsibility, but do not hide behind your legal mandate (i.e., do NOT say, "I don't really think it is abuse, but the law says I have to report it."). Tell the family what to expect and make a follow-up plan with the family, so they know that you will not abandon them.

24-2 A. *Learning objective:* **Describe the key historical issues in the assessment of intentional trauma, focusing on mechanism of the injury.** Infants who have not begun to walk rarely experience a fall that results in an injury or a fracture. Femur fracture is especially uncommon. You should obtain a thorough history regarding the activities leading up to the reported fall. You must identify the person(s) who witnessed the fall, where family members were at the time of the fall, how the baby reacted, and what the parental response was to the baby. Obtain a social history of the family, inquire about any family history of bone diseases and fractures, and obtain a feeding history for the baby. You must assess risk factors for rickets, osteogenesis imperfecta (OI), or other metabolic diseases.

24-2 B. *Learning objective:* **Outline the physical examination and imaging, and laboratory evaluation for a child with unexplained trauma.** The child must have a thorough physical examination to document all injuries. It is important to check the hair, mouth, palms, soles, and skin creases for injury and to look carefully for signs of diseases that can lead to pathologic fractures (e.g., abnormally blue sclera, large fontanel, and joint laxity, all of which occur in children with osteogenesis imperfecta). Injuries should be documented carefully and photographed. In addition, the child's overall level of care should be assessed. Growth parameters should be obtained and plotted. A skeletal survey must be done to detect or rule out occult fractures and to assess bone structure. Additionally, screening for bone mineralization can be done by measuring blood levels of calcium, phosphorus, and alkaline phosphatase. CT of the head and ophthalmologic examination are recommended if inflicted head trauma is suspected.

24-2 C. *Learning objective:* **Discuss the criteria used to decide whether a report should be made to child protective services.** If the evaluation yields *any* positive findings, such as an inconsistent history, presence of risk factors, additional injuries or fractures, or evidence of neglect, a report *must* be made to child protective services. If the evaluation is negative, it is still reasonable to report the matter to child protective services, given the child's young age and the knowledge that young infants are at greatest risk for inflicted fractures.

24-3 A. *Learning objective:* **Discuss the findings from the history and physical examination that raise concern about sexual abuse.** The child's history raises the concern of child sexual abuse and provides the key information. Always take a report by a child seriously. The child's unremarkable physical examination does not diminish the likelihood of sexual abuse. The majority of sexually abused children will have a normal genital examination when seen by a physician because (1) the child's genitals were never injured or (2) injuries to the child's genitals have healed by the time the examination is performed. Few genital findings are specifically diagnostic of sexual abuse.

24-3 B. *Learning objective:* **Discuss the responsibilities of the mandatory reporter concerning possible sexual abuse.** This case *must* be reported to both social services and the police. Remember that sexual abuse of a child is a crime, which mandates police involvement in the investigation. The physician's role is to identify the concern, not to make the final determination of abuse.

24-3 C. *Learning objective:* **Discuss the risks of sexually transmitted disease (STD) in cases of sexual abuse, and identify patients for whom cultures or other diagnostic tests should be performed.** Because she has no evidence of genital trauma and no signs of infection, cultures may not be needed for this patient. The need for STI screening should be based on clinical judgment. Universal screening is not recommended but it is more common now that nucleic acid amplification testing (NAAT) is available. In prepubertal children, cultures for *Neisseria gonorrhoeae* and *Chlamydia* should be obtained if there are symptoms or signs of an infection. If the child has no symptoms and the examination does not identify trauma or infection, the likelihood of identifying STI is low. After discussing the child's examination and reporting requirements with the family, the need for counseling should be discussed. Most children are thought to benefit from counseling after sexual abuse.

BIBLIOGRAPHY

DiScala C, Sege R, Li G, Reece RM: Child abuse and unintentional injuries: A 10-year restrospective, *Arch Pediatr Adolesc Med* 154:16, 2000.

Duhaime AC, Christian CW, Rorke LB, Zimmerman RA: Nonaccidental head injury in infants: the "shaken baby syndrome," *N Engl J Med* 338:1822, 1998.

Felitti VJ, Anda RF, Nordenberg D et al: Relationship of childhood abuse and household dysfunction to many of the leading causes of death in adults. The Adverse Childhood Experiences (ACE) Study, *Am J Prev Med* 14:245, 2998.

Reece R, Ludwig S, editors: *Child abuse: medical diagnosis and management*, Philadelphia, 2001, Lippincott, Williams & Wilkins.

Sedlak AJ, Broadhurst DD: *The Third National Incidence Study of Child Abuse and Neglect*, Washington, DC, 1996, US Department of Health and Human Services.

Sugar NF, Taylor JA, Feldman KW: Bruises in infants and toddlers: those who don't cruise rarely bruise, *Arch Pediatr Adolesc Med* 153:399, 1999.

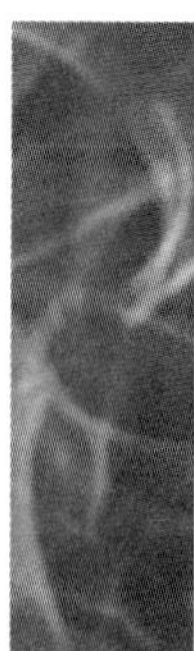

25

Cough

TIMOTHY D. STARNER and
ROBIN R. DETERDING

ETIOLOGY

What Is Cough?

Cough is a reflex to remove mucus and other material from the airways that is triggered by stimulation of receptors located between the pharynx and terminal bronchioles. Afferent signals from cough receptors are sent via the vagus and glossopharyngeal nerves to the cough centers in the brainstem and pons. Efferent signals travel through the vagus, phrenic, and spinal motor nerves to the larynx, diaphragm, and muscles of the chest wall, abdomen, and pelvic floor.

What Causes Acute Cough?

In children, acute cough (< 3 weeks) is usually the result of infection. Most of these are viral upper respiratory illnesses. The cough from a viral respiratory illness usually improves within 1 week. Asthma is the next most common cause of cough, but distinguishing between asthma and viral respiratory infections can be difficult initially because exacerbations of asthma in children are often associated with upper respiratory infections. Bronchiolitis or bronchopneumonia from respiratory syncytial virus and other viruses tends to occur in seasonal epidemics and affects young infants most severely. Bacterial pneumonias in infants and children are less common than viral infections, and the patient with bacterial pneumonia usually appears more ill and has crackles, higher fever, and more tachypnea.

What Causes Chronic Cough?

Chronic cough persists for more than 3 weeks in children (Table 25-1). Asthma is the most common cause. Many of these children will have chronic asthma, but even intermittent asthmatic patients can have a lingering cough from an acute exacerbation of asthma that lasts longer than 3 weeks. Infectious etiologies include bacterial or viral pneumonias,

Table 25-1

Causes of Chronic Cough in Children

Infant	Preschool	School Age/Adolescent
Congenital anomalies	Foreign body	Asthma
Tracheoesophageal fistula	Infections	Postnasal drip
Airway malacia	Viral	GERD
Infections	Mycoplasma	Infections
Viral	Pertussis	Viral
Chlamydia	Bacterial	Mycoplasma
Pertussis	Asthma	Cystic fibrosis
Asthma	Cystic fibrosis	Irritant (smoking)
Cystic fibrosis	Irritant (passive smoke)	Habit cough

GERD, Gastroesophageal reflux disease.

although most pneumonias cause acute cough. Both *Bordetella pertussis* (whooping cough) and *Mycoplasma* pneumonia (walking pneumonia) are particularly well known for causing cough that can last for more than 2 months. A history of exposure to adults who have chronic cough may suggest these two infections.

EVALUATION

What Are Key History and Examination Findings?

Table 25-2 lists pertinent history and physical examination findings for common causes of cough in children.

What Tests Help to Evaluate Cough?

Pulse oximetry should be obtained if there is concern for anything more than a mild viral upper respiratory illness. This quickly identifies hypoxia, which can result from ventilation-perfusion mismatch in asthma and pneumonia. A chest x-ray should be obtained in all patients with chronic cough and for selected patients with acute cough if they have either unusual or confusing history or significant physical examination findings. If a child is old enough to perform pulmonary function testing (usually about 5 to 6 years old), spirometry can detect airway obstruction. Forced vital capacity (FVC), forced expiratory volume in 1 second (FEV_1), and expiratory fraction from 25% to 75% of vital capacity ($FEF_{25\%-75\%}$) give the most useful information. The usual pattern for airway obstruction is that $FEF_{25\%-75\%}$ is more decreased than FEV_1, which is more decreased than FVC. In addition, the FEV_1/FVC ratio is > 0.80. If cystic fibrosis is suspected, a sweat chloride test should be obtained using the Gibson-Cooke pilocarpine iontophoresis method. The conductance-method screening test for sweat chloride *is not reliable.* A barium swallow or esophageal pH probe may be useful if gastroesophageal reflux disease (GERD) and aspiration are suspected.

Table 25-2

History and Physical Examination in the Evaluation of Cough

Cause	History	Examination
Asthma	Recent viral infection Similar episodes with past URIs Increased cough at night Wheezing or shortness of breath Cold/exercise aggravate cough Family or personal history of asthma, allergies, or eczema	Increased work of breathing (retractions, accessory muscle use, nasal flaring) Wheezing or coughing Prolonged expiratory time Difficulty completing sentences Hyperinflated chest
Bronchitis or pneumonia	Cough Rapid breathing Fever Poor feeding Acute onset Exposures to illness (daycare) Decreased energy/activity	Increased respiratory rate Increased work of breathing (retractions, accessory muscle use, nasal flaring) Crackles Diminished breath sounds
GERD	Coughing, gagging, or spitting up with or after meals Symptoms worse when supine	Back arching (infants) Frequent regurgitation or spitting up
Cystic fibrosis	Poor weight gain Frequent stools Sputum production	Protuberant abdomen (infants) Hepatomegaly Clubbing (advanced disease)

GERD, Gastroesophageal reflux disease; URIs, upper respiratory infections.

How Does a Therapeutic Trial Help with Diagnosis?

Empirical therapeutic trials can help identify the cause of a cough in children. If *asthma* is suspected, a trial with an adequate dose of oral corticosteroids should result in complete resolution of the cough within 10 days. If the cough does not fully resolve, other etiologies should be investigated. Response to a β-agonist, such as albuterol, is also suggestive of asthma but is less reliable than a steroid trial because it does not reverse inflammation. If GERD is suspected, an initial approach is to advise parents to give small, frequent feedings or to thicken formula with rice cereal; keep the child upright for at least 30 minutes after meals. Elevating the head of the bed to about 30 degrees is also useful, but pillows or car seats are not recommended because they can bend the infant at the waist and increase intraabdominal pressure on the stomach. If a therapeutic trial is chosen, either an H2-blocker or proton pump inhibitor may be used alone or in combination with a prokinetic agent (metoclopramide [Reglan]). The trial should last at least 1 month before assessing its impact. Of note, therapeutic trials in children can be more difficult than in infants, so adherence to the treatment plan must be assessed carefully, especially with oral steroids.

TREATMENT

How Do I Manage Acute Infectious Cough?

Most acute coughs are caused by viral illnesses and do not require antibiotic treatment. Community-acquired pneumonia should be treated with appropriate antibiotics.

What Medications Relieve Symptoms?

For asthmatic patients, a β-agonist bronchodilator such as inhaled albuterol should be prescribed first. Because airway inflammation is common in acute exacerbations and poorly controlled chronic asthma, oral steroids may be needed (see Chapter 69). If the cough is caused by GERD, proton pump inhibitors and prokinetic agents may be useful. Over-the-counter cough and cold medicines have not been shown to be effective in children (Paul et al., 2004) and may cause adverse outcomes (MMWR, 2007). The Food and Drug Administration is currently considering recommending that these preparations not be used in children, especially those younger than 2 years. Narcotic-containing cough suppressants, such as codeine, can be used for severe coughing at night but are contraindicated for use in infants younger than 6 months because of the increased risk of sudden infant death syndrome. An evidence-based guideline for managing chronic cough was recently published (Chang et al., 2006).

When Should I Refer a Patient to a Specialist?

There are no hard-and-fast rules about when to refer a patient for a persistent cough. Generally, a decision is based on the severity of the cough, its persistence, the physician's comfort level for management, and the family's level of concern. In general, patients are referred to a specialist when the cough does not respond to therapeutic trial of steroids or antibiotics, has been difficult to control, or the history is complicated and/or confusing.

KEY POINTS

- Most acute coughs are caused by viral upper respiratory infection.
- Asthma is a common cause of acute, chronic, and recurring cough.
- Viral upper respiratory infections often exacerbate asthma.
- Over-the-counter (OTC) cough suppressants are ineffective.

Case 25-1

A 2-year-old child presents to the clinic with a cough that started 5 weeks ago when he caught a bad cold from his 5-year-old brother. The cough is present all the time and sometimes is so bad that it makes him throw up. He has had two other similar coughing episodes with colds that cleared up slowly each time. There is no fever. His weight is following the curve at the 10th percentile. Otherwise, he has been healthy and has no complaints. On physical examination lung fields are clear.

A. What additional information from the history will assist you to narrow the differential diagnosis for this patient?
B. What is the most likely diagnosis for this patient?
C. What testing will assist with the diagnosis of this child's cough?
D. What treatment might be effective?

Case Answers

25-1 A. *Learning objective:* **Use the history to develop a differential diagnosis for cough.** Important additional information includes immunization status (specifically pertussis vaccine) and family history of asthma or atopic disorders. Exposure history such as siblings, other family members, and daycare often provides information about infections. Ask if the child's physical activity is limited by his cough. In addition, if any medications have been tried, such as "cough syrup" or albuterol, the child's response should be noted.

25-1 B. *Learning objective:* **Discriminate among the different causes of cough using history and physical examination.** Virally triggered asthma is the most likely diagnosis. Wheezing is not always present in such patients. Recurrent cough with upper respiratory infections and persistence of cough during and after such infections are common with this diagnosis. During a coughing episode you may see hyperinflation of the chest and use of abdominal accessory muscles. Other causes of cough are less likely. Viral infection without asthma does not usually last this long or recur so often. A child in daycare, however, may have frequent upper respiratory infections. Foreign body aspiration should be on the list of diagnoses, but the recurrent nature of the cough makes this less likely. Pertussis usually occurs in community-wide outbreaks among nonimmune or partially immune children. The cough is persistent and associated with posttussive vomiting but is not recurrent. Bacterial pneumonia usually has associated fever and crackles on examination of the lung. The child with pneumonia usually appears more ill.

25-1 C. *Learning objective:* **Use laboratory and imaging tests to evaluate cough.** In this particular case, no tests are needed. He is too young for pulmonary function testing. Chest radiograph is not likely to provide information that will aid management. A therapeutic trial in the office of an inhaled bronchodilator, such as albuterol, may result in reduction of cough, or occasionally will prompt appearance of wheezing, as air exchange improves to previously poorly ventilated parts of the lungs. Complete blood count, differential white blood cell count, or other tests are not helpful.

25-1 D. *Learning objective:* **Select medications to treat chronic cough.** This child likely has asthma. Because the cough has persisted for 5 weeks, airway inflammation must be considered and treated. A bronchodilator such as albuterol plus a 5- to 7-day course of steroids usually will provide relief from the cough.

BIBLIOGRAPHY

Chang AB, Glomb WB: Guidelines for evaluating chronic cough in pediatrics: ACCP evidence-based clinical practice guidelines, *Chest* 129 (1 suppl), 260S 2006.

MMWR: Infant deaths associated with cough and cold medications—two states, 2005. *Morb Mortal Wkly Rep*, 56(1):14, 2007.

Paul IM, Yoder KE, Crowell KR et al: Effect of dextromethorphan, diphenhydramine, and placebo on nocturnal cough and sleep quality for coughing children and their parents, *Pediatrics* 114:e85, 2004.

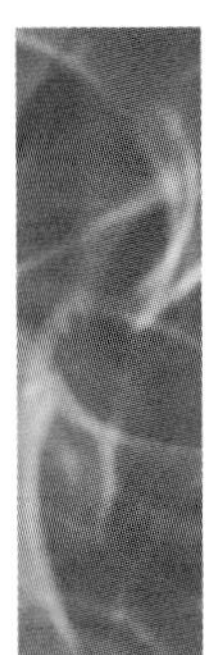

26

Dehydration/Fluids and Electrolytes

JEROLD C. WOODHEAD

ETIOLOGY

What Causes Dehydration and Electrolyte Imbalance?

Dehydration most commonly develops when diarrhea and/or vomiting cause excessive water and electrolyte loss. It may also develop from inadequate fluid intake or from other causes of excessive water and electrolyte loss (see Chapters 28, 33, 41, and 60). Severe dehydration can cause hypovolemic shock if fluid loss compromises the circulatory system. Disturbances of water and electrolyte balance may develop without dehydration, such as severe hyponatremia caused by excessive water intake ("water poisoning") and severe hypernatremia caused by excess sodium intake. Disturbances of acid/base balance may also accompany fluid and electrolyte disorders and are common in diabetic ketoacidosis.

What Are the Basics of Fluid and Electrolyte Management?

The total daily fluid requirement is the sum of maintenance + deficit + ongoing losses.

Maintenance fluids are required daily to replace p*hysiologic* fluid and electrolytes losses (Table 26-1). Holliday and Segar demonstrated that daily water and electrolyte needs depend on metabolic rate, which is highest in infants and young children. The healthy child's maintenance fluids are provided orally. Maintenance needs are increased by several mechanisms, including fever. A fluid deficit may result if adequate maintenance is not provided.

Deficit develops when a *pathologic* process, such as vomiting or diarrhea, causes excessive fluid loss, leading to dehydration. If a child does not drink an amount adequate to meet maintenance needs, a deficit develops. Fever can lead to a deficit because it causes an increase of insensible losses by approximately 13% for each degree above 38° C. Burns cause a marked loss of fluid from skin surfaces.

Ongoing losses from surgical drains or nasogastric tubes must be replaced regularly with fluid that has the appropriate water and electrolyte composition.

Table 26-1

Physiologic Fluid Losses

Fluid Loss	Component (% Maintenance)	
Sensible fluid loss (55%)	Urine (50%)	Stool (5%)
Insensible fluid loss (45%)	Skin (30%)	Lungs (15%)

How Is Dehydration Classified?

Dehydration is classified by the serum sodium concentration:

Isonatremic dehydration is defined by serum sodium between 130 to 150 mEq/L, although careful monitoring of serum sodium is important when it is below 135 mEq/L, especially in conditions that cause vascular contraction, metabolic stress, and pain, all of which stimulate antidiuretic hormone (ADH) secretion that promotes water retention and a further drop in serum sodium to dangerous levels. Isonatremia is identified in approximately 85% of dehydrated children. Water and sodium are lost in amounts equivalent to the serum concentrations.

Hyponatremic dehydration is defined by serum sodium below 130 mEq/L, although some use a cutoff of 132 mEq/L. Hyponatremia develops in approximately 10% to 15% of dehydrated children. As mentioned, conditions that stimulate ADH secretion promote hyponatremia. Infants with cystic fibrosis or salt-losing congenital adrenal hyperplasia are particularly likely to develop hyponatremic dehydration. Dehydrated patients with hyponatremia demonstrate a greater degree of vascular insufficiency than do those with isonatremic dehydration, and hypovolemic shock is common. Seizures may occur if serum sodium falls below 120 mEq/L. Hypoxemia may occur in severe hyponatremia and poses a high risk of brain dysfunction and damage. Severe hyponatremia requires prompt correction of the sodium deficit using a 3% solution of NaCl.

Hypernatremic dehydration occurs uncommonly but represents a medical emergency in many cases. When serum sodium concentration increases above 150 mEq/L, there is the potential for cerebral edema and central pontine myelinolysis. Fluid and sodium abnormalities associated with hypernatremia must be corrected slowly, usually over a 48-hour time span.

Diabetic ketoacidosis is a special case and demands careful assessment of dehydration, metabolic state, and mental status. Assessment of serum electrolytes, acid/base status, and glucose are key to successful management. Intravenous fluids and insulin must be administered with caution: Rapid rehydration and/or rapid correction of hyperglycemia may trigger development of cerebral edema.

EVALUATION

How Do I Determine Maintenance Fluid Needs?

Calculation of maintenance based on body weight most often suffices beyond the newborn period (> 28 days of age) (Table 26-2). In this formulation adapted from Holliday and Segar's work, age and weight reflect metabolic rate.

Table 26-2

Daily Maintenance Water and Electrolytes Beyond the Newborn Period

Body Weight (kg)	Water (ml/kg)	Sodium (mEq/kg)	Potassium (mEq/kg)
< 10	100 ml/kg	3	2
10-20	1000 ml + 50 ml/kg for each kg between 10–20 kg	3	2
> 20	1500 ml + 20 ml/kg for each kg > 20 kg	3*	2

*Maintenance sodium for patients > 20 kg is adequately provided with a solution containing 34 mEq/L of sodium (0.2% NaCl).

How Does the History Help Identify Dehydration?

Dehydration risk is estimated from information about the fluids consumed, the fluids lost, and the underlying illness. Knowledge of the child's maintenance fluid requirement helps you assess the adequacy of fluid intake. Remember that fever increases insensible water loss. The duration and severity of fever, diarrhea, and/or vomiting give clues to the potential severity of dehydration. History of decreased urine output suggests impending or actual dehydration. If a child has gone long periods without urine output, severe dehydration is likely. If a child has diarrhea, decreased fluid intake magnifies stool water loss and increases risk for hypernatremia. Loss of bicarbonate in diarrheal stool promotes metabolic acidosis. Persistent vomiting quickly depletes an infant's total body water, and the HCl loss from the stomach results in metabolic alkalosis and hypochloremia. Such vomiting is classically seen with pyloric stenosis. Burns, colostomy tubes, recent surgery, and diabetes all promote fluid and electrolyte loss.

Does the Physical Examination Detect Dehydration?

Acute water loss in a dehydrating illness results in an acute weight loss, but the amount of water lost is not exactly the same as the weight loss. For purposes of calculation, the three categories of dehydration are assigned percent values to estimate water loss. For *infants less than 20 kg*, dehydration is classified as mild (5%), moderate (10%), or severe (15%). An estimate of the severity of dehydration is based on physical findings (Table 26-3). In *mild* dehydration, physical evidence is usually lacking (or at most minimal). As dehydration worsens, physical findings become more obvious. ***Capillary refill is the most reliable and reproducible marker of hydration status.***

How Do I Know If Emergency ("Bolus") Fluids Are Needed?

Hypovolemic shock is the most common reason for emergency intravenous fluid. The presence of lethargy, prominent tachycardia, mottled and cool skin, delayed capillary refill, and prominent tenting indicate that an infant or child is in shock. A rapid infusion of isotonic fluid

Table 26-3

Physical Examination Findings for Dehydration

	Degree and Percent of Dehydration					
	Mild		**Moderate**		**Severe**	
	INFANT	*CHILD*	*INFANT*	*CHILD*	*INFANT*	*CHILD*
	< 20 kg (5%)	> 20 kg (3%)	< 20 kg (10%)	> 20 kg (6%)	< 20 kg (15%)	> 20 kg (9%)
Examination						
Neurologic status	Alert, consolable		Irritable		Lethargic/obtunded	
Pulse	Age appropriate		Slightly increased		Increased	
Oral mucosa and lips	Moist		Dry/tacky		Parched/cracked	
Eyes	Moist, not sunken		Slightly dry, deep-set		Dry, sunken	
Tears, if crying	Present		Present, reduced		Absent	
Fontanelle (if patent)	Flat		Soft, slightly depressed		Sunken	
Skin (touch)	Unremarkable		Dry		Clammy	
Skin turgor	Good		Tenting		Tenting or no turgor	
Capillary refill	< 2 sec		2–3 sec		> 3 sec	

Adapted from Stone B: Fluids and electrolytes. In Robertson J, Shilkofski N, editors: *The Harriet Lane handbook,* ed 17, St. Louis, 2005, Mosby.

supports the circulation and reverses signs of shock. Occasionally, a rapid infusion of isotonic fluid for a vomiting child who has only mild-moderate dehydration will reduce nausea and allow consumption of oral fluids without further vomiting.

Are Laboratory Tests Needed to Evaluate Dehydration?

If dehydration is severe, and especially if vomiting is prominent, serum sodium is particularly important to monitor. Other laboratory tests include serum electrolytes, bicarbonate or total CO_2, and creatinine. Arterial oxygen should be monitored in hyponatremia. Urinalysis is useful to assess specific gravity and presence of ketones. Additional tests such as blood glucose are ordered based on the illness history. Tests are usually not needed for mild-moderate dehydration.

TREATMENT

What Are the Steps to Treat Severe Dehydration?

This section emphasizes isonatremic dehydration. Calculations for hyponatremia, hypernatremia, and diabetic ketoacidosis are more complicated (see Bibliography).

- *Identify shock and administer emergency isotonic fluid.* This supports the circulation and corrects hypovolemic shock. Frequent reassessment of response to therapy is needed.
- *Determine* the nature of dehydration (isonatremic, hyponatremic, hypernatremic) based on electrolytes.
- *Calculate* water and sodium deficits.
- *Correct water and electrolyte deficit and provide for maintenance.*
- *Monitor for ongoing losses* and replace them as needed.

How Should I Administer Emergency Fluids in Shock?

A "bolus" of 20 ml/kg of isotonic crystalloid such as 0.9% saline (normal saline [NS]) or lactated Ringer's solution should be rapidly infused (in 30 minutes, if possible). Your *orders must specify the fluid, the volume, and the rate.* You must reassess clinical status continuously and may need to repeat the "bolus" therapy once or twice if signs of shock do not diminish. If tachycardia persists after several rapid infusions of isotonic fluid, administer a colloid such as Plasmanate, plasma, or blood. Shock associated with trauma and/or hypoxia will need much more aggressive resuscitation, usually with blood or blood products. Shock caused by infection will also require intensive management beyond fluid replacement.

What Fluid Does a Dehydrated Child Need?

The total fluid required is the sum of maintenance + deficit (+ ongoing losses, if any). ***You must not simply increase daily maintenance fluids in dehydration,*** as that will not provide adequate sodium. Intravenous fluids for a child with *isotonic dehydration* are calculated from the current, dehydrated weight, because a pre-illness weight is usually not available. This method is safe, effective, and less prone to calculation errors of more complex management schemes.

How Do I Calculate the Fluids for a Dehydrated Child?

- ***Maintenance water and sodium*** are calculated from body weight (Table 26-2).
- ***Deficit water*** is based on current body weight × dehydration % (Table 26-3).
- ***Deficit sodium*** is determined from the volume of the deficit × 140 mEq/L (standard serum sodium concentration).

As an example, water and sodium needs for a 10-kg child with severe (15%) isonatremic dehydration are determined as follows:

	Maintenance	Deficit	Total
Water	1.0 L (10 kg × 100 ml/kg)	1.5 L (10 kg × 15%)	2.5 L
Sodium	30 mEq (10 kg × 3 mEq/kg)	210 mEq (1.5 L × 140 mEq/L)	240 mEq

What Final Fluid Should I Infuse?

Calculate the final fluid needed to provide both deficit and maintenance, then choose a prepackaged fluid (Table 26-4) that most closely approximates the calculated electrolyte needs.

Intravenous fluids are prepackaged in liter volumes. Because the child in the previous example needs 2.5 L of fluid, three 1-liter bags of fluid will be required. A total of 240 mEq of sodium must be provided in 2.5 L of fluid, so the final sodium concentration will be 96 mEq/L (240 mEq ÷ 2.5 L). The closest commonly available fluid to the calculated sodium concentration is 0.45% NaCl ("half-normal saline"), which contains 77 mEq/L and would provide 192.5 mEq of sodium in 2.5 L. Because the kidneys of previously healthy children will correct dehydration if supplied adequate water and sodium, half-normal saline suffices for this patient. *Remember to monitor serum sodium during therapy to detect development of hyponatremia if any ADH-stimulating conditions, such as pain, are present.* Intravenous fluids commonly also contain 5% glucose to counteract catabolism in the acute phase of dehydration treatment. Potassium is ***not*** added until adequate urine output and renal function have been documented. The final calculated fluid is most practically infused at a stable rate over a 24-hour period, or 104 ml/hr (2.5 L ÷ 24 hours). The fluid order would be written: ***Infuse 2.5 L of D5 ½ NS at a rate of 104 ml/hour.***

Table 26-4

Standard Intravenous Fluid Solutions

Solution	Na^+ (mEq/L)	K^+ (mEq/L)	Cl^- (mEq/L)	Lactate (mEq/L)	Ca^{2+} (mEq/L)
Hypotonic solutions					
0.2% NaCl (1/4 NS)	34	—	34	—	—
0.33% NaCl (1/3 NS)	56	—	56	—	—
0.45% NaCl (1/2 NS)	77	—	77	—	—
Isotonic solutions					
0.9% NaCl (NS)	154	—	154	—	—
Lactated Ringer's (LR)	130	4	109	28	3
Hypertonic solution					
3% NaCl	513	—	513	—	—

NS, Normal saline.

Adapted from Stone B: Fluids and electrolytes. In Robertson J, Shilkofski N, editors: *The Harriet Lane handbook,* ed 17, St. Louis, 2005, Mosby.

What about Potassium?

Potassium deficit is typically not calculated except in complicated dehydration, such as diabetic ketoacidosis. ***Do not administer potassium intravenously to a patient with reduced urine output,*** because ***potassium is potentially dangerous.*** The inadequate circulating volume and poor renal perfusion that develop in moderate to severe dehydration cause reduced renal function, which manifests as reduced urine output. Thus urine output is a useful clinical marker of renal function in a previously healthy dehydrated infant or child. Once urine output has returned to appropriate rates, potassium may be added to intravenous fluids. In general, concentrations of potassium in intravenous fluids should not be greater than 20 mEq/L unless there is a specific need for higher concentrations.

How Do I Treat Serious Dehydration States?

Hyponatremia, hypernatremia, and diabetic ketoacidosis demand careful calculation of fluid and electrolyte deficits. Frequent reassessment of treatment progress is critical. See the bibliography at the end of the chapter for discussions of the fluid management of these problems.

How Do I Calculate Pre-illness Weight?

You can estimate the pre-illness weight using the dehydrated weight plus the estimated degree of dehydration:

Pre-illness weight = current weight ÷ (1 – % dehydration)

For a 10-kg child who has 15% dehydration, pre-illness weight is 11.8 kg = 10 kg ÷ (1 – 0.15). Maintenance and deficit calculations are then based on this pre-illness weight so that a "prescription intravenous fluid" can be administered to the patient. This approach is especially useful for management of diabetic ketoacidosis.

Can Dehydration Be Treated with Oral Fluids?

Oral rehydration solutions (ORSs) suffice for mild to moderate dehydration unless vomiting or other problems make oral rehydration dangerous or impractical. Commercial ORSs are easily found in pharmacies and grocery stores (Table 26-5). The Rehydration Project provides instruction on homemade ORSs *(http://rehydrate.org/index.html)*. ORS administration is based on severity of dehydration:

- Mild dehydration: 50 ml/kg of ORS over a 4-hour period
- Moderate dehydration: 100 ml/kg of ORS over a 4-hour period

Table 26-5

Oral Rehydration Solutions

Solution	CHO (g/dl)	Na^+ (mEq/L)	K^+ (mEq/L)	Cl^- (mEq/L)	Base (mEq/L)	mOsm per kg H_2O
WHO/UNICEF	2.0	90	20	80	30	310
Cerealyte	4.0	70	20	60	30	220
Infalyte	3.0	50	25	45	30	200
Naturalyte	2.5	45	20	35	48	265
Pedialyte	2.5	45	20	35	30	250
Rehydralyte	2.5	75	20	65	30	310

CHO, Carbohydrate; Cl^-, chloride; K^+, potassium; Na^+, sodium.

From Snyder JO: Evaluation and treatment of diarrhea, *Semin Gastrointest Dis* 5:47, 1994.

Start with small volumes (5 to 10 ml via syringe, spoon, or cup) every 5 to 10 minutes, then increase volume and extend intervals as tolerated. Persist with oral therapy even if vomiting occasionally occurs, but be prepared to use intravenous fluids if severe vomiting makes ORS therapy impossible. After completion of the 4-hour ORS therapy, resume the regular diet, if tolerated, to provide maintenance fluids. Calculate the maintenance need and provide parents with specific advice about how to give this quantity of fluid. Do *not* simply advise parents to "push fluids" or "make sure he drinks enough water." Remember to have parents monitor for ongoing losses, especially diarrhea or vomiting. Remind parents to call for assistance if they need it.

KEY POINTS

- Daily fluid requirement = maintenance + deficit + ongoing losses.
- Fever increases maintenance fluid need.
- Most children with moderate dehydration can be rehydrated orally.
- Use current weight to calculate intravenous fluids for most patients. This simplifies calculations.
- Do NOT add KCl to intravenous fluids until urine output has been documented.
- Hyponatremia may be associated with hypoxemia.

Case 26-1

A 6-month-old child weighs 7.5 kg.

A. What are his daily maintenance needs for water, sodium, and potassium?

Case 26-2

A 15-month-old child weighs 11 kg.

A. What are her daily maintenance needs for water, sodium, and potassium?

Case 26-3

A 9-month-old boy has had diarrhea and vomiting for the past 24 hours. He has taken only 10 ounces of formula over the past 24 hours. His diaper was dry this morning, which alarmed his mother because his diapers are usually "soaked" first thing in the morning. You note that he is fussy but can be consoled, but he has no tears. His fontanelle is slightly sunken, as are his eyes. His lips are dry and his skin is pale but not mottled. Pulse is 130 beats/minute, respirations are 40 breaths/minute, and the temperature is 36.3° C. Weight is 8.5 kg. Capillary refill is 2.5 seconds (upper limits).

A. Give an estimate of the percentage of dehydration, and determine if the dehydration is mild, moderate, or severe.
B. Would this child benefit from an infusion of isotonic fluid to expand the vascular space?
C. Write a prescription for the fluid (fluid type, volume, and time of infusion or rate in milliliters per minute).
D. What is his water deficit?
E. What is his sodium deficit?
F. What is his maintenance water?
G. What is his maintenance sodium?
H. Write a prescription for fluid replacement of water and sodium (deficit + maintenance).
I. Will you add potassium? When? How much?

Case 26-4

A 14-month-old boy has had vomiting and diarrhea for the past 36 hours. He has not urinated for the past 12 hours. In the office he weighs 9 kg and has clinical findings consistent with severe dehydration (15% water loss): heart rate 160 beats/minute, lethargy, parched mucous membranes, tenting, mottled skin, and capillary refill time of 4.5 seconds. Because he appears so ill, you draw blood to determine serum electrolyte and creatinine levels and elect to use his pre-illness weight rather than his current dehydrated weight to calculate fluid needs.

A. What is his pre-illness weight?
B. What fluid and quantity will you give as an emergency bolus?
C. During administration of emergency fluids, laboratory results return: Serum sodium is 135 mEq/L. Serum creatinine is 0.9 mg/dl. What do these results tell you about this patient?
D. What is his deficit water? Sodium deficit?
E. What is his maintenance water? Sodium maintenance?
F. Write a prescription for replacement of deficit and maintenance fluid.
G. What clinical clue will you use to determine when you can add potassium to the intravenous fluid?

Case Answers

26-1 A. *Learning objective:* **Determine daily maintenance fluid requirements for an infant ≤ 10 kg.**
Water: 7.5 kg × 100 ml/kg = 750 ml
Sodium: 7.5 kg × 3 mEq/kg = 22.5 mEq
Potassium: 7.5 kg × 2 mEq/kg = 15 mEq

26-2 A. *Learning objective:* **Determine daily maintenance fluid requirements for a child ≥ 10 kg.**
Water: 10 kg × 100 ml/kg = 1000 ml
1 kg × 50 ml/kg = 50 ml
Total = 1050 ml
Sodium: 11 kg × 3 mEq/kg = 33 mEq
Potassium: 11 kg × 2 mEq/kg = 22 mEq

26-3 A. *Learning objective:* **Identify dehydration from clinical findings.** This child has moderate (~10%) dehydration based on findings from history and physical examination (see Table 26-3).

26-3 B. *Learning objective:* **Use clinical findings and the estimate of dehydration to determine the need for emergency (bolus) fluid administration.** Tachycardia and tachypnea indicate decreased circulating volume and justify an infusion of isotonic fluid (either 0.9% saline—normal saline—or lactated Ringer's solution).

26-3 C to G. *Learning objective:* **Calculate fluid therapy for a dehydrated child, including maintenance and deficit fluids.**

Calculations: 9-month-old with moderate dehydration

		Total	
FLUID	CALCULATION	WATER	SODIUM
Emergency fluid*	8.5 kg × 20 ml/kg	170 ml	0.9% NaCl (infused over 30 minutes)
Deficit water	8.5 kg × 10% = 0.85 kg	850 ml	—
Deficit sodium	0.85 L × 140 mEq Na^+/L	—	119 mEq
Maintenance water	8.5 kg × 100 ml/kg	850 ml	—
Maintenance sodium	8.5 kg × 3 mEq/kg	—	25.5 mEq
Total (deficit + maintenance)	—	1700 ml	144.5 mEq

Final fluid: 144.5 mEq sodium in 1700 ml water or 85 mEq Na^+/L
Order for fluids: 1.7 L D5W + 85 mEq NaCl/L to run at 71 ml/hr for 24 hr
OR use D5W + 0.45% NaCl (D5W + 1/2 normal sodium)
*Emergency fluid is *not* subtracted from the final fluid volume.
Monitor urine output and add KCl, 20 mEq/L, to the fluids when urine output resumes.

26-3 I. *Learning objective:* **Recognize that potassium must not be added to intravenous fluids for the moderately to severely dehydrated child until evidence of appropriate renal function has been established.** Potassium should not be added to IV fluids until the child has established a steady urine output.

26-4 A to G. *Learning objective:* **Calculate fluid therapy, including maintenance and deficit fluid, using laboratory test results to guide the calculations.** The illness has resulted in severe isotonic dehydration with reduced renal function manifested by a serum creatinine of 0.9 mg/dl, when age-appropriate serum creatinine should be ~0.5 mg/dl. Pre-illness weight calculation and fluid calculations are shown in the table.

Calculations: 14-month-old with severe dehydration

Variable	Calculation	Total		
		WEIGHT	WATER	SODIUM
Pre-illness weight	9 kg ÷ (1.0 – 0.15)	10.59 kg	—	—
Emergency fluid*	10.59 kg × 20 ml/kg	—	212 ml	0.9% NaCl
Deficit water	10.59 kg × 15%	—	1589 ml	
Deficit sodium	1.589 L × 140 mEq/L	—	—	222.5 mEq
Maintenance water	10 kg × 100 ml/kg = 1000 ml + 0.59 kg × 50 ml/kg = 30 ml	—	1030 ml	—
Maintenance sodium	10.59 kg × 3 mEq/kg	—	—	32 mEq
Total deficit + maintenance		—	2610 ml	254.5 mEq

Final fluid: 254.5 mEq sodium in 2.6 L = 98 mEq/L

Order for fluids[†]: 2.6 L D5W + 98 mEq/L NaCl to run at 108 ml/H for 24 hr

OR

2.6 L D5W-0.45% NaCl (D5W 1/2 NS) at 108 ml/hr for 24 hr. *If you use the latter, you must monitor serum sodium carefully to avoid development of hyponatremia.*

*The emergerncy fluid is administered over 30 minutes. This may need to be repeated once or twice, depending on the response of heart rate to the fluid. Emergency fluid water volume and sodium content are not subtracted from the total maintenance + deficit.

[†]Do *not* add potassium to intravenous fluids until urine output has been documented. In severe dehydration, monitor electrolytes and serum creatinine.

BIBLIOGRAPHY

General information (including hpyo- and hypernatremia):

Stone B: Fluids and electrolites. In Robertson J, Shilkofski N, editors: *The Harriet Lane handbook,* ed 17, St. Louis, Mosby.

Holliday MA, Segar WE: The maintenance need for water in parenteral therapy. *Pediatrics*, 19:823–832, 1957.

Diabetic ketoacidosis:

Salikof D: Endocrinology. In Robertson J, Shilkofski N, editors: *The Harriet Lane handbook,* ed 17, St. Louis, Mosby.

Oral Rehydration Solutions:

Duggan C, Santoshan M, Glass RI: The management of acute diarrhea in children: oral rehydration, maintenance and nutritional therapy. Centers for Disease Control and Prevention, *MMWR*, 41(RR-16):1–20, 1992.

27

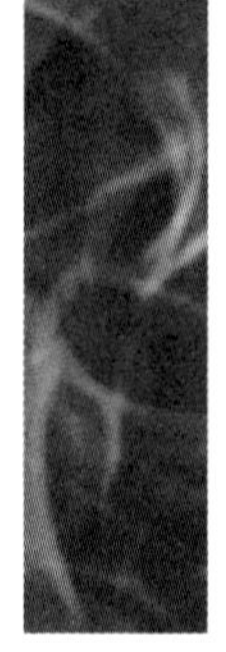

Developmental Delay: Suspected

DIANNE M. McBRIEN

"Doctor, shouldn't he be talking already?"
"Our daughter seems slower than her classmates. We're concerned."

ETIOLOGY

Is Developmental Delay a Major Child Health Problem?

Questions about child development commonly arise during the pediatric office visit. Family members may voice specific concerns, or the physician may be the first to suggest that a child is developing slowly. Each health supervision visit should include a brief assessment of developmental milestones. If the family or healthcare provider suspects a delay, however, a more thorough investigation is warranted. The causes of developmental delay are diverse, and systematic thinking through the classes of possible etiologies is needed to identify the cause of a child's problems. Many cases of developmental delay elude diagnosis, because most children with mild mental retardation have unremarkable prenatal and birth histories, normal laboratory profiles, and normal head imaging results. The likelihood of identifying a specific etiology tends to increase with the degree of developmental delay. Parents almost always ask, "How did this happen?"—a question that you may not always be able to answer.

What Functional Deficits Occur in Developmental Delay?

A child with developmental delay has deficits in one or more of the following functions:

- *Input,* or receiving information from the environment
- *Processing,* or breaking information into usable components
- *Output,* or using the components to interact with the environment

A problem in one area can affect ability in another. For example, the input problem of sensorineural hearing loss can diminish the processing ability to understand the nuance of spoken language, even after the loss is treated. A specific disability can cause deficits in all three functions: Cerebral palsy (Chapter 58), for example, may be associated with the input disorders of strabismus and sensorineural hearing loss; processing problems, including mental retardation and learning disabilities; and output problems of spasticity and contractures.

How Do I Determine the Cause of Developmental Delay?

Once you identify the functional deficits, you can begin to think about causes. Tables 27-1, 27-2, and 27-3 indicate the most common etiologies for input and processing deficits. These lists include general categories of disease and the most common causes of developmental delay.

- Most input problems consist of hearing loss (Table 27-1) or visual loss (Table 27-2).
- Processing disorders (Table 27-3) include mental retardation or learning disabilities. These disorders all represent some degree of static or progressive brain dysfunction.
- Output problems usually bring an infant or child with developmental delay to medical attention. Examples include difficulty with gross motor or fine motor movements, balance, and communication.

EVALUATION

What Questions Should I Ask the Family?

Genetic, prenatal, environmental, and many other factors can contribute to developmental differences. Your history must be as inclusive as possible. Where possible, information from each phase of the child's life should be recorded so that patterns may be identified. Conduct the interview in language that is easily understood by most families. For example, the question, "*Is there anyone related to your son who had a hard time learning to read, or reads with difficulty now?*" is much more likely

Table 27-1

Causes of Hearing Loss in Children

Genetic	Prenatal Insult	Infectious	Toxic	Trauma
Syndromic deafness (Alport's and Treacher Collins syndromes; neurofibromatosis) Nonsyndromic autosomal recessive deafness	TORCH infection Anoxic event Severe intraventricular hemorrhage	Recurrent otitis media (conductive) Meningitis (neurosensory)	Antibiotics Loop diuretics Cisplatin	Head injury

TORCH, Toxoplasmosis, other, rubella, cytomegalovirus, herpes simplex.

Table 27-2

Causes of Visual Loss in Children

Genetic	Metabolic	Degenerative	Prenatal	Postnatal	Infectious	Traumatic
Congenital glaucoma	Galactosemia	Tay-Sachs disease and other lipidoses	Cataracts from TORCH exposure	Retinopathy of prematurity	Meningitis	Retinal hemorrhage (shaken baby syndrome)
Inherited retinal dystrophy	Organic acidurias	Mitochondrial disorders	Fetal alcohol syndrome	Birth anoxia	Gonorrheal and chlamydial conjunctivitis	Accidental injury
Familial cataract syndrome		Peroxisomal disorders	Brain malformation related to in utero vascular insult	Severe IVH	Herpetic keratitis	
		Rett syndrome				

IVH, Intraventricular hemorrhage; TORCH, toxoplasmosis, other, rubella, cytomegalovirus, herpes simplex.

Table 27-3

Causes of Mental Retardation in Children

Genetic	Metabolic	Degenerative	Prenatal	Postnatal	Infectious	Traumatic
Down syndrome	Organic acidurias	Lipidoses	Fetal alcohol or substance exposure	Birth anoxia	Meningitis	Shaken baby syndrome
Prader-Willi syndrome	Urea cycle disorders	Peroxisomal disorders	Hydrocephalus associated with neural tube defect	Severe IVH	Encephalitis	Nonintentional head injury
Fragile X syndrome	Hypothyroidism	Mitochondrial disorders	Intrauterine vascular insult or infection			
Neurocutaneous disorders		Maternal coagulopathy				
X-linked hydrocephalus						
X-linked neuronal migration disorder						

IVH, Intraventricular hemorrhage.

to elicit useful information than the query, "*Do you have a family history of dyslexia?*" Certain elements of the history are standard in the structured workup of any child with suspected developmental delay. The following questions are by no means comprehensive, but including them in your history should help you screen for the most prevalent developmental disorders on a typical pediatric clerkship.

What Should I Ask about Prenatal Events?

A thorough prenatal history obtained using gentle, open-ended questions will lead you to areas that may require more probing. A brief inquiry into the ***mother's prepregnancy health*** will yield information about collagen vascular disease, diabetes, seizure disorder, and other potentially teratogenic health issues. Queries related to the ***pregnancy*** itself require particular care, because the mother of a developmentally delayed child often feels at fault for the child's problems; she may be exquisitely sensitive to any nuance of blame in the interview. In general, however, parents will talk freely if *you listen actively and encourage them to tell their story*. You can do so by asking about the clinical details outlined in Table 27-4 and about the quality of the pregnancy experience itself: If the mother has given birth before, was this pregnancy easier or harder than the other(s)? Did the mother have the "flu," a urinary tract infection, or other illnesses during her pregnancy? Did this baby move around more or less than her other babies? What tests did the doctor do? (You may or may not already have this information). Did the mother need to take any special medications or to rest in bed to prevent premature delivery of the baby? The prenatal history should also include inquiry about prescription drugs, over-the-counter medications, and vitamin supplements taken by the mother at any point during the pregnancy. Table 27-5 lists commonly used medications associated with developmental problems. Questions about alcohol, tobacco, and drug consumption during pregnancy should be carefully posed to avoid the appearance of casting blame. If you frame the inquiry neutrally you are more likely to learn what you need to know: "*I ask every parent about drinking and use of substances such as pot, cocaine, and meth during pregnancy. Did you use any? And if so, how much?*"

Table 27-4

Pregnancy-Related Historical Factors Associated with Developmental Delay

Maternal Health	Fetal Viability	Labor and Delivery
Diabetes mellitus	Multiple pregnancy	Premature delivery
Seizure disorder	"Vanishing twin" syndrome	Prolonged rupture of membranes
Antiphospholipid syndrome	Placental anomalies	Chorioamnionitis; other reproductive tract infection
		Evidence of fetal acidosis

Table 27-5

Prenatal Medications Associated with Developmental Delay

Medication	Developmental Anomaly
Anticonvulsants	
Phenytoin Trimethadione Valproic acid	In utero exposure to all of these drugs can cause anomalies, including craniofacial defects, microcephaly, mental retardation, facial and digital anomalies
Dermatologic agents	
Lindane	Mental retardation
Isotretinoin	Mental retardation and major birth defects
Anticoagulants	
Warfarin	Porencephalic cysts

What Should I Ask about Labor and Delivery?

Ask about length of labor, mode of delivery, any assistive methods such as forceps or vacuum, and any needed resuscitation. A simple way to ask about resuscitation is, "*Did [child's name] need help breathing right after he was born?*" You should also ask the mother if she had a fever or was treated for an infection during labor because studies have linked cerebral palsy to maternal reproductive tract infection. Look in the record for Apgar scores and notes about labor and delivery.

What Postnatal Events Should I Document?

Review any health problems identified in the nursery, such as respiratory distress, jaundice, hypoglycemia, anemia, and fever. If the infant underwent head ultrasound or other head imaging in the nursery, obtain the results. Note the recommendations made at discharge, including need for supplemental oxygen, apnea monitoring, and supplemented or nonoral feeding.

What about the Child's Health History?

History of the child's general health from birth to the time of the evaluation should identify any head injury, seizures, serious illness, hospitalizations, or surgeries. Medications and allergies should be reviewed. Any hearing or visual loss should be noted, as should results of hearing and vision screens. You should review the child's appetite, sleep habits, and bladder and bowel function.

How Can I Determine the Degree of Delay?

Many parents report their concerns about development in a general sense, stating, "She's just not where she should be." Work with them to clarify the problems, if possible: "She's not saying any words yet and she's almost 2 years old." Having a clear idea of the family's issues will help you address their needs efficiently. Chapter 9 discusses the timing of developmental milestones. More detailed lists of developmental stages are available in standard texts, the *Denver II*, and *Bright Futures* publications. Developmental screening tools that are often used in the primary care setting include the Cognitive Adaptive Test/Clinical Linguistic and Auditory Milestone Scale (CAT/CLAMS) and the Infant Motor Screen. Studies have shown, however, that parental perception of delay is generally as sensitive as results of more formal tests. In other words, listen to the parents.

What Kind of Developmental Delay Is Most Common?

Most young children with suspected delay present with *gross motor* or *language* concerns. Fine motor delays are less common. This chapter focuses on the recommended assessment of suspected gross motor or language delay. Delays of gross motor abilities in infants and toddlers, such as sitting and independent walking, are the most common developmental problems noted by parents and physicians. Families rarely bring a child for a first-time evaluation of significant gross motor delay after the preschool years *except if the child seems to be regressing*. Significant gross motor delay manifesting in infancy is most commonly related to cerebral palsy (see Chapter 58) or to mental retardation associated with a number of etiologies. Concerns about language and communication typically arise between the ages of 18 months and 4 years.

GROSS MOTOR DELAY

How Do I Assess Gross Motor Delay?

The family's daily observations of muscle tone, strength, and reflexes can be helpful to you. Ask whether the baby seems stiff or floppy. Some parents may describe *increased* muscle tone by commenting that the baby's legs are hard to move during a diaper change or that she is difficult to position in her car seat. Others may describe *decreased* muscle tone by stating that the child feels like a rag doll or a sack of flour when picked up. Inquire if the strength or tone of the child feels different on one side of the body. Ask too about a strong hand preference: Appearance of this trait before the second year of life suggests hemiplegia of the contralateral upper extremity. Review, as well, the presence of any abnormal movements, such as tremor, slow writhing movements, head bobbing, and ataxia.

What Problems Accompany Gross Motor Delays?

The motor-delayed child often has a history of feeding and bowel problems. Ask about oral-motor symptoms, including slow feeding, milk leaking out of the mouth, and difficulty with new textures. Then inquire about dysphagia or aspiration symptoms such as poor weight gain, coughing, gagging, "wet" breathing with feeding, vomiting or frequent "wet" burps, bruxism, frequent respiratory infections, and unexplained fevers. Constipation is common in children with developmental disorders, so stool frequency and consistency should be reviewed.

How Should I Start the Physical Examination?

The physical examination should pay particular attention to the neuromuscular elements, including muscle bulk, reflexes, tone, and quality of movements. Level of alertness should be noted, as well as any skeletal abnormalities, including scoliosis, leg-length discrepancy, or unstable hip. Observation is a key component of the examination.

How Do I Assess Muscle Tone?

Assessment of muscle tone is done first by observing the undressed child at rest on the examination table and then by suspending the child under the arms. Continue your assessment of tone by gently moving each joint through its full range of motion. Is the movement fluid and smooth or is it jerky, flaccid, or stiff? Do you meet resistance for most of the range, and then find that the joint abruptly "gives way?" This sign, known as the *clasp-knife reflex,* is a hallmark of spasticity and should prompt you to entertain concerns of cerebral palsy.

What Physical Findings Occur with Hypertonia?

The young child with ***hypertonia*** tends to display few spontaneous movements at rest or when lifted up. One or both hands may be fisted, and the feet may be extended with the toes pointed. The upper extremities may be held close to the body as well. The clasp-knife reflex mentioned previously is commonly identified. When lifted off the examining table, the hypertonic child may extend and occasionally adduct the hips—the legs will appear almost to cross and the child will point the toes, a movement known as "scissoring" (see Chapter 58).

What Will I Identify on Examination of a Hypotonic Infant?

The ***hypotonic*** infant tends to lie with hips flexed and abducted ("frog-leg position"). When you suspend the hypotonic infant under her arms, you will appreciate the sensation that she may slip through your hands ("scapular fall-through").

What Other Physical Findings Should I Identify?

While completing your neuromuscular examination, look for abnormal persistence of any primitive reflexes, such as Moro, asymmetrical tonic neck, positive supporting reaction, and the parachute response (see Chapter 58). Try to elicit deep tendon reflexes, and note any briskness or clonus—typical of the child with spasticity. Also look for extra movements, including tremors, head bobbing, fasciculations, and writhing movements. Look at the child's muscle bulk to identify relative atrophy or hypertrophy in certain muscle groups. Ambulatory boys with Duchenne's muscular dystrophy commonly have marked gastrocnemius hypertrophy. The rest of your physical examination should include a search for signs of neurocutaneous disorder, including café au lait spots, inguinal or axillary freckling, and hypopigmented areas. You should also search for dysmorphic facial and body features. Examples might include low-set ears, hypertelorism, webbed neck, or digital abnormalities. Screen especially for strabismus, which is common in children with cerebral palsy and brain malformations. Length, weight, head circumference, and body mass index (BMI) should be measured and plotted at each visit and carefully compared with past growth data, if available.

LANGUAGE AND COMMUNICATION DELAY

How Do I Assess Communication Delays?

Communication refers to the child's capacity to express himself or herself clearly. Parents usually express concern about language and communication in children between ages 18 months and 4 years, often comparing the child with a sibling, cousin, or playmate. The delay may occur by itself or as part of a global developmental problem. Ask which words the child uses, if any. If the child does not use words, inquire if she uses signs, pointing, or other attempts at communication. Become familiar with the speech and language milestones, and compare your patient's communication level with these. Review the medical history for frequent otitis media and for cleft palate repair. Look for documentation of audiologic evaluation. Review the family history for hearing loss as well. Because autism spectrum disorder is an important cause of communication delay in young children, discuss the child's social interactions, interests, and degree of flexibility (see Chapter 58).

How Do I Assess a Child with Communication Delay?

First, sit quietly and observe the child interacting with the family in order to gain information about eye contact, intent to communicate, size of vocabulary, appropriate usage, and articulation. A child with communication delay requires a complete neurologic examination plus a search for neurocutaneous and dysmorphic stigmata. Inspect the oral cavity, with special attention to the palate: An obvious cleft will be hard to miss, but look for a bifid or partially cleft uvula because it may indicate a submucous cleft palate, which is associated with middle ear dysfunction and conductive hearing loss. Careful assessment of the tympanic membranes may reveal middle ear effusion or other pathology.

How Should I Choose Diagnostic Studies?

Whether a child has gross motor, fine motor, or communication delays, the diagnostic evaluation must consider each procedure's yield, potential therapeutic benefits, and cost. Also bear in mind that most children with mild mental retardation have essentially normal chromosomal, metabolic, and radiographic profiles. Suggested diagnostic tests include

- Hearing and vision screens (if not previously done)
- Complete blood count (CBC) and blood lead level
- Genetic consultation: This should be considered for a child with dysmorphic features. Karyotype and molecular DNA studies for fragile X syndrome are indicated for a child of either sex with

significant delay, regardless of family history of mental retardation. Fluorescence in situ hybridization (FISH) probe for 15q11-q13 deletions may be appropriate in the floppy child (Prader-Willi syndrome) or in a child with significant delay and autistic features (Angelman syndrome).

- Metabolic evaluation: Thyroid functions, plasma amino acids, urinary organic acids, lactate, and plasma biotinidase. These tests may be indicated when symptoms of delay are accompanied by failure to thrive, recurrent vomiting, developmental regression, or positive family history.
- Infectious serologies: Toxoplasmosis, other agents, rubella, cytomegalovirus, herpes simplex (TORCH) titers or lymphocytic choriomeningitis virus (LCMV) IgM-enzyme-linked immunosorbent assay (ELISA) may be appropriate in a young child with significant microcephaly or cataracts or when a suggestive prenatal history is present.
- Creatine kinase level is useful in the floppy or weak child.
- Brain imaging is sometimes indicated to investigate for congenital malformations, atrophy, hydrocephalus, or space-occupying lesions. Magnetic resonance imaging (MRI) provides the best contrast between gray and white matter and helps delineate healed injuries or degenerative changes. MRI is also the tool of choice for examination of posterior fossa anatomy. Computed tomography (CT) is recommended to identify calcifications and to assess ventricular size.

TREATMENT

How Do I Talk to Parents about Developmental Delay?

The diagnosis of a developmental problem can devastate families. The manner in which the physician breaks the news sets the stage for management success or failure, and for future interactions with other medical providers. A physician perceived as abrupt or insensitive in this encounter can foster resentment by the family toward the entire medical community and its recommendations for years to come. News of the diagnosis should be delivered when both parents are present. If only one parent can be present, a grandparent, friend, or social worker should be there for support. If possible, pagers should be turned off during the interview. *News of the diagnosis should never be left on an answering machine, faxed, or sent as electronic mail.* Information about the diagnosis also should never be mailed before you arrange a personal discussion with the family. Assuring parents of your continued availability is important. In addition, you should provide the names of resources in the community and elsewhere, including the option for second opinions if desired by parents. The family may benefit from involvement with parent support groups, many of which can be accessed on the Internet. If you have established a working relationship with a multidisciplinary team skilled in the management of developmentally delayed children, your management task will be easier and more rewarding.

Can a Developmentally Delayed Child Be Managed in a Primary Care Office?

The primary care physician has a critical role in management of a child with developmental delay to coordinate care and provide ongoing health supervision. Once you have identified that a young child has delayed development, you should confer with the family about appropriate intervention. Consultation with subspecialty services such as pediatric neurology or otolaryngology may be indicated. If the diagnosis is in question, referral to a developmental pediatrician is in order for further clarification. Refer the child for needed services such as speech and language therapy, physical therapy, or occupational therapy. Hearing and visual status should be monitored carefully because new-onset sensory loss may be less clinically obvious in this developmentally delayed population. Bowel patterns should be followed because constipation and encopresis are extremely common. Be aware that many developmental disorders are associated with seizures, and keep a high index of suspicion for the onset of seizure disorder. Sleep disorders are also relatively common in this population, and chronic sleep deprivation will have a negative impact on developmental progress and on family function. Overnight sleep study may be indicated to investigate for apnea, nocturnal seizure, hypoventilation, and parasomnia; infants can be evaluated with the shorter "nap study."

What Specific Treatments Should I Recommend?

Many children with motor output problems such as cerebral palsy and myelomeningocele will need help maintaining appropriate body and joint position at rest and in motion. Some of the positioning therapies that help achieve this goal include orthotic splints, braces, casts, and appropriately customized wheelchair systems. Some children with significant spasticity benefit from the use of muscle relaxant medications. More information about treatment of cerebral palsy is available in Chapter 58.

Why Is Nutrition Important?

Careful attention should be paid to feeding and growth in the child with significant developmental delay, who may be at risk for oral-motor problems, neurogenic dysphagia, reflux, aspiration, and increased caloric needs. A feeding evaluation including swallow study may be indicated to see which textures, if any, the child can safely consume. Appropriate medications should be prescribed for any gastroesophageal reflux. The child with recurrent aspiration and/or impaired nutritional status may benefit from gastrostomy placement.

KEY POINTS

- Families often raise concerns about child development in the pediatric office.
- Your task is to determine if your patient is in fact delayed, to consider a variety of etiologies in that delay as you evaluate and diagnose, and to refer the patient and family to needed subspecialties and services.
- Family members are usually experts on the topic of their child. Respectfully use their input as you formulate plans of care together. In fulfilling this task, you will empower a family to help the child.

Case 27-1

A 9-month-old infant does not yet sit independently and has just begun to roll from the prone to the supine position. She coos occasionally but does not jabber or make consonant sounds. She does not seem to orient toward the faces of familiar people, although she does smile spontaneously. She does not yet reach for toys. The parents also report that she feeds very slowly, taking almost an hour to finish a bottle and chokes often while drinking. She was born at home following an unremarkable pregnancy and delivered by the local midwife, who recorded a spontaneous vaginal delivery at term. She weighed 2200 g at birth; head circumference and length were not measured. On physical examination, she is a thin infant girl with obvious microcephaly. Weight is 6.3 kg; length is 65 cm. Length-weight ratio is at the 10th percentile. Head circumference is 39 cm, far below the 3rd percentile for age (at the 50th percentile for a 3-month-old infant). She does not fix and follow with her eyes on examination, and the red reflex is absent bilaterally. In the supine position, she lies with hips moderately abducted, occasionally kicking her legs. Her arms lie limp beside her, but her right hand closes in a fist around your finger when you test palmar grasp. When you suspend her in mid air, she straightens her legs and points her toes. She has a strong and persistent asymmetrical tonic neck reflex. The remainder of the examination is significant for a liver edge descended to 2 cm.

A. This infant was referred for concerns of gross motor delay. In what other area(s) is she delayed? Based on the information given, provide a rough estimate of her current developmental age.
B. Does this infant have deficits in input, processing, or output?
C. What etiology(ies) do you suspect might have caused this infant's disability? Based on your suspicions, what workup would you plan?

Case Answers

27-1 A. *Learning objective:* **Assess the development of an infant or young child and identify any delay in the areas of motor and language development.** She has delays in all major areas of development—fine motor, language, social, and gross motor. Based on the information provided, her developmental age is about 3 months. At 9 months of age, a typical child should be jabbering (combining syllables into vocalizations that sound like words) and may be saying "mama" and "dada," although these expressions are probably not specific to the parents yet. Hallmarks of typical 9-month-old social development should include interactive gestures and games such as waving bye-bye and playing peek-a-boo. He or she should not only be reaching for toys but also be able to transfer toys from hand to hand; many will have developed a pincer (thumb-finger) grasp.

27-1 B. *Learning objective:* **Identify the functional deficits in a child with developmental delay, specifically assessing input, processing, and output.** Your history and physical examination suggest a child with a visual problem, which suggests an input deficit. You note several abnormalities on the neuromuscular examination, including persistent primitive reflexes and abnormal muscle tone, both of which create an output problem. She also has significant developmental delay and is at risk of later diagnosis of mental retardation, which is a deficit in processing.

27-1 C. *Learning objective:* **Use the history, physical examination, and diagnostic tests to develop a differential diagnosis of possible causes of developmental delay.** Birth weight was 2200 g at term, which suggests intrauterine growth retardation (IUGR). The infant is severely microcephalic, and head circumference appears to be increasing even more slowly than her height and her weight. Absent red reflexes indicates cataracts or some other bilateral anterior visual problem. She has hepatomegaly plus multiple abnormalities on neuromuscular examination suggestive of cerebral palsy (see Chapter 58). The combination of microcephaly, visual problems, and hepatomegaly with a history of IUGR is strongly suggestive of a child with intrauterine TORCH infection. Because of her pronounced microcephaly, consider obtaining a head CT. This study is preferable to MRI for viewing calcifications. In an infant with poor growth and developmental delay, the possibility of a metabolic disorder should also be considered. The presence of hepatomegaly and lack of red reflexes in this case should heighten your suspicion. Consider obtaining serum glucose, lactate, plasma amino acid, and urinary organic acid levels.

BIBLIOGRAPHY

Batshaw M, editor: *Children with disabilities*, Baltimore, 2002, Paul H. Brookes.

Developmental Behavioral Pediatrics Online: *www.dbpeds.org* includes self-assessment quizzes, articles, parent handouts, and research updates.

First Signs: *www.firstsigns.org* has a comprehensive Web site for parents and professionals, with links to screening tools, review articles on topics in developmental pediatrics, and lists of resources for parents and professionals.

Levine M, Carey W, Crocker A, editors: *Developmental–behavioral pediatrics*, Philadelphia, 1999, WB Saunders.

28

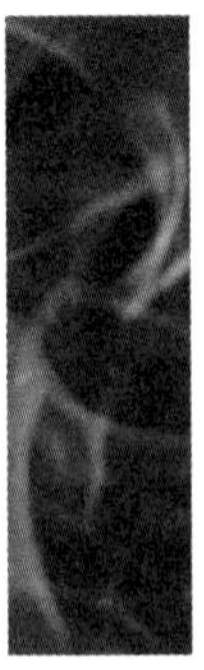

Diarrhea

WARREN P. BISHOP

ETIOLOGY

How Big a Problem Is Diarrhea?

Diarrhea is the most common cause of morbidity and mortality in the world, although in developed nations it has much less severe consequences. Acute diarrhea in North America is typically viral in etiology, is usually self-limited, and requires no diagnostic studies or specific therapy. When bacterial infection is suspected, stool testing should be done. Chronic or recurrent diarrhea has a much broader differential diagnosis, but most cases are not caused by serious underlying pathology. To diagnose and treat acute and chronic diarrhea, it is important to have a good understanding of its pathophysiology.

What Is Diarrhea?

Parents concerned about diarrhea usually describe stool that has a liquid texture. Sometimes they might mean excessively frequent stools, or are concerned with large-volume stools. The accepted medical definition of diarrhea is *excessive daily stool volume*, more than the normal upper limit of around 10 ml/kg/day. It is certainly possible to have diarrhea by this definition with stools that are at least partially formed or to not have diarrhea even with liquid bowel movements.

What Causes Diarrhea?

Physiologic mechanisms of diarrhea include excessive *secretion* of water and electrolytes (secretory diarrhea), and *malabsorption* (malabsorptive or osmotic diarrhea).
Etiology may be infectious, inflammatory, or neither.

What Is Secretory Diarrhea?

Secretory diarrhea may be stimulated by infection or inflammation. Cholera, the classic example of secretory diarrhea, is caused by a bacterial toxin that stimulates intestinal secretion of water and electrolytes. Intestinal inflammation, as in ulcerative colitis and Crohn's disease, is a much more common cause of secretory diarrhea. In this case, cytokines, prostaglandins, and enteric hormones are responsible for increased secretion. Regardless of the cause, secretory diarrhea yields watery stools with a relatively high electrolyte content. *Secretory diarrhea continues even when fasting.*

How Does Osmotic Diarrhea Develop?

Osmotic diarrhea commonly results from intestinal injury, dietary indiscretions, or specific defects in digestion leading to malabsorption. Celiac disease is a relatively common example of intestinal injury causing malabsorption. Cystic fibrosis causes diarrhea because of maldigestion of fats and proteins. Osmotic diarrhea can also be caused by the ingestion of nondigestible or nonabsorbable substances. Laxatives such as magnesium salts, polyethylene glycol, and lactulose all fit the latter category. When a single, specific digestive enzyme is lacking, as in lactose intolerance, osmotic diarrhea results only when the substrate of that enzyme (lactose) is eaten. Overindulgence of certain foods for which we have limited absorptive capacity can also cause diarrhea. A common example is the watery diarrhea seen with excessive intake of fructose in fruit juices or soft drinks. Stools in osmotic diarrhea have a relatively low electrolyte content because the osmolarity of the stool is largely accounted for by the malabsorbed material. *Osmotic diarrhea ceases when enteral intake is withheld.*

What Is "Toddler's Diarrhea?"

Toddler's diarrhea occurs when young children ("toddlers") drink large quantities of sweet, clear liquids. The watery, osmotic diarrhea results from the large fluid and carbohydrate load that exceeds the intestinal absorption capacity. These children have excellent growth and no evidence of generalized malabsorption. The loose stools are particularly evident when the toddlers are still in diapers, a messy and unpleasant situation.

EVALUATION

How Can I Distinguish the Types of Diarrhea?

History usually provides most of the information needed to decide if true diarrhea is present, to classify the diarrhea by type, and to consider the diagnostic approach (Table 28-1). It is seldom possible to determine the exact weight of stool in grams per day.

How Do I Determine the Cause of Acute Diarrhea?

Table 28-2 lists common causes of acute diarrhea. Stool cultures are seldom indicated unless fever or bloody diarrhea suggests bacterial etiology. Rotavirus is the most common infectious agent. This is seen mostly during the winter months and also is accompanied by vomiting. Stool odor is particularly offensive. Testing for rotavirus is seldom necessary, except for epidemiologic reasons.

Table 28-1

Types of Diarrhea

Classification	History
Secretory	Continues when NPO, high stool electrolyte content.
Osmotic (malabsorptive)	Diarrhea is worse with intake of malabsorbed substance and ceases when intake is withheld.
	Failure to thrive occurs when malabsorption is generalized.
	Stool has low electrolyte concentration.
Infectious	Fever, blood in stools (with invasive bacterial etiology).
	History of exposure, associated nausea and vomiting (rotavirus and other viral agents).
	Prior antibiotic use *(Clostridium difficile).*
Noninfectious	Lack of infectious history.
	History of dietary cause, history suggesting chronic inflammatory condition (see inflammatory classification).
Inflammatory	Long duration, associated signs of inflammatory disease (arthritis, rash, perianal lesions, etc.), failure to thrive.
Noninflammatory	Absence of inflammatory history.

NPO, Nil per os (nothing by mouth).

Table 28-2

Conditions Causing Acute Diarrhea

Lactose intolerance
Bacterial agents: *Campylobacter, Salmonella, Shigella,* pathogenic *Escherichia coli, Clostridium difficile, Vibrio cholerae*
Laxative ingestion
Parasites: *Giardia, Ameba, Cryptosporidium*
Allergy

What Causes Chronic or Recurrent Diarrhea?

Refer to Table 28-3 for common causes of chronic or recurrent diarrhea, which differ in important ways from those of acute diarrhea. The major clues to diagnosis are sometimes found in the dietary history, but some disorders have no association with particular foods, especially when inflammation, intestinal injury, or lack of multiple digestive enzymes (cystic fibrosis) is the cause. Many types of diarrhea have features of both malabsorption and secretion. For example, the cytokines released by lymphocytes in inflammatory bowel disease typically stimulate secretory diarrhea, while the associated bowel injury may lead to malabsorption.

Table 28-3

Common Causes of Chronic or Recurrent Diarrhea

Diagnosis	Symptoms
Toddler's diarrhea	Copious watery stools, large intake of sweet, clear liquid beverages. No weight loss.
Lactose intolerance	Watery stools and flatulence following ingestion of nonfermented dairy products. Often a temporary result of injury caused by viral enteritis. In older children, may simply be onset of primary lactase nonpersistence (adult lactose intolerance).
Pancreatic insufficiency (cystic fibrosis, Schwachman-Diamond syndrome)	Greasy, foamy, extremely foul-smelling stools due to maldigestion of fat and protein.
Short bowel syndrome	Generalized malabsorption because of diminished surface area. Stools typically acidic and watery with smaller fat and protein component than seen with pancreatic insufficiency.
Celiac disease	Similar to short bowel syndrome but typically less severe. Diarrhea not always present, depending on severity and extent of intestinal injury.
Laxative use	Watery stools because of osmotic action of laxative.
Parasite *(Giardia, Cryptosporidium)*	Watery, often foul-smelling stools with cramping. Strong secretory component—diarrhea persists when NPO.
Irritable bowel syndrome	Watery stools typical of secretory diarrhea, often alternating with more normal stools. Associated with crampy abdominal pain.
Inflammatory bowel disease	Watery stools, often with blood and mucus, associated with cramps. May have failure to thrive, arthritis, or other extraintestinal symptoms.
Allergic enteritis	Chronic diarrhea, often with blood and mucus. Presence of eosinophils on fecal smear and in biopsies of intestine. Symptoms gradually decrease on exclusion of offending antigen.

NPO, Nil per os (nothing by mouth).

How Do Osmotic and Secretory Diarrhea Differ Clinically?

The likelihood of toddler's diarrhea is high if a child is thriving despite the diarrhea and drinks lots of juice. Generalized malabsorption with impaired calorie absorption is suggested by weight loss, bloating, and foul-smelling or fatty stools. Both are forms of osmotic diarrhea. Secretory diarrhea, conversely, typically is not aggravated by or associated with the intake of any particular food. The simplest way to distinguish osmotic from secretory diarrhea is to stop all oral intake, provide intravenous fluids, and observe what happens. Osmotic diarrhea will cease but secretory diarrhea will persist. At home, parents can limit juice intake if toddler's diarrhea is suspected, with the expectation of greatly reduced stool volume. Similarly, when lactose intolerance is suspected, strict elimination of dairy products from the diet will decrease diarrhea.

What Does the Osmotic Gap Tell Me about Diarrhea?

All stools are isosmotic: fecal osmolarity is always the same as other body fluids (~280 mOsm/L). In osmotic diarrhea, the osmotic load comes from the maldigested nutrient(s), whereas in secretory diarrhea most of the osmolarity comes from Na^+, K^+, and associated anions. Measuring stool sodium and potassium allows calculation of the stool *osmotic gap*:

$$\text{Osmotic gap} = 280 - \{2 \times ([Na^+] + [K^+])\}$$

Osmotic gap is < 50 mOsm/L with secretory diarrhea and > 50 mOsm/L with osmotic diarrhea.

What Other Tests Should I Order?

Laboratory testing is not necessary for every child with diarrhea. When you suspect toddler's diarrhea in a thriving child with large juice intake, no test is indicated other than a trial of restricted clear liquid intake. Patients with severe acute diarrhea or chronic diarrhea require appropriate investigation, as listed in Table 28-4.

Table 28-4

Laboratory Investigation of Severe or Chronic Diarrhea

Clinical Information	Appropriate Test
Fever, bloody stools	Stool culture, complete blood count; consider radiologic investigation and referral for colonoscopy
Foul-smelling, fatty stools; poor weight gain	Sweat chloride, fecal fat analysis, Sudan stain
Weight loss, variable diarrhea, bloating	Antibody testing for celiac disease (antiendomysial antibodies, tissue transglutaminase antibody); consider referral for small bowel biopsy
Thriving child, watery stools, excessive liquid intake	None—trial of reduced liquid intake
Watery diarrhea and bloating, worse with dairy products	Trial of dairy restriction; consider antibody testing for celiac disease

TREATMENT

How Is Dehydration Prevented in Acute Diarrhea?

Young children with diarrhea should be given one of the oral rehydration fluids, *not* a juice or a carbonated beverage with high sugar and low electrolyte concentrations that promote worsening diarrhea. *Oral rehydration therapy* is discussed in Chapter 26. There is no justification for the old practice of continuing clear liquids for several days before restarting feedings. Early reinstitution of nutritional feedings results in more rapid resolution of diarrhea and better weight gain.

When Are Antibiotics Required to Treat Diarrhea?

Some bacterial diarrhea does not require antibiotic therapy, such as *Campylobacter* diarrhea, for which antibiotic therapy has a negligible effect. Agents that are markedly invasive should always be treated, including *Shigella* and *Entameba histolytica.* Treatment of *Giardia lamblia* and *Vibrio cholerae* markedly shortens the course of disease. Treatment of *Salmonella* infections is recommended only for immunocompromised hosts, children with sickle cell disease, infants, children with fever, and those with a positive blood culture. Severe or prolonged *Escherichia coli* diarrhea may benefit from antibiotic therapy, although recent evidence indicates that treatment of the O157:H7 serotype increases the risk of hemolytic uremic syndrome.

KEY POINTS

- Most diarrhea results from viral gastroenteritis or excessive intake of sweetened beverages.
- Secretory diarrhea *continues* during fasting.
- Osmotic diarrhea *stops* during fasting.

Case 28-1

A 3-year-old girl has had six watery stools per day for the last 3 months. All dairy products have been removed from her diet, and she is being given 24 ounces of fruit juice every day to avoid dehydration. She has had no fever or weight loss, does not seem ill, has had no abdominal pain, and no history of mouth sores, rash, arthritis, or perianal disease. She does not attend daycare and has not traveled outside the United States. She has not been taking laxatives and there are none in the medicine cabinet at home. No one else in the family has had diarrhea

A. What is her diagnosis and why are infectious causes of diarrhea unlikely?
B. What is the likely cause of the diarrhea?

C. How should she be managed?
D. What outcome would you expect from this management?

Case Answers

28-1 A. *Learning objective:* **Identify common causes of diarrhea using information from the history.** "Toddler's diarrhea" is the most likely diagnosis. She has no fever, weight loss, or blood in the stool. Her exposure history is minimal. Most importantly, her dietary history provides the key information.

28-1 B. *Learning objective:* **Discuss the dietary causes of diarrhea.** Excessive intake of carbohydrate from juice provides an excessive osmotic load and promotes water loss in the bowel.

28-1 C. *Learning objective:* **Discuss the evaluation and management of osmotic diarrhea.** You would order no tests. You should advise limiting juice to 4 ounces per day and resuming cow's milk.

28-1 D. *Learning objective:* **Discuss the expected outcome after restricting the offending dietary agent.** You would expect that after making dietary changes the parents would report marked decrease in diarrhea. The child should continue to follow the growth curve.

BIBLIOGRAPHY

Branski D: Chronic diarrhea and malabsorption, *Pediatr Clin North Am* 43:307, 1996.

DeWitt TG: Acute diarrhea in children, *Pediatr Rev* 11:6, 1989.

Duggan C: "Feeding the gut": the scientific basis for continued enteral nutrition during acute diarrhea, *J Pediatr* 131:801, 1997.

Kneepkens CM: Chronic nonspecific diarrhea of childhood: pathophysiology and management, *Pediatr Clin North Am* 43:375, 1996.

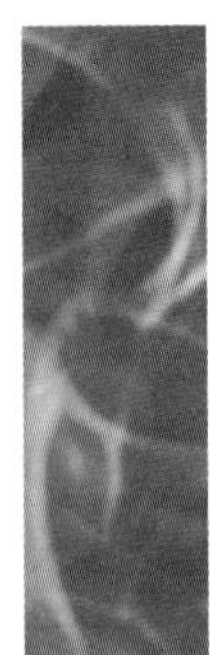

29

Dysuria, Urinary Frequency, and Urgency

LAVJAY BUTANI and BRUCE Z. MORGENSTERN

ETIOLOGY

How Are Dysuria, Frequency, and Urgency Defined?

Dysuria refers to painful or uncomfortable urination.

Frequency refers to a pattern of voiding at brief intervals, triggered by the sensation of bladder fullness. Although the voiding frequency can be quite variable in children, most children older than 7 years void between 3 and 8 times per day. This variability means that the term *urinary frequency* should be applied only after taking into consideration the baseline urinary habits of your particular patient.

Urgency refers to an exaggerated sense of needing to urinate.

What Causes These Symptoms?

Common causes of these three symptoms include conditions that lead to irritation of the bladder or urethral mucosa:

- Infections: bacterial or viral cystitis/urethritis
- Chemical irritation: bubble baths, hypercalciuria
- Mechanical trauma: bladder calculi, sexual abuse

Uncommon causes must be considered if none of the previous can be identified:

- Neurogenic: tethered cord that causes bladder spasms rather than true dysuria, but can also result in urinary tract infections (UTIs), which would then cause dysuria
- Psychological: pollakiuria—urinary urgency and frequency without dysuria, of uncertain etiology, but possibly triggered by emotional stress
- Diseases that cause polyuria such as diabetes mellitus, diabetes insipidus, diuretic use, and psychogenic polydipsia.

EVALUATION

How Do I Evaluate a Child with These Symptoms?

Obtain a complete history and perform a careful physical examination. Evaluate for signs and symptoms of UTI (Chapter 65). Ask about perineal hygiene and the use of bubble baths or the presence of a urethral/vaginal discharge. Consider a self-inserted vaginal foreign body in a young girl. Get details on the amount and type of fluids consumed by the child during a typical day. Obtain a sexual history, especially use of condoms, by adolescents. Ask about emotional stressors, such as the death of a family member, recent changes in school, and parental divorce. Investigate for possible sexual abuse and examine the external genitalia. Query the patient for a history of flank or abdominal pain and the family for a history of kidney stones in family members. Inspect the spine of the child for tufts of hair and sacral dimples. Perform a complete neurodevelopmental history and examination, especially of the lower extremities, rectal tone, and anal wink.

What Tests Should I Order?

The workup should be based on history and physical examination findings. Useful tests include:

- Urinalysis for specific gravity, glucosuria, cells, and bacteria
- Urine culture
- Urethral culture for *Chlamydia* and *Neisseria gonorrhoeae*
- Random urine for the calcium-to-creatinine ratio to detect hypercalciuria
- Abdominal x-ray (kidney, ureter, bladder) and renal and bladder ultrasound if you suspect stones or neurologic causes

TREATMENT

How Are Voiding Symptoms Treated?

Treatment depends on the underlying cause of the symptoms. General measures include frequent scheduled voiding during the daytime, improvement of perineal hygiene (girls should wipe from front to back after defecation and uncircumcised boys should clean under the foreskin when bathing), avoidance of chemical irritants such as bubble baths, identification of stressors and reassurance of children with pollakiuria that the condition is benign. A child with a neurogenic bladder should be referred to a pediatric urologist and neurosurgeon so that appropriate surgical and medical measures can be instituted to prevent deterioration of renal function.

KEY POINTS

- ◆ Dysuria, frequency, and urgency all result from irritation of the urethra or bladder.
- ◆ Psychoemotional stress and polyuria can present as urinary frequency.
- ◆ Urinary tract infections, chemical irritation, and hypercalciuria are common causes of dysuria.
- ◆ Sexual history must be obtained in children and adolescents with dysuria.
- ◆ The spine and lower extremities should be examined to look for neurologic causes, and the developmental history should be reviewed.

Case 29-1

An 8-year-old girl is referred to you for evaluation of dysuria that started 2 days earlier. She has also started wetting herself throughout the day. There is no history of fever or abdominal pain

A. What additional history would help in your evaluation?
B. What would you like to do next?

Case Answers

29-1 A. *Learning objective:* **Identify the likely causes of voiding symptoms from the history.** You should inquire about vaginal discharge, the use of bubble baths, and voiding habits. Obtain a detailed history regarding perineal hygiene, constipation, and encopresis. Ask about the past history of urinary tract infections (UTIs) and about the family history of kidney stones and UTIs. If trauma or other concerning findings are identified on physical examination and the parental history does not match physical findings, review the social history to investigate for possible abuse. Interview the child in the presence of a chaperone, with the parents out of the room.

29-1 B. *Learning objective:* **Describe the physical examination and laboratory evaluation of the patient who has urgency, frequency, or dysuria.** The most important part of the evaluation is a detailed physical examination focusing on the spine, lower extremities, and the external genitalia. A rectal examination to assess the tone of the rectal sphincter may be helpful if a neurogenic bladder is suspected. The initial laboratory tests should be a urinalysis with a microscopic evaluation of the urine sediment, and a urine culture to rule out urinary tract infection. Further investigations will be based on physical examination and urinalysis results.

BIBLIOGRAPHY

Langman CB, Moore ES: Hypercalciuria in clinical pediatrics: a review. *Clin Pediatr* 23:135, 1984.

Zoubek J, Bloom DA, Sedman AB: Extraordinary urinary frequency. *Pediatrics* 85:1112, 1990.

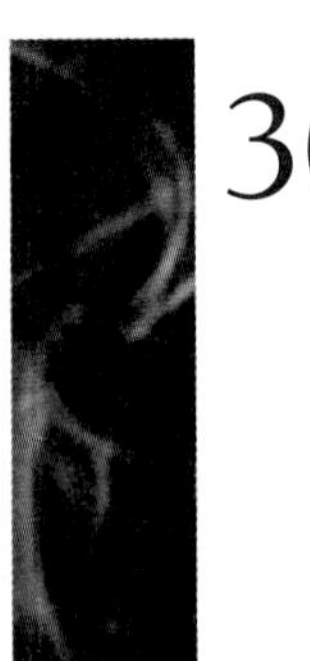

30

Ear Pain/Otitis Media

JEROLD C. WOODHEAD

ETIOLOGY

What Causes Ear Pain?

Ear pain is a frequent and persistent symptom of acute otitis media (AOM), the most common illness prompting a visit to a physician. Ear pain often develops *without* AOM in a child who has an upper respiratory infection with obstructed or poorly functioning eustachian tubes or during air travel when pressure change within the middle ear causes acute retraction or bulging of the tympanic membrane. Pain that worsens when the external ear is touched or moved usually reflects otitis externa, which often has an associated purulent discharge ("swimmer's ear"). An adolescent may have an inflammatory acne lesion within the ear canal that causes pain. Trauma to the ear canal or tympanic membrane by a cotton-tipped applicator or another foreign object can cause pain. Pain can be referred from teeth, a parotid gland, lymph nodes, or the temporomandibular joint and cause a child to describe "ear" pain or to rub or tug at the ear. Caries and dental abscesses are particularly common in children who have poor dental hygiene. Eruption of the first primary molars also can cause referred pain to the area of the ear. Mastoiditis is a rare but dangerous cause of ear pain and fever.

What Is Acute Otitis Media?

AOM represents infection of the middle ear cavity, usually before age 6 years, most often in the first 2 years of life. AOM is usually preceded or accompanied by viral upper respiratory infection. Children in daycare, preschool, play groups, school, or even large families have the highest risk for AOM. Rates of AOM are higher among children who live in homes where exposure to cigarette smoke occurs. Formula-fed infants have higher rates of AOM than do breast-fed infants, but any protective effect of breast-feeding is partial and lasts only as long as the infant is exclusively breast-fed. Other risk factors for AOM include prior episodes of AOM, antibiotic use in the previous 30 days, prolonged bottle feeding (especially beyond age 12 months), frequent use of a pacifier, and lower socioeconomic status. Children with Down syndrome and cleft palate have high rates of AOM, likely because of structural problems with the eustachian tubes. Immune deficiency may be first identified because of excessive or complicated episodes of AOM.

What Infectious Agents Cause Acute Otitis Media?

Viral infections produce inflammation, mucosal edema, and eustachian tube obstruction and dysfunction that promote bacterial infection of the middle ear and development of symptomatic AOM. Bacterial pathogens can be detected in 70% to 90% of children who have physical examination findings consistent with AOM. Bacteria identified include *Streptococcus pneumoniae* (~40%), nontypeable strains of *Haemophilus influenzae* (~30%), *Moraxella catarrhalis* (10% to 20%), and, much less commonly, *Streptococcus pyogenes* and *Staphylococcus aureus*. The precise bacterial cause of AOM for an individual patient must be inferred from community data because routine cultures are not recommended. The conjugate pneumococcal vaccine (PCV-7) has been shown to reduce the nasal carriage of *S. pneumoniae* and the incidence of AOM caused by the strains covered by this vaccine. *H. influenzae* type B is *not* a common cause of AOM, so the Hib vaccine has had little impact on AOM incidence.

How Often Does Antibiotic Resistance Occur?

Resistance to commonly used antibiotics has been increasing at an alarming rate worldwide for all of the major bacterial causes of AOM. Thirty percent to 50% of *S. pneumoniae* show resistance to one or more antibiotics, including penicillins, cephalosporins, macrolides, and trimethoprim-sulfamethoxazole. Up to 50% of *H. influenzae* are resistant to beta-lactam antibiotics, as are almost all isolates of *M. catarrhalis*, depending on the geographic region. Hence, resistant organisms have markedly altered treatment recommendations and have prompted reappraisal of the use of antibiotics for uncomplicated AOM.

EVALUATION

What Are the Diagnostic Criteria for Acute Otitis Media?

Diagnosis of AOM requires

- Acute onset of ear pain and fever, usually associated with upper respiratory infection (URI) symptoms.
- Bulging tympanic membrane, distorted tympanic membrane landmarks, erythema/inflammation of the membrane, middle ear effusion, and/or absent or reduced mobility to pneumatic otoscopic examination.

Does Ear Pain Always Mean Acute Otitis Media?

Ear pain is often overinterpreted by parents and physicians as indicating AOM. The diagnosis of AOM should only be made after careful assessment. AOM is a likely diagnosis when ear pain occurs in a child younger than 6 during an upper respiratory infection, especially when accompanied by fever. Occasionally a child will have ear pain followed by rapid resolution of pain at the time that a purulent drainage appears in the ear canal. This usually represents tympanic membrane rupture caused by AOM.

How Does History Help Identify the Cause of Ear Pain?

Ear pain is most evident when a verbal child tells you which ear hurts, when the pain started, and provides a description of the pain and what elicits it. The preverbal infant or toddler may cry, whimper, or rub and tug at the involved ear. Parents can describe the behavioral and sleep changes that they interpret as indicative of pain, especially if these symptoms have accompanied previous episodes of AOM in the child or a sibling. You need to identify details of the pain: onset, location, duration, and change over time. Ask about associated symptoms and signs, especially fever, upper respiratory infection, and otorrhea. ***It is important to document immunization status***, as widespread use of the conjugate vaccine for *S. pneumoniae* has reduced the rates of AOM. Inquire about risk factors such as exposure to tobacco smoke, attendance at daycare, any known trauma to the ear, and specific inciting causes such as swimming, air travel, acne, and insertion of cotton swabs in the ear canal. An "otitis-prone" child may have a past history of frequent AOM or of chronic middle ear effusion with accompanying conductive hearing loss and delayed language development. Listening to the child's speech will allow you to assess language development. You must understand development to interpret language skills, identify behaviors that might cause injury, and look for dental eruption as a cause of pain. Knowledge of risks associated with structural abnormalities (e.g., cleft palate) or syndromes will ensure that you consider appropriate issues during patient evaluation.

How Should I Examine a Child with Ear Pain?

Measure body temperature and look for "toxicity" (see Chapter 33). Identify patients who have high rates of AOM, including those with cleft palate, Down syndrome, and Treacher Collins syndrome. In addition, examine the nose, mouth, teeth, and lymph nodes. Finally, examine the ears. A successful examination of the ear requires assistance from the parent or caregiver to help stabilize the child's head and body (Figure 30-1). You must have experience with examination of the *healthy* ear, especially the examination of the tympanic membrane using a pneumatic otoscope (see Chapter 5). Use a checklist to guide your examination of the ears (Table 30-1).

What Physical Findings Are Associated with Ear Pain?

AOM is most likely if examination identifies an opaque, bulging, dull, inflamed, and poorly mobile tympanic membrane that has distorted or obscured anatomic landmarks. If you identify purulent otorrhea and if the child originally experienced acute ear pain but now has minimal

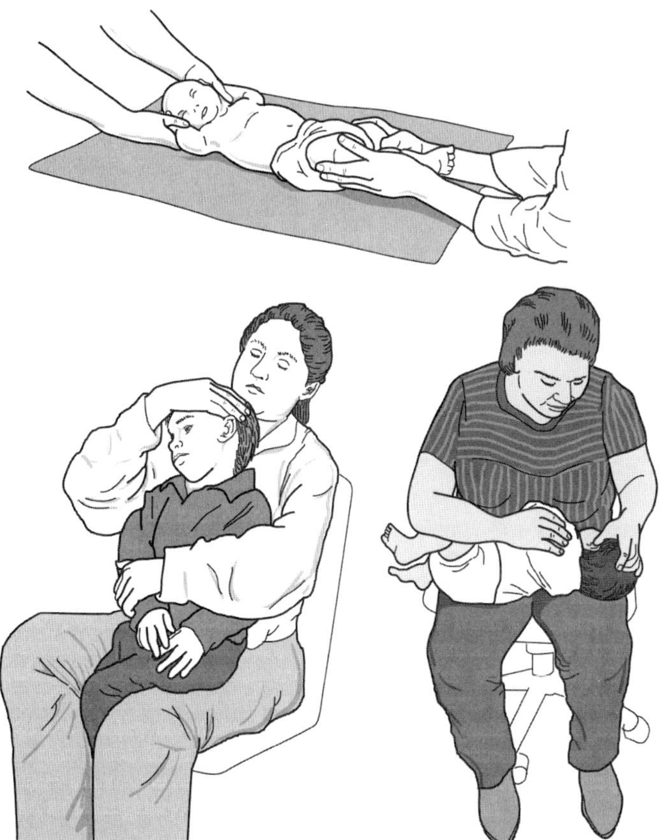

FIGURE 30-1 Three ways to position the infant or child for examination of the ear. (From Berkowitz CD: *Pediatrics: a primary care approach*, Philadelphia, 2000, WB Saunders, p 220.)

or no ear pain, the cause may be AOM with a perforated tympanic membrane. The perforation is usually difficult, if not impossible, to view with an otoscope because of the discharge. ***Otitis externa*** is suggested by pain with movement of the external ear along with a purulent discharge. A ***furuncle or inflammatory acne lesion*** should be evident in the ear canal. ***Mastoiditis*** causes pain behind the ear, classically with a "lop ear," in a febrile, toxic-appearing child who may also have AOM. ***Referred pain*** from a dental abscess, cervical lymphadenitis, temporomandibular joint dysfunction, or inflammation in the pharynx, parotid gland, or sinuses should be considered if examination identifies no problems of the external ear, the canal, or the tympanic membrane. An abscessed tooth is especially likely to cause "ear pain" if the child has poor dental hygiene, prominent plaque, and visible caries.

Table 30-1

Checklist for Examination of the Ears

	Healthy	Concerning
External ear	External ear anatomy (pinna canal); mastoid process	Pain with movement of external ear; "lop" ear; mastoid swelling, tenderness, and erythema
Canal	Patent; cerumen minimal	Cerumen occlusion; purulent discharge; foreign objects; furuncle
Tympanic membrane		
Landmarks	Malleus, umbo, pars tensa, pars flaccida, light reflection*	Obscured or distorted
Color	Pearly gray	Red, yellow, white, hemorrhagic
Physical appearance	Transparent/translucent, shiny	Opaque, dull; TM perforation or surgically implanted tympanostomy tubes
Position	Mid-position	Bulging or retracted
Movement (pneumatic otoscopy)	Movement with both positive and negative pressure	Diminished or absent motility
Other	Teeth; TMJ; sinuses; parotid gland; mastoid process	Dental caries and abscess; TMJ pain; sinus pain; parotid tenderness/ swelling; mastoid swelling or tenderness

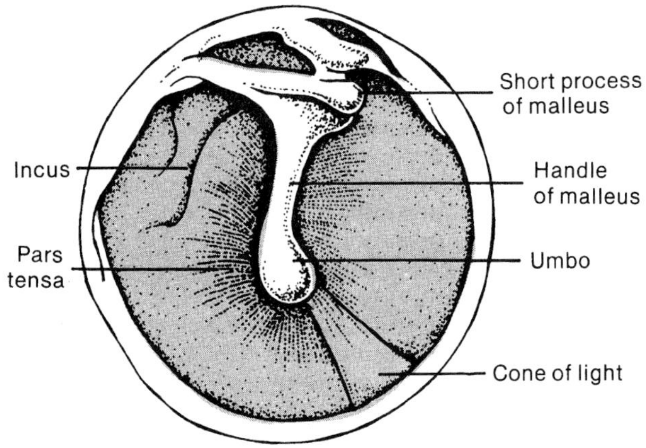

TM, Tympanic membrane; TMJ, temporomandibular joint.
*From Barness LA: *Manual of pediatric physical diagnosis*, ed 6, St Louis, 1991, Mosby–Year Book, p 66.

Are Laboratory Tests Necessary?

Most patients with ear pain or AOM do not require laboratory tests. Culture of middle ear fluid by tympanocentesis is *not* recommended for uncomplicated AOM. Failure of antibiotic treatment, especially if signs of toxicity are present, justifies tympanocentesis for culture. Complete blood count (CBC) with white blood cell (WBC) differential assists with the evaluation of the young, toxic-appearing patient. AOM in an infant or toddler with high fever (40° C) has a high association with bacteremia, especially if immunizations are lacking or incomplete for *S. pneumoniae*. In such cases, tympanocentesis and blood culture are appropriate, and a lumbar puncture with culture and fluid chemistries may be indicated. Culture of otorrhea is rarely recommended.

TREATMENT

Is Antibiotic Treatment Needed or Effective for Acute Otitis Media?

Long experience with antibiotic treatment of AOM has made this the standard of care in the United States. However, in Europe the standard of care no longer includes routine use of antibiotics. Complications previously associated with untreated AOM declined after routine antibiotic treatment was introduced. Antibiotic treatment of uncomplicated AOM reduces development of infection in the contralateral ear and may shorten duration of symptoms in some patients, but its efficacy otherwise has not been substantiated by careful study. Much evidence indicates that 70% to 90% of AOM resolves spontaneously, yet antibiotics have been identified as promoting resolution of infection. The discrepancy arises largely because studies have been poorly designed and have not included stringent definitions of AOM. Antibiotic treatment does not prevent development of subsequent episodes of AOM or of middle ear effusion and hearing loss 1 month after treatment. Treatment with antibiotics rapidly selects for resistant bacterial strains, a worldwide problem. Most pathogens that cause AOM have an increasing rate of β-lactamase production, and many have also developed resistance to trimethoprim-sulfamethoxazole and macrolides. Review of this topic by the American Academy of Pediatrics resulted in a Clinical Practice Guideline in 2004 that addressed the management of AOM.

What Does the AAP Recommend for AOM Treatment?

The American Academy of Pediatrics guidelines for treatment of AOM (see Bibliography and Table 30-2) include the *option to observe* a child older than 2 years for whom the diagnosis of AOM has been made from history and physical examination findings. The child must have fever < 39° C, only mild ear pain, and a family that will reliably return for further care if needed. Observation for 48 to 72 hours without antibiotic treatment includes pain management with appropriate doses of nonsteroidal antiinflammatory drugs (NSAIDs), plus education of the parents about monitoring symptoms. Follow-up at 48 to 72 hours is

Table 30-2

AAP Criteria for the Initial Management of Acute Otitis Media (AOM)

Age	AOM Diagnosis Certain*	AOM Diagnosis Uncertain
$<$ 6 months	Antibiotics	Antibiotics
6 months–2 years	Antibiotics	Antibiotics if severe illness Observation† if nonsevere
$>$ 2 years	Antibiotics if severe illness Observation† if nonsevere	Observation†

Adapted from American Academy of Pediatrics/American Academy of Family Physicians, Subcommittee on Management of Acute Otitis Media: Clinical practice guideline: Diagnosis and management of acute otitis media, *Pediatrics* 113:1451, 2004.

*"Diagnosis Certain" based on rapid onset of symptoms plus identification of middle ear effusion and tympanic membrane inflammation by otoscopic examination.

†Observation for nonsevere illness only: temperature $\leq$ 39° C, mild ear pain, not toxic-appearing.

recommended, although the physician may elect to provide a "rescue" antibiotic prescription for selected cases; parents would be instructed to use the antibiotic if symptoms fail to resolve or pain and fever worsen during the observation period. ***Children younger than 2 years, and children at any age with severe pain or fever $\geq$ 39° C should be treated with antibiotics at the time of diagnosis.*** When the diagnosis of AOM is uncertain, antibiotics should not be used.

Which Antibiotic Should Be Used?

Antibiotics for treatment of otitis media are listed in Table 30-3.

Can Acute Otitis Media Be Prevented?

Prevention efforts should focus on measures to prevent or reduce exposure to cigarette smoke, encourage breast-feeding, and discourage prolonged use of nursing bottles beyond 12 months of age. Pacifier use by infants and toddlers with frequent AOM should be discouraged. Promotion of hand washing in daycare and other places where children congregate can reduce spread of infection. Immunization against *S. pneumoniae* with the pneumococcal conjugate vaccine (PCV-7) protects against invasive disease and reduces the rate of AOM.

How Do I Treat Chronic Middle Ear Effusions?

Children with chronic middle ear effusions (also known as *otitis media with effusion* [OME]) may have ear pain when pressure change within the middle ear distorts the tympanic membrane. These children have conductive hearing loss, often experience language developmental delay, and also have high rates of AOM. Prophylactic antibiotic treatment does reduce the frequency with which AOM recurs, but it is also

Table 30-3

Antibiotic Choice for Patients with Certain Diagnosis of Acute Otitis Media (AOM)*

	Antibiotic Treatment Options					
	Initial Treatment at Diagnosis		**Treatment Failure# after 48–72 Hours of Observation**		**Treatment Failure# 48–72 Hours after Initial Treatment**	
Clinical Findings	**Recommended**	**Alternative for Penicillin Allergy**	**Recommended**	**Alternative for Penicillin Allergy**	**Recommended**	**Alternative for Penicillin Allergy**
AOM and fever < 39° C and mild otalgia	Amoxicillin (80–90 mg/kg/day)	*Type I:* Azithromycin, Clarithromycin *Non-Type I:* Cefdinir Cefuroxime Cefpodoxime	Amoxicillin (80–90 mg/kg/day)	*Type I:* Azithromycin Clarithromycin *Non-Type I:* Cefdinir Cefuroxime Cefpodoxime	Amoxicillin-clavulanate (90 mg/kg/day amoxicillin with 6.4 mg/kg/day clavulanate)	*Type I:* Clindamycin *Non-Type I:* Ceftriaxone for 3 days
AOM and fever ≥39° C and/or severe otalgia	Amoxicillin-clavulanate (90 mg/kg/day amoxicillin with 6.4 mg/kg/day clavulanate)	Ceftriaxone for 1 or 3 days	Amoxicillin-clavulanate (90 mg/kg/day amoxicillin with 6.4 mg/kg/day clavulanate)	Ceftriaxone for 1 or 3 days	Ceftriaxone for 3 days	Tympanocentesis and clindamycin

*AOM is defined as the acute onset of middle ear effusion with signs of inflammation. This typically occurs in a patient with acute fever and/or otalgia who has a bulging, inflamed tympanic membrane.

#Persistence or worsening of fever and/or otalgia.

(Adapted from American Academy of Pediatrics/American Academy of Family Physicians, Subcommittee on Management of Acute Otitis Media: Clinical Practice Guideline: Diagnosis and management of acute otitis media. *Pediatrics*, 113:1451–1465, 2004) associated with appearance of resistant organisms. Consequently, routine antibiotic prophylaxis can no longer be recommended for OME. Reserve this treatment for those children with OME whose AOM episodes recur more often than three times in 6 months or four times in 12 months. Neither a single course nor long-term administration of antibiotics causes resolution of OME. Children with persistent OME, especially if they have associated hearing loss and/or language delay, may be candidates for surgical implantation of tympanostomy tubes.

How Are Other Causes of Ear Pain Treated?

Treatment must be based on a specific diagnosis. In all cases, appropriate attention to pain control is important. NSAIDs have somewhat better efficacy than acetaminophen because of their antiinflammatory activity. Decongestants do not improve eustachian tube dysfunction. Otitis externa does not need systemic antibiotic treatment, although eardrops such as Cortisporin otic (hydrocortisone/polymyxin/neomycin) reduce pain, inflammation, and discharge. Refer children with caries and abscesses to a dentist.

KEY POINTS

- Acute otitis media has a high rate of spontaneous resolution, so a short trial of an NSAID may be advisable before starting antibiotics in children older than age 2 years.
- Antibiotics should be prescribed if the child is younger than 2 years, highly febrile, or ill appearing.
- Resistant bacteria are more common in children who attend daycare or have a past history of acute otitis media treated with antibiotics.

Case 30-1

An 18-month-old child is brought to the office with fever and fussiness. He did not sleep well last night, crying intermittently. Temperature was 101° F this morning. He has been well up until now

A. What information from the history will assist you to develop a differential diagnosis for this patient?
B. What would you expect to find on examination of the tympanic membrane if this child has AOM?
C. How would you treat this patient if you identified AOM? On what would you base your treatment decision?

Case Answers

30-1 A. *Learning objective:* **Identify the key risk factors for development of otitis media.** Details of the illness must be ascertained, including upper respiratory infection symptoms and their duration. It is important to identify exposures, such as ill siblings, daycare attendance, and environmental tobacco smoke. Ask about the child's past history of illness, immunization status, and the presence of middle ear effusions, eustachian tube dysfunction, and/or cleft palate. Ask about prior use of antibiotics because this is associated with infection by resistant organisms.

30-1 B. *Learning objective:* **Use an otoscope to identify the physical findings of acute otitis media.** The tympanic membrane would be inflamed and bulging and have few or no visible landmarks. The tympanic membrane would not move with insufflation (pneumatic otoscopy).

30-1 C. *Learning objective:* **Discuss management of the young child who has acute otitis media.** Use knowledge of common bacterial pathogens to guide treatment decisions. The choice of treatment depends on the clinical findings and the risk factors. Because of this child's age (< 2 years), fever, and discomfort, you should treat with antibiotics. Amoxicillin at a dose of 40 to 50 mg/kg would be the choice if he is not in daycare; high-dose amoxicillin (70 to 90 mg/kg) or amoxicillin plus clavulanate would be the choice if he is in daycare. *Streptococcus pneumoniae* is the most common bacterial pathogen identified in acute otitis media. Other organisms include *Moraxella catarrhalis* and *Haemophilus influenzae* (nontypeable strains). Antibiotic resistance is a growing problem with all of these organisms. In addition, control of pain and fever should be an important part of management. While the child is awake, parents may give acetaminophen (15 mg/kg/dose every 4 hours) or ibuprofen (10 mg/kg/dose every 6 hours).

BIBLIOGRAPHY

American Academy of Pediatrics/American Academy of Family Physicians: Subcommittee on Management of Acute Otitis Media: Clinical practice guideline: diagnosis and management of acute otitis media, *Pediatrics* 113:1451, 2004.

Wald E: Acute otitis media: More trouble with the evidence, *Pediatr Inf Dis J* 22:103, 2003.

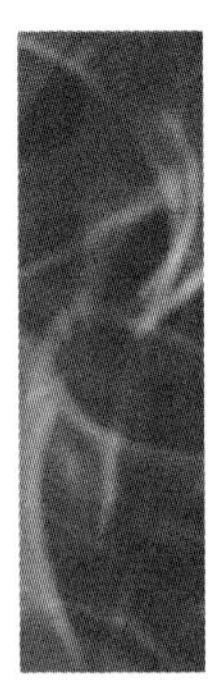

31

Emergencies and Trauma: An Initial Approach

CHARLES A. JENNISSEN and STEVEN Z. MILLER[†]

ETIOLOGY

What Causes Most Life-Threatening Emergencies?

Infants: infection, trauma (particularly child abuse), metabolic disorders, and congenital defects.
Toddlers and older children: trauma, either unintentional or inflicted.
Adolescents: trauma, especially when alcohol and automobiles mix.

As discussed in Chapter 11, preventable trauma must be addressed at all health supervision visits with attention to developmental risks, the potential for abuse, domestic violence, and high-risk situations. Specific emergency situations are discussed in Chapter 59.

EVALUATION

How Do I Recognize Life-Threatening Emergencies?

Your first task is to determine whether the child is critically ill, which is perhaps the most important skill that you learn in the pediatric clerkship. Your goal should be to use history, physical examination, and diagnostic tests consistently and reproducibly to determine if a problem is potentially life-threatening.

How Do I Identify the Critically Ill Patient?

A critically ill patient has a process that interferes with the delivery of oxygen and nutrients to the end organs. History and observation help you assess oxygenation and perfusion of critical organs because even subtle signs of organ dysfunction can provide clues to a critical illness.

Brain. Assess the patient's mental status. Start with an open-ended question such as, "How he is acting and behaving?" The parent's observations are likely to provide reliable information. Avoid questions that require parents to interpret a term, such as "Is he lethargic?" Parents may not think of lethargy in the same way that you do.

[†]Deceased.

Skin. Assess skin color, as it may suggest serious illness: blue—cyanosis; pale—anemia; gray—acidemia; mottled—shock; yellow—jaundice.

Kidneys. Make it a habit to ask about fluid intake and urine output in every history. Decreased urine output is a sign of dehydration and shock.

Respiratory System. Assess respiratory rate and effort. Parents may note tachypnea and increased work of breathing. Tachypnea is a sign of both ventilatory problems and shock. Even minor problems with oxygenation or perfusion of any organ will cause the respiratory system to compensate. Respiratory rate increases in an effort to enhance oxygen intake in hypoxia or to decrease CO_2 concentration in metabolic acidosis.

Cardiovascular System. A patient or a parent might notice that the child's "heart seems to be racing." Don't ignore this subtle sign. Tachycardia is the cardiovascular system's earliest defense in compensating for end organ perfusion problems caused by dehydration or shock.

Which Patient Presentations Should Cause Concern?

Certain scenarios may reflect a potentially life-threatening condition, despite the child's initial appearance, and almost always require additional diagnostic studies:

- Fever in an infant younger than 2 months may be caused by a serious bacterial infection in up to 10% of cases, even when the examination does not identify a focus for the fever.
- Fever in an immunocompromised patient, including conditions such as sickle cell disease and neutropenia, may also reflect serious bacterial infection.
- Fever and petechiae could be early signs of meningococcemia.
- Paroxysmal cough in the first year of life could be a sign of pertussis, and the infant may appear intermittently well.
- Bilious vomiting in an infant could be a sign of malrotation and volvulus. The examination and appearance could be intermittently normal.
- Syncope could be a sign of a potentially fatal cardiac lesion or dysrhythmia.
- Unexplained lethargy or altered level of consciousness has many potentially life-threatening causes, including abusive head trauma, seizures, and intussusception.

How Should I Structure the Physical Examination?

Use the primary survey for all patients. This initial physical examination is known as the ABCs but is often extended to include "D" and "E," as described in the next section. The primary survey must be followed in an unvarying sequence to ensure that you will identify life-threatening illnesses or injuries. Only after the ABC(DE)s are completed do you perform a careful head-to-toe examination, the *secondary survey.*

What Are the ABC(DE)s and How Do I Perform Them?

The ABC(DE)s are performed in the following unvarying sequence:

- *Airway.* Go to the head of the bed. Open the airway by extending the neck. For infants, this means placing a blanket under the shoulders to slightly extend the neck and tilt the head into a "sniffing" position. If you hyperextend the neck of an infant, the airway may collapse. For older children, the neck must be extended more to open the airway. You can also use a jaw thrust to move soft tissue structures and further open the airway. To do this, place your index fingers behind the posterior portion of the mandible and push forward. Administer 100% oxygen if needed. If any concern exists about cervical spine injury, use *only* the jaw thrust to open the airway and maintain cervical spine immobilization.
- *Breathing.* Look at the chest wall to assess respiratory rate, adequacy of chest rise, and work of breathing. Generally, newborn infants have respiratory rates of about 50 breaths/min, but by 1 year, the respiratory rate declines to 30 breaths/min. Respiratory rate above 60 breaths/min may signal respiratory distress in an infant. Rates slowly decrease to adult levels after age 1 year. Listen to the chest bilaterally, preferably almost at the axilla to avoid confusion with sounds from the opposite lung. Obtain a pulse oximetry reading. If ventilation is inadequate, you may need to provide bag-valve-mask (BVM) support with 100% oxygen.
- *Circulation.* To determine whether the patient is in shock, start by checking the pulses. Find the femoral or brachial pulse in an infant or young child (the carotid pulse is often difficult to find). Next, feel for a peripheral pulse (radial is usually best). Determine the heart rate, remembering that tachycardia is an early sign of shock. Newborn infants have heart rates up to 160 beats/min. By 1 year, the heart rate slows to 120 beats/min, then slows further as the child grows. Check capillary refill by pressing a finger tip or toe. Keep the extremity at or above the heart so you are not checking venous refill. Look for active bleeding and stop it if possible. Finally, obtain a blood pressure; if you are alone this can be deferred, but not left out.
- *Disability.* This mini-neurologic assessment ascertains mental status and the risk for central nervous system herniation:
  - Check pupils for size and responsiveness to light. Abnormalities will help make an early diagnosis of brain stem herniation and poisonings.
  - Establish the level of alertness. Look at the eyes for response when the patient is stimulated. All but the youngest neonates should at least look back at you. The "AVPU" scale is often used:
    A = Alert
    V = Responds to verbal stimuli
    P = Responds to pain only
    U = Unresponsive
- *Exposure/Environment.* Undress the patient so that you can complete a thorough physical examination. Then think about the environment and take measures to prevent hypothermia.

What Tools Can Help Me Identify a "Sick" Infant or Child?

A number of scales are used to quantify severity of illness in infants and young children, but they are mostly used as research tools. The Yale Observation Scale (Table 33-1) can help you learn to identify the "sick" or "toxic" appearing child.

What Diagnostic Tests Should I Order for the Initial Evaluation?

Order diagnostic tests only after the ABCs are completed and the patient has been stabilized.

- Arterial blood gas measurement provides information about oxygenation, ventilation, and acid-base status.
- Serum chemistries give information about renal function, sodium and potassium levels, blood glucose, and acid-base status.
- Inflammatory markers such as white blood count (WBC) with differential and C-reactive protein (CRP) can provide information about infection, as will cultures of blood, urine, and cerebrospinal fluid (CSF).
- Radiographs, ultrasound, and computed tomography (CT) scanning evaluate pulmonary, cardiac, and abdominal problems and trauma.

TREATMENT

What Initial Supportive Treatment Is Used?

The ABCs incorporate initial management to support oxygenation, ventilation, and perfusion:

- Administer 100% oxygen, with a nonrebreather mask if possible.
- Assist ventilation if necessary using a BVM.
- Give intravenous fluids to replenish the circulating volume. If a peripheral intravenous line cannot be established, insert an intraosseous line (a needle placed in the bone marrow, usually in the proximal tibia).
- *Reassess the adequacy of your initial interventions*—this is a must!
- Consider broad-spectrum antibiotics, preferably after cultures have been obtained.
- When the patient is stable, perform diagnostic tests.

What Should I Do If the Patient Stops Breathing?

After you call for assistance, use a BVM to ventilate the patient. You must make a good seal between the mask and the patient's face by forming the letter "C" with your thumb and ring finger on the mask and an "E" with your other fingers under the jaw; then press down. Squeeze enough air with the bag to cause a gentle rise in the chest. You may need to insert a nasogastric tube to remove air from the stomach if the patient requires bagging for any appreciable time. Proper use of the BVM is an essential skill that you should master before residency.

What Causes Problems with Bag-Valve-Mask Ventilation?

Difficulty ventilating with the BVM is almost always because of a mechanical problem:

- Air will not enter the airway. Inadequate or excessive neck extension may be collapsing the airway. Repositioning of the head will be required. Airway adjuncts such as an oropharyngeal or nasopharyngeal airway may overcome obstruction from the tongue or other soft tissues.
- The reservoir bag does not fill with oxygen, so you cannot ventilate the patient. You may need to increase the oxygen flow rate to keep the reservoir taut with oxygen.
- The BVM does not make a good seal with the patient. If you cannot maintain the seal with one hand and compress the bag with the other, have someone else make the seal with the mask while you bag.
- The BVM may have a hole in it. Check this by squeezing the BVM into your hand and listening for air coming out somewhere else. You may need to get another BVM.
- The pop-off valve on the BVM does not allow you to generate enough pressure to ventilate stiff lungs (as in a drowning victim). You may need to close the pop-off valve.

How Can I Tell If the Patient Is in Shock?

Shock occurs when oxygen and nutrients are not adequately delivered to the end organs. If uncorrected, shock will damage cells—often irreversibly. *Tachycardia* is one of the earliest signs of shock. Other signs include weak pulses, sluggish capillary refill, and poor urine output. Remember that a child can be in shock and still have "normal" blood pressure because vasoconstriction acts as a compensatory mechanism. Blood pressure is the last parameter to change in shock.

How Do I Manage the Different Types of Shock?

Distributive Shock. Mechanisms include sepsis, anaphylaxis, spinal trauma, and barbiturate poisoning. Management priorities include infusion of fluids and use of pressor medications to promote vasoconstriction.

Hypovolemic Shock. Mechanisms include hemorrhage and fluid loss. Management priorities include infusion of fluids and stopping the bleeding or fluid loss.

Cardiogenic Shock. Mechanisms include dysrhythmias, cardiomyopathies, structural heart lesions, and obstructive conditions such as cardiac tamponade and tension pneumothorax. Management priorities include extremely careful fluid resuscitation and treatment of the underlying cause, often with afterload reduction. The signs of cardiogenic shock can be quite subtle, and excessive fluid resuscitation may worsen the patient's condition. Always ask yourself, "How do I know that this is not cardiogenic shock?" when making management decisions.

Neurogenic Shock. This is rare. Management is with fluid resuscitation.

Which Fluids Should I Choose for a Child in Shock?

Treatment of shock requires refilling the intravascular space with an *isotonic* fluid such as normal saline (NS) or lactated Ringer's solution. Hypotonic solutions are inappropriate for vascular resuscitation. Isotonic crystalloids are most often used because they are readily available and have been documented to be effective. Colloids, including albumin, dextran, and blood products, are rarely used as the first choice because they have limited clinical advantage and cost more. They may be needed if a patient does not show adequate response to crystalloid infusion, especially if there has been blood loss. A general discussion of fluid management is found in Chapter 26.

What Do I Need to Know about Trauma Management?

The primary survey (ABCs), supportive management, and need for reassessment are the mainstays for all emergencies. Important considerations specific to trauma patients include:

- *Cervical spine immobilization.* Keep the neck immobilized while performing the airway assessment. Do not use neck extension to open the airway—use the jaw thrust.
- *Internal injury from trauma.* A "normal" external examination does not rule out internal injuries. In particular, physically abused children commonly have absence of external findings. All victims of trauma could be bleeding internally and have impending hypovolemic shock, even if they are well-appearing. The single biggest mistake in the management of a trauma patient is underestimating the injuries.

What Is the Secondary Survey for a Trauma Patient?

Immediately after the ABCs and initial supportive management, perform the secondary survey. This includes a thorough physical examination and selected tests, such as radiographs of the cervical spine, chest, and pelvis; urine evaluation (including urinalysis and pregnancy testing in a postmenarchal female); and blood tests called a "trauma panel." This panel may include hemoglobin/hematocrit, arterial blood gas, liver function tests, alcohol level, serum lactate, coagulation studies, and serum amylase or lipase. You will need to familiarize yourself with the specifics of the "trauma panel" at your medical center. An ultrasound evaluation of the abdomen called a FAST examination is also routinely done in many emergency departments primarily to look for internal bleeding.

What Does It Mean to "Clear the Cervical Spine"?

Any patient with trauma above the clavicles requires cervical spine immobilization. "Clearance" of the cervical spine generally requires radiographs before immobilization can be removed. However, evidence shows that immobilization can be removed safely when the patient demonstrates *all* of the following:

- Can communicate with you.
- Is totally alert.
- Has no neck tenderness.
- Has no distracting injuries or pain, such as a long bone fracture.
- Did not experience any neurologic symptoms—even transient ones.

Does Cervical Spine Management for Children Differ from That for Adult Trauma Victims?

More than half of all pediatric spinal cord injuries fit the description of SCIWORA: "Spinal Cord Injury Without Radiographic Abnormalities." *Transient neurologic symptoms* are a hallmark for this diagnosis. The cervical spine cannot be "cleared" if a child with cervical spine trauma has had transient neurologic symptoms, even with a "negative" radiograph. Such a patient must be referred for neurosurgical consultation and will need additional imaging studies.

KEY POINTS

- Learn the findings that indicate critical illness or "toxicity."
- Start every emergency intervention with the ABCs.
- Reassess the effectiveness of your interventions.
- Immobilize the cervical spine for trauma above the clavicles.

Case 31-1

A 17-year-old girl with fever and several days of diarrhea comes to the emergency department. Her mother is worried because the girl is not acting like herself today. Questioning reveals that she has not urinated in more than 24 hours and that she was difficult to wake up this morning.

A. Why are you concerned about this patient?
B. On physical examination, she is very sleepy, has temperature of 104° F, heart rate of 130 beats/min, respiratory rate of 30 breaths/min, blood pressure of 140/90 mm Hg, and O_2 saturation of 91%. The rest of the initial physical examination shows a generalized scarlatiniform rash without other specific findings. How would you interpret this examination?
C. What should be your initial management steps?

Case 31-2

An unrestrained 4-year-old girl was involved in a motor vehicle crash and hit her head against the windshield, causing a frontal scalp laceration. According to the emergency medical technician, she was alert and had stable vital signs at the scene. She was also noted to be in severe pain with what appeared to be a fractured femur. In the emergency department, she is alert and complains of leg pain but has no neck tenderness or neurologic symptoms.

A. What should be your initial management steps?

Case 31-3

A 7-year-old girl is brought by ambulance to the emergency department after falling from her bicycle. She was not wearing a helmet. On arrival, the child is unconscious with rapid, shallow respirations. She is wearing a cervical collar and has a splint on her right arm. Oxygen saturation is 97% in room air. Pulse is 120 beats/min, respiratory rate is 26 breaths/min, and blood pressure is 75/46 mm Hg. Her capillary refill is sluggish.

A. What are the first steps in the emergency management of this child?
B. After the patient's airway, breathing, and circulation are stabilized, what are the next steps in the emergency assessment?
C. What comprises the secondary survey for this patient?

Case Answers

31-1 A. *Learning objective:* **Identify the information from history that suggests a diagnosis of shock.** The change in behavior and the decreased urine output are worrisome. This patient likely has shock, either from infection or hypovolemia (or both). If a parent telephoned you in the middle of the night, you would arrange to have the patient seen immediately.

31-1 B. *Learning objective:* **Interpret the physical findings that commonly accompany shock.** The primary survey identifies many concerning issues:

- She is hypoxemic—91% is a key number because patients are at the steep portion of the oxygen saturation curve at this level and will have a PO_2 of 60 to 70 mm Hg. Any further decrease in oxygenation results in marked desaturation and impaired oxygen delivery to the end organs.
- She is difficult to arouse—suggesting poor end organ perfusion (the brain).

- She is tachycardic—this may be the most important and subtle sign of severe illness. Never overlook the heart rate. Unexplained tachycardia is the most often missed finding in patients who return to the ER severely ill after being seen earlier.
- She is tachypneic—which could mean compensation for metabolic acidosis resulting from poor perfusion and anaerobic metabolism.
- She is mildly hypertensive—patients in early shock can sometimes be slightly hypertensive as a compensatory response to poor perfusion. Do not be fooled by this.
- The scarlatiniform rash could be a sign of toxic shock syndrome—other rashes that could be a hint of sepsis include petechiae and purpura, as seen in meningococcemia.

31-1 C. *Learning objective:* **Develop a plan for the immediate management of shock.** First, administer 100% oxygen and monitor oxygen saturation. Then initiate supportive management for shock, including rapid infusion of isotonic crystalloid (lactated Ringer's or normal saline) via a large-bore intravenous catheter. Assess the response to the initial fluid bolus and repeat fluid infusions as necessary to restore circulating volume. Finally, because the patient may have toxic shock syndrome, administer antibiotics that will provide coverage for *Staphylococcus aureus* and group A beta-hemolytic streptococci after obtaining blood cultures.

31-2 A. *Learning objective:* **Recognize the potential for cervical spine injury in a trauma patient.** Before any further assessment is started, this patient must have her cervical spine stabilized with a collar. She also needs a full radiographic workup of the cervical spine, even though she is alert and has no neck tenderness or neurologic symptoms. The pain from the femur fracture could be distracting her from perceiving any neck pain. Therefore you cannot use clinical criteria to "clear" the cervical spine.

31-3 A. *Learning objective:* **Perform a primary survey (ABCs) on an injured patient and identify problems needing urgent intervention.**

Airway and breathing: This child is unconscious. She must have her airway stabilized and the cervical spine immobilized (imperative given the injury above the clavicles). The usual method of extending the neck to open the airway must be avoided. Instead, you should do a jaw thrust—in which you push the posterior part of the mandible forward using your fingers. She should be administered 100% oxygen by a nonrebreather face mask (or via an endotracheal tube if needed). Evaluate breathing effort by looking at the chest for retractions and symmetrical movement. Count the respiratory rate. Auscultate the chest (in the axilla, not close to the sternum) to assess the breath sounds. Monitor the oxygen saturation with pulse oximetry and continue to reassess the adequacy of ventilation.

Circulation: Her low blood pressure, rapid pulse, and sluggish capillary refill indicate shock, possibly related to occult hemorrhage. She should have large-bore intravenous lines inserted and be given intravenous isotonic fluid. Monitor the vital signs closely to assess adequacy of your intervention.

31-3 B. *Learning objective:* **Discuss the assessment of disability and environment/exposure.** The initial assessment after the ABCs would include undressing the child completely to assess for other trauma, protecting the patient from hypothermia, and performing a quick neurologic evaluation. This includes checking the pupils and mental status. Assessment of the level of consciousness, in this case, would include determination of the Glasgow Coma Scale score during the secondary survey. Evidence of herniation would include asymmetrical pupils, an unresponsive/posturing patient, and the presence of Cushing's triad—hypertension, bradycardia, and irregular respirations. Infuse mannitol and consider hyperventilating the patient if there are signs of herniation.

31-3 C. *Learning objective:* **Discuss the secondary survey, describe its content, and outline the sequence of events.** The secondary survey of this child includes a meticulous physical examination plus laboratory and imaging studies based on the results of the examination once the patient is stabilized. This child will need CT of the head. The concern for hypovolemia and possible occult bleeding should also prompt an abdominal and pelvic CT. The secondary survey for any patient with significant trauma includes urine evaluation, a "trauma panel" of blood tests and radiographs of the cervical spine, chest, and pelvis. Because she has a broken right arm, a radiograph of the arm will eventually be needed as well. In general, the purpose of the secondary survey is to look for specific injuries, especially occult bleeding, central nervous system injury, and cervical spine injury. The biggest error in trauma evaluation is underestimating the possibility of occult injury.

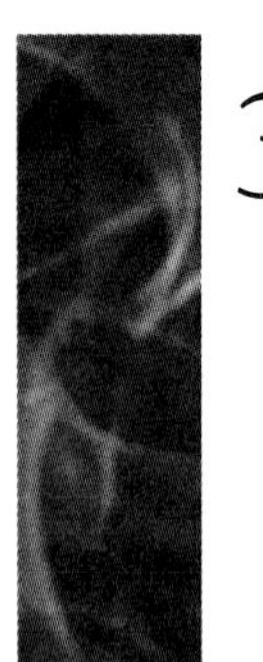

32

Enuresis/Urinary Incontinence

LAVJAY BUTANI and BRUCE Z. MORGENSTERN

ETIOLOGY

Should I Be Concerned If a 5-Year-Old Wets the Bed?

Bedwetting is common among 5-year-olds and is a form of *incontinence*, which is defined as the involuntary voiding of urine into clothing or bedding. This is also referred to as *enuresis*. Although often used interchangeably, the two terms are not synonymous. Incontinence refers to all potential causes of wetting. Enuresis refers to incontinence that has neither an anatomic nor a neurologic cause. Fifteen percent to 20% of 5-year-olds and 7% of 7-year-olds have not yet achieved bladder control at night, whereas almost all will be dry during the day. Enuresis and incontinence can be classified as *primary* when the child has never been continent, or *secondary* if wetting begins after at least a 6-month period of continence.

What Causes Incontinence?

Table 32-1 lists causes of primary and secondary incontinence. Primary enuresis, especially primary nocturnal enuresis, is thought to result from a physiologically immature bladder and resolves with time. Incontinence, either primary or secondary, can be caused by anatomic abnormalities of the urinary tract or spine or by other serious conditions that cannot be excluded without further evaluation, including functional abnormalities of the bladder, bladder inflammation, or polyuric states. History and physical examination provide critical information regarding the distinctions between these conditions. Secondary enuresis that results from psychological stressors is a diagnosis of exclusion.

What History Identifies the Cause of Incontinence?

A detailed history must focus on the child's voiding pattern and frequency. The pattern of incontinence is also important: diurnal, nocturnal, or both; constant dribbling or intermittent enuresis. Constipation often accompanies enuresis. Specific inquiry about social stressors should be made. History suggestive of diabetes (Chapter 60) or urinary

Table 32-1

Causes of Incontinence

Primary Incontinence	Secondary Incontinence
Physiologic (primary enuresis)	Psychological stressors (secondary enuresis)
Anatomic abnormalities (ectopic ureter, neurogenic bladder)	Anatomic abnormalities (neurogenic bladder)
	Bladder irritation (urinary tract infection, hypercalciuria)
	Polyuria (diabetes mellitus, diabetes insipidus, polydipsia, diuretic use)
	Bladder dysfunction (bladder sphincter dyssynergia)

tract infection (Chapter 65) will direct specific investigations. Urgency, dysuria, or family history of kidney stones will prompt evaluation for hypercalciuria. Family history is often positive in primary enuresis. Physical examination must include careful evaluation of the back for sacral or spine abnormalities, including hair tufts, masses, or deep sacral dimples. Genitourinary abnormalities, and neurologic problems, especially of the lower extremities, must be identified if present. Rectal examination to assess tone and presence or absence of constipation is important.

What Testing Is Needed?

Testing should be based on the information obtained by history and physical examination. Testing is generally not needed if your patient has primary nocturnal enuresis with a positive family history of enuresis but no associated urinary symptoms, no abnormal voiding during the day, and no abnormalities on physical examination. Some physicians elect to perform urinalysis and a clean-catch midstream urine culture for all patients with primary enuresis. If you suspect nonphysiologic incontinence, consider the following tests in addition to urinalysis and culture:

- Random urine specimen for calcium-to-creatinine ratio for hypercalciuria
- Blood glucose concentration for diabetes
- Kidney-ureter-bladder (KUB) radiograph and kidney and bladder ultrasound for spine abnormalities and neurogenic bladder
- Voiding cystourethrogram and intravenous pyelogram to look for bladder and ureteral anomalies

TREATMENT

How Do I Treat Incontinence?

Incontinence is a symptom and not a disease. Therefore management must address the underlying cause. For children with primary nocturnal enuresis, continued reassurance to the child and the family is imperative. Enuresis will resolve with time as the bladder matures. Motivated children whose quality of life is significantly hampered by their bedwetting may benefit from a commercially available enuresis alarm (Figure 32-1). Alarms are associated with a sustained reduction in enuresis even after they are discontinued. While awaiting spontaneous resolution, the intermittent use of nasal or oral desmopressin will allow older children to participate in overnight social outings without embarrassment. This is purely a symptomatic treatment and does not hasten bladder maturation; most children relapse when the medication is stopped.

KEY POINTS

- Primary nocturnal enuresis is usually physiologic and resolves with time.
- Some children with incontinence may have anatomic abnormality of the urinary tract or spine.
- A detailed examination of the lower extremities and spine is essential.
- Enuresis alarms reduce bedwetting in motivated children with primary nocturnal enuresis.

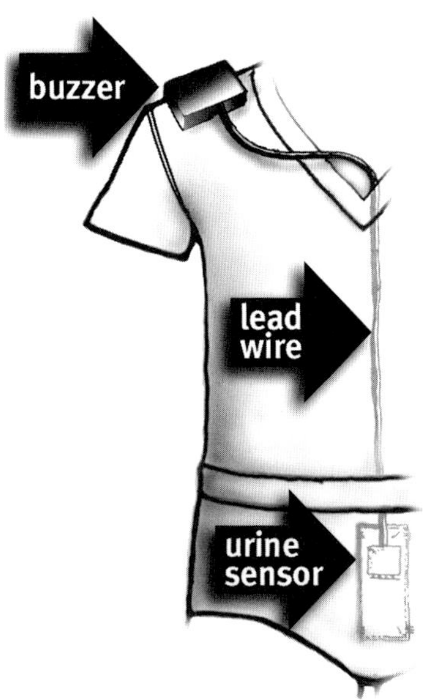

FIGURE 32-1 Schematic of an enuresis alarm.

Case 32-1

A 4-year-old girl is brought to your office for evaluation of constant dribbling of urine. She has never been continent of urine or stool.

A. What additional information from history and physical examination will you obtain?
B. What are the possible causes of her incontinence?
C. What further tests do you want to obtain?

Case 32-2

A 10-year-old boy is brought in by anxious parents because of new onset of diurnal and nocturnal incontinence. The family has recently moved into town. On direct questioning he and his parents note that his thirst and appetite have both increased since the move. His physical examination is completely unremarkable except for body mass index (BMI) > 95th percentile.

A. What are the possible causes of your patient's incontinence?
B. What further questions would you like to ask him?
C. How would you proceed with his evaluation?

Case 32-3

An 8-year-old girl has developed daytime and nighttime urinary incontinence. She has a history of constipation and has recently begun to complain of abdominal pain. On physical examination you find a firm tubular mass in the left lower quadrant. Rectal examination demonstrates lax rectal tone and firm stool in the rectal vault.

A. Why does this constipated patient have urinary incontinence?
B. What history and physical examination should you do to evaluate this patient?
C. Are any diagnostic tests indicated?

Case Answers

32-1 A. *Learning objective:* **Discuss the history and physical examination that are important in the evaluation of a child with urinary incontinence or enuresis.** You should ask about trauma to the spine at birth or later, lower extremity weakness, recurrent urinary tract infections (UTIs), and constipation. Physical examination should look for sacral deformities and assess lower extremity tone and strength. Test for anal wink and rectal sphincter tone, and perform a rectal examination.

32-1 B. *Learning objective:* **List the differential diagnosis of urinary incontinence or enuresis.** Causes include neurogenic bowel and bladder because of spinal bifida, behavioral enuresis, and constipation with or without encopresis. The possibility of physical abuse or emotional deprivation as a cause of behavioral enuresis should be considered if the history does not fit with the physical findings.

32-1 C. *Learning objective:* **Outline the imaging evaluation of a child with continuous urinary incontinence (daytime and nocturnal).** Imaging studies should include a KUB to look at the spine and a renal and bladder ultrasound. Also consider a voiding cystourethrogram to identify vesicoureteral reflux, magnetic resonance imaging of the spine to identify spina bifida, and an intravenous pyelogram to look for ureteral ectopia.

32-2 A. *Learning objective:* **Outline the causes of incontinence of recent onset.** Causes include diabetes mellitus, diabetes insipidus, psychogenic polydipsia, and urinary tract infection. Psychosocial stressors should also be considered in the absence of findings to support physical causes.

32-2 B. *Learning objective:* **Use the history to develop a differential diagnosis of acute urinary incontinence.** You need to inquire about the symptoms that accompany the changed voiding pattern. You should also review growth and medical records from his previous physician. Fever, abdominal pain, urgency, and dysuria usually accompany UTI, especially in boys. Weight loss, fatigue, excessive thirst, increased fluid intake, and increased urine output point to diabetes mellitus or insipidus. A variety of stressors at home and school may trigger enuresis; this boy's obesity and the recent move might be contributing to stress.

32-2 C. *Learning objective:* **Select appropriate laboratory tests to evaluate incontinence.** The most important test is the urinalysis to look for glucosuria, white blood cells, red blood cells, and bacteria. Urine specific gravity helps in the assessment of diabetes insipidus. Urine culture is important if infection is likely. If urinalysis is abnormal, further workup should be done as needed for the suspected condition. If all tests are negative, you can reassure the patient about the absence of a disease process but must schedule follow-up to address weight and stressors. A diary can help the child and parents identify stressors and eating patterns.

32-3 A. *Learning objective:* **Identify causes of urinary incontinence in constipated patients.** Children with chronic constipation often have urinary incontinence. A large fecal mass in the rectosigmoid distorts the bladder and also results in a reflex relaxation of both the rectal and urinary sphincters. Chronic constipation is usually the result of behavioral and dietary factors. Occasionally, the coexistence of constipation and enuresis is identified in children under emotional stress such as that associated with dysfunctional families or abusive situations. Neurogenic bowel/bladder may also cause these problems.

32-3 B. *Learning objective:* **Use the history and physical examination to assess a child with incontinence; in particular, recognize the psychoemotional antecedents of incontinence.** Ask about her urinary and bowel habit pattern and any changes that preceded the onset of urinary incontinence. Developmental history should review achievement of developmental milestones, especially toilet training. A careful physical examination should include neurologic and rectal examinations. The presence of stool in the rectal vault confirms chronic constipation. The history and physical examination may occasionally identify findings suggestive of physical and/or sexual abuse. Interview the patient and family separately if any suspicion exists for abuse.

32-3 C. *Learning objective:* **Discuss the diagnostic evaluation of a patient with incontinence.** Consider a KUB radiograph to determine extent of fecal impaction. Renal and bladder ultrasound may be indicated if suspecting neurogenic bladder. A comprehensive psychosocial evaluation may assist with the behavioral component of this problem. A skeletal radiographic screen is indicated if abuse is suspected.

BIBLIOGRAPHY

Matos V et al: Urinary phosphate/creatinine, calcium/creatinine, and magnesium/creatinine ratios in a healthy pediatric population, *J Pediatr* 131:252, 1997.

Rushton HG: Nocturnal enuresis: epidemiology, evaluation, and currently available treatment options, *J Pediatr* 114:691, 1989.

Wojcik LJ, Kaplan GW: The wet child, *Urol Clin North Am* 25:735, 1998.

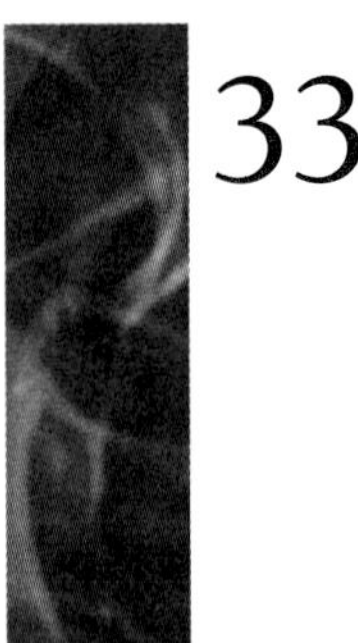

33 Fever

JEROLD C. WOODHEAD

ETIOLOGY

What Is Fever?

Fever is usually defined as a temperature above 38.0° C to 38.4° C (100.4° F to 101° F). Parents or other caregivers usually become aware of fever because a child looks "flushed" or feels "hot," which then leads to use of a thermometer that detects the elevated temperature. Most fever is associated with acute viral or bacterial infection and is self-limited, both in degree and duration. Fever less commonly results from malignancy, rheumatologic, or other diseases. "Teething" does not cause fever. Parents and medical professionals sometimes demonstrate "fever phobia," the worry that any level of fever always represents a serious infection or that it may rise without limit and cause "brain damage." This fear often prompts excessive concern, overuse of medical care, and overtreatment. Understanding the mechanism of temperature regulation, the nature of fever, and the range of "normal" body temperatures at different ages may reduce "fever phobia."

What Mechanism Causes Fever?

Fever is a *regulated* elevation of body temperature that results from alteration of the set point in the hypothalamic temperature regulatory center. In health, this center maintains temperature in a narrow range around 37° C (98.6° F), although between 12 and 36 months, healthy children have temperatures that may exceed 37.5° C (99.5° F). Temperature has a diurnal pattern that is lowest in the early morning and highest in the evening. Fever develops when a stimulus, such as infection, triggers release of *endogenous pyrogens* (cytokines, interleukins 1α and 1β) that reset the hypothalamic set point upward. This promotes vasoconstriction that results in heat retention, plus shivering and increased metabolic rate that increase heat production. Even when elevated during fever, body temperature remains regulated by the hypothalamus and rarely exceeds 41.5° C (106° F). Disappearance of pyrogens or treatment with an antipyretic resets the "thermostat" set point downward and temperature declines.

How Does Hyperthermia Differ from Fever ?

Hyperthermia is unregulated and, unlike fever, can cause temperature to rise well above 42° C (107° F) with risk of central nervous system (CNS) damage. Hyperthermia results from prolonged exposure to excessive environmental heat, physical conditions that prevent the body from removing heat, metabolic disorders such as malignant hyperthermia that cause excessive heat production, and CNS disorders that disrupt the hypothalamic center. Hyperthermia must be identified and managed promptly to minimize morbidity and prevent mortality.

What Is "Fever without Source?"

Fever without source refers to the situation when history and physical examination can find no obvious cause for fever. Most such patients have a viral illness, but when fever is above 40° C (104° F), *immunizations are incomplete,* and the child appears "toxic," the risk of a serious bacterial illness is high. The differential diagnosis includes urinary tract infection, bacteremia, pneumonia, osteomyelitis, and meningitis, all of which may be difficult to diagnose in the infant and young child. The risk that the fever represents bacteremia and meningitis has fallen dramatically since introduction of the conjugate vaccines for *Haemophilus influenzae* type B (Hib) and *Streptococcus pneumoniae* (PCV-7) (see Chapters 12 and 64). Urinary tract infection (Chapter 65) is the most common bacterial cause of fever without source in young children, especially girls. Osteomyelitis may be challenging to diagnose early in its course. Fever may be the first manifestation of Kawasaki disease, a malignancy, or a rheumatologic disorder.

What Is Fever of Unknown Origin?

Fever of unknown origin (FUO) refers to fever that persists longer than 2 weeks, most often *without* associated signs of acute "toxicity." FUO is much less common than fever without source. The differential diagnosis, evaluation, and management are discussed in other resources.

EVALUATION

How Should I Evaluate a Febrile Child?

First, use history to elicit symptoms and to characterize the illness pattern, duration, and perceived severity. Ask parents about their observations and concerns. Review the child's risk factors, especially *immunization status* and exposures such as daycare. Consider any past history of fever, infection, antibiotic treatment, and recurrent or chronic disease. *Observe* the ill child before beginning the hands-on physical examination to identify signs of toxicity (Table 33-1). Perform a careful physical examination with the goal of identifying a source of infection or a disease that can explain the findings. Use laboratory tests and imaging judiciously.

Table 33-1

Yale Observation Scale

	Healthy	Moderately Ill	Toxic
Cry	Strong or content	Whimpering or sobbing	Weak, moaning, high-pitched
Reaction	Cries briefly or content	Cries off and on	Continual or little response
State	Awake or awakens easily	Drowsy	Not arousable
Color	"Pink" or appropriate for ethnicity	Pale extremities	Ashen, mottled, cyanotic, pale
Hydration	Moist mucosa Good skin turgor	Dry mouth	Dry mucous membranes Tenting
Response	Smiles (alerts if <2 mo)	Brief smile or reaction	No reaction

Adapted from McCarthy et al: Observation scales to identify serious illness in febrile children, *Pediatrics* 70:802, 1982.

What Increases the Risk of Serious Bacterial Infection?

- *Age*: The highest risk of serious infection is in the newborn period (birth to 1 month). Premature infants have higher risk than full-term infants. Infections may result from birth-related events, so history must ask about maternal infections (especially group B *Streptococcus*), pregnancy, labor, delivery, and the postnatal period. The next highest risk period is from 1 to 3 months, especially before immunizations begin. Risk decreases from 3 months to 3 years, even though fever is most common in this age group. Risk of serious bacterial illness declines further after age 3 years, but meningococcal disease does occur sporadically in children and adolescents.
- *Toxicity:* This clinical appearance (see below) correlates with serious bacterial illness, but the *absence of toxicity in a highly febrile infant or young child is no guarantee that infection is absent.* Other risk factors such as age and immunization status should be taken into account.
- *Height of the fever:* Before introduction of Hib and PCV-7 vaccines, fever > 40° C (> 104° F) was highly correlated with serious bacterial infection. Although the risk of infection with *H. influenzae* type b and *S. pneumoniae* is now < 1% in immunized children, high fever plus concerning clinical findings should always be taken seriously and prompt a careful evaluation. Invasive tests may be less necessary now than in the past, however, if the child is fully immunized.
- *Immunizations*: Children who have not received Hib and PCV-7 immunizations are at highest risk for serious infection. In addition, immunization against influenza virus helps prevent this extremely contagious infection in children and reduces disease in adults. The new conjugate meningococcal vaccine should reduce this disease in adolescents.

- *Exposure or other risk factors:* Daycare, school, and home are common sites for exposure to infection. The family history of acute illnesses and immune deficiencies should be addressed. In addition, a child with an underlying disease such as sickle cell anemia may be predisposed to infection.
- *Previous infections* and previous *treatment with antibiotics* increase the risk of infection with antibiotic-resistant organisms.
- *Epidemiology:* Infections present in the community, such as viral influenza and *Neisseria meningitidis*, may explain fever. Knowledge of infectious disease activity in the community can focus the differential diagnosis, evaluation, and treatment.

What Should I Look for on Physical Exam?

Observe for toxicity, assess all systems thoroughly, and be alert for signs of dehydration, such as prolonged capillary refill. If the child appears toxic but a source for the fever is not found, do not attribute high fever to upper respiratory infection or otitis media, especially if immunizations are incomplete. Keep searching for signs of specific, serious infections such as meningitis, pneumonia, pyelonephritis, and osteomyelitis. Be aware that you may need to look for findings of a malignancy or rheumatologic disease. Kawasaki disease should be considered if fever persists more than 4 to 5 days and findings such as conjunctival injection, oral mucosal inflammation, and swollen hands and feet develop.

What Is Toxicity and How Do I Identify It?

Toxicity refers to the clinical appearance associated with the sepsis syndrome. The Yale Observation Scale provides clues to identify the toxic child (see Table 33-1). Tachycardia and increased work of breathing may also be identified in a highly febrile, toxic-appearing infant or young child.

How Do I Decide Whether Laboratory Tests Are Needed?

Specific signs such as a bulging fontanelle, petechial rash, foul-smelling urine, or bloody diarrhea will trigger a specific evaluation. Careful assessment of risk factors, especially immunizations, can reduce the rates of invasive tests, but skill and experience are needed to make this assessment. A toxic child with concerning risk factors who has fever without source must be evaluated to identify occult bacterial illness such as urinary tract infection (UTI) or bacteremia. Urine culture is important for all girls who have fever without source. Uncircumcised infant boys also have an increased rate of UTI. High fever in an infant younger than 3 months presents special challenges, and often prompts a "sepsis workup."

What Is a Sepsis Workup?

Sepsis workup is the complete evaluation for serious bacterial illness. It includes complete blood count (CBC) with differential leukocyte count,

C-reactive protein (CRP), blood culture, urine culture, and often lumbar puncture. Chest radiograph is advisable if a young child has fever without source, appears toxic, and also has tachypnea, respiratory distress, or a markedly elevated white blood count (WBC) or CRP.

Do Laboratory Tests Help Identify Serious Infection?

Now that the rate of bacterial infection has fallen because of widespread use of Hib and PCV-7 immunizations, the risk of bacteremia is below 1% and the need for CBC, CRP, and blood cultures for *immunized* febrile infants and young children has been questioned. Before these immunizations were widely used, bacteremia rates were 4% to 15% in patients who had high fever without source, and laboratory tests were recommended routinely to detect bacterial infection. WBC and differential were justified because of the frequency and severity of infections. These tests had high sensitivity and specificity for serious bacterial illness, but low positive predictive value. Some physicians still "screen" all febrile children with a CBC, but it is more logical to use a history of *incomplete immunizations* plus fever and toxicity as the trigger for ordering CBC, differential, and blood culture (and possibly CSF culture). Urine culture should be obtained for all febrile girls regardless of immunization status. Rapid influenza antigen test may be useful in the appropriate season. Remember that an extremely low WBC with *neutropenia* may indicate sepsis.

How Often Does a Urine Culture Help?

UTI is the most common serious bacterial infection in children younger than 3 years if another source of infection cannot be found. Urinalysis can assist with diagnosis of UTI, but *culture of an appropriately collected urine specimen* is a must. Catheterization is the best method to obtain urine for culture (see Chapter 65).

When Should a Lumbar Puncture Be Done?

A lumbar puncture for CSF analysis and culture should be done whenever concern is high for meningitis. You must have a high index of suspicion for meningitis when evaluating a febrile infant between birth and 6 months because clinical signs are often subtle.

TREATMENT

Should Fever Be Treated with an Antipyretic?

As a general rule, fever per se does not need to be treated unless the patient is uncomfortable. An uncomfortable febrile infant or young child may be fussy and may have decreased appetite or fluid intake. The verbal child may describe pain such as headache or myalgia. Acetaminophen (10 to 15 mg/kg/dose every 4 hours) or ibuprofen (5 to 10 mg/kg/dose every 6 to 8 hours) helps relieve discomfort and also lowers temperature. The antiinflammatory activity of ibuprofen provides an added advantage when fever and pain are caused by conditions such as acute otitis media, streptococcal pharyngitis, or influenza. Routine recommendation of antipyretic treatment of all fever risks reinforcement of fever phobia. Alternating doses of ibuprofen and acetaminophen are commonly used by physicians and parents, and one recent study suggests that this practice may produce more effective control of fever. All febrile children need additional water and electrolytes because elevated temperature increases insensible fluid loss (Chapter 26).

Are Antibiotics Needed When a Child Has Fever without Source?

The decision to administer antibiotics to a febrile infant or child relies on history to identify risk factors, observation to assess toxicity, physical examination to detect a focus for the fever, and perhaps screening laboratory tests. UTI is treated as discussed in Chapter 65.

- *High-risk infants younger than 3 months.* These infants have fever without source, often appear toxic, may have a history of health problems at or after birth or exposures to illnesses, and will be unimmunized with Hib and PCV-7 vaccines if younger than 2 months. High-risk infants should undergo a sepsis workup that will often reveal elevated WBC with a "left shift." These infants typically require hospital admission and management with intravenous antibiotics, such as a third-generation cephalosporin or amoxicillin plus gentamicin, until culture results confirm presence or absence of infection. If bacterial infection is not identified, infants will usually be discharged to home after 2 or 3 days. When infection is documented, treatment will be continued for the specific organism.
- *Low-risk infants younger than 3 months.* These infants have fever but do not appear toxic and have been previously healthy, including a benign neonatal course and no exposures to known infections. They also will be unimmunized with Hib and PCV-7 vaccines if younger than 2 months. Physical examination of such patients shows no concerning findings, and laboratory test results do not cause concern. Blood cultures are usually drawn, but a lumbar puncture may be omitted. Most of these low-risk infants are treated empirically with intramuscular ceftriaxone (50-75 mg/kg) pending culture results. Observation may be at home, if conditions allow. Follow-up within 24 hours is mandatory.
- *Between 3 months and 3 years.* Fever without source is treated according to risk factors and findings. If immunizations are complete for age, and if the child is not toxic-appearing, sepsis workup and empirical antibiotic treatment are not necessary, although it may be prudent to obtain a urine culture. If clinical findings suggest the need for antibiotics on an outpatient basis, blood culture and urine culture must be done. Treatment is generally administered as a single intramuscular injection of ceftriaxone (50 to 75 mg/kg) with outpatient follow-up the next day. If risk factors and clinical findings suggest the need for a complete sepsis workup and empirical antibiotic therapy, management may need to be in hospital.

- *Older children and adolescents.* This age group uncommonly has fever caused by occult infections. Diagnosis and management use the same principles as those discussed previously.

KEY POINTS

- Immunization against *H. influenzae* type B and *S. pneumoniae* has greatly reduced the incidence of invasive bacterial infection.
- Risk of serious bacterial infection is greatest when a young child has fever $\geq$ 40° C and toxicity.
- Toxicity is the clinical picture associated with sepsis.

Case 33-1

The mother of a 9-month-old girl telephones because her daughter has had fever and diarrhea for 24 hours. Temperature has been as high as 104° F, but acetaminophen reduces fever to 101° F. The child's appetite is decreased and she has been increasingly fussy. When her fever is high, her breathing seems "panting." According to the mother, this is the most ill that the child has ever been.

A. What information from the history worries you?
B. What conditions could cause this clinical picture?
C. What additional information do you need?
D. When seen in the office, the child has temperature 38.7° C; pulse 160 beats/min; and respiratory rate 36 breaths/min, unlabored. How do you interpret the vital signs in light of the above history?

Case 33-2

A 12-month-old boy with 2 days of fever up to 104° F is irritable, has pale mottled skin, cries inconsolably, and has dry lips and a sunken fontanelle. Pulse is 160 beats/min. Respiratory rate is 36 breaths/min, with prominent abdominal respirations.

A. What is toxicity? Is he toxic?
B. What will be your diagnostic approach to this child?
C. What criteria would you use to make the decision for treatment?

Case Answers

33-1 A. *Learning objective:* **Identify the factors in the history of the acute illness that point to a serious bacterial illness as the cause of fever in an infant or young child.** Worrisome features are level of fever (104° F), irritability, decreased appetite, and tachypnea. In addition, the mother's observation that this is the most ill that the child has ever been should raise concerns.

33-1 B. *Learning objective:* **List the causes of high fever in an infant or young child; include serious bacterial infections.** Serious bacterial infections include bacterial sepsis, meningitis, osteomyelitis, pneumonia, and urinary tract infection. Influenza is a seasonal viral infection that causes high fever, but many others may also do so.

33-1 C. *Learning objective:* **Obtain information from the history to develop a differential diagnosis for fever in an infant or young child.** Details of the acute illness are important, as are details of exposures (especially daycare attendance), family illnesses, and general health. Always assess the history of immunizations (Hib and PCV-7, specifically). In addition, you should ask about the child's past medical history.

33-1 D. *Learning objective:* **Identify physical findings that are concerning in a febrile child and that suggest the possibility of a serious bacterial illness.** Temperature is elevated. Heart rate and respiratory rate are rapid. Lack of respiratory distress is somewhat reassuring because pneumonia and shock often have associated respiratory distress manifested by retractions and use of accessory muscles. A more detailed physical examination may identify a focus of infection. In the absence of a focus, laboratory tests will be needed to further develop the diagnosis.

33-2 A. *Learning objective:* **Define toxicity and discuss the physical findings that accompany this condition.** Toxicity represents the clinical manifestations of the "sepsis syndrome." Its clinical findings develop from inadequate circulating volume to support vital functions. In this case, the child does manifest toxicity, which is evident from the high fever, the degree of respiratory distress, dehydration, and irritability.

33-2 B. *Learning objective:* **Use history and physical examination to evaluate a toxic-appearing child.** A thorough history will identify risks of serious bacterial illness. A careful physical examination must be done to identify a source for the fever. In many cases, no source will be identified, in which case screening laboratory tests should be done, including a white blood cell count with differential and blood culture. A febrile girl must have urine culture performed; boys may also have UTI, so urine culture should be considered. This particular child demonstrates dehydration as one of the manifestations of toxicity.

33-2 C. *Learning objective:* **Interpret laboratory tests to develop a management plan for a toxic-appearing febrile infant or young child.** The management of the febrile infant or young child depends on whether toxicity is present and whether the history identifies factors that place the child at high risk for serious bacterial infection. In this case, irritability and lethargy are concerning, and the presence of dehydration would prompt administration of intravenous fluids and a reassessment after the infusion. Ongoing management and decision making are aided by laboratory tests, including the CBC. Concern would be raised with WBC > 15,000 and "left shift" with "bands" > 1500. Hospitalization with administration of empirical antibiotic therapy is likely for this child, just based on the brief clinical picture presented previously. Specific therapy will depend on culture results and further diagnostic studies.

BIBLIOGRAPHY

Baraff LJ: Management of fever without source in infants and children, *Ann Emerg Med* 36:602, 2000.

Crocetti M, Moghbeli N, Serwint J: Fever phobia revisited: have parental misconceptions about fever changed in 20 years? *Pediatrics* 107:1241, 2001.

Hsiao AL, Chen L, Baker MD: Incidence and predictors of serious bacterial infections among 57–180-day-old infants, *Pediatrics* 117:1695, 2006.

Levine OS, Farley M, Harrison LH, et al: Risk factors for invasive pneumococcal disease in children: A population-based case-control study in North America, *Pediatrics* 103:e28, 1999.

McCarthy PL, Sharpe MR, Spiesel SZ, et al: Observation scales to identify serious illness in febrile children, *Pediatrics* 70:802, 1982.

Sarrell EM, Wielunsky E, Cohen HA: Antipyretic treatment in young children with fever, *Arch Pediatr Adol Med* 160:197, 2006.

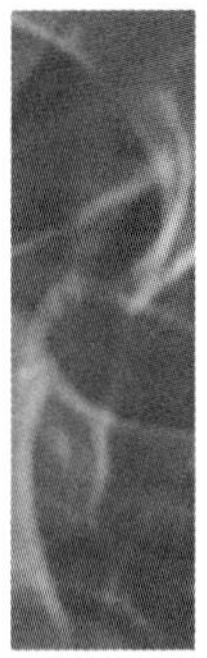

34 Growth Problems

NICHOLAS JOSPE

ETIOLOGY

What Growth Problems Am I Likely to Encounter?

Growth problems can be discussed in four broad categories: stature, weight, neural, and maturation. Growth in each category generally reflects the family pattern and usually falls within the population-based ranges that are described in growth charts and tables of maturation. Growth outside of expected ranges may result from a primary, usually irreversible, process that has a genetic or congenital basis or from a secondary acquired disease or condition in which poor growth is often reversible. Parents and children express concerns about short stature (but not usually tall stature), excessive or inadequate weight gain, head size that is too large or too small, or pubertal maturation that is earlier or later than expected. Very rarely, a newborn will have ambiguous genitalia, an emergency that demands immediate referral.

What Causes Growth Problems?

Heredity, genetic syndromes, nutritional deficiencies or excesses, and endocrine disorders are among the more common causes of growth problems. Table 34-1 lists some of the conditions, diseases, and disorders that you might encounter in patients with abnormal growth patterns. Obesity is the most common growth problem in children and adolescents. It results most commonly from chronic calorie excess caused by an imbalance between intake and expenditure. A persistent daily excess of 100 calories will result in weight gain of > 10 lb per year above the expected age-appropriate gain.

EVALUATION

How Do I Determine the Cause of Stature Problems?

The growth chart helps identify concerning growth patterns if growth measurements have been plotted regularly and accurately. Statural growth typically "follows the curve" parallel to percentile lines and does

Table 34-1

Causes of Growth Problems

Category	Problem	Cause
Stature	Short stature	Heredity* (including constitutional delay)
		Down and Turner syndromes
		Renal insufficiency and renal tubular acidosis
		Inflammatory bowel disease and celiac disease
		Hypothyroidism
		Cushing syndrome
		Growth hormone deficiency
	Tall stature	Heredity*
		Exogenous obesity
		Marfan and Klinefelter syndromes
		Homocystinuria
Weight	Obesity	Excessive calories*
		Hypothyroidism, hyperinsulinism, glucocorticoid excess (Cushing syndrome)
		Prader-Willi syndrome
	Poor weight gain	Inadequate calories*
		Failure to thrive ("nonorganic")
		Congestive heart failure
		Cystic fibrosis
		Hyperthyroidism
Neural	Microcephaly	Heredity*
		In utero infections
		Syndromes (e.g., Down syndrome)
	Macrocephaly	Heredity*
		Hydrocephalus
		Neurocutaneous diseases
Maturation	Early puberty	Girls: Heredity,* excessive estrogen (exogenous or endogenous)
		Boys: Heredity,* excessive testosterone
	Delayed puberty	Girls: Heredity,* Turner syndrome, thyroid disease, calorie deficiency (eating disorder)
		Boys: Heredity* (including constitutional delay)
	Ambiguous genitalia	Fetal developmental abnormalities
		Congenital adrenal hyperplasia
		Partial androgen insensitivity syndrome

*Most common.

not cross more than one line upward or downward. A truly "flat" curve crosses the percentile lines and is often a clue that a child has an underlying cause for poor statural growth. It is important to ask parents about their growth patterns during childhood (they may need to ask their own parents). If you include information about the stature of both parents in the medical record, you can calculate the predicted adult height using mid-parental stature (see Chapter 8).

How Should I Evaluate the Short Child?

Consider an evaluation if growth is flat, crosses percentile lines downward, or does not appear adequate to result in a final adult height close to that predicted from mid-parental stature. Review the family growth patterns for early or late development. Ask about signs and symptoms that suggest underlying gastrointestinal (GI) disease or hypothyroidism. Look carefully for physical findings of Turner syndrome in short girls (short, webbed neck; low-set, rotated ears; wide chest; nevi; nail dysplasia) and for the findings of Cushing syndrome or hypothyroidism. The child with Down syndrome or achondroplasia will be short, as may the child with cyanotic heart disease and chronic kidney disease. Laboratory testing should include screening for anemia, renal function, renal tubular acidosis, hypothyroidism, malabsorption, celiac disease, and growth hormone deficiency. Patients with inflammatory bowel disease usually have a positive stool test for blood.

When Should I Worry about Tall Stature?

Most tall stature is hereditary and is viewed positively in Western societies. Although few families express concern when a child is taller than peers, you should monitor growth to be certain that tall stature is consistent with the family growth patterns and does not reflect a pathologic process. Tall stature is associated with exogenous obesity, which should prompt a nutritional and behavioral history. A careful physical examination should discover findings consistent with Klinefelter or Marfan syndrome, homocystinuria, or pituitary gigantism. Look carefully for signs of early pubertal development in children with tall stature.

How Should I Evaluate the Obese Child?

Most obesity is exogenous and results from chronic excessive calorie intake and inadequate calorie expenditure. The most effective approach to evaluation and management of obesity involves the patient and family as active, willing participants. First ask for permission to discuss the topic, then encourage self-directed approaches to identify behaviors that contribute to the problem. A detailed history of the nutritional and exercise habits of the child and family is critical. It is important to establish whether obesity "runs in the family" and whether family members have the metabolic syndrome, type 2 diabetes mellitus, or early cardiovascular disease. The child with exogenous obesity almost always has tall stature. A waist circumference-to-height ratio (WC:Ht) of > 0.5 is associated with long-term adverse metabolic outcomes of obesity for children as well as for adults. Acanthosis nigricans may reflect insulin resistance and signal development of type 2 diabetes. Older children and adolescents with exogenous obesity should be evaluated for the metabolic syndrome (Table 34-2) and monitored closely for development of hypertension and type 2 diabetes. Cholesterol and lipid levels should be monitored.

Table 34-2

Criteria for the Metabolic Syndrome in Adolescence

Triglycerides (mg/dl)	$\geq$ 110
HDL-cholesterol (mg/dl)	
Male	$\leq$ 40
Female	$\leq$ 40
Abdominal obesity (waist circumference)	
Male	$\geq$ 90th percentile or WC:Ht > 0.5
Female	$\geq$ 90th percentile or WC:Ht > 0.5
Fasting glucose (mg/dl)	$\geq$ 110
Blood pressure	$\geq$ 90th percentile

HDL, High-density lipoprotein; WC:Ht, waist circumference-to-height ratio.
Adapted from Cook S et al: Prevalence of a metabolic syndrome phenotype in adolescents, *Arch Pediatr Adol Med* 157:821, 2003.

When Do I Need to Evaluate for Endocrine Causes of Obesity?

Endocrine disorders account for only a tiny fraction of all childhood obesity. Short stature is an important clue to this rare cause of obesity. Endocrine causes of obesity include hypothyroidism, glucocorticoid excess (Cushing syndrome), and hyperinsulinism. Review of the growth curve plus a careful history and thorough physical examination will identify most of the endocrine causes of obesity and direct the selection of laboratory tests needed to confirm the diagnosis. The physical examination will also identify uncommon syndromes that have obesity as a key feature, such as Prader-Willi syndrome, Laurence-Moon-Biedl syndrome, and Down syndrome.

How Do I Determine the Cause of Failure to Thrive?

Failure to thrive (FTT) is usually a problem in the first 2 years of life. It results from chronic calorie insufficiency caused by inadequate food intake, loss of calories from the GI tract because of mechanical problems or malabsorption, or from excessive metabolism. Severe, prolonged calorie insufficiency during early infancy can cause slowed growth in length. Table 34-3 lists findings that help identify the cause of FTT.

How Do I Assess Growth of the Head?

The head grows as the brain grows, and most commonly head circumference is genetically determined. Parental head circumference provides clues to the ultimate head size of their children. Careful measurement of head circumference is needed to monitor growth and to detect abnormalities. Head shape may confound head measurement or may be the major problem if premature fusion of sutures or torticollis causes asymmetrical head growth. Head size that reflects a pathologic process often is associated with developmental, neurologic, or other physical examination

Table 34-3

Failure to Thrive

Mechanism	Findings That Point to the Cause
Inadequate intake	Diet history. Insufficient nursing or inadequate quantity of formula or food. Dilute formula. Inexperienced parents. Fatigue and pallor (chronic renal failure).
Mechanical loss from gastrointestinal tract	Vomiting, diarrhea, disordered swallowing. Acute weight loss from pyloric stenosis.
Malabsorption	Vigorous appetite. Fatty stools (cystic fibrosis, celiac disease). Parasites such as *Giardia lamblia.*
Excessive metabolism	Signs of congestive heart failure. Irritability (hyperthyroidism).

findings. Microcephaly may reflect brain pathology and may be associated with numerous syndromes and with delayed development. Macrocephaly is a key finding in hydrocephalus, neurofibromatosis, and tuberous sclerosis, all of which have characteristic physical findings.

How Should I Assess a Child with the Early Onset of Puberty?

Familiarity with Development and Sexual Maturity Rating is important for evaluation of growth and puberty (see Chapter 15). You must also have a good understanding of growth patterns and of the physical changes that accompany pubertal development. Although puberty that starts before 8 years of age may be within physiologic limits, parents often have concern about girls between 7 and 10 who have physical changes of puberty. Breast development and rapid growth make them stand out from their elementary school peers. Boys less commonly have early puberty, but when they do they are taller than peers and often are the "star" athletes in elementary and junior high school. In most cases such children do not have worrisome conditions. The key to the benign nature of these findings is that although the features of puberty may be "early," their progression is not unduly rapid.

What Findings Indicate Early Puberty?

Parents commonly express concern about breast development (thelarche) in young girls or about adult body odor and appearance of axillary and pubic hair. Both may be isolated findings or may reflect the true onset of puberty. Thelarche may be an isolated finding or may be caused by exogenous estrogen, such as ingestion of birth control pills by a toddler. Axillary and pubic hair may appear if triggered by adrenal hormones without gonadal hormone production (adrenarche). Early thelarche and adrenarche are most often benign and isolated unless accompanied by other signs of puberty and growth acceleration. In this latter case, the findings indicate true pubertal onset caused by gonadal hormone secretion (gonadarche).

How Do I Distinguish Adrenarche from Gonadarche?

Adrenarche in both boys and girls is identified by physical changes such as adult body odor, acne, and axillary and pubic hair that are triggered by adrenal hormones without gonadal hormone production.
Gonadarche reflects gonadal hormone secretion, estrogen from the ovary and testosterone from the testis. When severe and progressive, it may lead to true pubertal development, early growth spurt, early fusion of epiphyses, and ultimate short stature. You should suspect gonadarche in a young patient who has physical findings of puberty when a growth spurt is evident from the growth chart. To confirm the diagnosis, measure levels of testosterone in males, or estradiol and progesterone in females, and do radiographic studies to look for advanced bone age. Table 34-4 compares adrenarche and gonadarche.

How Do I Evaluate a Patient with Delayed Puberty?

Delay of puberty most often occurs in boys as a reflection of a familial growth pattern and usually does not require an extensive workup. In contrast, delayed puberty in girls causes greater concern because it may indicate an underlying condition such as Turner syndrome. Pay special attention to the history of diet, exercise, stress, and symptoms of inflammatory bowel disease. Ask about the family growth history and the timing of puberty for family members. A helpful question is to inquire about the ability to detect odor because in Kallmann syndrome, anosmia is linked to hypogonadotropic hypogonadism. Carefully review the growth curve and document the physical findings that indicate lack of pubertal development. You must have familiarity with the sequence and timing of pubertal changes to interpret your findings. The distinction between gonadarche and adrenarche remains important (Table 34-4). Perform a thorough physical examination to identify clues to thyroid disease, suspicion for underlying organic disease, and presence of such conditions as Turner syndrome. Patients with delayed puberty typically have delayed bone age.

Table 34-4

Premature Puberty—Adrenarche Versus Gonadarche

Condition	Gender	Findings
Adrenarche	Male and female	Pubic hair, acne, axillary hair, body odor, oily hair and skin. *No* breast, genital, or growth changes.
Gonadarche	Male	Growth spurt, muscular development, increase in the size of the penis, attainment of full masculinization, advanced bone age, elevated testosterone.
	Female	Breast development, growth spurt, attainment of the female habitus, increase in the size of the uterus, menarche, advanced bone age, elevated estrogen and progesterone.

How Do I Evaluate the Newborn with Ambiguous Genitalia?

Ambiguity of the external genitalia is identified when a newborn's genitalia do not appear male or female. Infants with ambiguous genitalia may be genetically female with virilization, or genetically male with inadequate virilization. Virilization in newborn girls may include a large clitoris plus partial or complete posterior fusion of the labia majora. A full-term newborn who appears phenotypically male but has a short penis, severe hypospadias, or absent testes may be a virilized female. A phenotypically female infant who has a mass in the labia may be an incompletely virilized male; the mass may be a testis. These must all be investigated. The most frequent endocrine causes of ambiguous genitalia are congenital adrenal hyperplasia (CAH) and partial androgen insensitivity syndrome. Identification of ambiguous genitalia in a newborn should be considered an "emergency" and requires prompt referral to a center with a capable team of pediatric endocrinologists, urologists, surgeons, and geneticists. CAH is associated with life-threatening adrenal insufficiency.

TREATMENT

How Should I Manage Statural Growth Problems?

Short stature that is a primary manifestation of a congenital, hereditary, or syndromic condition rarely has any treatment. Diagnosis, counseling, and long-term follow-up are the key management principles. If a treatable disease such as growth hormone deficiency or hypothyroidism causes short stature, then treatment of that condition improves growth. Girls who have Turner syndrome benefit from growth hormone therapy throughout childhood and require estrogen and progesterone to stimulate menarche and maintain menses.

Can Obesity Be Treated?

The rare child whose obesity is caused by an endocrine disorder should be treated appropriately to control the disease. Exogenous obesity is best "treated" by prevention, which includes early and continued discussions of nutrition, exercise, and family habits at health supervision visits (see Chapters 10 and 11). Obesity is not easily managed once established. An obese patient may benefit from early and ongoing advice from a certified dietitian who is familiar with child nutrition. Family meal and cooking habits and ethnic or cultural patterns that contribute to excessive calorie intake must be identified. The child and family activity patterns must be discussed. Sedentary behaviors should be replaced by regular physical activity. Before puberty, weight stabilization rather than weight loss is part of the management program, unless weight is markedly above the 97th percentile. If excessive weight gain is identified in early childhood, parents can modify the young child's food intake and increase physical activities to slow the rate of weight gain, which will allow the child to "grow into" his or her weight. Excessive juice or sweetened beverage intake is a common "theme" among overweight children and often accounts for the offending excess calorie consumption. The school-aged child and adolescent need to participate actively in any weight management plan because access to food and decisions about activity both may be out of the control of parents. Replacing sedentary activities, such as watching television, playing video games, and prolonged use of computers, with regular physical activity can aid weight management. Adolescents who participate in support groups, such as Shape Down, have a much greater likelihood of successful weight management. Management of obesity requires involvement of the entire family to avoid stigmatizing the individual. Often the obese child or adolescent is a member of an obese family, so family management is crucial.

Can Maturational Problems Be Treated?

Patients with pathologic problems of pubertal maturation and those with ambiguous genitalia require the management expertise of a pediatric endocrinologist. Careful diagnosis, effective counseling, and long-term follow-up are key management principles.

KEY POINTS

- Measure growth parameters including body mass index (BMI) and plot them on the growth chart accurately.
- Look for flat growth curves or curves that cross more than one centile line (up or down).
- Exogenous obesity is the most common growth problem.
- Failure to thrive represents poor weight gain because of chronic caloric insufficiency.
- Familiarity with sexual maturity staging is needed to evaluate adolescent growth.

Case 34-1

Parents of an 11-month-old girl request an appointment to discuss her growth. They are concerned because she is smaller than her 1-year-old cousin. She was last seen in the office at age 9 months, at which time she was at the 25th percentile for both weight and length. Measurements today show that weight is now at the 5th percentile and length is at the 25th percentile.

A. What are the important changes in her growth parameters, and what information do you need to interpret them?
B. If this child's length had previously been at the 5th percentile and has now fallen below the 5th percentile over the preceding 2 months, how would your evaluation differ, and what conditions would be in the differential diagnosis?

Case 34-2

At the 7-year health supervision visit you note that a child has had a weight increase from the 75th to > 97th percentile, and that BMI is now > 97th percentile. Height is at the 90th percentile and WC:Ht is > 0.5. His mother tells you that he "does not eat a lot" and wonders why you are concerned.

A. How will you begin your evaluation of this child?
B. What information will assist you to plan management?

Case Answers

34-1 A. *Learning objective:* **Identify growth problems by assessing weight, length, and head circumference.** Weight has fallen on the curve from 25th to 5th percentile, while length has remained stable. This suggests that there has been a decrease in calories available to maintain weight gain. You need to find out about her eating habits, especially the kinds and quantities of food consumed. Additional questions should focus on illnesses that might result in loss of calories (e.g., vomiting, diarrhea) or chronic health conditions that waste calories (e.g., malabsorption, hyperthyroidism). True failure to thrive results from conditions listed in Table 34-3. In practical terms, asking about the child's development might identify that she has begun walking recently and has greatly increased her energy expenditure while decreasing her food intake because she is "too busy" to eat. A child with this history does not have failure to thrive and usually resumes growth along the curve.

34-1 B. *Learning objective:* **Identify the infant or young child with short stature, and list the conditions that must be considered in the evaluation.** Concern about a chronic illness or a genetic disorder would be increased. Careful physical examination to identify characteristic features of a disease or genetic syndrome is important. Laboratory tests should be done to assess renal function, look for metabolic derangements, and assess the possibility of chromosomal abnormalities. In particular, Turner syndrome is high on the differential diagnosis list of short infant girls. Chronic renal failure in infancy also causes growth failure.

34-2 A. *Learning objective:* **Discuss an approach to management of obesity.** Because the mother seems resistant to consider your findings as a problem, you must invite her to discuss the physical findings and also engage the child in the process. Success will depend on participation by the child and his family. Use of growth charts to demonstrate the changes in body weight may assist your discussion.

34-2 B. *Learning objective:* **Identify the causes of obesity.** Information about eating habits, meal patterns, and physical and leisure activities should be sought. Because chronic calorie excess (intake > expenditure) causes excessive weight gain, the impact of small daily calorie imbalance will need to be identified. At this age, stabilization of weight may be the best approach, allowing the child to "grow into his weight" by maintaining a flat weight curve while growing in height. A change from two 8-ounce glasses of whole cow milk (20 kCal/oz) to skim milk (13 kCal/oz) will reduce daily calorie intake by more than 100 kCal. This change may produce weight stabilization if the calories are not replaced in the diet by other foods. Regular follow-up, encouragement, and ongoing support will be needed.

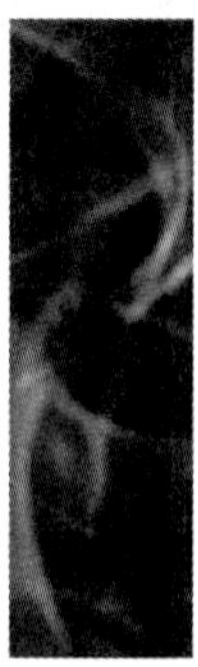

35

Headache

ADAM HARTMAN

ETIOLOGY

How Common Are Headaches in Children?

Headaches occur from infancy through adolescence, and prevalence increases with age. Headaches may be difficult to diagnose in the preverbal child. The most common causes of acute headache in children include febrile upper respiratory infections, sinusitis, and migraine. Up to 11% of adolescents have migraine headaches. Chronic headaches represent a significant reason for a neurology consultation.

How Are Headaches Classified?

Frequency and time course are used to classify headache patterns, with many different etiologies in each pattern (Table 35-1).

EVALUATION

How Do I Evaluate the Patient with Headache?

History should focus on timing, location, character, and quality of pain and should identify exacerbating and relieving factors. A diary of the headaches can be extremely useful in delineating the type(s) and patterns of headache suffered by the patient, as outlined in Table 35-1. The location of the headache can help differentiate one type of headache from another. A sleep history should be obtained (because some children with obstructive sleep apnea complain of headaches). It is sometimes helpful for a patient to draw what the headaches "look like," especially when he or she is too young to articulate their character (Figure 35-1). Careful general and neurologic examination may identify findings characteristic of specific headache types, including optic disc edema seen with pseudotumor cerebri. The first diagnostic priority should be the consideration of etiologies known to cause sudden morbidity, followed by a reasonable investigation for underlying causes.

Table 35-1

Headache Patterns and Their Causes

Headache Pattern	Possible Causes
Acute	Self-limited minor infections, acute sinusitis, migraine, meningitis, intracranial hemorrhage, trauma, toxic ingestions, post-lumbar puncture headache
Acute, recurrent	Migraine, tension-type headache, cluster headaches, toxic ingestions, mitochondrial disorders, trigeminal autonomic cephalgia, seizures
Chronic, nonprogressive	Tension-type headache, muscle contraction, chronic daily headaches, and analgesic withdrawal
Chronic, progressive	Tumors, abscesses, vascular malformations, pseudotumor cerebri, and hydrocephalus

What Are the Characteristics of Acute Headache?

Acute headaches have a sudden or rapid onset. Fever and constitutional symptoms such as rhinorrhea or myalgias usually accompany headaches associated with viral infections. A patient with meningitis usually appears "toxic" (see Chapter 33) and has physical examination findings that may include meningismus, Kernig's sign, or Brudzinski's sign. Sinus tenderness accompanies headache caused by sinusitis. Bleeding from arteriovenous malformations, berry aneurysms, and subdural hemorrhages often present suddenly with severe pain after seemingly minor head trauma. Depending on the history obtained from the patient and others who witnessed the patient's behavior, workup may include

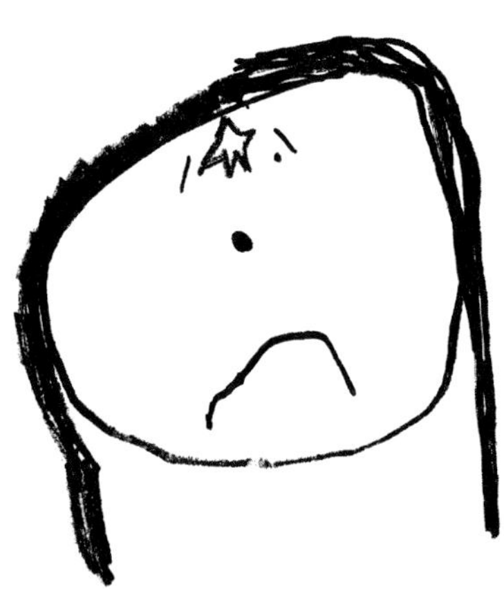

FIGURE 35-1 Depiction of a migraine headache by a 5-year-old girl who suffers from severe migraines.

imaging, a lumbar puncture, or other laboratory studies. Hypertension, bradycardia, and irregular respirations ("Cushing's triad") in a patient with acute headache signals impending brain herniation and is a medical emergency.

How Are Acute, Recurrent Headaches Evaluated?

Acute, recurrent headaches typically have the characteristic features of migraine or cluster headaches. Migraines are the result of overly excitable neurons, which then affect cranial neurovascular structures. History identifies an intermittent, throbbing headache that is often associated with constitutional symptoms such as nausea, vomiting, photophobia, or phonophobia. Migraines can occur with or without auras, are relieved by rest, and can run in families. Focal neurologic findings are only rarely associated with migraines. There are now specific diagnostic criteria for migraines in children. Some precursors of migraines in children include benign paroxysmal vertigo and abdominal migraine. Migraine variants include hemiplegic migraine and ophthalmoplegic migraine. Headache may also follow toxic ingestions or seizures, and the history and physical examination will allow the diagnosis.

How Should I Evaluate Chronic, Nonprogressive Headache?

Chronic, nonprogressive headaches are identified by careful history and a physical examination that excludes neuropathologic processes. Patients with this headache type typically are in their early teens and many are academic "overachievers." They describe their headaches as chronic tension-type headaches, usually characterized by frontal pressure that is worse at the end of the day. Pain may be throbbing, but not as intensely as a migraine, and may be associated with nausea or vomiting. A thorough history of the home, school (including the number of days missed because of headaches), substance use, analgesic use, and psychiatric comorbidities should be obtained from the patient and parents. It is wise to discuss the history with the patient and caregivers together *and* separately. Patients typically report headaches related to school attendance on at least 15 days of the month, with some relief during activities that the patient enjoys, or on weekends. Symptoms can be highly variable, and this headache type often coexists with migraine headaches, so it is important to ask if the patient has more than one type of headache. Most cases are either idiopathic or have psychosocial associations. The differential diagnosis includes caffeine or analgesic withdrawal and carbon monoxide poisoning. The physical examination should be thorough. In the absence of findings that point to a specific diagnosis, a headache diary can be useful to delineate pain frequency, severity, and possible triggers. Imaging is rarely useful. Psychometric testing may be extremely useful because it can identify problems such as anxiety, depression, or learning disabilities

How Do I Evaluate Chronic, Progressive Headache?

Chronic, progressive headache is caused by increased intracranial pressure. Approximately 60% of children with brain tumors have headache. The classic history for a brain tumor headache includes early morning vomiting and occipital headache. These patients have varying additional findings, including nausea, personality changes, changes in academic performance or speech, stiff neck, diplopia, pupillary abnormalities, papilledema, hypoactive deep tendon reflexes, anesthesia, hypesthesia, ataxia, and coma. Cushing's triad—hypertension, bradycardia, and irregular respirations—may develop with brain tumor and signals impending brain herniation. Neuroimaging studies in a patient with findings of increased intracranial pressure may identify a tumor or may be "normal." The latter result suggests pseudotumor cerebri, which is associated with medications, including steroids and oral contraceptives; systemic disorders, such as lupus and malnutrition; and disorders of thyroid, parathyroid, and adrenal glands. Pseudotumor cerebri may cause papilledema, sixth nerve palsy, and ataxia. It most likely is caused by impaired cerebrospinal fluid resorption.

Is Neuroimaging Needed to Evaluate All Headache?

Neuroimaging should be ordered for patients with the symptoms and signs of increased intracranial pressure discussed in the previous section. Imaging is also recommended if severe headache has a sudden onset, suggesting intracranial hemorrhage, and for headache that seems to be refractory to therapy. Computed tomography (CT) is widely available and is the study of choice to look rapidly for a midline shift, dilated ventricles, or an acute hemorrhage. Magnetic resonance imaging (MRI) is better for looking at detail, particularly in the posterior fossa, so it is used if cerebellar or brainstem pathology is suspected. If the CT is negative but abnormalities in the rest of the brain are suspected, consider an MRI.

TREATMENT

What Treatment Is Used for Acute Headache?

Most acute headaches are transient and respond to analgesics. Treatment with antibiotics may be needed for bacterial infection that causes headache. Treatment of the underlying disorder is needed for headache associated with more serious illness such as meningitis or an intracranial hemorrhage. Acute migraine is treated with triptans, nonsteroidal antiinflammatory drugs (NSAIDs), and metoclopramide.

How Are Acute-Recurrent Headaches Treated?

Successful treatment requires that the physician understand patient and family concerns. A careful explanation of migraine and other headache types will greatly enhance patient adherence to a treatment regimen that includes counseling, medication, and biofeedback. Counseling, often in the form of a sympathetic ear by a primary care provider, can provide advice for coping mechanisms and address the patient's or caregivers' expectations. If the history identifies exacerbating circumstances or triggers, these need to be addressed.

What Are the Treatment Options for Migraines?

Treatment of migraine involves triptans and other drugs to abort an episode, acetaminophen or NSAIDs to treat pain, metoclopramide to reduce vomiting, and anticonvulsants, antidepressants, antihypertensives, antihistamines, or NSAIDs to prevent an attack. Few of these medicines have been rigorously studied in young children in large clinical trials, so the choice of agent is guided in large part by personal preference, experience, and side effect profiles. Patients whose symptoms cause prolonged suffering should receive prophylaxis. Recommendations vary, but most agree that prophylaxis is indicated when a patient has more than four migraine attacks per month or has single attacks that cause school absence for more than 5 days a month. Girls who have migraine associated with menses (catamenial headaches) should be referred to a neurologist because their treatment can be complex.

How Do I Treat Chronic Nonprogressive Headache?

It is useful to consider prevention/prophylaxis and to have a plan for treatment if prophylaxis fails. A "no-absence" school attendance goal and a plan to redirect the patient's attention to self-paced activities such as athletics can be useful. Psychological care can be extremely useful to provide support for the patient and family with this often unpredictable but incapacitating chronic pain condition. A patient who has analgesic withdrawal headaches or medication overuse headaches may benefit from referral to a neurologist.

How Is Pseudotumor Cerebri Treated?

Such patients are typically referred to a neurologist who treats medically with either acetazolamide or (paradoxically) steroids or with serial lumbar punctures. An ophthalmologist should perform formal visual field testing. The most important goal of treatment is preservation of the visual fields, which may require surgery.

KEY POINTS

- Most acute headaches are caused by infectious diseases or migraine.
- When acute headache recurs, migraine is a common cause.
- Chronic nonprogressive headaches usually reflect "tension" or muscle contraction.
- If a headache becomes progressively worse, consider increased intracranial pressure.

Case 35-1

An 8-year-old girl presents to the emergency department with the sudden onset of a headache on the right side of her head for the last hour. She was playing in the backyard when the headache began. An aunt had a similar event when she was a teenager. She has no significant past medical history. On examination, her temperature is 36.5° C, pulse is 50 beats/min, respiratory rate is 10 breaths/min, and blood pressure is 145/90 mm Hg. She responds to some questions and is somewhat combative during the examination. She is holding her head and crying. Her pupils constrict consensually from 4 to 3 mm bilaterally. Strength and reflexes are symmetrical. Her toes are down-going but she is uncooperative with the cerebellar and gait examinations.

A. What type of headache is this (i.e., acute, acute recurrent, chronic progressive, chronic nonprogressive)?
B. What is the differential diagnosis of his headache? Do her vital signs give you a clue?
C. What are the priorities for further diagnosis and management?

Case 35-2

An 11-year-old girl has a headache that has lasted 3 days. Her mother says that her daughter gets the headaches every week. The patient describes them as throbbing, bifrontal, lasting 4 to 8 hours. Loud noises and bright lights bother her during the headaches. She has some vomiting associated with the headaches. They are relieved by going to bed and occasionally by ibuprofen. There is no other significant past medical history. Her mother gets monthly "sinus headaches" just before her menstrual cycle. On examination, the patient is lying curled up quietly on your examining table. Her vital signs include temperature of 37.2° C, pulse 92 beats/min, respiratory rate 16 breaths/min, and blood pressure 110/70 mm Hg. Her head and neck examination is unremarkable, as is her neurologic examination, including funduscopy, cranial nerves, strength, cerebellar examination, and gait.

A. What type of headache is this (i.e., acute, acute recurrent, chronic progressive, chronic nonprogressive)?
B. What is the differential diagnosis of her headache?
C. What are the priorities for further diagnosis and management?

Case Answers

35-1 A. *Learning objective:* **Identify the chronologic pattern that characterizes an acute-onset headache.** This is an acute-onset headache.

35-1 B. *Learning objective:* **Discuss the clinical features of an acute-onset headache that point to the need for emergent intervention.** The differential diagnosis includes infection, intracranial hemorrhage, trauma, and toxic ingestions. There is no history of infectious or toxic etiologies. Her vital signs demonstrate Cushing's triad of increased intracranial pressure (ICP)—hypertension, bradycardia, and irregular respirations. This is a surgical emergency.

35-1 C. *Learning objective:* **Outline the immediate evaluation plan for a patient who has severe headache and signs of increased intracranial pressure.** Because of Cushing's triad, the patient should have emergent CT to rule out a hemorrhage and signs of increased ICP. If that is normal, she should have blood and cerebrospinal fluid (CSF) studies to look for infection. Imaging for this child showed a ruptured arteriovenous malformation.

35-2 A. *Learning objective:* **Identify the chronologic pattern that characterizes acute, recurrent headache.** The history is characteristic for an acute, recurrent headache.

35-2 B. *Learning objective:* **List the differential diagnosis for acute, recurrent headaches in childhood and adolescence.** The differential diagnosis includes migraine headaches, tension-type headaches, or toxic ingestions. For the headache pattern described in the case, the most likely diagnosis is migraine headache.

35-2 C. *Learning objectives:* **Discuss an evaluation and management plan for migraine headache or other acute, recurrent headaches.** These headaches are not life threatening. A headache diary can be very useful to elaborate further in the history. Once the frequency and severity (including number of school days missed) have been elucidated, the discussion about therapy can begin. Options for therapy will include acute treatment with each episode (if infrequent), and prophylactic medications if the headaches are frequent. Identifications of the headache triggers may also allow suggestions for behavioral, environmental, or other modifications.

BIBLIOGRAPHY

Childhood Brain Tumor Consortium: The epidemiology of headache among children with brain tumor, *J Neurooncol* 10:31, 1999.

Lewis DW: Toward the definition of childhood migraine, *Curr Opin Pediatr* 16:628, 2004.

Lewis D et al: Practice parameter: pharmacological treatment of migraine headache in children and adolescents: report of the American Academy of Neurology Quality Standards Subcommittee and the Practice Committee of the Child Neurology Society, *Neurology* 63:2215, 2004.

Medina LS et al: Children with headache: clinical predictors of surgical space-occupying lesions and the role of neuroimaging, *Radiology* 202:819, 1997.

Rothner AD: Classification, pathogenesis, evaluation, and management of headaches in children and adolescents, *Curr Opin Pediatr* 4:949, 1992.

Winner P, Gladstein J: Chronic daily headache in pediatric practice. *Curr Opin Neurol* 15:297, 2002.

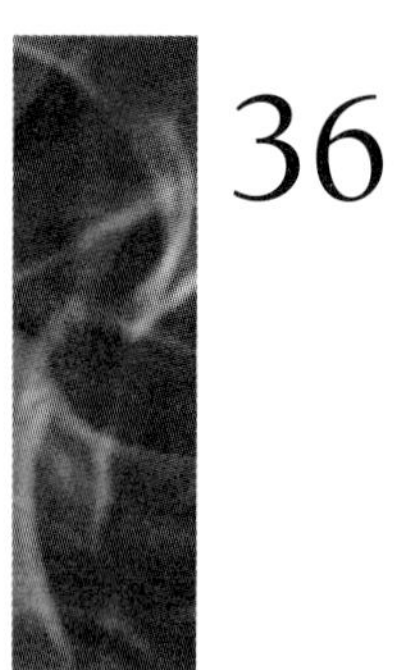

36 Pharyngitis

WILLIAM V. RASZKA

ETIOLOGY

What Are the Common Causes of Pharyngitis?

Pharyngitis, or inflammation of the pharynx, is a frequent complication of upper respiratory tract infections. The principal bacterial organism that causes pharyngitis is *Streptococcus pyogenes,* although *Mycoplasma, Neisseria gonorrhoeae,* and *Arcanobacterium haemolyticum* may cause infections in adolescents. Viruses, however, cause the vast majority of pharyngeal infections. Some viruses, particularly Epstein-Barr virus (EBV) and adenovirus, also commonly cause exudative pharyngitis, a condition in which tonsils and pharynx have a white exudate and inflammation. Distinguishing viral causes from *S. pyogenes* is important, because untreated *S. pyogenes* tonsillopharyngeal infection may lead to nonsuppurative complications such as acute rheumatic fever.

EVALUATION

How Do Viral and Streptococcal Pharyngitis Differ?

Patients with viral pharyngitis and streptococcal pharyngitis may present with similar signs and symptoms. Generally, viral pharyngitis begins gradually, often associated with rhinorrhea and other signs of upper respiratory tract infection. Streptococcal pharyngitis usually has a more sudden onset and higher fever than most viral illnesses, with the notable exception of EBV infection. In addition, headache, sore throat, and abdominal upset often accompany strep infection, but *not* cough or rhinorrhea. The likelihood that the patient may have streptococcal tonsillopharyngitis is highest if pharyngeal pain is associated with fever but without cold symptoms; age younger than 2 years decreases the likelihood. Patients with streptococcal pharyngitis usually have prominent pharyngeal erythema, palatal petechiae, tonsillar exudates, and tender anterior cervical lymph nodes. A rapid antigen test or culture of the tonsils or pharynx that is positive for group A β-hemolytic streptococci (GABHS) confirms the diagnosis.

How Do I Detect Viral Causes of Pharyngitis?

Although many patients with viral pharyngitis present with nonspecific findings, some have features characteristic of specific infections. Herpangina, a Coxsackie virus infection, is associated with vesiculoulcerative lesions on the soft palate. Patients with EBV infection ("mononucleosis") may be difficult to distinguish from those with streptococcal pharyngitis based on the history and physical examination. They often complain of sore throat, malaise, and fever. Physical examination reveals diffuse lymphadenopathy, particularly of the anterior and posterior cervical chains, exudative pharyngitis, and splenomegaly. Laboratory findings in patients with EBV infection include atypical lymphocytosis and mild hepatic transaminase changes. In children older than 5 years, a positive IgM heterophile antibody test (Monospot) is highly suggestive of EBV infection. Specific EBV titers can confirm the diagnosis in children of all ages.

TREATMENT

What Is the Treatment for Streptococcal Pharyngitis?

Streptococcal pharyngitis should be treated with penicillin for 10 days. A macrolide antibiotic or first-generation cephalosporin can be used for those patients who are penicillin allergic. Treatment minimizes the likelihood of acute rheumatic fever, a nonsuppurative complication of GABHS pharyngitis, but does not prevent poststreptococcal glomerulonephritis.

How Is Mononucleosis Treated?

Treatment is supportive. In those patients with marked tonsillar hypertrophy and imminent airway obstruction, corticosteroid therapy may be useful. Children may complain of fatigue for weeks. Children should refrain from participating in contact sports until their splenomegaly resolves. Treatment with antibiotics often results in a diffuse rash.

KEY POINTS

- Patients with streptococcal pharyngitis usually do not have "cold" symptoms.
- Mononucleosis and streptococcal pharyngitis have similar clinical findings during the early stages of disease.
- Treatment of group A β-hemolytic streptococcal pharyngitis shortens the duration of illness and prevents acute rheumatic fever.

Case 36-1

A 5-year-old boy is brought to the physician because of fever, malaise, and sore throat for the past 3 days. He appears mildly ill but not toxic. His temperature is 38.2° C, pulse 120 beats/min, and respiratory rate 20 breaths/min. Physical examination reveals pharyngeal erythema, mild tonsillar hypertrophy, and bilateral, 2-cm, tender anterior cervical lymph nodes. The rest of the examination is normal.

A. What is the most likely diagnosis in this patient?
B. What would you be most concerned about?
C. What diagnostic steps, if any, are indicated in this patient?

Case Answers

36-1 A. *Learning objective:* **Discuss the differential diagnosis of pharyngitis in children and adolescents and identify the most common etiologies.** In the majority of patients with sore throat, the most likely etiologic agent is a virus. This patient has none of the characteristic findings associated with some viruses, such as the vesiculoulcerative lesions in patients with herpangina. The differential diagnosis includes streptococcal pharyngitis and EBV infection.

36-1 B. *Learning objective:* **Describe the natural history of pharyngitis.** Most viral processes will resolve spontaneously without sequelae. Patients with untreated *Streptococcus pyogenes* pharyngitis, however, may develop nonsuppurative complications such as rheumatic heart disease.

36-1 C. *Learning objective:* **Select the appropriate diagnostic tests to evaluate pharyngitis, recognizing that laboratory tests are not indicated for most common viral infections.** Because most pharyngitis is viral in etiology, no laboratory or other diagnostic tests are needed. If there is a suspicion that the patient may have streptococcal pharyngitis, the usual approach (in the United States) is to look for *S. pyogenes.* Most physicians will use a rapid antigen test to detect *Streptococcus.* If this is positive, the patient is given antibiotics. If negative, the specimen is cultured. The patient is treated with antibiotics only if the culture grows *S. pyogenes.* Pharyngitis caused by EBV (mononucleosis) is often diagnosed clinically. The presence of increased reactive lymphocytes in the white blood cell differential, a positive heterophile antibody test in children older than 5 years, or specific EBV serologies can be used to confirm the diagnosis.

BIBLIOGRAPHY

Ebell MH: Epstein-Barr virus infectious mononucleosis, 70:1279, 2004.
Gerber MA: Diagnosis and treatment of pharyngitis in children. *Pediatr Clin North Am* 52:729, 2005.

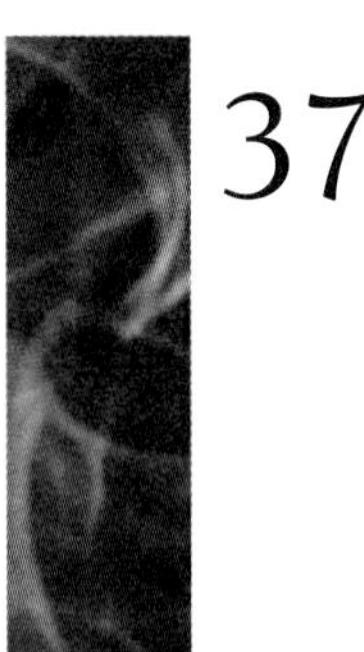

37 Seizures

ADAM HARTMAN

ETIOLOGY

How Common Are Seizures in Children?

Seizures occur in 3% to 5% of children. Febrile seizures occur in 2% to 4%. Epilepsy, the tendency to have recurrent unprovoked seizures, occurs in roughly 1% of children, making it one of the most common neurologic disorders in this age group.

How Are Seizures Classified in Children?

Seizures can be classified as focal or primarily generalized. In *focal seizures,* the first signs of neurologic dysfunction are noted in one anatomic location, then may spread to other regions of the brain. *Primarily generalized seizures,* in contrast, seem to affect global neurologic function from the onset. Examples of focal seizures in children include benign epilepsy with centrotemporal spikes and temporal lobe epilepsy. Examples of generalized seizures in children include febrile seizures, benign neonatal familial convulsions, infantile spasms, and childhood absence epilepsy. These are also classified as "developmentally determined" because they only appear in childhood. The differential diagnosis of seizures includes migraines, strokes, gastroesophageal reflux, breath-holding spells, dystonias, narcolepsy, night terrors, and syncope.

What Is Status Epilepticus?

Status epilepticus (SE) is currently defined as seizure activity that lasts more than 30 minutes or recurrent seizures without a return to a baseline of normal mental status for more than 30 minutes. Because 75% of seizures last less than 10 minutes, however, the definition of SE will probably be changed. Prolonged status epilepticus is dangerous for the developing brain and must be treated aggressively.

What Causes Seizures in Childhood?

The most common causes of pediatric seizures vary by age group. In the *newborn* period, hypoxic-ischemic encephalopathy is a common cause of seizures in the first 24 hours of life. Central nervous system (CNS) hemorrhage, infection, cerebral malformations, metabolic disorders, and drug withdrawal can also cause neonatal seizures. In *infants and older children,* common causes include idiopathic generalized seizures, febrile seizures, infections, tumors, strokes, hemorrhages, and neurocutaneous disorders. Some seizure types are specific to childhood.

Is There a Molecular Basis for Seizures in Children?

Studies have identified abnormal sodium or γ-aminobutyric acid (GABA) channels in some families who suffer from febrile seizures and mutations in voltage-gated potassium channels in benign familial neonatal convulsions, the so-called fifth-day fits.

What Is a Febrile Seizure?

Febrile seizures are developmentally determined seizures that occur primarily between 6 months and 5 years of age. The fever is usually high and associated with an acute infection. Febrile seizures often run in families. They need to be distinguished from seizures caused by meningitis and metabolic disorders and from underlying seizure disorders triggered by fever. *Simple* febrile seizures occur only once in a febrile illness, are generalized, and last less than 15 minutes. *Complex* febrile seizures occur more than once in a febrile illness, last longer than 15 minutes, or are focal. Approximately 30% of children will have a recurrence of febrile seizures, with 90% within 1 year after the initial seizure. Risks for recurrence include young age, family history of febrile seizures, low temperature at the time of the seizure, illness frequency, and occurrence of the seizure early in the illness episode. Children at risk for developing epilepsy include those who are developmentally abnormal, those with complex febrile seizures, or those with a family history of epilepsy.

What Are Infantile Spasms?

Infantile spasms usually start within the first year of life. These seizures may be flexor, extensor, or mixed in nature. The classic description is a "salaam" attack, during which the infant extends the arms and flexes at the neck, trunk, hips, and knees. Seizures tend to occur in clusters, particularly on awakening. Symptomatic infantile spasms have an underlying cause, including a host of structural and metabolic abnormalities, and represent about 80% of the total. Cryptogenic seizures have no identifiable underlying cause and represent about 20% of the total. The electroencephalographic pattern is highly disorganized *(hypsarrhythmia)*. Many infants have recurrent seizures. The prognosis for normal neurologic development with symptomatic infantile spasms is poor. The differential diagnosis includes an exaggerated startle response, colic, hypnagogic jerks, the myoclonic epilepsies, and benign myoclonus.

How Do Absence Seizures Differ from Complex Partial Seizures?

Absence seizures usually occur during school age, are brief (< 30 seconds), may occur more than 20 times a day, can be induced by hyperventilation, and are characterized by an electroencephalogram (EEG) with 3-Hz spike and wave complexes. Complex partial seizures can occur at any age. They are usually longer than 1 minute, only occur a few times during the day, cannot generally be induced by hyperventilation, are associated with postictal lethargy, and show focal abnormalities on EEG.

EVALUATION

How Do I Know If a Child Had a Seizure?

The patient's history is the best way to make a diagnosis. A precise description of the event may suggest the diagnosis. For example, an infant whose eyes suddenly rolled back, began shaking, lost consciousness for 2 minutes, then fell asleep for 15 minutes most likely had a seizure. In contrast, a toddler who was frustrated, exhaled, held his or her breath, then fell to the ground with perioral duskiness most likely had a breath-holding spell. Seizures are more likely than other paroxysmal disorders if there are focal movements (e.g., limb, face, or eye), depressed level of consciousness, and postictal paralysis ("Todd's paralysis") or sleep. Other important factors in the history include the length and timing of the episode, color changes (e.g., cyanosis), and associated or triggering symptoms. Review past medical, birth, and family histories, and perform a complete developmental assessment. The differential diagnosis includes gastroesophageal reflux, breath-holding spells, vasovagal episodes, migraine, stroke, tics, and dystonias. Abnormal developmental history, focal neurologic findings, or neurocutaneous findings generally mandate further workup.

When Are Laboratory Tests Needed?

Measure blood glucose in any seizing child. Choice of additional testing depends on the type of seizure, the history, and the physical examination. The American Academy of Neurology recommends an EEG after the first unprovoked seizure, but not all neurologists agree. It is important to note that EEG is most sensitive for certain conditions such as absence seizures and infantile spasms. If the diagnosis of seizurelike activity is uncertain, a normal EEG during a typical episode rules out epilepsy. EEG may identify a specific epilepsy syndrome such as juvenile myoclonic epilepsy in a teenager with occasional early morning jerks. EEG also can localize a seizure focus, which may make the patient a candidate for surgery if medicines do not work. Continuous EEG with video recording of behavior is currently used to evaluate complex patients. Imaging is recommended for the patient with focal neurologic findings to rule out a focal lesion, such as a tumor. Laboratory studies are best guided by the history and physical exam. Emergency management of seizures is discussed in Chapter 59.

What Evaluation Is Needed for Febrile Seizures?

Lumbar puncture should be done in infants younger than 6 to 12 months with a first-time febrile seizure to rule out meningitis. Infants aged 12 to 18 months with simple febrile seizures should also be considered for lumbar puncture, but it is generally easier to detect signs of meningitis in this age group. In experienced hands, children older than 18 months with simple febrile seizures do not require lumbar puncture routinely. Imaging is not routinely recommended for simple febrile seizures. EEG is not routinely recommended unless the history is atypical or there is a family history of epilepsy.

TREATMENT

What Do I Do If I See a Patient Having a Seizure?

If the patient has a generalized convulsion, remember the ABCs described in Chapter 59. Make sure the patient will not be injured: move dangerous objects if possible, roll the patient on the side to prevent aspiration, and loosen clothing that might constrict the airway. Do NOT put anything in the patient's mouth. Typically, most convulsions last less than 1 minute. Patients usually have shallow breathing during the convulsion, then take a big gasp when it is over. Note any movements of eyes, face, or limbs at the onset and record the length of the episode, as this may be the only clue of a focal onset. As the child recovers, be reassuring and pay attention to the ABCs. If the seizure just involves a momentary lapse in attention, try to engage the patient in questions while noting movements of the face or limbs and timing the event.

What Medicines Are Used to Treat Seizures?

Treat any underlying cause such as meningitis, hypoglycemia, or hypocalcemia. If a child has one "unprovoked" or idiopathic generalized seizure, most experts recommend observation without medication because the chance of recurrence is low (< 40%). If a child has epilepsy, anticonvulsant therapy is usually initiated. For status epilepticus, lorazepam or diazepam can be used as initial therapy. After status epilepticus has been controlled, other medications (listed later) may be prescribed for seizure prophylaxis in patients who have a risk of developing epilepsy. Phenobarbital, although fairly effective in preventing and treating seizures, is associated with learning delays or behavioral disorders if used chronically. Similarly, phenytoin can cause a number of adverse sequelae with chronic use, although fosphenytoin is a valuable agent to use acutely. Second-generation anticonvulsants, such as carbamazepine and valproic acid, are useful in treating partial and generalized seizures and often are the first agents tried. Although most patients tolerate them, their use may be limited by adverse side effects, including bone marrow suppression, liver toxicity, possible effects on long-term bone health, and teratogenicity. The newest generation of anticonvulsants includes oxcarbazepine, levetiracetam, topiramate, lamotrigine, zonisamide, gabapentin, and felbamate. They are used both as adjunctive therapy with other anticonvulsants, and occasionally as monotherapy. They have fewer medication interactions than older anticonvulsants and also have fewer side effects.

When Can I Stop the Anticonvulsant Therapy?

The timing for stopping an anticonvulsant depends on the cause of the seizures. If the child's seizures were caused by an acute event, such as a metabolic derangement that has been treated, or an encephalopathy, many experts recommend stopping the anticonvulsant shortly after the underlying disorder has been addressed or resolves. If the child has symptomatic epilepsy or a disorder such as tuberous sclerosis or juvenile myoclonic epilepsy that has a long-term risk of seizures, then prolonged anticonvulsant therapy will likely be needed. Children with idiopathic seizure disorders can stop anticonvulsants 2 years after the last seizure.

Do Children with Febrile Seizures Require Treatment?

Treatment of the acute, simple febrile seizure is not necessary. Rectal diazepam gel can be administered to arrest a prolonged, complex febrile seizure. Seizure prophylaxis is not recommended for simple febrile seizures, but might be indicated for complex febrile seizures. Oral diazepam administered at the start of fever may prevent febrile seizures. Phenobarbital cannot be used acutely to prevent a febrile seizure.

Do Specific Forms of Epilepsy Have Specific Treatment?

Acetazolamide is used to treat absence epilepsy. Adrenocorticotropic hormone (ACTH) is used for infantile spasms. A dietary regimen known as the ketogenic diet is used for treating medically intractable seizures. Resection of a seizure focus in the brain and vagus nerve stimulation are occasionally done for refractory epilepsy.

How Are Infantile Spasms Treated?

ACTH is the primary medication used to treat infantile spasms. Unlike the response of other types of seizures to treatment, ACTH either works or does not. Vigabatrin, valproic acid, or clonazepam have also been used. The etiology of the spasms is not a great predictor of response to treatment. The only etiology for which there *seems* to be a successful therapy is tuberous sclerosis, for which vigabatrin has excellent success. Before starting ACTH, test for tuberculosis with purified protein derivative (PPD), as steroids can unmask a latent infection. During ACTH therapy, monitor blood pressure, serum electrolytes, and blood glucose.

Do Patients with Epilepsy Have Problems in Addition to Seizures?

Any child with a chronic illness, including epilepsy, is at higher risk for abuse. The incidence of psychiatric diagnoses, such as depression and anxiety, are increased in children with all forms of epilepsy. Patients with epilepsy also have lower marriage and employment rates. Only some of these problems are related to medication. Adolescent women need to be counseled about pregnancy. All patients need to be counseled about safety during recreational activities. Driving laws for patients with epilepsy vary by state.

What Resources Are Available for Families of Children with Epilepsy?

The Abilities Network (*www.abilitiesnetwork.org/*) can provide information to families of children with epilepsy. A number of excellent books have been written for parents.

KEY POINTS

- Seizures occur in 3% to 5% of children.
- The most common seizure type is the febrile seizure.
- A detailed description of a paroxysmal event helps determine whether the event was a seizure.
- Atypical seizures, focal seizures, and prolonged seizures all require thorough evaluation.

Case 37-1

A 19-month-old boy is brought to your office after an episode of unresponsiveness, with arm and leg shaking that lasted about 1 minute. He has had a runny nose and cough for the last 2 days, and his mother thinks he feels warm. He has had three episodes of otitis media in the past. On examination, he is alert and curious about your office. Temperature is 38° C, heart rate is 130 beats/min, and respiratory rate is 20 breaths/min. He has some mild rhinorrhea and a right otitis media. The examination is otherwise unremarkable, including his neurologic examination.

A. Was this a seizure?
B. If so, what type of seizure was it?
C. What evaluation would be useful to help you answer these questions?
D. What treatment, if any, would you recommend for him?

Case 37-2

A 9-month-old girl is brought to the emergency department by ambulance after her parents discovered her shaking her arms and legs after she awakened from a nap. About 25 minutes have elapsed since her parents first discovered her. She was born prematurely at 30 weeks and was in the neonatal intensive care unit for 8 weeks after having multiple infections and "breathing problems." She has never had a seizure before. Her arms and legs are still shaking and she is unresponsive to your voice. Temperature is 36.5° C, heart rate is 120 beats/min, and respiratory rate 22 breaths/min.

A. What are your priorities in approaching this infant?
B. What additional information would you like, once she is stable?
C. What further evaluation would you like to do?
D. What treatment will she likely require?

Case Answers

37-1 A. *Learning objective:* **Identify a seizure using the history, physical examination, and if possible, observation of the patient during an episode.** From the history presented, it sounds like a seizure. The differential diagnosis includes a breath-holding spell, a seizure induced by a metabolic derangement, or a drug ingestion.

37-1 B. *Learning objective:* **List the common types of seizures in childhood, and differentiate among them using clinical information.** It sounds most like a febrile seizure, but he might have had an idiopathic generalized tonic-clonic seizure induced by a fever.

37-1 C. *Learning objective:* **Select the appropriate diagnostic workup to arrive at a final diagnosis for a child who has had a seizure.** History and physical examination should guide choice of laboratory and imaging tests. Further history about his development and the family history can help distinguish what caused this event. If it sounds like a febrile seizure, no further workup is indicated. If the features do not suggest a simple febrile seizure, consider obtaining basic chemistries, blood glucose, complete blood count, urinalysis, cultures (including blood and urine), and an EEG. If he had meningeal signs, a lumbar puncture would be done.

37-1 D. *Learning objective:* **Develop a management plan for common seizures.** If this child were diagnosed with his first simple febrile seizure or first idiopathic generalized tonic-clonic seizure, he would not be treated. The brief nature of the seizure and his unremarkable history and physical examination argue against the need for medications. The most important management step would be a detailed explanation of your diagnosis and its prognosis. If this seizure represented one of a series of recurrent seizures, he would likely be started on an anticonvulsant medication, with medication choice dependent on the ictal pattern.

37-2 A. *Learning objective:* **Identify status epilepticus, and recognize that it is a medical emergency.** The patient is in status epilepticus. This is a medical emergency. Initially, attention should be directed to her airway, breathing, and circulation (including placement of an intravenous line). Blood glucose should be determined and if hypoglycemia is identified it should be treated with intravenous glucose. Lorazepam should be prepared for intravenous administration.

37-2 B. *Learning objective:* **Discuss the approach to evaluation of status epilepticus after the patient is stabilized.** After the patient has been stabilized, additional history should be directed toward looking for signs of infection, trauma (including nonaccidental), medication overdoses or toxic ingestions (e.g., caffeine), and other etiologies discussed in the chapter.

37-2 C. *Learning objective:* **Select laboratory and other diagnostic tests to evaluate status epilepticus.** Additional testing should include blood glucose, serum electrolytes, complete blood count, urinalysis, and cultures (including blood and urine). Depending on the history, examination, and initial testing, studies such as imaging, lumbar puncture, EEG, drug screen, and metabolic testing might also be indicated.

37-2 D. *Learning objective:* **Discuss the treatment options for a patient with status epilepticus.** Depending on the results of tests, treatment might include antibiotics, anticonvulsants, or observation. If there is evidence of maltreatment, child protection services should be contacted. If the seizure was caused by a stroke, the patient might require rehabilitative services.

BIBLIOGRAPHY

Committee on Quality Improvement, Subcommittee on Febrile Seizures: The long-term treatment of the child with simple febrile seizures, *Pediatrics* 103: 1307, 1999.

Guerinni R: Epilepsy in children, *Lancet* 367:499, 2006.

Hirtz D et al: Practice parameter: evaluating a first nonfebrile seizure in children: report of the quality standards subcommittee of the American Academy of Neurology, The Child Neurology Society, and The American Epilepsy Society, *Neurology* 55:616, 2000.

Hirtz D et al: Practice parameter: treatment of the child with a first unprovoked seizure: report of the Quality Standards Subcommittee of the American Academy of Neurology and the Practice Committee of the Child Neurology Society, *Neurology* 60:166, 2003.

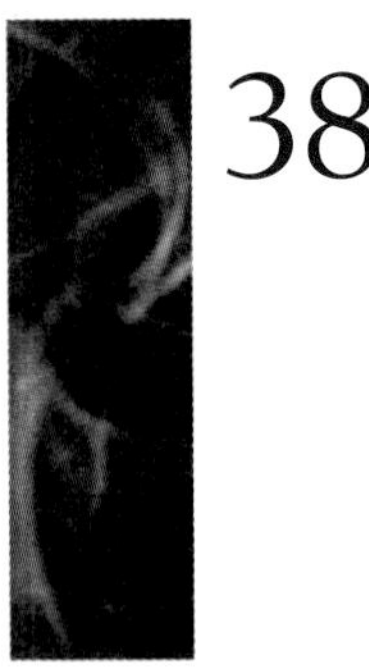

38 Stridor

TIMOTHY D. STARNER and
ROBIN R. DETERDING

ETIOLOGY

What Is Stridor and What Causes It?

Stridor is a continuous whistlelike noise during *inspiration*. This contrasts with wheezing, which occurs during *expiration*. Anything that causes edema or obstruction in the larynx or the upper trachea can produce stridor. Table 38-1 lists common causes of stridor.

Table 38-1

Causes of Stridor
Edema of the upper airway
Croup (common)
Epiglottitis (rare)
Endotracheal tube trauma
Airway malacia (softening of airway cartilage)
Laryngomalacia
Tracheomalacia
Foreign body
Vocal cord dysfunction

EVALUATION

How Do I Determine If a Foreign Body Causes Stridor?

The history provides the clues to diagnosis. Most older patients have a clear history of choking or gagging if a foreign body (FB) causes stridor. In contrast, when a toddler aspirates an FB, the aspiration episode is commonly unwitnessed and an accurate history can be difficult to obtain. Knowledge of development should make you suspect an FB aspiration if a toddler has the sudden onset of stridor or unexplained cough without prior symptoms. An FB in the esophagus can also cause stridor by compressing the trachea.

What Findings Are Important?

Table 38-2 shows key historical findings for some of the most common causes of stridor. Croup and laryngomalacia are discussed in Chapter 69. Children with croup usually have signs of a viral illness, such as rhinorrhea, cough, and fever. In airway malacia, vocal cord dysfunction, and FB aspiration, the patient usually otherwise appears healthy.

What Tests Help Determine the Cause of Stridor?

Bronchoscopy is the most useful test to determine if airway malacia, FB, or vocal cord dysfunction is present. A chest film can reveal a radiopaque FB (e.g., coin) or show a narrowed upper trachea (steeple sign) in croup. The flow-volume loop on pulmonary function tests can be useful to show the presence of a fixed airway obstruction.

TREATMENT

When Is Stridor Considered a Medical Emergency?

Stridor should be considered a medical emergency when there is severe respiratory distress. Increased $PaCO_2$ or hypoxia are late findings and are signs of impending respiratory failure. In FB aspiration, even patients who are stable are at risk of acute respiratory failure if cough moves the FB from one mainstem bronchus to the other or lodges it in the trachea, causing complete airway obstruction.

Table 38-2

Key Historical Findings for Most Common Causes of Stridor

Cause	History
Croup	"Barky," seal-like cough Viral syndrome prodrome Worse at night Age < 3–4 years
Foreign body	Possible aspiration episode (toy, food) Coughing or choking while eating Sudden onset
Vocal cord dysfunction	Teenager Abrupt onset and resolution Competitive or type A personality
Airway malacia	Present since early infancy Daily symptoms without resolution No response to medical therapies Worse with viral upper respiratory infection

What Medications Can Be Used to Treat Acute Stridor?

Nebulized racemic epinephrine can decrease swelling in mucosal tissue and temporarily relieve stridor. Careful monitoring is critical because the improvement will be relatively short-lived and treatment may need to be repeated. *Dexamethasone* produces a much longer-lasting reduction of tissue swelling, but clinical improvement will not be apparent for at least 6 to 12 hours after administration.

How Do I Manage Stridor Caused by a Foreign Body?

Careful airway management is crucial. It is important to transport the patient to a center where rigid bronchoscopy and removal of the FB can be performed. An emergent tracheostomy may not protect the airway because it may be above the level of the FB obstruction and may not alleviate the symptoms. Keeping the patient as calm as possible will decrease the likelihood that the FB will be coughed into the trachea or the other main stem bronchus, an event that could precipitate respiratory failure. Dexamethasone is often given to reduce airway swelling, which may improve stridor and aid in the subsequent removal of the FB by bronchoscopy.

KEY POINTS

- Stridor is an inspiratory noise.
- Stridor is caused by obstruction of the upper trachea.
- Stridor along with upper respiratory symptoms is likely to be croup.
- Think of foreign-body aspiration when onset of stridor is abrupt.

Case 38-1

A previously healthy 24-month-old child is seen in the emergency department in the early morning hours for marked shortness of breath, stridor, rhinorrhea, and a brassy cough. She has a low-grade fever and appears to be in moderate distress. Her oxygen saturation is 93% in room air.

A. What is the most likely cause of this child's respiratory distress?
B. What would be the most effective immediate therapy for this patient?

Case Answers

38-1 A. *Learning objective:* **Recognize upper airway obstruction and list common and uncommon but dangerous causes.** This child most likely has croup, which is caused by a viral infection of the larynx and trachea creating swelling in the subglottic space. Stridor is the characteristic sound created by upper airway swelling and obstruction. The classic history in croup includes worsening symptoms at night and low-grade fever. Less common but more serious conditions include tracheitis, which is usually associated with high-grade fever, and a toxic-appearing patient. Epiglottitis is a potentially life-threatening, but fortunately rare, condition that is not usually associated with cough. The child with epiglottitis is toxic appearing and has high fever. Vocal cord dysfunction as a cause of stridor is not seen in young children.

38-1 B. *Learning objective:* **Select appropriate management for a child with croup, based on the severity of symptoms.** The majority of children with croup need only supportive therapy, including cool mist, ibuprofen or acetaminophen, and calming efforts. Often, a child with mild croup will have a marked reduction in symptoms during the drive to the emergency department. However, when symptoms persist, the child may be in need of more aggressive therapy. Because the child described in the case is in respiratory distress and has low oxygen saturation, she would benefit from nebulized epinephrine and intramuscular injection of dexamethasone. Nebulized epinephrine has been shown to reduce symptoms rapidly, but the patient should be observed for at least 3 hours after treatment because rebound symptoms may occur. Dexamethasone has been shown to reduce airway swelling and obstruction, but the onset of action would not occur for hours. Intubation may be required if the patient worsens despite treatment. Albuterol does not treat croup.

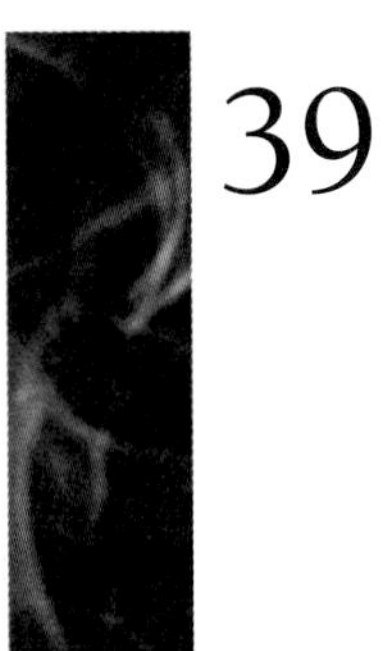

39 Syncope

NORMAN B. BERMAN

ETIOLOGY

What Is Syncope and How Common Is It?

Syncope is the sudden loss of consciousness and posture and is common, particularly in adolescents. Syncope accounts for 3% of visits to emergency departments, but many episodes of syncope never come to medical attention. *Presyncopal symptoms* of dizziness and lightheadedness without loss of consciousness are even more common. Syncope is generally benign; the clinical importance of syncope relates to the risk of associated injury and of underlying heart disease as the cause.

What Causes Syncope?

Neural mediated hypotension causing a transient decrease in cerebral blood pressure is the most common cause of syncope. Neurally mediated syncope often begins with decreased systemic venous return from prolonged standing. This causes an adrenergically driven increase in heart rate and contractility. In susceptible individuals, this can lead to stimulation of a vagally mediated reflex bradycardia, a drop in blood pressure and cerebral perfusion, and then syncope. Vagal stimulation is also the cause of syncope that occurs with painful stimuli, carotid sinus sensitivity, and other variants. Direct orthostatic hypotension is a common cause of presyncopal symptoms but less commonly causes frank syncope.

What Are the Cardiac Causes of Syncope?

There are relatively few primary cardiac causes of syncope. Anything causing severe left ventricular outflow obstruction can cause syncope, such as aortic stenosis or hypertrophic obstructive cardiomyopathy. Rare cardiac causes of syncope include congenital coronary artery anomalies, cardiac tumors, and pulmonary hypertension. Cardiac arrhythmias are another important cause of syncope. Any arrhythmia causing profound bradycardia (sinus node dysfunction, complete atrioventricular block) or tachycardia (supraventricular tachycardia,

Wolf-Parkinson-White syndrome, ventricular tachycardia) can cause syncope. Ventricular tachycardia is uncommon in children, but when present, associated problems such as long QT syndrome and cardiomyopathies must be considered.

What Are Neurologic Causes of Syncope?

Neurologic problems, specifically seizures, are often considered in the differential diagnosis of syncope but in fact are quite rare. Seizures (Chapter 37) can appear similar to a syncopal event, but generally can be differentiated from syncope with a detailed history of the event. Seizures causing a loss of tone are rare. Generalized tonic seizures can appear similar to syncope but are differentiated by the history of stiffening.

EVALUATION

What Happens in Syncope?

Children describe the symptoms leading to a syncopal event in remarkably similar terms: An initial feeling of dizziness or lightheadedness is followed by a sensation of warmth, then progresses to visual disturbances, such as blurring or graying of the vision, and then to completely "blacking out" while maintaining the ability to hear things. Patients often do not remember beyond this point and will next remember awakening on the ground. Observers will report that the child or adolescent looked pale and was unresponsive to verbal stimuli, then slumped limply or fell to the ground. Typical syncope is brief, lasting only seconds after the patient loses posture and falls to the ground. Occasionally the patient may be observed having tonic-clonic type movements at the time of loss of consciousness.

How Do I Evaluate Syncope?

A good history is key to the evaluation. It is important to first determine if the child actually lost consciousness and posture, as presyncopal symptoms may be called "fainting." The events prior to the syncopal event are critical to evaluate. Typical syncope occurs most often with the patient standing, less often while sitting. Syncope that occurs while supine should not be considered benign. There is often a history of meal skipping or inadequate fluid intake prior to a syncopal event. In adolescent girls, syncope may be associated with menstruation. Patients often do not present to the physician with their first episode of syncope, so a history of prior syncopal events and the setting in which they occurred is important to obtain. The past medical history and family history are pertinent and may suggest one of the specific cardiac causes of syncope listed earlier.

What Concerning Factors Are Associated with Syncope?

Syncope associated with exertion must be considered ominous and always requires further evaluation. Most often, a pediatric cardiologist will guide this evaluation. Hypertrophic cardiomyopathy is the most common cause of sudden death in young athletes and may first present with an episode of exertional syncope. Other dangerous causes of exertional syncope include coronary artery anomalies, other cardiomyopathies, and exercise-induced arrhythmias.

What Are Key Physical Examination Findings?

Although a good physical examination is important for a child with syncope, it is generally unrevealing. Orthostatic blood pressures are good to obtain but are neither sensitive nor specific. A heart murmur in a child with syncope should raise concern about possible structural heart disease and may warrant further evaluation. An irregular rhythm should raise concern about a possible arrhythmia.

How Should I Approach Diagnostic Testing?

Diagnostic testing in patients with syncope should always include an electrocardiogram (ECG). This simple, inexpensive study is a good screening tool for some of the dangerous causes of syncope: hypertrophic cardiomyopathy, long QT syndrome, Wolf-Parkinson-White syndrome, and other arrhythmias. In patients with exertional syncope, echocardiography is mandatory. A chest radiograph may be considered but is unlikely to be of diagnostic or therapeutic value.

TREATMENT

How Is Syncope Treated?

A patient with an isolated episode of syncope occurring in a characteristic setting may not have further episodes, so prophylactic therapy is not warranted. Patients should be encouraged to eat regular meals and to avoid dehydration. Many patients with syncope learn to prevent further episodes simply by lying down when presyncopal symptoms develop. Patients with more frequent syncope that interferes with daily activities may benefit from medical therapy. Fludrocortisone is the most commonly used first-line medication.

KEY POINTS

- Most syncope results from neurally mediated mechanisms that reduce cerebral blood pressure.
- The history of events leading up to, during, and after neurally mediated syncope is characteristic and helps make the diagnosis.
- Syncope uncommonly results from seizures or primary cardiac causes.

Case 39-1

A 14-year-old girl was brought to the emergency department after losing consciousness during a wedding in which she was a bridesmaid. According to witnesses, she "passed out" during the ceremony and fell to the ground. She was unconscious briefly and remembers feeling dizzy before passing out. She has never fainted previously.

A. What is the most likely cause of this patient's syncopal episode?
B. What are the other important causes of syncope to consider?
C. What evaluation is needed for a child with typical syncope?
D. How does the evaluation differ if the child had exertional syncope?

Case Answers

39-1 A. *Learning objective:* **Identify the most common cause of syncope.** Syncope is most often caused by a neurally mediated (vasovagal) mechanism. A characteristic finding in this form of syncope is the history of lightheadedness and blurring of vision immediately preceding the episode.

39-1 B. *Learning objective:* **Discuss the cardiac and neurologic causes of syncope.** Syncope could be a sign of an arrhythmia, structural heart disease, cardiomyopathy, or seizures. Syncope occurring during exertion is concerning for cardiac disease.

39-1 C. *Learning objective:* **Discuss the evaluation of syncope.** History should focus on the presyncopal events and on the past history of syncope. Family history may give clues to cardiac or neurologic diseases. The physical examination should be directed to an evaluation of cardiac rate and rhythm and to a complete neurologic assessment. Any patient with a history of syncope should have an electrocardiogram.

39-1 D. *Learning objective:* **Discuss the reasons that syncope associated with exertion must be thoroughly evaluated.** Any child with exertional syncope should undergo evaluation by a cardiologist, including an echocardiogram. In this latter instance, hypertrophic cardiomyopathy should be strongly suspected. During the athletic preparticipation examination, it is key to inquire about exertional syncope by asking if the individual has ever lost consciousness during exercise. A positive history should exclude the athlete from all participation until the syncope can be completely evaluated.

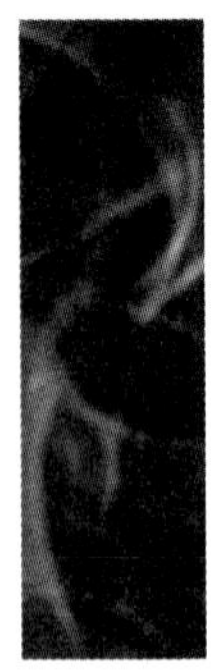

40

Upper Respiratory Tract Infections

WILLIAM V. RASZKA

ETIOLOGY

What Causes the "Common Cold"?

Upper respiratory tract infection (URI) is the most common acute minor illness diagnosed in a pediatrician's office. Generally, the child has rhinorrhea and mild irritability and may also have earache or sore throat. The physician must decide if the child's symptoms and signs are caused by a viral infection or are indicative of a bacterial infection such as otitis media, sinusitis, or even pneumonia. More than 200 viruses cause colds, although rhinoviruses comprise more than one-third of this number. Viral infection confers serotype-specific, lifelong immunity, but more than 100 serotypes of rhinovirus exist, so the chance of sequential infections with different serotypes is great. Parainfluenza, metapneumovirus, and respiratory syncytial viruses also cause URI.

EVALUATION

How Does a "Cold" Present?

Children initially present with mucoid ("clear") rhinorrhea, pharyngeal irritation, and some systemic complaints such as malaise. Fever occurs variably. Infants and younger children may present only with nasal discharge and irritability. After 2 or 3 days, the nasal discharge thickens and becomes cloudy and discolored from the shedding of epithelial cells and white blood cells; the color change does not necessarily indicate a bacterial infection. In patients with a cold, the physical examination is generally unremarkable except for reactive cervical lymphadenopathy and nasal discharge. Bacterial complications such as otitis media, sinusitis, or pneumonia are suggested by specific findings related to the system involved. Otitis media is diagnosed when the tympanic membrane is bright red or yellow, bulges, and has loss of landmarks and mobility (see Chapter 30). Sinusitis and pneumonia are discussed in Chapter 64. The signs and symptoms of the usual cold last 5 to 14 days. Parents are often concerned that their child has had a persistent cold for weeks or even months. The most likely explanation for the parent's observation is that the child has experienced sequential viral infections rather than one persistent infection. On average, a child may experience 6 to 8 colds in a year. This number may be higher with daycare attendance.

TREATMENT

What Treatment, If Any, Is Recommended for a Cold?

No medications have been shown to effectively decrease viral shedding or the duration of symptoms. In most situations, the most appropriate therapy is to maintain good fluid intake and manage symptoms such as fever and myalgia with acetaminophen or ibuprofen. Nonpharmacologic interventions such as mist, application of normal saline nose drops, bulb suctioning of the nostrils, and elevation of the head of the bed may be beneficial in some patients. Pharmacologic interventions, such as antihistamines, decongestants, expectorants, and cough suppressants, generally trade one set of symptoms for another. The most common complications of pharmacotherapy are irritability and sedation. In older children and adults, decongestants (sympathomimetics) may be helpful. Antibiotics are not useful in viral infections.

KEY POINTS

- The clinical findings of the "common cold" include nasal congestion, nasal discharge, and vague systemic complaints.
- A discolored nasal discharge does not indicate that the patient has a bacterial infection.
- There is no effective treatment for the "common cold."

Case 40-1

An 18-month-old boy is brought to the physician's office because of thick nasal discharge and low-grade fever for the past 3 days. He has been drinking fluids but not eating well, and he has been waking often during the night. He is on no medications. Sitting comfortably in his mother's lap, his temperature is 38° C, pulse 140 beats/min, and respiratory rate 24 breaths/min. He has thick green nasal discharge. The left tympanic membrane is pink, has visible landmarks, and is mobile. The rest of the examination is unremarkable.

A. What is the most likely explanation for the patient's findings?
B. Are antibiotics likely to be beneficial in this patient?
C. Are over-the-counter preparations likely to be useful?

Case Answers

40-1 A. *Learning objective:* **Describe the clinical history and physical findings of upper respiratory infection and list the common causes.** The most likely explanation is that this patient has a viral upper respiratory illness. Two lines of evidence support this. One is that his illness is consistent with a viral upper respiratory infection. The second is that he has no evidence of a bacterial complication such as otitis media or sinusitis. Yellow, green, or thick nasal discharge in itself does not indicate a bacterial complication.

40-1 B. *Learning objective:* **Discuss the use of antibiotics as treatment for upper respiratory infections.** Antibiotics are not likely to be useful for this patient because he most likely has a viral illness. The color of the discharge has not been shown to indicate a bacterial process. Although antibiotics are commonly prescribed in such situations, this practice has helped lead to the increasing prevalence of antibiotic-resistant bacteria. The American Academy of Pediatrics has published guidelines for the diagnosis and management of sinusitis.

40-1 C. *Learning objective:* **Select over-the-counter medications for management of upper respiratory infections, recognizing their limitations and side effects.** Little data exist to support the use of over-the-counter cough and cold preparations in the pediatric population. Most products contain antihistamines that may help children sleep but only because of a common side effect of the medication, namely sedation. Pseudoephedrine occasionally provides relief, if nasal congestion is a major symptom, but irritability and sleeplessness are common side effects that limit its usefulness. Use of an antipyretic medication such as acetaminophen or ibuprofen will aid in management of fever or myalgia. Some patients may benefit from the use of saline nose drops, bulb suctioning of the nostrils, and elevation of the head of the bed.

BIBLIOGRAPHY

Herendeen NE, Szilagy PG: Infections of the upper respiratory tract. In Behrman RE, Kliegman RM, Jenson HB, editors: *Nelson textbook of pediatrics,* ed 16, Philadelphia, 2000, WB Saunders.

Turner RB: New considerations in the treatment and prevention of rhinovirus infections, *Pediatr Ann* 34:53, 2005.

41

Vomiting and Gastroesophageal Reflux

WARREN P. BISHOP and
DINESH S. PASHANKAR

ETIOLOGY

What Is Vomiting?

Vomiting is a highly coordinated reflex process that results in forceful expulsion of gastric contents through the mouth. Vomiting is a common problem in children and can be a symptom of many disorders affecting different organ systems. The many causes of vomiting in children can usually be distinguished with a thorough history and a complete physical examination. Vomiting must be distinguished from gastroesophageal reflux.

What Is Gastroesophageal Reflux?

Most parents of young infants us the term "spitting up" to describe gastroesophageal reflux, which is the *effortless regurgitation* of stomach contents, usually after feeding. Reflux occurs when the lower esophageal sphincter relaxes transiently and allows stomach contents to enter the esophagus. This process differs from vomiting because it is not forceful. In most cases, reflux causes no problems for infants, although parents are often alarmed. In older children, reflux can present as vomiting or heartburn. Persistent reflux can lead to esophagitis, a condition known as gastroesophageal reflux disease (GERD) that can result in irritability, poor weight gain, and sometimes cough or concerning behaviors.

How Do I Categorize Causes of Vomiting?

It is useful to classify causes of vomiting depending on the age of children. Table 41-1 lists some common and uncommon causes of vomiting in three different age groups. Remember that regurgitation or spitting up is common in infants and indicates physiologic gastroesophageal reflux, not true vomiting. Viral gastroenteritis and gastroesophageal reflux are common causes at all ages, although they tend to occur predominantly in infants and younger children. Infections outside the gastrointestinal tract (extraintestinal infections), such as otitis media, pneumonia, and urinary tract infection, are more likely to cause vomiting in younger

Table 41-1

Causes of Vomiting According to Age

Infant (< 1 yr)	Child (1–12 yrs)	Adolescent (> 12 yrs)
	Common	
Gastroesophageal reflux	Gastroesophageal reflux	Gastroesophageal reflux
Gastroenteritis	Gastroenteritis	Peptic disorders
Viral (rotavirus)	Viral (rotavirus)	Duodenal ulcer
Bacterial	Bacterial	Gastritis *(Helicobacter)*
Anatomic obstruction	Extraintestinal infections	Gastroenteritis
Pyloric stenosis	Otitis media	Toxic/medications
Intestinal atresia	Urinary tract infection	Extraintestinal infections
Intussusception	Sinusitis	Sinusitis
Malrotation	Pneumonia	Pyelonephritis
Extraintestinal infections		
Otitis media		
Urinary infection		
Pneumonia		
	Uncommon	
↑Intracranial pressure	Anatomic obstruction	↑Intracranial pressure
Meningitis	Malrotation	Meningitis
Hydrocephalus	↑Intracranial pressure	Brain tumor
Inborn errors of metabolism	Meningitis	Pancreatitis
Milk protein intolerance	Brain tumor	Appendicitis
	Pancreatitis	Cancer chemotherapy
	Appendicitis	Cyclic vomiting syndrome
	Cancer chemotherapy	Pregnancy
	Cyclic vomiting syndrome	Migraine
	Motion sickness	Motion sickness
	Psychogenic	

children than in adolescents. Persistent vomiting in neonates or infants should raise suspicion about anatomic obstructions in the gastrointestinal tract such as intestinal atresia, malrotation, or pyloric stenosis. Peptic disorders such as *Helicobacter* gastritis or duodenal ulcer are seen most often in adolescents. Raised intracranial pressure is an important condition that can cause vomiting at any age. The likely causes of raised intracranial pressure are meningitis and hydrocephalus in infants and brain tumors in older children. Motion sickness can cause vomiting in children and adolescents. Cyclic vomiting syndrome is an uncommon disorder characterized by recurrent episodes of vomiting separated by symptom-free intervals, without any obvious organic cause.

What Is Pyloric Stenosis?

Pyloric stenosis is a condition unique to the young infant in the first 2 to 6 months of life. Hypertrophy of the pyloric muscle at the stomach outlet prevents stomach emptying and causes persistent vomiting that can eventually result in severe dehydration with hypochloremic metabolic alkalosis. The cause is unknown, but it is *not* congenital. Unlike intestinal atresia or malrotation that present with vomiting in the first days to weeks of life, pyloric stenosis takes time to manifest symptoms because the hypertrophic pylorus develops after birth.

EVALUATION

How Does the Nature of Vomiting Help with Diagnosis?

Details about the nature of vomiting can provide important diagnostic clues that help you focus your history and examination. Start with an open-ended question, such as "Tell me more about the vomiting." Then, ask specific questions to identify duration, temporal pattern, relation with meals, color, and intensity of vomiting. Table 41-2 provides some diagnostic clues for the nature of vomiting. It is important to remember that bilious vomiting indicates intestinal obstruction unless proven otherwise.

What Symptoms Are Associated with Vomiting?

Location and quality of abdominal pain may lead you to specific intraabdominal organ pathology. Painless "vomiting" in a happy, growing infant is usually gastroesophageal reflux. Epigastric pain is suggestive of peptic disorders such as duodenal ulcer, gastritis, or reflux esophagitis. Pain

Table 41-2

Diagnostic Clues to Vomiting

Clue	Causes
Duration	
Acute	Gastrointestinal infection, extraintestinal infection
Acute, progressive	Anatomic obstruction, intraabdominal pathology
Chronic, mild	Gastroesophageal reflux, peptic disorders
Cyclic, intermittent	Migraine, cyclic vomiting syndrome
Temporal Association	
Postprandial	Gastroesophageal reflux, peptic disorders
Early morning	Raised intracranial pressure, pregnancy
Color	
Bloody	Active bleeding in upper gastrointestinal tract (e.g., esophagitis, duodenal ulcer, Mallory-Weiss tear)
Coffee ground	Recent-onset bleeding in upper gastrointestinal tract
Bilious	Intestinal obstruction (beyond pancreatic ampulla)
Intensity	
Effortless regurgitation	Gastroesophageal reflux (common in infancy)
Projectile	Obstruction in upper gastrointestinal tract (e.g., pyloric stenosis)

of acute pancreatitis is also in the epigastrium, often radiating to the back. Pain of acute appendicitis is initially periumbilical, then moves into the right lower quadrant. Diffuse severe acute abdominal pain may indicate peritonitis, perforated viscus, or intestinal obstruction. ***Nausea*** is a common symptom in gastrointestinal causes of vomiting, although it is absent in patients with raised intracranial pressure. ***Headache*** with vomiting should raise suspicion of neurologic causes, such as brain tumor or central nervous system (CNS) infection with elevated intracranial pressure, but is also seen in sinusitis. ***Weight loss*** may indicate chronic vomiting, as in pyloric stenosis. ***Other symptoms*** associated with vomiting may include fever, which signifies an infection that could be gastrointestinal or outside the gastrointestinal tract. Diarrhea along with vomiting is suggestive of gastroenteritis.

What Else Helps Identify the Cause of Vomiting?

Consider the possibility of a toxic ingestion or a side effect of a medication. Nausea and vomiting are adverse effects of many prescribed medications, including cancer chemotherapy. Over-the-counter medications such as nonsteroidal antiinflammatory drugs can cause gastric irritation, vomiting, and even hematemesis. Ask about herbal and "alternative" treatments. If a child has both vomiting and diarrhea, you should ask about travel, daycare, exposure to contaminated water, or similar illness in family or friends. Pregnancy should be considered in sexually active adolescent girls. Psychogenic vomiting may be seen in adolescents with anxiety or bulimia.

What Should I Look for on Physical Examination?

First evaluate vital signs and general appearance to identify the acutely ill child who is likely to require urgent therapeutic intervention. Vomiting can lead to dehydration that manifests as tachycardia, dry mucous membranes, and low urinary output. Surgical conditions such as peritonitis or a perforated viscus can lead to septic shock with poor capillary refill and hypotension. In the abdominal examination, you should assess for tenderness, bowel sounds, organomegaly, and masses. Guarding and rebound tenderness indicate acute abdomen or significant intraabdominal pathology, such as peritonitis. Epigastric tenderness suggests pancreatitis or peptic disorders. A child with acute vomiting plus localized right lower quadrant tenderness and guarding has acute appendicitis until proven otherwise. Bowel sounds are sluggish in paralytic ileus and may be hyperdynamic in mechanical intestinal obstruction. Children with gastroesophageal reflux and gastroenteritis may not have any abnormal findings on physical examination. If increased intracranial pressure is suspected, you should look for bulging fontanelle in infants and papilledema by funduscopy in older children.

When Are Diagnostic Tests Indicated?

After a thorough history and physical examination, laboratory workup should be ordered with a specific focus on possible causative disorders.

Ill-appearing child: A child who has vomiting and acute abdominal pain and who also appears to be sick should be admitted to the hospital for surgical evaluation. Tests including complete blood count (CBC) with differential, electrolytes, amylase, lipase, and studies of liver and renal function are useful. Imaging studies can identify intraabdominal pathology: Plain x-ray of the abdomen should be ordered if bowel obstruction is suspected. Contrast study of the gastrointestinal tract is useful to diagnose intussusception, partial bowel obstruction, and anatomic abnormalities. Ultrasound is especially useful to diagnose pyloric stenosis and, along with computed tomography (CT) scan, is used to diagnose other intraabdominal pathology, such as appendicitis or pancreatitis.

Well-appearing child: Infants with uncomplicated physiologic gastroesophageal reflux rarely require any investigations. Rotavirus antigen test and stool cultures may be obtained in a child with vomiting that is followed by diarrhea. For children with possible peptic disorders, endoscopy with biopsy and 24-hour pH study are useful tests. A well-appearing child with chronic vomiting can be evaluated as an outpatient, but consider brain imaging by CT or magnetic resonance imaging (MRI) scan for a child with chronic headache and vomiting. Children with cyclic vomiting syndrome require extensive metabolic, neurologic, and gastrointestinal workup.

TREATMENT

How Do I Treat a Vomiting Child?

Treatment of vomiting is directed at the underlying disorder. Hospitalization and intravenous fluid resuscitation may be necessary for dehydration. Surgical intervention is necessary for conditions of acute abdomen, such as acute appendicitis, intussusception, and intestinal obstruction. An infant with pyloric stenosis must first have fluid and electrolyte abnormalities corrected before undergoing the surgical procedure to relieve the pyloric hypertrophy. Gastroenteritis is usually a self-limiting illness, and most children do not require any specific treatment except for oral rehydration. For growing infants with physiologic gastroesophageal reflux, no treatment is usually required, except for reassurance; older children with significant gastroesophageal reflux may benefit from acid suppression treatment, such as proton pump inhibitors. Adolescents with *Helicobacter* gastritis and duodenal ulcer require antibiotics specific for *Helicobacter*, plus treatment with proton pump inhibitors. Raised intracranial pressure and extraintestinal infections require specific treatment depending on the cause.

What Is the Role of Antiemetic Medications?

Avoid use of antiemetic agents unless you have a clear understanding of the underlying cause of vomiting. The antiemetic agents include medications such as antihistamines, phenothiazines, and selective serotonin inhibitors (e.g., ondansetron). These medications are useful in patients who have chemotherapy-induced vomiting, motion sickness, or cyclic vomiting syndrome. However, they are contraindicated in surgical emergencies and in situations in which specific treatment for the underlying cause is available.

KEY POINTS

- Vomiting is a forceful expulsion of stomach contents.
- Vomiting may result from infection, obstruction, or other conditions.
- Reflux is effortless regurgitation.
- Pyloric stenosis is a condition unique to the first few months of life.

Case 41-1

A 2-year-old boy has had vomiting, diarrhea, and a low-grade fever for the past 3 days. He vomits three or four times a day, and the vomitus consists of recently ingested food and fluid, without any bile or blood. He has also had six loose stools per day for the past 3 days. His 8-year-old brother had similar problems last week. On examination, he is afebrile and well hydrated. His abdomen is soft and nontender without any organomegaly or masses.

A. What is the likely diagnosis?
B. What investigations would you like to do?
C. How would you treat him?

Case 41-2

A 10-year-old boy is brought to the emergency room (ER) with severe abdominal pain and vomiting for 1 day. He was healthy until yesterday. His abdominal pain is in the right lower quadrant and is getting worse. He vomited four times today, without any bile or blood. He was unable to walk from the car to the ER. His temperature is 101° F, he has a pulse rate of 120 beats/min, and his blood pressure is 90/50 mm Hg. On examination he appears ill and apprehensive and is very uncomfortable. He complains of severe abdominal pain whenever he is moved. He is reluctant to let you examine his abdomen.

A. What is the differential diagnosis?
B. His abdominal examination reveals localized tenderness in the right lower quadrant, along with involuntary guarding. What would be your next steps for evaluation and management?

Case Answers

41-1 A. *Learning objective:* **Develop a differential diagnosis for vomiting, with or without diarrhea, taking age and exposure history into account.** The likely diagnosis is acute gastroenteritis. The presence of diarrhea and fever along with history of similar illness in a sibling is strongly suggestive of gastrointestinal infection. Obstruction is unlikely because of the absence of bile and abdominal pain. Similarly, the relatively mild symptoms and lack of progression argue against acute appendicitis or other inflammatory intraabdominal process.

41-1 B. *Learning objective:* **Select diagnostic tests to identify the cause of vomiting, with or without diarrhea.** The appropriate investigation would be stool test to look for infection. Because rotavirus infection is the most common cause of vomiting and diarrhea at this age, stool rotavirus test should be ordered. The bacterial infections are uncommon and often are accompanied by high fever and blood and mucus in stools. The parasitic infections such as giardiasis usually present as chronic diarrhea with weight loss but without vomiting or fever.

41-1 C. *Learning objective:* **Discuss management options for the common causes of vomiting, with or without diarrhea.** Specifically, recognize that acute viral gastroenteritis requires only supportive therapy. Viral gastroenteritis is a self-limiting illness and needs no specific treatment. In fact, medications such as antiemetics or antidiarrheal drugs are not recommended. The important management approach is to prevent dehydration by maintaining adequate intake of fluids, such as oral rehydration solution. Use the child's age, weight, and hydration status to determine his fluid needs for the next 24 hours, then instruct the parents about ways to administer this quantity of fluid.

41-2 A. *Learning objective:* **List the common causes of acute abdominal pain, recognizing the pathophysiology of acute bacterial infections such as acute appendicitis.** The occurrence of acute, severe abdominal pain, fever, and progressive vomiting in a previously healthy child should raise the suspicion of surgical causes of "acute abdomen." The differential diagnosis should include acute appendicitis or intestinal obstruction. The presence of right lower quadrant pain would favor the diagnosis of acute appendicitis.

41-2 B. *Learning objective:* **Interpret the findings on abdominal examination of a patient with acute appendicitis, and select laboratory and imaging studies to confirm the diagnosis.** The next steps should be intravenous fluid resuscitation, surgical consultation, and admission to the hospital. You would likely obtain a complete blood count with differential, a urinalysis, and a blood culture. Imaging studies such as plain radiograph, ultrasound, and/or computed tomographic scan would be required to diagnose intraabdominal pathology and to plan further management with the surgical team.

BIBLIOGRAPHY

Li BUK, Sferra JJ: Vomiting. In Wyllie R, Hyams JS, editors: *Pediatric gastrointestinal disease,* ed 2, Philadelphia, 1999, WB Saunders.

Murray KF, Christie DL: Vomiting, *Pediatr Rev* 19:337, 1998.

Orenstein SR: Gastroesophageal reflux, *Pediatr Rev* 13:174, 1992.

42

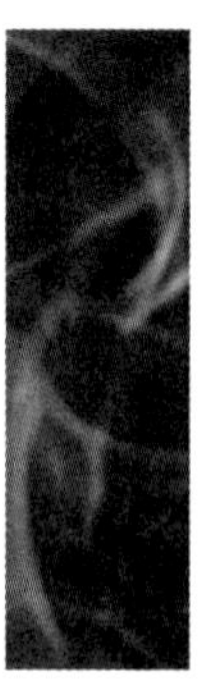

Weakness

ADAM HARTMAN

ETIOLOGY

What Causes Weakness in Infants and Children?

The differential diagnosis may be approached anatomically (i.e., cerebral hemispheres, spinal cord, and neuromuscular junction) or temporally (i.e., prenatal exposures to toxins, postnatal infections). The emphasis in this section is anatomic diagnosis. Table 42-1 lists the causes of weakness by anatomic location.

What Causes Muscular Dystrophy?

Muscular dystrophy (MD) is a group of disorders involving different muscle proteins. *Duchenne MD* is an X-linked recessive disorder that results from a deficiency of dystrophin. It usually presents in males in the first decade and progresses to respiratory failure in the second or third decade. *Becker MD* becomes clinically apparent in the first or second decade and is a milder form of X-linked dystrophin abnormality. *Facioscapulohumeral MD* is an autosomal dominant disorder with findings of facial weakness, winged scapulae, and lower limb weakness after the first decade. *Limb-girdle MD* is a family of disorders caused by abnormalities of sarcolemmal membrane proteins that has autosomal recessive or dominant inheritance. Symptoms appear in the first or second decade with slow disease progression.

What Causes Spinal Muscular Atrophy?

Spinal muscular atrophy (SMA) is the most common fatal neuromuscular disease of infancy. The three clinical forms all represent a deficiency of the *SMN1* gene (survival motor neuron 1) on chromosome 5, which produces the SMN protein. An identical gene, *SMN2,* also produces SMN protein but not as effectively as *SMN1*. Hence, the clinical forms of SMA represent variable production of functional SMN from the *SMN2* locus. Patients with certain forms of SMA may have extra copies of *SMN2*. All forms of SMA involve atrophy of the anterior horn cells. Type 1, also known as

Table 42-1

Etiology of Weakness by Anatomic Location

Systemic
Endocrine (thyroid, parathyroid, adrenal)
Heavy metal intoxication
Sepsis
Inborn errors of metabolism (maple syrup urine disease, glycogen storage disease, type II)

Cerebral Hemispheres and Cerebellum
Cerebral palsy (especially extrapyramidal)
Migrational abnormalities
Cerebral malformations (e.g., schizencephaly)
Benign congenital hypotonia
Chromosomal abnormalities (e.g., trisomy 21, Prader-Willi syndrome)
Stroke

Spinal Cord
Spinal muscular atrophy, types 1–3
Occult dysraphism
Trauma
Poliomyelitis
Transverse myelitis
Spinal cord tumors or abscesses

Peripheral Nerve
Hereditary peripheral neuropathies
Guillain-Barré syndrome
Refsum disease
Bell's palsy
Trauma
Critical illness polyneuropathy

Neuromuscular Junction
Myasthenia (neonatal, congenital, and juvenile forms)
Eaton-Lambert syndrome
Botulism
Aminoglycoside antibiotics (usually in combination with other disease processes)

Muscle
Muscular dystrophy
Myotonic dystrophy
Congenital myopathies
Metabolic myopathies (including storage disorders, mitochondrial diseases, periodic paralyses, and iatrogenic)
Inflammatory myopathies (including dermatomyositis)

Werdnig-Hoffman disease, has its onset early in infancy. Affected children rarely survive the first year of life. Infants affected with type 2 develop abnormalities after 6 months of life and have a slower progression of disease. Type 3, also known as Kugelberg-Welander disease, usually appears only after 18 months and has a very slow disease progression.

What Is Guillain-Barré Syndrome?

Guillain-Barré syndrome (GBS) is a polyneuropathy with acute ascending weakness, areflexia, paresthesias and/or dysesthesias, and autonomic dysfunction. Symptoms typically plateau over the course of a few weeks. One motor form of the disease has been associated with *Campylobacter jejuni* infection. A variant, known as *Miller-Fisher syndrome,* consists of ataxia, ophthalmoplegia, and areflexia. The differential diagnosis of GBS includes botulism, transverse myelitis, myasthenia gravis, spinal cord trauma, toxin ingestion, inflammatory and metabolic myopathies, and tick paralysis.

How Does Botulism Present at Different Ages?

Infant botulism is the result of botulinum toxin expressed by ingested spores, whereas botulism in older children and adults is because of ingestion of the toxin itself. Infants typically present with constipation and weakness; cranial nerve dysfunction and hyporeflexia may appear later. Infant botulism is more common in Pennsylvania, Utah, and California. Older children and adults more commonly present with bulbar symptoms (e.g., cranial nerve abnormalities) and descending weakness.

EVALUATION

How Do I Know Whether an Infant Is Floppy?

An infant is floppy if decreased tone or muscle strength is evident on examination. Easy fatigability and joint laxity may also be seen. The infant may have a significant head lag, may have a positive "slip-through" test in vertical suspension, or may be easily draped over the examiner's hand when examined in the prone position (horizontal suspension).

What History Is Needed to Evaluate a Floppy Infant?

It is important to note prenatal complications, intrauterine movement, intrauterine infections, amniotic fluid levels, and length of pregnancy. Review the birth history for presentation at delivery, Apgar scores, and abnormalities such as contractures. Ask about poor feeding and acquisition of developmental milestones. Also ask parents about their impression of the infant's tone and strength. The family history is crucial, especially a history of consanguinity, similar findings in any relatives, inborn errors of metabolism, or early infant deaths. Examination of family members can yield a diagnosis of myotonic dystrophy or myasthenia.

What Physical Findings Are Found in Weakness?

The patient's general appearance can yield important clues. A healthy full-term infant rests with arms and legs flexed; in contrast, a hypotonic infant rests in the so-called frog-leg position. Facial features, especially a tented upper lip, can be a sign of myotonia. Watch the child walk into the office and play: A gait that is waddling or clumsier than expected for age can suggest hypotonia. Evaluate different muscle groups for tone, power, bulk, and fasciculations. Remember that chubby limbs may be the result of fat rather than muscle. Fasciculations are a sign of denervation. Older children can be asked to perform Gowers' maneuver: lie prone on the floor and get up to the standing position. A patient with a *positive Gower's sign* will "walk" with hands up the extremities and trunk to stand, a sign of proximal muscle weakness. Difficulty hopping, walking on heels and toes, and climbing onto the table all can suggest muscle weakness. Myopathies tend to affect proximal musculature, whereas neuropathies tend to affect distal motor function. Myasthenic processes tend to be evident in bulbar musculature such as muscles in the face, and may show some diurnal variation. Hyperreflexia and dysmorphic features suggest central nervous system disease. Hyporeflexia, muscle atrophy, and fasciculations suggest peripheral nervous system disease.

Which Laboratory Tests Are Useful?

Creatine kinase level may be elevated in primary muscle disease or in denervating disease but it does not definitively rule in or out neuromuscular disease. In infants, electrolyte levels may show hypocalcemia, hypermagnesemia, acidosis, or alkalosis. A thyroid panel may be useful. Testing for inborn errors of metabolism is indicated if other testing is normal or if the presentation includes emesis, hypoglycemia, failure to thrive, or other signs of metabolic derangement. Imaging of the central nervous system is useful if a central etiology is considered. In children and adolescents, nerve conduction studies (NCS) and electromyography (EMG) can show characteristic patterns of certain disorders (e.g., myotonic discharges in myotonia). Muscle biopsies (with the attendant metabolic and enzyme studies) can be performed on patients for whom the diagnosis of primary muscle disease or denervation is likely.

Is Genetic Testing Helpful for Diagnosis of Weakness?

Testing through commercial and reference or research laboratories is the preferred method of testing for SMA and some other disorders. Genetic counselors should be consulted for prenatal testing and evaluation of asymptomatic patients.

What Tests Are Useful in the Diagnosis of Guillain-Barré Syndrome?

Classically, 1 week after the onset of GBS symptoms, the cerebrospinal fluid (CSF) has a higher protein concentration than expected for a given CSF white blood cell count (known as *albuminocytologic dissociation*). If the lumbar puncture is done earlier, this abnormality might not yet be evident. Earlier diagnosis can be made using NCS, which shows absent F-waves.

How Do I Diagnose Botulism?

EMG is usually the first test to show abnormalities. A rectal swab is useful to detect the organism in an infant's stool. In other forms of botulism, toxin can be detected in the serum or a wound.

TREATMENT

What Therapy Is Available for Muscular Dystrophy?

MD cannot be cured at present. Prednisone may delay progression of the signs in Duchenne MD but does not alter the ultimate outcome. Patients eventually need bracing, physical therapy, and wheelchairs. Supportive medical care includes early detection of respiratory infections and insufficiency. Ventilatory support might be required in the later stages of the disease. In all cases of MD, genetic counseling and family support systems are available and highly recommended.

How Is Guillain-Barré Syndrome Treated?

GBS is an autoimmune process and therapy typically includes either intravenous immune globulin (IVIG) or plasma exchange. Both are equally efficacious, but children have fewer morbidities with IVIG. The most important indicators to follow are the patient's respiratory vital capacity and vital signs. Dysautonomias in patients with GBS can be life threatening and require intensive monitoring. Supportive care is needed to manage the airway and maintain blood pressure in the acute phase and to provide physical therapy, occupational therapy, and speech/language therapy during recovery. Neuropathic pain should also be addressed.

How Do I Treat Botulism?

Human botulism immune globulin is used to treat infants. Trivalent equine botulism immune globulin is used in older children and adults. Supportive care with close monitoring is critical. Because the clinical picture in infants often resembles sepsis, antibiotics may be administered, but aminoglycosides should be avoided because they may affect neuromuscular transmission.

KEY POINTS

- Hypotonic infants have frog-leg posture and "slip through" your hands when lifted.
- Boys with Duchenne MD demonstrate a positive Gowers' sign.
- Guillain-Barré syndrome can develop after minor viral illnesses and may have life-threatening complications.
- Honey should never be given to young infants because of the risk of botulism.

Case 42-1

A 5-year-old boy is brought for an evaluation because he does not walk as well as the other children in daycare and also has trouble playing on the jungle gym. His mother cannot understand why walking should be difficult because the boy's legs appear to be "muscular." The boy did not walk until age 18 months but had no other medical problems in infancy. On examination, he has a positive Gowers' sign. His calves look very large. His strength is reduced (4/5) in the proximal muscle groups, but his tendon reflexes are 2+. He is uncooperative with the sensory examination. His toes are down-going.

A. What is the most likely diagnosis?
B. What testing is indicated?
C. How should you counsel his parents about therapy?

Case 42-2

A 10-year-old boy has refused to walk for the last 4 days. He has also had low-grade fever and mild cold symptoms. There is no significant past medical history. His development was normal. His father thinks he is "faking it." On examination, his cranial nerves are normal. He is able to swallow and speak without difficulty. He has decreased power in his legs. The reflexes in his arms are 2+, but you cannot elicit them in his legs. No plantar response can be elicited. Sensation is intact. He is unable to bear weight on his legs, even when supported.

A. What is the most likely diagnosis?
B. What tests would you like to do?
C. How should he be treated?

Case Answers

42-1 A. *Learning objective:* **Discuss the causes of weakness in a child.** Based on the history and physical examination, the most likely diagnosis is Duchenne MD. Key findings are proximal muscle weakness, pseudohypertrophy of the calf muscles, and a positive Gowers' sign.

42-1 B. *Learning objective:* **Select diagnostic tests to evaluate a child with weakness.** This patient's history and physical examination provide important diagnostic clues, but he should have blood drawn for serum creatine kinase level and genetic testing for Duchenne MD (dystrophin analysis). Expect highly elevated creatine kinase levels if he has Duchenne MD. Electromyography and muscle biopsy are occasionally needed for diagnosis of some cases of weakness. Additional tests might include thyroid studies, serum chemistries, and glucose. Central nervous system imaging may be useful in certain instances, but not in this case.

42-1 C. *Learning objective:* **Discuss the treatment and prognosis of Duchenne muscular dystrophy.** Prednisone may be useful to help improve strength and function. He should be referred for physical therapy to maintain his current functional status. He might eventually need orthoses for his feet, a wheelchair, or surgery for scoliosis. Respiratory support will be needed in the late stages of the disease, commonly in late adolescence. Most patients die before age 20. The parents should be referred to a support group for Duchenne MD.

42-2 A. *Learning objective:* **Use the history and physical examination to identify the cause of acute weakness.** The most likely diagnosis based on the information presented is Guillain-Barré syndrome. The absence of a "sensory level" makes a spinal cord process (e.g., transverse myelitis, spinal cord trauma, or tumor) unlikely. His history is not really consistent with myasthenia gravis, botulism, toxin ingestion, an inflammatory myopathy (which is usually associated with a rash, high fevers, or joint symptoms), or tick paralysis.

42-2 B. *Learning objective:* **Select diagnostic tests to evaluate a patient who has the acute onset of weakness.** The diagnosis is initially a clinical one, but nerve conduction studies would demonstrate characteristic findings (e.g., an absent F-wave). If he were symptomatic for more than 1 week, a lumbar puncture would likely show an albuminocytologic dissociation. Laboratory studies to exclude other diagnoses (e.g., thyroid function studies to rule out a metabolic myopathy) might be indicated, depending how confident the clinician is of the diagnosis.

42-2 C. *Learning objective:* **Discuss management of Guillain-Barré syndrome.** IVIG would be a good first-line choice for therapy. Vital capacities should be measured at least three times a day, and oral intake should be closely followed because Guillain-Barré syndrome can progress to life-threatening cranial nerve involvement. Also monitor for the potential autonomic complications, such as large swings in blood pressure or dysrhythmias. Physical therapy can help with function and to prevent contractures. There are support groups that can be helpful for the parents, as well.

BIBLIOGRAPHY

Crawford TO: Clinical evaluation of the floppy infant, *Pediatr Ann* 21:348, 1992.

Dinolfo EA: Evaluation of ataxia, *Pediatr Rev* 22:177, 2001.

Fox CK, Keet CA, Strober JB: Recent advances in infant botulism, *Pediatr Neurol* 32:149, 2005.

Kovacs J, Sankar R: Evaluation of hypotonia and weakness in infants and children, *Family Pract Recertif* 22:21, 2000.

Ryan MM: Guillain-Barré syndrome in childhood, *J Paediatr Child Health* 41:237, 2005.

Section 3

Patients Presenting with Physical Findings

43

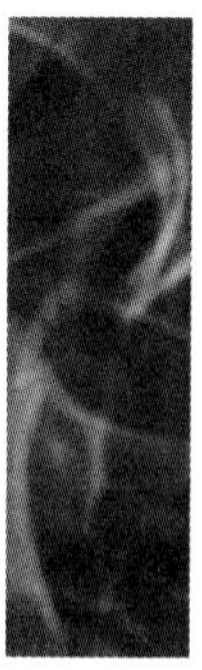

Abdominal Masses

ROGER BERKOW

ETIOLOGY

A mass in the abdomen can be caused by a wide variety of conditions and may present varying signs and symptoms depending on the organ or tissue involved, the age of the patient, and whether the mass is cystic or solid, malignant, or benign. The tendency of cancerous tissue to metastasize will also affect the presentation.

What Abdominal Masses Occur in Newborns?

The most common abdominal mass in the newborn period results from obstruction within the renal collecting system, leading to hydronephrosis. Complete obstruction would be detected during pregnancy because of oligohydramnios. Other nonmalignant abdominal masses include teratomas (most specifically in the sacrococcygeal area), duplication of the gut, and choledochal duct cyst. Hepatomegaly and splenomegaly result from storage diseases, portal vein thrombosis, viral and bacterial infections, hemolytic processes, and malignant infiltration.

What Malignancies Are Found in the First Year of Life?

Neuroblastoma is the most common malignant abdominal mass of newborns and in the first year of life. Most arise in the adrenal gland, but enlarged liver and lymph nodes can also be seen in metastatic disease. Neuroblastoma in this age group has a generally good prognosis and can often be treated with surgery alone if localized. Adrenal neuroblastoma with metastatic disease in the liver, spleen, skin, or bone marrow (but *not* in the bone) is termed stage 4S ("special"). This seemingly advanced disease has the potential for spontaneous regression with no or minimal therapy. More aggressive neuroblastoma may have biologic markers such as amplification of the N-*myc* oncogene. Wilms' tumor is the other common malignant abdominal mass in the first year of life. The incidence of this embryonic renal malignancy begins to increase during the second 6 months of life. Other malignancies causing abdominal masses in this age group include germ cell tumors, soft tissue sarcoma, and hepatoblastoma. Lymphomas are rare.

What Masses Are Found in Toddlers and Young Children?

Noncancerous masses in children between ages 1 and 6 include hepatomegaly and splenomegaly caused by infection or storage disease. Ovarian cysts are rarely seen at this age. Malignant lesions include neuroblastoma, Wilms' tumor, and lymphoma; hepatoblastoma, rhabdomyosarcoma of the vagina, bladder, or retroperitoneum, and ovarian germ cell tumors are seen less often. Constipation can sometimes be confused with an abdominal mass.

Is Neuroblastoma More Aggressive in Older Children?

Neuroblastoma beyond the first year of life often presents with bony pain, pallor, and an abdominal mass plus disseminated disease involving the bone and bone marrow. A child older than 2 years with disseminated neuroblastoma has poor prognosis despite aggressive multimodal therapy (surgery, chemotherapy, and radiotherapy). Paravertebral neuroblastoma may have intraspinal extension and cause spinal cord compression and paralysis of the legs. This medical emergency requires rapid treatment by those familiar with neuroblastoma.

What Is Wilms' Tumor?

Wilms' tumor is the second most likely cause of a malignant abdominal mass in the 1- to 6-year-old child. Parents often find a flank swelling during bathing or changing of diapers. Wilms' tumor is usually localized at diagnosis but can metastasize to lymph nodes, lungs, and liver. The prognosis is excellent, even with advanced disease. The "classic triad" of abdominal mass, hematuria, and hypertension is rare.

What Other Malignancies Cause Abdominal Masses?

Lymphoma occurs less often than neuroblastoma or Wilms' tumor. It can present with intussusception, especially in children older than 5 years, or hepatomegaly/splenomegaly. In these situations the metabolic problems associated with "tumor lysis syndrome" (hyperuricemia, hyperkalemia, hyperphosphatemia, hypocalcemia) must be anticipated. Rhabdomyosarcoma in the bladder or vagina can present with hematuria or vaginal bleeding, respectively, along with a pelvic or abdominal mass. It can also present as a retroperitoneal mass with or without obstruction of renal outflow or crampy abdominal discomfort. The extent of disease and the specific pathologic subtype of the rhabdomyosarcoma determine prognosis. Hepatoblastoma, ovarian germ cell tumors, and Ewing's sarcoma of the retroperitoneum or pelvis must also be considered in the differential diagnosis of abdominal masses in this age group.

What Causes Abdominal Masses in School-Aged Children?

Lymphoma is the most common abdominal mass in children ages 6 to 12 years. Neuroblastoma and Wilms' tumor occur less often. Bowel wall lymphoma must be considered as a cause of intussusception in this age group. Less common malignancies include primitive neuroectodermal tumor (PNET)/Ewing's sarcoma in the retroperitoneum or the pelvis; rhabdomyosarcoma in the bladder, prostate, vagina, or retroperitoneum; ovarian tumors, most commonly of germ cell origin; and hepatic malignancies. Constipation is probably the most common nonmalignant cause of a palpable mass in a school-aged child.

What Masses Are Found in Adolescents?

The most common malignant abdominal masses from 12 to 20 years of age include lymphoma (hepatosplenomegaly or ascites), rhabdomyosarcoma, PNET/Ewing's sarcoma, and ovarian germ cell tumors. In late adolescence, ovarian carcinoma, bowel cancer, renal cell carcinoma (especially in the presence of a family history), and hepatocellular carcinoma must be considered but are rare. Pregnancy is a common cause of a pelvic or abdominal mass in a sexually active girl.

EVALUATION

What Are the Important Points in the History?

Close attention should be paid to the location, onset, and rate of growth of the mass. Ask about the presence or absence of abdominal pain, vomiting, diarrhea, hematuria, and vaginal bleeding. Premature pubertal development may be caused by hepatoblastoma if the tumor produces androgen. If a mass is accompanied by bone pain, weight loss, and night sweats or fevers, consider the possibility of malignancy. In the adolescent, a detailed sexual and menstrual history must be obtained. In neonates, a careful prenatal history about maternal oligohydramnios or other problems with the pregnancy can give clues to the cause of the lesion. Family history should include malignancies in close relatives to help evaluate for familial cancer syndromes. The history of a parent or grandparent who had splenic enlargement or removal may give clues to a hemolytic process or a storage disease.

What Should I Look for on Physical Examination?

Physical examination should include the patient's general status and the state of nutrition. Neuroblastoma is often associated with weight loss, bruising, and an ill-appearing child, whereas Wilms' tumor often presents in an otherwise well-appearing child. The location of the mass and its apparent association with different organ structures often help diagnosis. Perform a vaginal examination if there is a pelvic mass or vaginal bleeding. Do a rectal examination if blood is present in stool or if there is a pelvic mass. The presence or absence of lymphadenopathy will provide clues about dissemination of some malignancies. Congenital anomalies should be noted, especially aniridia (lack of the iris) or hemihypertrophy, both of which are associated with Wilms' tumor.

Where Should I Start with Laboratory Tests?

Initial laboratory evaluation includes a complete blood count with differential leukocyte count to assess the integrity of the bone marrow and the possibility of blood loss. Assessment of electrolytes, renal function, hepatic function, uric acid, calcium, and phosphorus can evaluate for organ infiltration and look for tumor lysis syndrome. Urinalysis to detect hematuria is important in the evaluation of suspected Wilms' tumor. Urine homovanillic (HVA) acid and vanillylmandelic acid (VMA) levels help in the diagnosis of neuroblastoma. Serum alpha-fetoprotein and beta-human chorionic gonadotropin can be elevated in hepatoblastoma and germ cell tumors. Pregnancy evaluation must be done in any female of childbearing age with a pelvic mass.

What Imaging Studies Should I Order?

Abdominal ultrasound will help identify the organ of origin, whether the mass is solid or cystic (or has components of both), the presence or absence of ascites, and the patency of abdominal blood vessels. Ultrasonography can be done safely in an adolescent if pregnancy is a concern. The chest radiograph should be done next to identify pulmonary metastasis or mediastinal adenopathy. These studies are then followed by a computed tomographic analysis of the chest, abdomen, and pelvis to further define the location and extent of the lesion and to more completely evaluate for metastasis. This evaluation should be done with and without contrast and is important for proper surgical planning. Other imaging studies such as magnetic resonance imaging, bone scan, gallium scan, and positron emission tomographic scan can be done based on the suspected diagnosis.

TREATMENT

How Are Abdominal Masses Treated?

The approach to treatment depends on the cause of the mass. Nonmalignant masses may require either medical or surgical treatment (or both, especially in the case of renal obstruction in the newborn or young infant). Masses that have a high likelihood of malignancy will require biopsy and/or surgical removal. Confirmation of malignancy will be followed by a multidisciplinary approach to treatment coordinated by a pediatric oncologist, in cooperation with the pediatric surgeon, and radiation oncologist.

KEY POINTS

- An abdominal mass must be considered in the context of the child's age, the location of the tumor, and the associated findings.
- A coordinated approach involving a multidisciplinary team including the pediatric oncologist, pediatric surgeon, pediatric radiologist, and radiation oncologist is essential for correct diagnosis and treatment.

Case 43-1

A 2-year-old child was noted to have a swelling in the abdomen when her grandmother was bathing her 3 or 4 days ago. The mass was noted in the right flank, and pushing on it did not cause pain. She has been well, with no loss of appetite, nausea, or vomiting. She has had no bruising, bleeding, or fever. No constipation or diarrhea was noted. No weakness in the legs and no difficulty walking are appreciated. No pain in the arms or legs is noted. Physical examination shows a heart rate of 110 beats/min and temperature of 37° C. Height and weight are at the 25th percentile. A 4 × 5 cm mass is noted in the right flank; no pain is noted. The extremities are all equal in size and the eyes are normal. No bruising or petechiae are seen.

A. What are the two most likely malignant disorders to present in this fashion?
B. What laboratory data would you obtain to help in management and diagnosis?
C. What imaging study would you do first?

Case Answers

43-1 A. *Learning objective:* **Recognize that abdominal masses vary by cause according to the patient's age and that certain malignancies are more common in early childhood.** Wilms' tumor and neuroblastoma are the two most likely malignancies. The child's age, abrupt appearance of the mass, prior good health, and absence of systemic illness all point to an early stage of these malignancies. If the mass had been present for a longer time, then systemic signs caused by progression of these malignancies would develop. Hepatomegaly or splenomegaly might cause a mass in a 2-year-old child, but systemic illness would usually be present. If a mass had been detected earlier in infancy, obstructive lesions such as hydronephrosis would have been more common.

43-1 B. *Learning objective:* **Identify the appropriate laboratory tests for the evaluation of an abdominal mass in a child.** The initial laboratory assessment should include complete blood count, reticulocyte count, urine studies for vanillylmandelic acid (VMA) and homovanillic acid (HVA), urinalysis, and serum chemistries.

43-1 C. *Learning objective:* **Identify the appropriate imaging studies for evaluation of an abdominal mass.** The initial imaging study should be abdominal ultrasonography (US), to identify the origin of the mass, its consistency (cystic or solid), presence of ascites, and patency of vascular structures. If a solid mass is found, computed tomography (CT) of the chest, abdomen, and pelvis should be performed. Further imaging studies depend on results of the US and CT.

BIBLIOGRAPHY

Pizzo PA, Poplack DG, editors: *Principles and practice of pediatric oncology,* ed 4, Philadelphia, 2002, Lippincott-Raven.

Ries LAG et al, editors: *Cancer incidence and survival among children and adolescents: United States SEER Program, 1975–1995* (NIH Publication No. 99-4649), Bethesda, MD, 1999, National Cancer Institute.

44

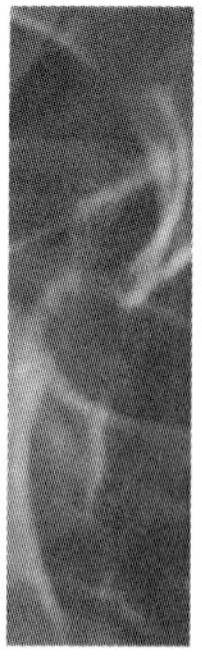

Bleeding and Bruising

ROGER BERKOW

ETIOLOGY

What Causes Bruising and Bleeding?

A bruise is a collection of blood under the skin, usually from trauma to superficial blood vessels. Bruising and excessive bleeding *without obvious trauma* point to a disorder in one or more components of the hemostatic mechanism: platelets, coagulation proteins, and blood vessels.

How Does the Hemostatic Mechanism Stop Bleeding?

When blood vessels are damaged, circulating platelets are exposed to blood vessel collagen and connective tissue. Platelet interaction with these tissues and with other platelets causes release of platelet granules that stimulate adherence and aggregation of platelets. Platelets and damaged vessels also release tissue factors that initiate the conversion of prothrombin to thrombin. Once formed, thrombin interacts with fibrinogen to form fibrin monomers. Factor XIII stimulates the monomers to form fibrin polymers, which interact with the adhering platelets to form a fibrin plug that prevents further bleeding. Platelet plug formation plus contraction of the blood vessel make up the primary hemostatic mechanism.

What Platelet Problems Cause Bleeding?

Platelets may fail to function properly or may be decreased in number. Increased destruction and decreased production both result in a decrease in platelets (Table 44-1). Most disorders in both categories occur infrequently, but all must be considered carefully.

What Causes a Decreased Platelet Count?

Immune-mediated platelet destruction, also called immune-mediated thrombocytopenia (idiopathic thrombocytopenic purpura, ITP), is the most common cause of a decreased platelet count. An antiplatelet antibody develops, usually after a viral illness, and attaches to the platelets,

Table 44-1

Disorders Associated with Decreased Platelet Count
Increased Destruction
Immune mediated (ITP, isoimmune)
Disseminated intravascular coagulation (DIC)
Sepsis
Hemolytic uremic syndrome (HUS) or TTP
Kasabach-Merritt syndrome (hemangiomas)
Hypersplenism
Decreased Production
Viral illness
Medications (prescription and OTC)
Leukemia or infiltrative malignancy
Chemotherapy drugs
Thrombocytopenia with absent radii
Amegakaryocytic thrombocytopenia
Wiskott-Aldrich syndrome
Aplastic anemia
Congenital marrow failure syndromes

ITP, Idiopathic thrombocytopenic purpura (immune-mediated thrombocytopenia); OTC, over the counter; TTP, thrombotic thrombocytopenic purpura.

which are then removed from the circulation by macrophages within the spleen. In children, 80% of cases of ITP are acute, resolving within 6 months with or without treatment; 20% will become chronic, persisting longer than 6 to 12 months. Older children with ITP, especially those in whom the disorder becomes chronic, may have an autoimmune disorder.

Do Newborn Infants Develop Thrombocytopenia?

A unique variety of ITP occurs when maternally derived antiplatelet IgG crosses the placenta, leading to destruction of fetal platelets. This thrombocytopenia can occur if the mother has ITP or an autoimmune disorder, or if she lacks the PLA-1 antigen on the fetal platelets. This latter situation is termed *isoimmune thrombocytopenia.* The mother becomes sensitized by fetal platelets that enter into her circulation. She forms antiplatelet antibodies that cross the placenta and bind to fetal platelets, shortening their survival. Thrombocytopenia develops in the fetus, which makes vaginal delivery dangerous owing to the possibility of intracranial bleeding. The newborn's platelet count usually begins to increase several weeks after birth as the antiplatelet antibody level falls.

What Congenital Conditions Cause Thrombocytopenia?

Thrombocytopenia caused by an isolated defect of marrow platelet production may present at birth with the syndrome of megakaryocytic thrombocytopenia and the thrombocytopenia with absent radii syndrome. When reduced platelet production from congenital disorders appears later, it is often accompanied by decreases in other blood cell lines. Fanconi's anemia has bone marrow failure, absent radii and thumbs, short stature, and increased risk of leukemia; dyskeratosis congenita is a syndrome of bone marrow failure with cutaneous and ectodermal dysplasia; and Bloom's syndrome includes short stature, bone marrow failure, and increased risk of leukemia. Thrombocytopenia is also associated with the Wiskott-Aldrich syndrome, an immunologic deficiency characterized by eczema, recurrent infections, T-cell function abnormalities, altered antibody response to antigens, and small platelets.

What Acquired Conditions Decrease Platelet Production?

Platelet production is reduced in aplastic anemia, leukemia, and infiltrative malignancy (e.g., neuroblastoma). Bone marrow aspirate and biopsy will identify pathology of other cell lines. Viral infections or sepsis can also suppress platelet production, as can chemotherapy and prescription and over-the-counter medicines.

What Congenital Disorders Cause Platelet Dysfunction?

von Willebrand's disease (VWD) is an autosomal dominant disorder with variable penetrance and is the most common congenital abnormality of platelet function that is associated with increased bleeding. Bleeding occurs because the quantity or function of von Willebrand's factor (VWF) is too low to promote the platelet-platelet and platelet-tissue interactions and the stabilization of factor VIII necessary to form a platelet plug. Another platelet disorder that causes bleeding results from congenital inability to secrete stored platelet granules, either because of a deficiency of platelet granules or because of a deficiency of arachidonic acid production. This prevents the platelet plug from forming or increasing in size.

What Causes Acquired Platelet Dysfunction?

Salicylate decreases the platelet's ability to release granules by inhibition of the cyclooxygenase pathways and by decreased production of arachidonic acid and is the most common cause of acquired platelet dysfunction. Other drugs that inhibit platelet adherence and aggregation include ethanol, antihistamines, and dextran. Cardiopulmonary bypass also inhibits platelet function.

What Coagulation Problems Must I Consider?

Anything that disrupts either the intrinsic or extrinsic coagulation pathway (Figure 44-1) will result in bruising and bleeding. Congenital deficiency of factors VIII and IX are commonly referred to as *hemophilia A* and *B,* respectively. These X-linked disorders are the most common congenital abnormalities of the fluid phase of coagulation.

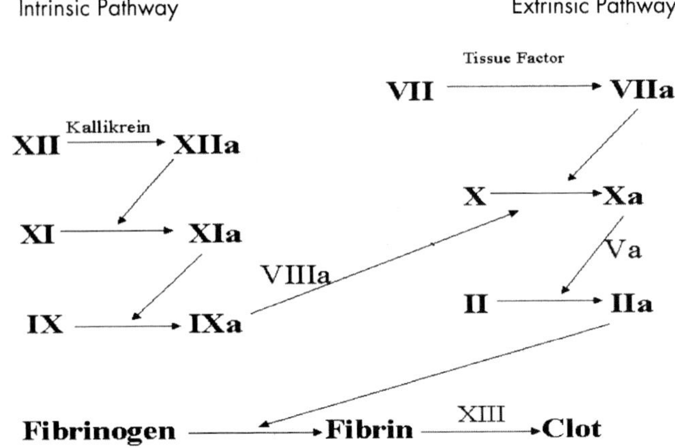

FIGURE 44-1 Coagulation pathways.

What Are Some Acquired Abnormalities of Coagulation?

Newborns are all deficient in the vitamin K–dependent coagulation factors because the gastrointestinal tract lacks the bacteria that synthesize vitamin K. Breastfed newborns have an additional risk because human milk has a low vitamin K concentration. To prevent vitamin K–deficiency bleeding (*hemorrhagic disease of the newborn*), vitamin K must be administered at birth. Bleeding is most commonly seen in newborns who were born at home and who did not receive vitamin K. Parents occasionally refuse vitamin K for hospital-born babies and must be made aware of the risk of serious bleeding. A similar bleeding problem can develop in older children if prolonged administration of antibiotics depletes the gut flora and vitamin K production falls. Sepsis can cause *disseminated intravascular coagulation,* which activates the hemostatic mechanism and depletes coagulation factors. Severe hepatic dysfunction can lead to decreased production of factors II, VII, IX, and X (the hepatic or vitamin K–dependent factors). Rarely, antibodies against coagulation factors develop in collagen vascular diseases and viral illnesses with resultant bleeding; paradoxically, these antibodies can also inhibit naturally occurring anticoagulants and increase the likelihood of venous thrombosis.

What Inflammatory Problems Cause Bleeding?

Collagen vascular disorders are the most common inflammatory processes that cause bruising and bleeding despite appropriate platelet function and number and an intact coagulation mechanism. Henoch-Schönlein purpura often presents with joint or abdominal pain plus a purpuric rash on the legs and buttocks. Deposition of IgA in blood vessels disrupts the integrity of the vessel wall and results in bleeding. Platelet count and function and coagulation proteins are normal.

EVALUATION

How Should I Evaluate Bruising or Bleeding?

The history must identify the age at onset, frequency of bleeding episodes, known triggers of bleeding (e.g., trauma or tooth brushing), and the location of the bleeding or bruises. Ask about fever, rash, abdominal pain, joint swelling, and headache. Review the family history. Consider the developmental stage of the child: Bruising is infrequent before crawling and walking develop; conversely, the toddler often has bruises on the shins and forehead. Remember to consider child abuse if bruising is seen in nonambulatory infants, in unusual locations, or in patterns that resemble objects that might have been used to strike the child (see Chapter 24).

What Laboratory Tests Help the Evaluation?

The laboratory workup for all patients with bruising or bleeding must consider factors that affect the hemostatic process:

- Platelet number and function
- Concentrations of coagulation factors and presence of inhibitors of these proteins
- Blood vessel contractility or inflammation

The initial step is to check the platelet count in relation to the complete blood count (CBC): If the platelet count alone is decreased, then a process isolated to the platelets is likely; if more than one cell line is decreased, then a process affecting the bone marrow must be considered; if all cell lines in the CBC are present in appropriate numbers, then the functional status of the platelets must be tested with bleeding time or the PFA-100 test. Bleeding time measures the integrity of the microvasculature and the ability of platelets to form the initial platelet plug. It is prolonged with decreased numbers of platelets and when the platelets have abnormal adherence or aggregation. PFA-100 is increasingly used as a substitute for the bleeding time. Coagulation proteins are assessed with the activated partial thromboplastin time (aPTT) that measures the coordinated activation of the *intrinsic pathway* of coagulation, and the prothrombin time (PT) that measures the *extrinsic pathway*. Plasma concentrations of the coagulation factors should also be assayed, especially factors VIII and IX. More specific tests will depend on history and the initial screening results.

What Findings Indicate Idiopathic Thrombocytopenic Purpura?

A typical patient is 2 to 8 years of age and develops bruising and petechiae 10 days to 2 weeks after a minor viral illness or occasionally after immunizations. Physical examination shows petechiae and ecchymoses but no pallor, hepatosplenomegaly, lymphadenopathy, or bone or joint pain. Thrombocytopenia and large platelets is the prominent laboratory abnormality, with platelet count usually less than 10,000/mm^3. The CBC otherwise shows normal white blood cell count and differential, hemoglobin, and hematocrit. If a bone marrow aspirate is performed, increased megakaryocytes are seen.

How Is von Willebrand's Disease Identified?

VWD often presents with recurrent nosebleeds or menorrhagia. Family history reveals increased bleeding in first-degree relatives. The aPTT is usually normal or mildly prolonged and bleeding time is usually prolonged. VWF, ristocetin cofactor, and factor VIII levels are all usually mildly to moderately decreased. VWF levels may be variable owing to release of stores from the endothelium, so repeat levels may be necessary to document VWD if the nature of the bleeding and the family history make the disease likely.

What Clues Point to Acquired Platelet Dysfunction?

These patients typically have been healthy before the appearance of increased bruising and nosebleeds, or occasionally more severe mucosal bleeding. The bleeding may be episodic and associated with a specific medication such as aspirin. A thorough history of prescribed and over-the-counter medications will often discover the cause of the bleeding.

What about Leukemia or Another Malignancy?

Leukemia (Chapter 63) typically has prominent thrombocytopenia with bruising and bleeding, plus fever, lymphadenopathy, splenomegaly, and joint swelling. CBC reveals abnormalities of all cell types. Bone marrow aspiration or biopsy will be necessary, as will other diagnostic tests appropriate to the diagnosis under consideration.

When Should I Consider Hemophilia?

A typical patient with hemophilia is a male infant who develops excessive bruising plus joint swelling at age 4 to 10 months. The family history often reveals males in the maternal lineage with similar problems. Approximately 20% to 25% of hemophiliacs have no family history and the initial presentation may be prolonged bleeding with circumcision. Hemophiliacs commonly have painful joint swelling caused by spontaneous bleeding or bleeding after minimal or unrecognized trauma. Inflammation of the affected joints is absent. Suspect hemophilia if a patient has an isolated prolongation of the aPTT. Factor VIII and IX levels will identify the missing factor. If levels of these factors are normal, then measure factors XI and XII. Patients with bleeding and isolated prolongation of PT should have factor VII levels measured.

How Do I Detect Inflammation of Blood Vessels?

Conditions that produce inflammatory changes in the microvasculature, such as Henoch-Schönlein purpura, cause a purpuric rash with or without joint and abdominal pain. The platelet count is normal. It is important to test the urine for blood and protein and the stool for blood. Close follow-up of the blood pressure is also important.

TREATMENT

How Is Idiopathic Thrombocytopenic Purpura Treated?

Most cases spontaneously remit and require no therapy. More severe cases may require corticosteroids or intravenous immunoglobulin (IVIG). Bone marrow aspirate to rule out a malignancy such as leukemia is wise before corticosteroids are administered. Patients who are Rh positive will benefit from intravenous anti-D antibodies. *Transfusion of platelets is contraindicated,* except in the face of life-threatening bleeding, because transfused platelets will be rapidly coated with circulating antibody and removed from the circulation.

How Is Isoimmune Thrombocytopenia Treated?

The newborn with isoimmune thrombocytopenia should be transfused with platelets isolated from the mother, because maternal platelets lack the PLA-1 antigen to which the antibody is directed. IVIG and corticosteroids are also used.

How Do I Treat Abnormal Platelet Function?

Treatment of VWD involves either the infusion of specific purified concentrates to replace the missing VWF or the administration of desmopressin, which triggers release of both stored VWF and factor VIII. If acquired platelet function abnormalities result from drug exposure, cessation of the medication will reverse the problem after approximately 7 days, the life span of circulating platelets.

How Are Coagulation Abnormalities Treated?

If a male patient has bleeding, characteristic clinical findings, and a markedly prolonged aPTT, fresh frozen plasma should be infused empirically while awaiting results of factor VIII and IX levels. Once the diagnosis of hemophilia has been established, management should emphasize prevention of trauma, with infusion of recombinant factor VIII or IX when needed to control bleeding. Repeated episodes of hemarthrosis, if not treated early, will lead to permanent joint damage. Intracranial bleeding can be life threatening and should be promptly and aggressively treated. In hepatic dysfunction, administration of factors II, VII, IX, and X (the hepatic or vitamin K–dependent factors) will restore hemostatic function.

KEY POINTS

- Platelet count, aPTT, PT, and bleeding time screen for problems with the primary components of the hemostatic mechanism.
- Measurement of platelet production and function or of specific coagulation factors should be based on the clinical and family histories and on the results of the screening tests.

Case 44-1

A 9-month-old white male is brought for evaluation of easy bruising. His mother states that he has been generally well but began bruising easily when he started to crawl at about age 6 months. The bruising has gotten worse as he has begun to pull up to a stand over the last week. The child has shown steady, appropriate development and has had no other illnesses. Family history reveals that the maternal grandfather had easy bruising and chronic arthritis. Examination of the child shows numerous bruises on the buttocks, legs, and forehead.

A. What additional history is helpful?
B. What physical findings should you look for to assess this child's bruising?
C. What is the differential diagnosis at this point?
D. What laboratory studies will help in the diagnosis?
E. Screening laboratory test results: CBC and platelets are within the appropriate ranges for age. The PT is 12 seconds (normal) and the aPTT is $>$ 100 seconds (prolonged). What additional laboratory tests will help establish a final diagnosis?
F. If specific test results demonstrate that the factor VIII is $<$ 1% (low) and the factor IX is 100%, what is the patient's diagnosis?

Case Answers

44-1 A. *Learning objective:* **Obtain appropriate historical information to evaluate bruising and bleeding in a child.** Ask about bleeding in the neonatal period (specifically with circumcision). Determine whether the child has had skin rash (petechiae), has been ill-appearing, or had a recent febrile illness (to suggest disseminated intravascular coagulation or immune-mediated thrombocytopenia). Inquire about the family history of bleeding (especially along the maternal side). The maternal grandfather's bruising and arthritis are important historical clues in this case.

44-1 B. *Learning objective:* **Identify physical findings important in the assessment of a child with a suspected bleeding disorder.** You must look for the presence or absence of petechiae, lymphadenopathy, hepatosplenomegaly, joint swelling or effusion (suggestive of hemophilia), and apparent fractures or other suspicious marks (to suggest nonaccidental trauma). Careful examination of large joints will establish whether intraarticular bleeding has occurred.

44-1 C. *Learning objective:* **Outline the differential diagnosis of bruising and bleeding in childhood.** The differential diagnosis is still quite broad for this patient and includes abnormalities of both the fluid phase and platelet phase of coagulation and the possibility of nonaccidental trauma. Infectious causes seem less likely because of the absence of fever and other symptoms and signs. The family history points to the possibility of a hereditary bleeding disorder, such as hemophilia.

44-1 D. *Learning objective:* **Select laboratory tests for the initial evaluation of bruising and bleeding.** In this situation, CBC with platelet count, PT, and PTT are the appropriate initial screening tests.

44-1 E. *Learning objective:* **Interpret screening laboratory tests and obtain specific tests to establish a diagnosis.** Factor VIII and factor IX levels should be ordered.

44-1 F. *Learning objective:* **Interpret specific laboratory tests to establish a diagnosis.** This boy has hemophilia A, factor VIII deficiency.

BIBLIOGRAPHY

Behrman RE, Kliegman RM, Jenson, HB, editors: *Nelson's textbook of pediatrics,* ed 17, Philadelphia, 2004, WB Saunders.

Hoekelman RA et al, editors: *Primary pediatric care,* ed 4, St Louis, 2001, Mosby-Year Book.

Lanzkowsky P, editor: *Manual of pediatric hematology and oncology,* ed 4, New York, 2005, Elsevier.

Nathan DG et al, editors: *Nathan and Oski's hematology of infancy and childhood,* ed 6, Philadelphia, 2003, WB Saunders.

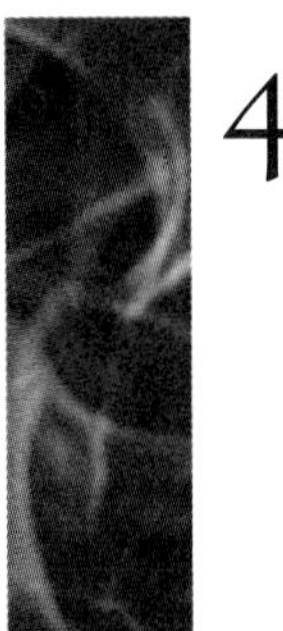

45

Edema

LAVJAY BUTANI and BRUCE Z. MORGENSTERN

ETIOLOGY

What Does Edema Signify?

Edema may be localized or generalized. This discussion focuses on generalized edema, which is a physical manifestation of the expansion of the body's extravascular fluid compartment (usually by > 10%), observed as soft tissue swelling. Generalized edema accompanied by fluid in the peritoneal cavity is referred to as *anasarca.*

What Causes Edema?

Three basic mechanisms cause generalized edema:

1. *Increased hydrostatic pressure,* which forces fluid from the intravascular space into the extravascular space (e.g., congestive heart failure, constrictive pericarditis, and acute or chronic renal failure).
2. *Decreased oncotic pressure* resulting from hypoalbuminemia, which promotes the movement of fluid into the extravascular tissues because of diminished protein binding within the vascular space (e.g., hepatic failure, nephrotic syndrome, protein malnutrition, hypercatabolic state, and malabsorption syndromes).
3. *Increased capillary permeability,* which allows fluid to "leak" into extravascular tissues (e.g., capillary endothelial damage because of endotoxemia in the sepsis syndrome).

EVALUATION

How Can I Evaluate a Child with Edema?

Some clues from the history and physical examination that point toward the cause of edema, and the suggested basic initial laboratory workup for these conditions, are presented in Table 45-1. For more details on the specific disease processes, refer to the appropriate sections elsewhere in the text.

Table 45-1

Evaluation of a Child with Edema

Disease Process	Historical Clues	Physical Examination	Basic Workup
Renal failure	Decreased urine output, failure to thrive	Short stature, hypertension	Serum creatinine, urinalysis
Nephrotic syndrome	Puffy eyes, worst in the morning	Generalized edema, anasarca, ascites	Serum albumin, urinalysis
Liver disease	Jaundice, abdominal pain	Icterus, hepatomegaly, ascites	Hepatic transaminases, serum albumin, prothrombin time
Malnutrition	Food faddism, anorexia	Growth failure, loose skin folds, thin brittle hair, protuberant abdomen	Serum albumin, diet record, psychosocial evaluation
Malabsorption	Frequent loose stools, oily stools	Abdominal distention, pallor, abdominal pain	Serum albumin, complete blood count, iron studies, stool studies
Sepsis	Fever, symptoms suggestive of an infectious process such as cough (for pneumonia), altered mental status	"Toxic" appearance, hypotension, skin rash	Blood culture; culture body fluid where infection is suspected
Anaphylaxis	Bee sting, recent exposure to medication/food known to cause allergic reactions (e.g., peanuts)	Oropharyngeal edema, stridor or wheezing, urticaria	Skin testing, provocative food challenge, RAST test

RAST, Radioallergosorbent test.

Where Might I Find Edema on Physical Examination?

Sites where edema might be detected include the distal tibia (pretibial edema), the periorbital region (periorbital edema), the lower back (sacral edema), and the abdomen (ascites). Sacral and pretibial edema can be detected by pressing the skin for a few seconds and observing for an indentation (pitting edema). Clues that ascites might be present include

- Visible abdominal distention with bulging flanks
- Stretching of the umbilicus in the horizontal direction or bulging of an umbilical hernia

- Dullness to percussion in the flanks when supine; the dullness resolves when the patient rolls to the lateral position (shifting dullness)
- Fluid wave (place one hand on the flank and tap sharply on the other flank)

TREATMENT

How Do I Manage a Patient with Generalized Edema?

Management depends entirely on the underlying cause. While awaiting the results of the diagnostic workup or the response to a specific treatment, consider diuretics for a patient who has intravascular volume expansion (e.g., acute renal failure). When hypoalbuminemia causes massive ascites or large pleural effusions that compromise respiration, a patient may benefit from intravenous albumin infusions combined with diuretics. Albumin infusions are not without risk, and they need to be carefully considered and administered. A low-salt diet is also generally recommended to limit sodium and water retention by the kidney.

KEY POINTS

- Generalized edema is a sign of significant extravascular volume expansion.
- Many disease processes result in edema; management depends on the underlying disease.
- A low-salt diet and diuretic treatment, with or without intravenous albumin, might be of benefit.

Case 45-1

A 12-month-old girl is brought to your office because her shoes have been getting progressively tighter for the past 2 weeks. She also "looks pale" and has been having looser bowel movements since her mother weaned her off the breast 1 month ago. This morning, her face, abdomen, and legs also looked swollen. Weight is at the 90th percentile; length is 50th percentile. On examination, her heart rate is 110 beats/min, her respiratory rate is 18 breaths/min, and her blood pressure is 105/65 mm Hg. Her conjunctiva are pale. She has periorbital and pedal edema and also has a markedly distended abdomen with a fluid wave.

A. What are the possible causes of this child's problem?
B. How would you proceed with her evaluation?

Case Answers

45-1 A. *Learning objective:* **List the likely causes of edema in childhood.** The likely causes of edema in childhood include nephrotic syndrome, renal failure, malabsorption syndrome, and liver disease.

45-1 B. *Learning objective:* **Discuss the evaluation of edema by history, physical examination, and laboratory testing.** Detailed history is outlined in Table 45-1. Laboratory tests should include urinalysis, serum albumin, complete blood count with red blood cell indices, iron studies, stool studies, serum electrolytes, and serum creatinine. Further testing to be based on the previously mentioned screening tests.

BIBLIOGRAPHY

Haws RM, Baum M: Efficacy of albumin and diuretic therapy in children with nephrotic syndrome, *Pediatrics* 91:1142, 1993.

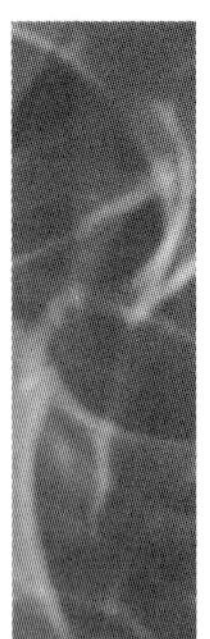

46

Hypertension

LAVJAY BUTANI and BRUCE Z. MORGENSTERN

ETIOLOGY

What Is Hypertension in a Child?

Ideally, blood pressure (BP) should be less than the 90th percentile for age. Hypertension is defined as BP that is above the 95th percentile for the child's age, gender, and height, measured on at least three separate occasions. For example, a 4-year-old boy with BP 120/80 mm Hg is above this cut-off: Even if his height is at the 95th percentile, his BP should not be above 115/71 mm Hg. (See Table 46-1 for the 95th percentile ranges of BP for children between the 5th and 95th percentiles for height.) For complete tables of BP values in children see *www.nhlbi.nih.gov/guidelines/hypertension/child_tbl.htm* or *Pediatrics* 114:555, 2004.

Why Is Hypertension of Concern?

Hypertension is uncommon in infants and young children but is identified with some regularity in older children and adolescents. The prevalence of hypertension is approximately 1% in children, compared with 30% in adults. Persistently elevated BP in childhood is somewhat predictive of adult hypertension, with the associated risks for coronary artery disease and stroke.

What Causes Hypertension in a Child?

In some children and in most adults, elevated BP that does not result from identifiable pathology in a single organ system is labeled *primary hypertension* (formerly called "*essential*"). Hypertension that results from a pathologic process in one organ or organ system is labeled *secondary hypertension*. BP elevation also may be caused by medications, such as over-the-counter cold preparations, which often are vasoconstrictors. Acute elevations in BP may be seen with emotional or physical stress, including that associated with a visit to a physician's office ("white-coat" hypertension). Systolic pressure may be elevated for a period after

Table 46-1

95th Percentile for Blood Pressure (BP) Readings in Children and Adolescents

	Boys*		Girls*	
Age	**Systolic BP**	**Diastolic BP**	**Systolic BP**	**Diastolic BP**
1	98–106	55–59	101–107	57–60
2	101–110	59–63	102–109	61–65
3	104–113	63–67	104–110	65–68
4	106–115	66–71	105–111	67–71
5	108–116	69–74	107–113	69–73
6	109–117	72–76	108–114	71–75
7	110–119	74–78	110–116	73–76
8	111–120	75–80	112–118	74–78
9	113–121	76–81	114–120	75–79
10	114–123	77–82	116–122	77–80
11	116–125	78–83	118–124	78–81
12	119–127	79–83	120–126	79–82
13	121–130	79–84	121–128	80–84
14	124–132	80–85	123–130	81–85
15	127–135	81–86	124–131	82–86
16	129–138	83–87	125–132	83–86
17	132–140	85–89	126–132	83–86

Adapted from Gajewski KK: Cardiology. In Robertson J, Shilkofski N, editors: *The Harriet Lane handbook,* ed 17, Philadelphia, 2005, Mosby, pp 164–167.

*95th percentile BP for children from 5th to 95th percentile height.

vigorous exercise, an important fact to consider in sports physical examinations. Transient elevations in BP are also common with smoking, alcohol or caffeine consumption, and the use of illicit drugs such as cocaine and amphetamines. These personal habits should be addressed routinely at health supervision visits for older children and adolescents and should be specifically included in the history designed to identify causes of elevated BP. Obesity is an important cause of hypertension that defies classification into a particular category. Elevated BPs can normalize with weight loss. Table 46-2 lists specific causes of hypertension.

EVALUATION

How Should I Evaluate Blood Pressure?

Because hypertension is clinically silent, the routine measurement of BP in all children older than 3 years is strongly recommended to enable early detection and intervention. BP should also be measured in children younger than 3 years who have an underlying disorder such as renal, cardiac, or endocrine disease. If BP is elevated, *repeat the BP measurement yourself* to ensure the accuracy of the recorded value and that the correct size BP cuff was used. Next, repeat BP measurements over

Table 46-2

Causes of Hypertension in Children

PRIMARY HYPERTENSION

SECONDARY HYPERTENSION

Renal causes (80% of all secondary hypertension)
- Renal parenchymal diseases (80% of all renal causes)
  - Acute and chronic renal failure
  - Acute and chronic glomerulonephritis
  - Renal scarring/reflux nephropathy
  - Structural malformations: renal hypodysplasia, polycystic kidneys
  - Tumors (rare as a cause of hypertension)
- Renovascular hypertension
  - Fibromuscular dysplasia
  - Neurofibromatosis
  - Williams syndrome

Cardiac causes (10% of all secondary hypertension)
- Coarctation of the aorta
- Aortoarteritis (rare in North America)

Endocrine causes (2% of all secondary hypertension)
- Cushing disease
- Mineralocorticoid excess
  - Conn syndrome, licorice ingestion, glucocorticoid use
  - Congenital adrenal hyperplasia (certain subtypes)
  - Syndrome of apparent mineralocorticoid excess
  - Glucocorticoid-remediable aldosteronism
- Hypothyroidism and hyperthyroidism
- Pheochromocytoma (rare as a cause of hypertension in children)

Miscellaneous causes
- Central nervous system tumors or other space-occupying lesions
- Liddle syndrome
- Autonomic neuropathy (Guillain-Barré syndrome)
- Acute intermittent porphyria
- Stimulant use such as Ritalin

time to document persistence of the elevation. The time span over which repeat measurements are done depends on the degree of BP elevation and presence or absence of other symptoms and signs. Pay attention to any BP determination that is above the range expected, but use the term *hypertension* only if BP persistently exceeds the 95th percentile for age, gender, and height.

How Do I Measure Blood Pressure in Children?

Because BP measurements are easily affected by extraneous factors, strict adherence to proper technique is crucial. Any standard sphygmomanometer can be used with a cuff of the correct size and with proper technique. The bladder of the BP cuff should completely encircle the arm, preferably without overlap, and it should cover two-thirds of the arm from axilla to antecubital fossa. The arm should be raised to the level of the atrium during auscultation.

How Do I Start the Evaluation of Hypertension?

If the patient's BP is persistently above the 95th percentile for age, gender, and height, the history and physical examination should search for possible causes of hypertension, evidence of end-organ damage, and comorbid conditions such as dyslipidemia, diabetes, and obesity. The laboratory workup should be based on the data obtained by history and physical examination (Table 46-3).

Table 46-3

Diagnostic Evaluation for Secondary Hypertension

Causes of Hypertension	Clues from History, Physical Examination, and Screening Laboratory Tests	Imaging and Second-Line Tests
Renal parenchymal		
Renal failure/GN	H/o oliguria, hematuria, proteinuria, edema, elevated serum creatinine	Renal ultrasound C3 and C4 complement
Renal scarring	H/o UTIs/unexplained fevers	DMSA renal scan/VCUG
Anatomic (polycystic kidneys)	Palpable kidneys Family history of renal disease	Renal ultrasound or CT
Renovascular		
Renal artery thrombosis	H/o umbilical catheterization as neonate	Renal arteriogram (gold standard)
Fibromuscular dysplasia	Dysmorphic facies (Williams syndrome) Neurofibromas, axillary freckling, café au lait spots Abdominal bruits Hypokalemia Elevated plasma renin level	Alternative imaging (not standardized in children) Captopril renal scans MRA and Duplex ultrasound of renal arteries
Cardiac (coarctation)	Cardiac murmur BP elevated in arms	Chest radiograph and echocardiogram
Endocrine		
Cushing disease	H/o exogenous steroid use, weight gain, acne, moon facies, abdominal striae Hyperglycemia	Elevated urine and serum cortisol
Conn syndrome	H/o muscle weakness Hypokalemia	Increased serum aldosterone

(continued)

Table 46-3

Diagnostic Evaluation for Secondary Hypertension (Continued)

Causes of Hypertension	Clues from History, Physical Examination, and Screening Laboratory Tests	Imaging and Second-Line Tests
Congenital adrenal hyperplasia	H/o amenorrhea, hirsutism Ambiguous genitalia	Abnormal urinary corticosteroid profile
Pheochromocytoma	Episodes of flushing, palpitation, tremors, panic attacks, palpable abdominal mass	Urinary catecholamines
Thyroid abnormalities	Change in bowel habits, heat or cold intolerance, tremors Tachycardia, myxedema, exophthalmos	Thyroid function tests (T3, T4, and TSH)
GRA/AME	Family history of hypertension, hypokalemia Low plasma renin level	Abnormal urinary steroid profile: 18 oxo-cortisol (GRA), cortisol/cortisone metabolites (AME)

AME, Apparent mineralocorticoid excess; BP, blood pressure; CT, computed tomography; DMSA, dimercaptosuccinic acid; GN, glomerulonephritis; GRA, glucocorticoid-remediable aldosteronism; H/o, history of; MRA, magnetic resonance angiography; T3, triiodothyronine; T4, thyroxine; TSH, thyroid-stimulating hormone; UTI, urinary tract infection; VCUG, voiding cystourethrogram.

Further investigation will depend on factors unique to you and your patient:

- How significantly elevated is the BP? Is it life threatening?
- How difficult is it to control your patient's BP medically?
- What evidence do you have that your patient has a treatable cause of hypertension?
- How aggressive do you and the family want to be in the workup?
- What do you plan to do if you identify a specific cause for the hypertension?
- Do the benefits of investigation or treatment outweigh the risks?

What Findings Suggest Secondary Hypertension?

Secondary hypertension is generally thought to be likely if elevated or labile BP is identified in a young child who has no family history of hypertension but has findings of end-organ damage, such as left ventricular hypertrophy or hypertensive retinopathy. At least one recent study, however, does not support the validity of these factors. Therefore all children and adolescents with hypertension should be screened for secondary hypertension with the following:

- BP measurement in all four extremities to look for coarctation of the aorta (Chapter 56)
- Urinalysis and serum creatinine concentration to screen for renal disease (Chapter 65)
- Echocardiogram (ventricular hypertrophy reflects severity and duration of BP elevation)
- Additional tests may include
  - Renal ultrasound with Doppler study of the renal arteries
  - Serum cholesterol and triglyceride
  - Plasma renin level

What If a Cause Is Not Identified?

Often a detailed history, physical examination, and initial diagnostic tests may not identify a cause for hypertension. If the child has a mildly elevated BP, you may elect to skip additional workup and focus on management. If you decide on further testing, you should look for renal disorders, which are statistically the most common causes of secondary hypertension (Table 46-2). A comprehensive workup for endocrine or neurologic causes is not cost effective in the absence of signs and symptoms.

TREATMENT

How Do I Manage a Hypertensive Child?

The care of a child with hypertension is best undertaken by a multidisciplinary team that includes a pediatric nephrologist/hypertension specialist, a dietitian, and often a counselor/social worker. Management should be based on the specific underlying cause of hypertension. Dietary changes may include reduced dietary salt, saturated fats, and refined carbohydrates and increased dietary fiber, all of which will aid weight control. Cardiovascular conditioning promotes fitness and may reduce BP. There is no evidence to support exclusion of a child with hypertension from participation in sports. Frequent monitoring of BP is important. Consider home BP monitoring or ambulatory BP monitoring, especially if you suspect white-coat hypertension.

When Are Antihypertensive Medications Needed?

The decision to use medications to control hypertension should be made only after considering the risk-benefit ratio of the therapeutic agent and the potential short-term and long-term consequences of untreated hypertension in your particular patient. Table 46-4 lists antihypertensive drugs and the dosages commonly used in children.

Table 46-4

Commonly Used Oral Antihypertensive Drugs in Children

Drug	Dosing Guidelines (mg/kg/day)
Propranolol (beta-blocker)	1–8
Nifedipine XL (calcium channel blocker)	0.25–3
Enalapril (ACE inhibitor)	0.2–0.4
Hydralazine (vasodilator)	1–8

ACE, Angiotensin-converting enzyme.

KEY POINTS

- Hypertension is persistence of BP above the 95th percentile for age, gender, and height.
- A detailed history and physical examination are essential to look for the cause of hypertension, to evaluate for end-organ damage, and to identify comorbid conditions that might also increase later cardiovascular and cerebrovascular disease.
- Management of a child with hypertension should be undertaken by a multidisciplinary team

Case 46-1

A 14-year-old athletic boy comes to your office immediately after soccer practice for a sports physical examination. BP in the right arm while sitting is 144/80 mm Hg. His height and weight are both at the 95th percentile for his age and body mass index (BMI) is at the 90th percentile. His physical examin- ation shows a prominent abdominal fat pad but is otherwise unremarkable.

A. What would you do to determine if your patient has hypertension?
B. What further information do you need?
C. What tests, if any, would you obtain?

Case 46-2

A 17-year-old girl has had increasing fatigue for the past 3 months. She recently saw her pediatrician, who found elevated BP. Her past history is significant for recurrent episodes of acute pyelonephritis, with the last infection occurring 7 years ago. Today she has BP of 150/90 mm Hg. Her height and weight are at the 50th percentile for her age. The physical examination is otherwise unremarkable.

A. What are the possible causes of your patient's hypertension?
B. What would your next step(s) be in evaluating your patient?

Case Answers

46-1 A. *Learning objective:* **Identify elevated BP using appropriate resources.** This boy's systolic BP is > 95th percentile for age and height (Table 46-1). BMI is at the 90th percentile for age, which places him at risk for development of obesity. Repeat BP three times yourself at the current visit, using appropriate technique and cuff size. Let the patient sit quietly for 30 to 60 minutes if at all possible so that the effects of vigorous exercise might abate.

46-1 B. *Learning objective:* **Use the history and physical examination to distinguish between primary and secondary hypertension.** Ask questions to identify possible causes of elevated BP. In this case, vigorous exercise may explain the BP, but ask about cold medications, smoking, caffeine consumption, and illicit drug use. Further questions should address symptoms and signs of renal, cardiac, and endocrine diseases (Table 46-3). Review the medical record for previous BP readings and any evidence of disorders associated with elevated BP. Family history of hypertension, cardiovascular disease, diabetes, and obesity should be sought. Physical examination should include the ocular funduscopic assessment to look for end-organ damage. If BP remains elevated after the effects of exercise have resolved, and if the history and physical examination do not identify specific disorders, schedule repeat BP measurements over the next week and consider laboratory and imaging tests.

46-1 C. *Learning objective:* **Use laboratory and imaging studies to assess elevated BP. Recognize when observation alone is appropriate.** Look for secondary hypertension: four-extremity BP readings, urinalysis, serum creatinine, and echocardiography. Consider renal ultrasound with Doppler studies and lipid analysis, especially if there is a FHx of cardiac disease or diabetes. Plasma renin studies may also be helpful. Observation, with repeat BP measurements over a period of weeks to months is a reasonable approach, depending on the degree of BP elevation and the test results. Discuss weight management with physical activity and appropriate food intake.

46-2 A. *Learning objective:* **Identify diseases and disorders that cause hypertension.** Recurrent pyelonephritis, sustained elevation of BP, and symptoms point to the possibility that hypertension is caused by renal scarring and/or reflux nephropathy. She may also have reduced renal function.

46-2 B. *Learning objective:* **Select laboratory and imaging tests to evaluate hypertension in a symptomatic patient.** Obtain four-extremity BP readings, urinalysis, serum creatinine, and echocardiography.

Consider renal ultrasound and Doppler, plasma renin, and serum cholesterol. Consider VCUG and DMSA renal scan.

BIBLIOGRAPHY

National High Blood Pressure Education Program Working Group On High Blood Pressure In Children and Adolescents: The fourth report on the diagnosis, evaluation, and treatment of high blood pressure in children and adolescents, *Pediatrics* 114(2 Suppl 4th Report):555, 2004.

47

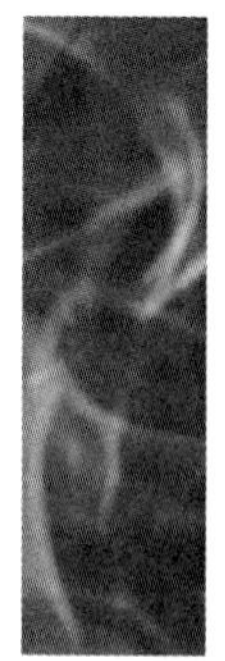

Lymphadenopathy and Lymphadenitis

WILLIAM V. RASZKA

ETIOLOGY

Do Lymphadenopathy and Lymphadenitis Differ?

Parents often express concern when a child has visible or palpable lymph nodes, especially if they are large, tender, or persistent. Small, nontender ("shotty") lymph nodes are commonly palpable in the anterior cervical chain of healthy, immunologically intact children and generally do not represent a concerning finding. ***Lymphadenopathy*** refers to nontender swelling of the lymph node, usually to greater than 10 mm in size. ***Lymphadenitis*** implies enlargement and inflammation of a lymph node, often accompanied by tenderness. In many patients, the distinction between the two may be blurred.

What Causes Lymphadenopathy?

Viral infection commonly causes bilateral enlarged, minimally tender, mobile anterior cervical nodes without other lymph node involvement. Systemic viral infections, such as Epstein-Barr virus, usually cause more diffuse involvement of lymphoid tissue that includes nodes in the anterior and posterior cervical chains, and axilla, plus the spleen. Malignancy such as leukemia may cause lymphadenopathy (see Chapter 63).

What Causes Lymphadenitis?

Acute bacterial lymphadenitis is usually caused by infections with *Staphylococcus aureus* or *Streptococcus pyogenes*. Chronic cervical lymphadenitis may be caused by anaerobic bacteria in patients with poor oral hygiene, *Bartonella henselae* (the agent of cat scratch disease), or nontuberculous mycobacteria. Children with Kawasaki disease may have cervical node enlargement, along with fever and other manifestations of the disease.

EVALUATION

What Findings Accompany Acute Lymphadenitis?

A child with acute staphylococcal or streptococcal lymphadenitis typically has had several days of fever and an increasingly tender, swollen lymph node by the time medical attention is sought. Examination typically demonstrates a unilateral, enlarged, tender, warm, and red, solitary node or tightly matted group of lymph nodes. Although treatment is often started empirically, aspiration of a suppurative node for Gram staining and culture confirms the microbiologic diagnosis and can identify methicillin-resistant *S. aureus,* which has become prevalent. Occasionally, Kawasaki disease with cervical lymphadenitis may cause diagnostic confusion, but these patients do not respond to antibiotic treatment, continue to have persistent fever, and develop additional findings, including eye, mucous membrane, and extremity changes. Children with cat scratch disease or nontuberculous mycobacterial infection may be difficult to distinguish from patients with staphylococcal or streptococcal infection early in the disease course.

How Do I Identify Cat Scratch Disease?

Most patients with cat scratch disease have had exposure to a young cat or kitten. The clinical course is more indolent and prolonged than with staphylococcal and streptococcal infections and usually does not have prominent fever. The enlarged node is often in the neck region but may also be in the axilla or the epitrochlear area. The lymph node may become quite enlarged and may suppurate, but it does not have the same degree of tenderness and overlying erythema as occurs with other more acute infections. Cat scratch disease may be diagnosed clinically, but serologic tests and histopathologic examination of the node may sometimes be required.

TREATMENT

How Should I Treat Lymphadenitis?

Viral lymphadenopathy or adenitis requires no treatment. For patients with suspected acute bacterial adenitis, treatment typically consists of antibiotics active against *S. aureus* and *S. pyogenes*. Occasionally, a large suppurative lymph node may need surgical incision and drainage, in addition to antibiotic treatment. Referral to a pediatric dentist may be needed when dental abscesses are identified. Antibiotic therapy is not necessary for cat scratch disease. Patients with nontuberculous mycobacterial lymphadenitis should have the node removed. The lymphadenopathy associated with Kawasaki disease disappears after treatment with intravenous immunoglobulin.

KEY POINTS

- Most acute cervical lymph node swelling results from viral infections and does not require treatment.
- *Streptococcus pyogenes* and *Staphylococcus aureus* are the most common causes of acute bacterial cervical lymphadenitis.
- Consider cat scratch disease or nontuberculous mycobacterial disease if the unilateral lymph node swelling is chronic.

Case 47-1

A 3-year-old boy is brought to the physician because of right-sided neck swelling for the past week. He has been afebrile, active, and has not appeared ill to his parents. The family owns several dogs and cats. His heart rate is 100 beats/min and respirations are 20 breaths/min. Physical examination demonstrates a 4.0-cm, mobile, soft, minimally tender lymph node without overlying erythema, in the right anterior cervical chain. Pharyngeal mucosa is pink and moist; tonsils are not inflamed or enlarged. The rest of the examination demonstrates no other adenopathy. He has scratches on his arms and legs.

A. What are the most common causes of unilateral lymphadenopathy in children?
B. What is the most likely diagnosis in this patient?
C. How would you go about making a diagnosis in this patient?

Case Answers

CERVICAL LYMPHADENITIS

47-1 A. *Learning objective:* **Discuss the common causes of acute cervical lymphadenitis, distinguishing between unilateral and bilateral adenopathy.** In a child, the causes of unilateral lymph node swelling include acute bacterial lymphadenitis *(Staphylococcus aureus* and *Streptococcus pyogenes),* cat scratch disease *(Bartonella henselae),* and nontuberculous mycobacteria. Patients with Kawasaki disease also may have unilateral cervical adenopathy. Viral infections most typically cause bilateral anterior cervical lymph node swelling. Systemic viral infections such as Epstein-Barr virus (EBV) commonly cause enlargement of posterior chain nodes, in addition to those in the anterior chain.

47-1 B. *Learning objective:* **Identify the history and physical findings typical for common causes of lymphadenitis.** Onset and duration of swelling, nature of symptoms, immunization status, and exposure history are important to elicit. In this patient, the unilateral lymph node enlargement with few local or systemic signs and exposure to cats or kittens should make cat scratch disease most likely. Acute bacterial lymphadenitis seems less likely given the absence of fever, overlying erythema, or tenderness of the involved node. Nontuberculous adenitis is common in children aged 1 to 4 years and must be part of the differential diagnosis. He might also have a viral infection, but the week-long unilateral swelling without other clinical findings argues against this diagnosis.

47-1 C. *Learning objective:* **Know the diagnostic tests used to detect common infectious agents.** Serologic testing is useful in the diagnosis of cat scratch disease. Occasionally, the diagnosis is confirmed histologically. If streptococcal pharyngitis is suspected, a rapid streptococcal antigen test or culture from swab of the pharynx can be used to confirm or exclude infection. In the case of a fluctuant, tender node in a febrile child, a Gram stain and culture of material aspirated from the node may be used to confirm staphylococcal or streptococcal infection.

BIBLIOGRAPHY

Leung AK, Robson WL: Childhood cervical lymphadenopathy, *J Pediatr Health Care* 18:3, 2004.

Peters TR, Edwards KM: Cervical lymphadenopathy and adenitis, *Pediatr Rev* 21:399, 2000.

48

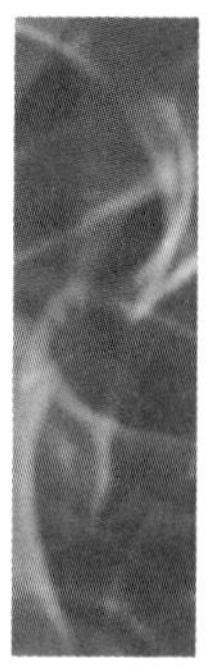

Murmurs

NORMAN B. BERMAN

ETIOLOGY

What Is an Innocent Heart Murmur?

Heart murmurs are present at some point in more than half of all healthy children. By far the most common murmur in a child is a Still's murmur, which is an innocent or functional murmur most commonly heard in toddlers and preschool-aged children. A Still's murmur does not suggest the presence of any underlying heart disease or abnormality and eventually goes away. Peripheral pulmonary stenosis is a common benign murmur most often first noted near 1 to 2 months of age. This murmur is simply caused by blood flow through a young infant's small pulmonary arteries. It requires no treatment. ***Innocent murmurs are always systolic. Diastolic murmurs are always pathologic.***

What Heart Diseases Cause Murmurs in Infants and Children?

A heart murmur in a child could also be caused by a congenital heart defect. The most common congenital heart defect is a ventricular septal defect (VSD), which is typically diagnosed in infancy but occasionally first noted in an older child. Atrial septal defect (ASD) is also common and typically is not noted until a few years of age. Coarctation of the aorta is a less common but important cause of a systolic murmur. Coarctation is difficult to detect when it is mild, but it typically progresses over the first few years to a more severe coarctation. Aortic stenosis and pulmonic stenosis are also seen in children and cause murmurs. In previous years rheumatic fever and rheumatic heart disease were common causes of murmurs. These are rarely seen now in the United States.

Does a Heart Murmur in a Newborn Mean Heart Disease?

A systolic heart murmur is common in a newborn infant because of the transition from fetal to newborn circulation (dropping pulmonary vascular resistance, closing patent ductus arteriosus, closing patent foramen ovale). These transitional murmurs should resolve within the first few days of life. A murmur first noted in the newborn period (< 1 month of age) is much more likely to be pathologic than is a murmur first noted in a school-aged child. Many congenital heart defects are not detected in the newborn nursery and will be diagnosed when a murmur is first heard in the first few weeks or months of life. Often, the presence of the murmur is the only sign of the heart defect. The other signs of heart defects (cyanosis, congestive heart failure) can be either very subtle, delayed, or absent, because milder heart defects should not cause symptoms.

EVALUATION

How Do I Know If a Murmur Is Innocent or Pathologic?

When assessing a murmur in a child without a history of heart disease, ask the following questions. If the answers are all positive, the murmur is likely to be innocent.

Is the child otherwise healthy? A murmur in a child with failure to thrive or other chronic illness causes concern and raises the question of a congenital heart defect.

Is the precordium quiet? Or is there a lift or heave suggesting cardiac enlargement? This is particularly important in infants younger than 1 month, in whom other signs of a heart defect can be absent.

Is the second heart sound physiologically split? The second heart sound should be split with inspiration and single with expiration. This is sometimes difficult to determine, but a fixed, widely split S2 is pathognomonic for an ASD and may be the only significant physical finding.

Are the pulses easily palpable? Femoral pulses must be checked during the well-child examination at all ages and particularly in a child with a murmur. Decreased femoral pulses suggest the presence of coarctation of the aorta.

Is the murmur in systole? Diastolic murmurs are always pathologic. A venous hum is an innocent sound heard continuously throughout systole and diastole. This is not a diastolic murmur.

Is the murmur grade I–II/VI? A loud murmur (grade III/VI or higher) is much more likely to be pathologic. Innocent murmurs are usually grade II/VI or less.

The other important criterion used to diagnose an innocent murmur is the quality of the murmur. A Still's murmur has a distinctive vibratory or musical quality and is heard best at the left lower sternal border in the supine position.

What Tests Help Evaluate a Murmur?

Electrocardiogram (ECG). An ECG can be very helpful, but a normal ECG does not prove that the murmur is innocent, nor does an abnormal ECG prove that it is pathologic. A preschool child with a new murmur may have a Still's murmur or an ASD. The ECG should be normal with a Still's murmur and should show right ventricular hypertrophy in > 95% of patients with ASD. However, many congenital heart defects, even when moderate to severe, can present with a normal ECG. The

ECG also has a significant false-positive rate, particularly for diagnosing ventricular hypertrophy.

Chest radiograph. A chest radiograph is *not* a useful diagnostic test for evaluation of a heart murmur. It is unlikely that any heart defect will be detected that was not already discovered by examination or ECG. The positive predictive value of a chest radiograph in this setting is only 40%.

Is an Echocardiogram Needed to Evaluate Heart Murmurs?

Echocardiography is *not necessary in the routine assessment of children with a murmur.* Physical examination by a skilled examiner is highly accurate at differentiating an innocent from a pathologic murmur. Echocardiography is useful to define cardiac anatomy when a pathologic murmur is suspected. The strategy of referring a child with a concerning murmur to a pediatric cardiologist has been shown to be more cost effective than the strategy of obtaining an echocardiogram.

TREATMENT

Does a Child with a Murmur Need Treatment?

An innocent murmur is "normal" and requires no treatment or special precautions. Many children are inappropriately restricted from sports participation because of an innocent murmur. Parents should be reassured that the murmur is a "normal" finding that does not imply heart disease. This should be described in clear and certain terms to avoid creating the impression that there may be something abnormal causing the murmur. Information about murmurs caused by congenital heart diseases is found in Chapter 56.

KEY POINTS

- Innocent murmurs are heard in more than 50% of healthy young children.
- Innocent murmurs are always systolic and most often grade I-II/VI.
- Diastolic murmurs are always pathologic.

Case 48-1

At a routine health-supervision visit, you detect a systolic heart murmur in a 5-year-old child. A heart murmur has not been noted previously. She is a healthy child, with no symptoms referable to the cardiovascular system

A. What is the most likely cause of her murmur?
B. What are some of the important things to look for when assessing a child with a murmur?
C. What evaluation is needed for a child with a murmur?

Case Answers

48-1 A. *Learning objective:* **Identify the common murmurs heard in children.** The Still's murmur is particularly common in preschool-aged children and is overall the most common murmur in childhood. An atrial septal defect or even coarctation of the aorta might have escaped notice, but physical examination findings will help you distinguish these pathologic causes from a Still's murmur.

48-1 B. *Learning objective:* **Use history and physical examination to determine whether a heart murmur represents a physiologic or pathologic process.** You should review the history to assess the child's overall state of health, including growth and development. Look at the vital signs: pulse rate, respiratory rate, and blood pressure. Focus your physical examination on precordial activity, the location, intensity, and timing of the murmur, the splitting of the second heart sound, and the presence of pulses. A Still's murmur is systolic, is vibratory and "musical" in quality, has low intensity (which may change with position), and is associated with a physiologically split second heart sound. A systolic murmur associated with a fixed-split second sound is characteristic of an atrial septal defect. If the systolic murmur is prominent in the back, consider coarctation of the aorta. Listen carefully to the diastolic phase of the cardiac cycle: A diastolic murmur is pathologic. If you hear a continuous sound, in both systole and diastole, you may be listening to a venous hum—another benign sound often associated with a Still's murmur. A 5-year-old child is less likely to have a patent ductus arteriosus that has gone unrecognized.

48-1 C. *Learning objective:* **Select appropriate diagnostic tests to evaluate a heart murmur, recognizing the patient who does not need further evaluation.** Evaluation depends on the nature of the murmur and other physical findings. A child who has no abnormalities in the areas listed above does not necessarily need further evaluation. A child who has any abnormalities in these areas will need a cardiac evaluation, including an electrocardiogram and referral to a cardiologist.

BIBLIOGRAPHY

Birkebaek NH et al: Chest roentgenogram in the evaluation of heart defects in asymptomatic infants and children with a cardiac murmur: reproducibility and accuracy, *Pediatrics* 103:E15, 1999.

Danford DA: Cost-effectiveness of echocardiography for evaluation of children with murmurs, *Echocardiography* 12:153, 1994.

49

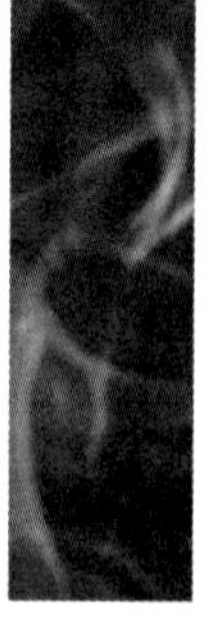

Rashes and Skin Lesions: Diagnostic Approach

DANIEL P. KROWCHUK

ETIOLOGY

Surveys indicate that 10% to 20% of visits by pediatric patients to outpatient facilities are associated with a dermatologic problem as the primary reason, a secondary concern, or an incidental finding. Dermatology is a visual discipline and with experience, most common problems and many subtle variations can be recognized. An atlas, text, consultant, or other resource can be used to aid in identification of uncommon problems. This chapter's approach to the diagnosis of skin problems in children is based on the morphology of the patient's lesions. The appropriate history and a careful description of what you see will overcome a major obstacle to diagnosis.

EVALUATION

Although dermatology relies heavily on recognition of skin lesions, an appropriate, problem-oriented history is the first step in diagnosis. Some questions that may be useful and their rationale are presented in the following sections.

What Should I Ask about the Present Illness?

When did the rash begin? Has it gotten better or worse? Has it occurred in the past?

Conditions such as atopic dermatitis are chronic and recurrent, whereas others such as viral exanthems are acute and self-limited.

Are there associated symptoms?

A generalized erythematous macular eruption associated with fever, nasal congestion, and cough suggests the presence of a viral exanthem. Fever, petechiae, and purpura in an ill-appearing child may indicate a serious bacterial infection such as meningococcemia. Atopic or contact dermatitis and scabies characteristically produce pruritus.

Is the patient using any medications?

The onset of wheals in a child receiving an oral antibiotic might represent urticaria as a manifestation of drug allergy. Lithium can worsen acne, and minocycline may cause hyperpigmentation. Topical therapies also may be relevant to the patient's problem; neomycin, diphenhydramine, and certain anesthetics may induce a contact dermatitis when applied topically.

Are there factors that worsen or precipitate the rash?

The malar rash of systemic lupus erythematosus is worsened by sun exposure. For many children with atopic dermatitis, reduced humidity during colder months is associated with an exacerbation of disease.

What treatment has been tried? What was its effect?

It is helpful to know which therapies have been used, if they were used appropriately, and if they were effective. Treatment for head lice infestation, for example, may fail if the product is used incorrectly.

What Does the Family History Add?

Is there a family history of skin disease or other health problems?

In children with atopic dermatitis, often there is a history of atopic disease, including atopic dermatitis, allergic rhinitis, or asthma. If a child is found to have multiple café au lait macules and a diagnosis of neurofibromatosis type 1 is being considered, determining if there are affected first-degree relatives is vital. Whether other family members are similarly affected is relevant when cutaneous infections or infestations are suspected. Impetigo, tinea capitis, scabies, and head lice often are transmitted within families.

Why Is the Social History Important?

Does the patient work after school?

Occupational exposure to greases or oils (e.g., in a fast-food restaurant or car repair shop) may worsen acne.

Has the patient ever been involved in a sexual relationship?

A confidential sexual history may be important. Secondary syphilis and disseminated gonococcal infection, for example, have cutaneous manifestations. Molluscum contagiosum, infestation with pubic lice, and scabies may be transmitted through sexual contact.

How Do I Describe What I See?

Recognizing and describing skin lesions accurately are essential to diagnosis. The first step is to identify the primary lesion, defined as the earliest lesion and the one most characteristic of the disease. Next, it is important to note the distribution, arrangement, and color of primary lesions, along with any secondary change, such as crusting or scaling.

What Are the Types of Primary Lesions?

Flat lesions include macules and patches. A *macule* is a small, circumscribed area of color change without elevation or depression, such as a café au lait macule. A *patch* is a large macule, although specific size criteria are lacking.

Elevated lesions may be solid or fluid filled. *Solid lesions* include *papules* (< 0.5 cm in diameter), *nodules* (≥ 0.5 cm in diameter), *wheals* (a pink, rounded or flat-topped elevation because of edema in the skin), and *plaques* (plateau-shaped structures often formed by the coalescence of papules). Elevated *fluid-filled lesions* may be *vesicles* (< 0.5 cm in diameter and filled with serous fluid), *bullae* (≥ 0.5 cm in diameter and filled with serous fluid), *pustules* (< 0.5 cm in diameter and filled with purulent material), and *cysts* (≥ 0.5 cm in diameter that represent sacs containing fluid or semisolid material).

Depressed lesions include *erosions,* which reflect superficial loss of epidermis with a moist base, or *ulcers,* deeper lesions extending into the dermis or below.

Why Is the Distribution of Lesions Important?

Certain disorders have unique patterns of distribution that can be useful for diagnosis. For example, seborrheic dermatitis commonly involves the scalp, eyebrows, and nasolabial folds. Psoriasis also affects the scalp, but lesions are often seen in areas that are traumatized, such as the elbows and knees. Acne is limited to the face, back, and chest, sites of the highest concentrations of pilosebaceous follicles.

How May Lesions Be Arranged?

- Linear array (e.g., vesicles in contact dermatitis resulting from poison ivy)
- Grouped or clustered (e.g., vesicles in herpes simplex virus infection)
- Dermatomal (e.g., vesicles in herpes zoster)
- Annulus or ring (e.g., papules in granuloma annulare or a patch in erythema migrans)

How Do I Describe the Color of Skin Lesions?

Although the color of a lesion may be obvious, terms that may be helpful include

- Skin colored
- Erythematous (pink or red)
- Hyperpigmented (tan, brown, or black)
- Hypopigmented (pigment is decreased but not entirely absent)
- Depigmented (all pigment is absent, as occurs in vitiligo)
- Violaceous (purplish)

When erythematous lesions are observed, it is important to note if they blanch. If red blood cells are within vessels (e.g., as occurs in urticaria), compression of the skin forces the cells into deeper vessels and blanching occurs. However, if the cells are outside vessels, as occurs in forms of vasculitis, blanching will not occur; nonblanching lesions are termed *petechiae*, *purpura*, or *ecchymoses*.

What Are Secondary Changes?

Secondary changes are alterations in the skin that may accompany primary lesions and may be valuable in differential diagnosis.

- *Crusting* represents dried fluid. It is commonly seen following the rupture of vesicles or bullae, as occurs with the "honey-colored" crust of impetigo.
- *Scaling* represents epidermal fragments that are characteristic of several disorders, including fungal infections (e.g., tinea corporis) and psoriasis.
- *Atrophy* is an area of surface depression because of absence of the dermis or subcutaneous fat. Atrophic skin often appears thin and wrinkled.
- *Lichenification* is a thickening of the skin that results from chronic rubbing or scratching (e.g., as occurs in atopic dermatitis); as a result, normal creases appear more prominent.

How Do I Put It All Together?

Once you have identified the primary lesions, along with the distribution, arrangement, color, and secondary changes, your observations can be formulated into one or two sentences. For example, "Erythematous, scaling papules, and plaques are located on the extensor surfaces of the extremities. There is scaling of the scalp and pitting of the nails." This description assists in differential diagnosis: By identifying scaling papules and plaques, you have placed the patient's condition into the category of papulosquamous (elevated and scaling) diseases and have eliminated countless other disorders from consideration. In children, the most common papulosquamous disorders are chronic atopic or contact dermatitis, tinea corporis, and pityriasis rosea; less common causes are psoriasis, secondary syphilis, lichen planus, dermatomyositis, and lupus erythematosus. Given the location of the lesions on extensor surfaces and involvement of the scalp and nails, psoriasis becomes a primary consideration.

Tables 49-1 and 49-2 are provided to assist in differential diagnosis based on the morphology of lesions and list the disorders you are most likely to encounter, plus a few less common ones. When the physical findings are unclear, you will need a textbook or atlas of dermatology, a consultant, or another resource.

TREATMENT

Treatment can be planned only after you have determined the diagnosis. Details of treatment for specific rashes are outlined in Chapter 57.

Table 49-1

Differential Diagnosis of Rashes in Neonates

Elevated Lesions

Papules

Common

Erythematous
- Erythema toxicum
- Miliaria rubra
- Acne
- Candidiasis
- Scabies

White
- Milia

Yellow
- Sebaceous gland hypertrophy

Skin colored
- Epidermal nevus
- Skin tags

Uncommon

Yellow
- Juvenile xanthogranuloma
- Mastocytosis

Nodules

Common

Erythematous
- Hemangioma

Uncommon

Skin colored
- Condylomata acuminata
- Dermoid cyst

Yellow
- Mastocytosis

Plaques

Common

Skin colored or yellow
- Nevus sebaceus

Skin colored
- Epidermal nevus

Vesicles or Bullae

Common

Erythema toxicum
Miliaria crystallina
Sucking blisters
Bullous impetigo
Herpes simplex virus infection

Uncommon

Incontinentia pigmenti
Aplasia cutis congenita
Varicella
Epidermolysis bullosa
Bullous ichthyosiform erythroderma

Pustules

Common

Erythema toxicum
Transient neonatal pustular melanosis
Miliaria pustulosa
Herpes simplex virus infection
Folliculitis
Acne
Candidiasis
Scabies

Uncommon

Acropustulosis of infancy

(continued)

Table 49-1

Differential Diagnosis of Rashes in Neonates (Continued)

Flat Lesions	Depressed Lesions
Macules	***Erosions***
Common	**Common**
Hypopigmented	Bullous impetigo
Prehemangioma	Neonatal herpes simplex virus infection
Postinflammatory hypopigmentation	Staphylococcal scalded skin syndrome
Hyperpigmented	**Uncommon**
Transient neonatal pustular melanosis	Aplasia cutis congenita
Café au lait macule	Acrodermatitis enteropathica
Postinflammatory hyperpigmentation	Epidermolysis bullosa
Congenital melanocytic nevus	Bullous ichthyosiform erythroderma
Uncommon	
Hypopigmented	
Ash leaf macule	
Patches	
Common	
Erythematous	
Salmon patch (nevus simplex)	
Hemangioma (early)	
Port wine stain	
Atopic dermatitis	
Seborrheic dermatitis	
Diaper dermatitis (irritant or seborrheic)	
Hyperpigmented	
Mongolian spot	
Lentigo	
Uncommon	
Erythematous	
Acrodermatitis enteropathica	
Hyperpigmented	
Linear and whorled hypermelanosis	
Hypopigmented	
Hypomelanosis of Ito	
Nevus depigmentosus	

Table 49-2

Differential Diagnosis of Rashes in Older Infants, Children, and Adolescents

Elevated Lesions

Papules without Scaling

Common

Erythematous
Viral exanthems
Scarlet fever
Insect bites
Scabies
Urticaria
Papular urticaria
Acne
  Early lesions of guttate psoriasis
  Erythema multiforme
Skin colored
  Keratosis pilaris
  Molluscum contagiosum
  Flat warts
Hyperpigmented
  Nevus (intradermal)

Uncommon

Yellow
  Mastocytosis

Plaques without scaling

Common

Skin colored
  Nevus sebaceous
  Epidermal nevus
Hyperpigmented
  Congenital melanocytic nevus

Papules or Plaques with Scaling (papulosquamous diseases)

Common

Tinea corporis
Pityriasis rosea
Chronic atopic or contact dermatitis
Psoriasis

Uncommon

Dermatomyositis
Lupus erythematosus
Lichen planus

Nodules

Common

Erythematous
Pyogenic granuloma
Skin colored
Wart
Callus
Corn
Epidermal cyst
Granuloma annulare

Uncommon

Erythematous
  Angiofibroma
Skin colored
  Neurofibroma
Yellow
  Mastocytosis

Vesicles or Bullae

Common

Contact dermatitis
Bullous impetigo
Varicella
Herpes simplex virus infection
Hand, foot, and mouth disease
Erythema multiforme

Uncommon

Polymorphous light eruption
Linear IgA dermatosis

Pustules

Common

Folliculitis
Scabies
Acne
Perioral dermatitis

Uncommon

Associated with systemic bacterial infection (e.g., disseminated gonococcal infection)

(continued)

Table 49-2

Differential Diagnosis of Rashes in Older Infants, Children, and Adolescents (Continued)

Flat Lesions	
Macules	***Patches***
Common	**Common**
Erythematous	Erythematous
Viral exanthems	Salmon patch (nevus simplex)
Drug eruptions	Port wine stain
Hypopigmented	Atopic dermatitis
Pityriasis alba (postinflammatory hypopigmentation)	
Tinea versicolor	Hyperpigmented
Vitiligo	Mongolian spot
Halo nevus	Becker's nevus
Hyperpigmented	Lentigo
Freckles	**Uncommon**
Postinflammatory hyperpigmentation	Erythematous
Tinea versicolor	Toxic shock syndrome (diffuse macular erythema)
Café au lait macules	Hyperpigmented
Melanocytic nevus	Linear and whorled hyperpigmelanosis
Uncommon	Incontinentia pigmenti
Hypopigmented	
Lichen sclerosus et atrophicus	
Scleroderma	
Ash leaf macule	
Piebaldism	

Depressed Lesions
Erosions
Common
Bullous impetigo
Herpes simplex virus infection
Staphylococcal scalded skin syndrome
Uncommon
Epidermolysis bullosa

(continued)

Table 49-2

Differential Diagnosis of Rashes in Older Infants, Children, and Adolescents (Continued)

Hair Loss	
Congenital	***Acquired***
Localized	**Localized**
Nevus sebaceous	Friction alopecia
Epidermal nevus	Tinea capitis
Aplasia cutis congenita	Traction alopecia
Diffuse	Trichotillomania
Hair shaft abnormalities	Alopecia areata
Hypothyroidism	Psoriasis
	Secondary syphilis
	Scleroderma
	Diffuse
	Telogen effluvium
	Chemotherapy
	Hypothyroidism
	Acrodermatitis enteropathica

KEY POINTS

- Diagnosing rashes and skin lesions depends on your ability to describe their morphology, color, arrangement, and location.
- Time course, progression, and associated symptoms give important clues about the cause.
- Treatment can be successful only if the diagnosis is correct.

Case 49-1

You are evaluating a previously healthy 8-year-old girl with a 2-day history of a pruritic rash. On physical examination you observe erythematous papules and vesicles located on the arms. Some lesions are distributed in a linear array.

A. What are the most common causes of a vesicular eruption in a child?
B. What is the most likely cause of the child's rash?

Case 49-2

A 6-year-old boy has had a spot on his right arm for 2 weeks. It is mildly pruritic and is gradually enlarging. Physical examination is remarkable only for a 3-cm erythematous circular lesion on the right arm. The border of the lesion is elevated and scaling; there is some central clearing.

A. What is the differential diagnosis of scaling elevated lesions?
B. What is the likely diagnosis?

Case 49-3

A 6-year-old girl has a 2-day history of sore throat, headache, and fever. Today she developed a rash on her face and trunk. Physical examination reveals an alert girl with a temperature of 38.5° C who appears mildly ill. Her pharynx is erythematous, there is exudate on the tonsils, and she has enlarged, tender anterior cervical lymph nodes. Fine erythematous papules are located on the face, trunk, and extremities. The rash is concentrated in the axillary folds.

A. What conditions could be responsible for this girl's illness?
B. What is the most likely diagnosis?

Case 49-4

A 1-day-old healthy neonate develops erythematous macules concentrated on the trunk. In the center of several macules is an erythematous papule or vesicle.

A. What are the common causes of a vesicular eruption in newborns?
B. What is the most likely cause in this infant?

Case 49-5

A 5-year-old boy has had a patch of hair loss of 3 weeks' duration. He has been well and there is no history of trauma to the scalp or hair. On physical examination you observe a 3- to 4-cm area of alopecia within which are scale and broken hairs.

A. What are the common causes of acquired hair loss in children?
B. What is the likely cause of this child's alopecia?

Case Answers

49-1 A. *Learning objective:* **Discuss the differential diagnosis of vesicular eruptions.** Disorders that are most likely to cause vesicles in children include contact dermatitis; varicella; herpes simplex virus infection; hand, foot, and mouth disease; and erythema multiforme (Table 49-2).

49-1 B. *Learning objective:* **Recognize the importance of the arrangement and distribution of lesions in the differential diagnosis.** The child presented in the case has a pruritic eruption that is limited to the arms. It is composed of erythematous papules and vesicles, some of which have a linear arrangement. These findings are most consistent with a diagnosis of contact dermatitis caused by poison oak, ivy, or sumac. The keys to the diagnosis are the location of the rash on exposed body surfaces (sites not protected by clothing), the presence of vesicles (suggesting an acute dermatitis caused by a potent antigen), and the linear arrangement of some lesions (the result of brushing against and damaging the plant). Other disorders that commonly produce vesicles are not characterized by a linear arrangement of lesions nor would the distribution of lesions be limited to the arms.

49-2 A. *Learning objective:* **Discuss the differential diagnosis of papulosquamous disorders.** Papulosquamous disorders are characterized by elevated lesions (e.g., papules or plaques) that have associated scale. The most common of these in children are tinea corporis, pityriasis rosea, chronic dermatitis (e.g., atopic or contact), and psoriasis (Table 49-2).

49-2 B. *Learning objective:* **Recognize tinea corporis.** The child described in the case has a single erythematous circular lesion (e.g., an annulus). The border is elevated, erythematous, and scaling. These findings suggest the diagnosis of tinea corporis. Unlike other papulosquamous disorders that occur commonly in children, tinea corporis generally produces one or a few lesions and is not generalized or widespread in its distribution. In addition, individual lesions often exhibit central clearing.

49-3 A. *Learning objective:* **List disorders that cause an acute illness characterized by fever and rash.** The girl presented in the case has a febrile illness characterized by pharyngitis, fever, headache, and a generalized rash that is concentrated in flexural areas. The rash is composed of fine erythematous papules. The most likely causes of these findings, particularly in a child who is mildly ill-appearing, are a viral respiratory infection (many viruses cause a rash along with other symptoms, although the rash often is composed of pink macules) or an infection with a bacterial agent that produces a toxin that affects the skin (as might occur with scarlet fever, staphylococcal scarlet fever, or toxic shock syndrome).

49-3 B. *Learning objective:* **Identify scarlet fever.** The most likely explanation for the girl's symptoms is scarlet fever. Pharyngeal infection with *Streptococcus pyogenes* causes pharyngitis with fever, headache, and abdominal pain. Some strains of the organism elaborate an erythrogenic toxin that causes a rash composed of fine erythematous papules that are concentrated in skin flexures (e.g., the axillae and groin). On palpation, the rash feels rough, giving it a so-called sandpaper texture. There also may be erythema or petechiae located in the antecubital creases (Pastia's lines).

49-4 A. *Learning objective:* **Discuss the differential diagnosis of vesicular eruptions in newborns.** Common causes of vesicles in newborns are erythema toxicum, miliaria crystallina, and herpes simplex virus infection. Sucking blisters and bullous impetigo result in bullae, fluid-filled lesions that are larger than vesicles.

49-4 B. *Learning objective:* **Recognize erythema toxicum.** In a healthy newborn, the most likely explanation for this rash is erythema toxicum, a benign and self-limited condition of unknown cause. Erythema toxicum can be distinguished from other disorders that produce vesicles clinically. For example, miliaria crystallina produces very fragile vesicles without surrounding erythema. The lesions of herpes simplex virus infection typically are clustered (not individual) vesicles on an erythematous base.

49-5 A. *Learning objective:* **List the causes of acquired localized hair loss in children.** The child presented in the case has developed a patch of hair loss. Common causes of this acquired localized alopecia include tinea capitis (a fungal infection), traction alopecia (loss of hair often resulting from tight braiding), friction alopecia (caused by rubbing the head on another surface [seen primarily in very young infants]), trichotillomania (pulling or twisting the hair), and alopecia areata (an autoimmune condition).

49-5 B. *Learning objective:* **Identify tinea capitis.** The cause of this child's alopecia is tinea capitis, a fungal infection of the scalp. This is the most common cause of acquired localized alopecia and, for reasons unknown, is a particular problem for African-American children. The fungus invades and reproduces within hair shafts. As a result, the hairs are weakened and break at the scalp, leaving remnants of infected hairs within the follicles ("black dot" hairs). As is typical for fungal infections on the skin, there often is associated scaling. Other causes of localized alopecia would not result in scaling or "black dot" hairs.

BIBLIOGRAPHY

Textbooks

Cohen BA: *Pediatric dermatology,* ed 3, Philadelphia, 2005, Elsevier Mosby.

Paller AS, Mancini AJ: *Hurwitz clinical pediatric dermatology,* ed 3, Philadelphia, 2005, Saunders Elsevier.

Weston WL, Lane AT, Morelli JG: *Color textbook of pediatric dermatology*, ed 4, St Louis, 2002, Mosby.

Electronic Textbooks

Habif TP: *Clinical dermatology*, ed 4, Philadelphia, 2004, Mosby. Available via MD Consult.

Electronic Atlases

http://dermatlas.org Dermatlas. It contains more than 7900 images of pediatric dermatologic disorders. Each image is accompanied by a brief case history. One may search by diagnosis, disease category, or body site involved. There is a quiz to test your knowledge. This is a useful resource.

http://tray.dermatology.uiowa.edu/DermImag.htm. An atlas of general dermatology maintained by the University of Iowa Department of Dermatology. Images of conditions are listed alphabetically.

www.dermis.net. A dermatologic online image atlas maintained by the University of Erlangen, Germany. It contains more than 4500 images of adult and pediatric dermatologic disorders. Conditions may be searched alphabetically or by body area. There is a quiz to test your knowledge.

Section 4

Patients Presenting with Abnormal Laboratory Test Results

50

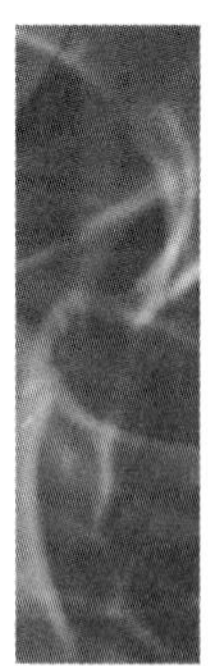

Anemia

ROGER BERKOW

What Is Anemia?

Anemia is defined by a hemoglobin and/or hematocrit more than two standard deviations below the mean for age. Anemia is also classified according to red blood cell (RBC) size, as measured by mean corpuscular volume (MCV). Other RBC indices that may also be abnormal in anemia include mean corpuscular hemoglobin (MCH), a measure of the amount of hemoglobin in each RBC, and mean corpuscular hemoglobin concentration (MCHC), a measure of the concentration of hemoglobin within each RBC. This chapter provides a general discussion of anemia. Chapter 63 discusses specific anemias.

How Do Hemoglobin and Red Blood Cell Size Change with Age?

The newborn's hemoglobin varies with gestational age, timing of umbilical cord clamping, and clinical condition at the time of birth. Hemoglobin concentration is high at birth for a healthy term infant. It then decreases during the first 2 months, after which it slowly increases until adult levels are achieved during adolescence. RBCs also change in size with advancing age: At birth, RBCs are large, with MCV of 110 to 120 fl. MCV decreases over the first 6 months of life to 70 to 79 fl and then slowly rises to adult levels (80-95 fl) during late childhood and adolescence. Table 50-1 gives the age-associated ranges for expected hemoglobin and MCV. Values for MCH and MCHC are available in standard references.

What Causes Anemia?

Anemia can be caused by RBC loss, destruction, or lack of production. The causes of anemia vary, based on the age of the child. Causes of anemia are discussed in the Evaluation section and listed in Tables 50-2 and 50-3.

Table 50-1

Age-Related Values for Hemoglobin and Mean Corpuscular Volume

Age	Hemoglobin (g/dl) ($\pm$ 2 SD)	Mean Corpuscular Volume (fl) ($\pm$ 2 SD)
Newborn (full term)	16.5 (3)	108 (10)
1 mo	13.9 (3.2)	101 (10)
2 mo	11.2 (1.8)	95 (11)
6–24 mo	12.0 (1.5)	78 (8)
2–6 yr	12.5 (1.0)	81 (6)
6–12 yr	13.5 (2.0)	86 (9)
12–18 yr male	14.5 (1.5)	88 (10)
12–18 yr female	14.0 (2.0)	90 (12)

Adapted from Brunetti M, Cohen J: Hematology. In Robertson J, Shilkofski N: *The Harriet Lane Handbook,* ed 17, Philadelphia, 2005, Mosby, p 337.

Table 50-2

Anemia with Decreased Reticulocyte Index (RI < 2)

Decreased MCV	Normal MCV	Increased MCV
Iron deficiency	Chronic infection	Vitamin B_{12} deficiency
Thalassemia	Recent blood loss	Folate deficiency
Lead ($>$ 50 μg/dl)	Marrow failure	Metabolic disease
Copper deficiency	Malignancy	Chemotherapy
Chronic infection	Aplastic anemia	EtOH
	Transient erythroblastopenia	Hypothyroidism
	Diamond-Blackfan syndrome	Myelodysplasia
	Renal failure (chronic)	Drugs

EtOH, Ethanol; MCV, mean corpuscular volume.

EVALUATION

How Do I Assess Anemia in a Young Infant?

In the first 6 months after birth, consider the length of gestation because most neonatal iron stores are deposited in the last trimester of pregnancy. A premature infant has high risk for early development of anemia. Review the newborn and maternal records to identify possible incompatibility of the ABO or Rh blood groups that might have caused hemolysis. Neonatal jaundice may also suggest underlying hemolytic disease. A newborn who had a complex postnatal course and spent time in the neonatal intensive care unit may be anemic because of the large amounts of blood drawn. If the patient is a twin, in utero twin-to-twin transfusion may have caused anemia. Perinatal problems, such as placental abruption or placenta previa, lead to excessive blood loss from

Table 50-3

Anemia with Increased Reticulocyte Index (RI > 3)

RBC Membrane Causes			
Extrinsic	**Intrinsic**	**Hemoglobin**	**Cytoplasm**
Autoimmune	Hereditary spherocytosis	Sickle cell disease	G-6PD deficiency
Isoimmune	Hereditary elliptocytosis	Unstable hemoglobins	Pyruvate kinase deficiency
Infection		Thalassemia	Other glycolytic enzyme deficiency
Microangiopathic HUS/TTP DIC Heart valves			
Vitamin E deficiency			
Congenital dyserythropoietic anemia			

DIC, Disseminated intravascular coagulation; G-6PD, glucose-6-phosphate dehydrogenase; HUS, hemolytic uremic syndrome; RBC, red blood cell; TTP, thrombotic thrombocytopenic purpura.

the mother and the newborn. Did the mother take prenatal vitamins or experience any infections during the pregnancy?

How Do I Evaluate an Anemic Older Infant or Child?

A careful history should search for fever, bruising, or bleeding that might indicate a malignancy, such as leukemia or neuroblastoma, or marrow dysfunction, such as aplastic anemia. Lymphadenopathy or hepatosplenomegaly might suggest an infiltrative process or perhaps certain types of storage disease. Recent infections such as Epstein-Barr virus or parvovirus could have suppressed RBC production. Has the child experienced episodes of pallor, unexplained episodes of pain (particularly in the hands and feet, as is seen in young children with sickling disorders), or episodic jaundice (which would support a hemolytic cause for anemia)? Has there been blood loss in the stool, urine, or sputum that might indicate particular areas to evaluate?

How Do I Detect Nutritional Anemia?

A careful assessment of the child's diet is important in the evaluation of anemia. Iron deficiency is the most common nutritional anemia, so ask about sources of iron in the current diet (see Chapter 63). Also inquire about feeding during infancy: When was the child switched from breastfeeding or infant formula to cow milk, which is both a poor source of iron and a cause of gastrointestinal bleeding in infants younger than 12 months? Does the child drink goat milk, which is deficient in folic acid? Does the child take a strictly vegetarian diet, which is deficient in vitamin B_{12}? Does the child currently take vitamins with or without iron? Does the child eat non-food items (pica), which suggests iron deficiency and increases the risk of lead intoxication?

Do Medications Ever Cause Anemia?

Inquire about *all* medications, whether prescribed, over-the-counter, alternative, or herbal. Cephalosporins, penicillins, and others can cause the development of antibodies to RBCs. Sulfonamides may suppress red and white blood cell production as well as induce hemolysis in children with glucose-6-phosphate dehydrogenase (G-6PD) deficiency. Anticonvulsants may be associated with a macrocytic anemia.

How Does Family History Help in the Evaluation?

A family history of anemia, jaundice, splenectomy for reasons other than trauma, or cholecystectomy in young relatives could indicate hemolysis or hemoglobinopathy. If the ethnic background of the family members is African, Asian, or Mediterranean, the child's anemia might be related to sickle cell diseases, G-6PD deficiency, thalassemia, or hemoglobin E.

How Do Vital Signs Change in Anemia?

Tachycardia reflects the body's effort to compensate for anemia by increasing the delivery of oxygen to the tissues through increased circulation. Fever may indicate infection, which may be the primary cause of anemia or a complication of another anemia-causing process. Blood pressure may be elevated in chronic renal disease, which often has associated anemia from decreased erythropoietin. Acute renal insufficiency may present with pallor and elevated blood pressure, especially when microangiopathic hemolytic anemia and thrombocytopenia occur in hemolytic uremic syndrome.

What Is Found on Physical Examination?

Examination of the conjunctivae and nail beds will confirm presence of pallor. *Pallor* means a pale complexion of the skin. Anemia is the most common medical cause of pallor, but it can also result from a lack of exposure to sunlight, a familial tendency toward pale skin color, vasoconstriction (e.g., shock), or exposure to cold. Look for jaundice, bruising, petechiae, lymphadenopathy, hepatosplenomegaly, abdominal masses, or hemangiomas. A cardiac flow murmur generally accompanies tachycardia. Presence of congenital abnormalities can give clues to many disorders that can be associated with anemia. Fanconi's anemia, for example, is often associated with abnormalities of the radial side of the hand, short stature, mental retardation, and bone marrow failure. Rectal examination will identify gross or occult blood in the stool.

How Do I Interpret the Complete Blood Count ?

If hematocrit and hemoglobin identify anemia, the RBC count, MCV, MCH, MCHC, and platelet count will provide more information. The white blood cell count, the differential leukocyte count, and a review of all cell lines on the peripheral blood smear will help determine if the process causing the anemia affects only the RBCs or other marrow elements as well.

What Is the Value of the Reticulocyte Count?

The reticulocyte count is essential in the evaluation of anemia. It gives information about the ability of the bone marrow to produce the RBCs needed to correct anemia. *Increased reticulocyte count is the expected physiologic response to anemia.* A healthy bone marrow provided with adequate substrates (iron, vitamin B_{12}, folic acid, globin chains) can rapidly increase RBC production in response to anemia by releasing reticulocytes into the peripheral circulation. An *absent or inadequate reticulocyte response* to anemia indicates (1) a lack of substrates for the production of RBCs, (2) a problem intrinsic to the bone marrow, or (3) inadequate erythropoietin. A *markedly elevated reticulocyte count* demonstrates that substrates are available but suggests that anemia results from destruction of RBCs. It is important to correct the reticulocyte count for the degree of anemia. This "corrected reticulocyte count" is also called the *reticulocyte index* (RI):

- *RI > 3* (elevated) means that RBCs are being produced by the marrow in response to anemia, most often as a result of hemolysis.
- *RI = 2–3* is the expected response to a nonhemolytic anemia.
- *RI < 2* (decreased) indicates an inadequate marrow response for the degree of anemia, usually seen with inadequate substrate levels or decreased production of erythropoietin.

Anemias associated with decreased RI are listed in Table 50-2. Anemias with elevated RI are listed in Table 50-3. Specific anemias are discussed in Chapter 63.

How Does Red Blood Cell Size Vary in Different Anemias?

RBC size (MCV) is especially important in evaluation of anemia with a decreased reticulocyte count (see Table 50-2). Small RBCs, with MCV below the expected range for age, result when substrates or cofactors are inadequate. Large RBCs, with increased MCV for age, result from a decrease in the substrates needed for division of RBC precursors. Anemia with normal MCV occurs with recent blood loss or with inadequate erythropoietin stimulation of marrow RBC production in chronic disease. Disorders associated with hemolysis will most often have normal MCV but will have an elevated RI. These disorders are covered in Chapter 63.

What Additional Tests Should I Order?

No additional tests may be needed if simple dietary iron deficiency is suspected in a patient with anemia and low MCV. A therapeutic trial with iron will confirm the diagnosis. However, if the diagnosis is less evident, it is appropriate to measure serum iron, total iron binding capacity, serum ferritin level, and a blood lead level. Use of hemoglobin electrophoresis or globin chain synthesis studies will detect thalassemia.

When the MCV is normal, a bone marrow aspirate can aid the diagnosis of marrow failure syndromes or malignancy. When the MCV is elevated, vitamin B_{12} and folic acid levels, thyroid function tests, and appropriate metabolic studies will help to identify the cause of macrocytic anemia. In the presence of an elevated RI, a review of the peripheral blood smear may lead to the identification of an abnormal appearance to the RBCs, such as the changes seen in hereditary spherocytosis, sickling disorders, or microangiopathic hemolytic anemias. Coombs' test (direct and indirect) will identify antibody-mediated hemolysis, and analysis of specific activity of RBC enzymes will identify the most common causes of hemolytic anemia.

TREATMENT

How Is Anemia Treated?

Treatment depends on the cause. Details for specific types of anemia are provided in Chapter 63. In general, because iron deficiency is the most common cause of anemia in the otherwise healthy child, a trial of iron therapy is appropriate when history, physical examination, and laboratory findings are consistent with such a diagnosis. Rapid increase in the reticulocyte count within days of the start of iron therapy supports the diagnosis of iron deficiency. Hemoglobin rises more slowly, and replenishment of the iron stores even more slowly, so a total of 3 to 4 months of therapeutic iron is needed to treat iron-deficiency anemia. Failure of reticulocytosis indicates the need for further evaluation. Other causes of anemia may require other nutritional treatments, such as folic acid and vitamin B_{12}. Malignancy-associated anemia or the anemia of renal disease will be treated along with the underlying disease.

KEY POINTS

- Anemia can be caused by the decreased production, increased destruction, or loss of RBCs from the circulation.
- The history, physical examination, and selected laboratory tests help make the diagnosis of anemia straightforward.

Case 50-1

A 15-month-old male comes for a routine health supervision visit. He was last seen at 9 months of age and has had no major problems since that time. He is walking without difficulty and says about 10 words. He puts everything in his mouth. The mother indicates that he has been less active than usual over the last several weeks and that a friend thought that the boy looked pale last week. He is a good eater and takes five 8-ounce bottles of whole milk daily.

He was switched to cow's milk at age 9 months. He eats some baby food. He has no significant past illnesses, and the family history is negative for any major illness. There have been no changes at home. Physical examination reveals heart rate of 150 beats/min, temperature of 37° C, weight at the 75th percentile, and height at the 50th percentile. He is pale but has no evidence of bruising, hepatomegaly or splenomegaly, lymphadenopathy, or masses.

A. Why do you suspect anemia, and what information from the history assists you to develop the differential diagnosis for this child?
B. What laboratory tests will you select to evaluate the anemia?
C. Based on the following screening laboratory test results, what is the differential diagnosis, and which among the list is most likely?

White blood cell count 5000/mm^3
Red blood cell count 2.5 million/mm^3
Hemoglobin 5 g/dl
Hematocrit 15%
Mean corpuscular volume 63
Reticulocyte count 0.5%

D. What additional laboratory studies might support the diagnosis?

Case 50-2

R.B. is a 1-month-old black male who is coming for his first health supervision visit. He was born at term to a G1 P1 mother who had no problems with her pregnancy. Birth weight was 3 kg. He was discharged from the nursery at 2 days of age and had no complications in the nursery. He is nursing well from the breast every 2 to 3 hours and has four or five yellow stools per day and 8 to 10 wet diapers per day. His newborn screen revealed hemoglobin FS. He has not had any follow-up tests.

A. What additional history do you need?
B. Why does this child have a high risk for morbidity and mortality? What medication will decrease those risks?
C. What will you discuss with the family about sickle cell disease?

Case Answers

50-1 A. *Learning objective:* **List the key issues in the history for the evaluation of anemia in infancy and childhood.** The patient was switched from infant formula to whole milk before 12 months of age, which increases the risk of occult blood loss from the gastrointestinal tract and also reduces the iron intake from the diet. Hence, iron deficiency should be strongly considered in the differential diagnosis. Inquire specifically about a family history of anemia and about a personal history of pain, fever, bruising, or bleeding. Information about ethnicity would be helpful to assess the possibility of a hemoglobinopathy (e.g., thalassemia is more common in patients of southern European/Mediterranean descent). Exposure to environmental lead is another key item in the history.

50-1 B. *Learning objective:* **Select appropriate laboratory tests for the initial evaluation of anemia.** Complete blood count and reticulocyte count should be done initially. Testing for occult blood in the stool may also provide important information.

50-1 C. *Learning objective:* **Interpret laboratory test results to arrive at a diagnosis.** The differential diagnosis includes iron-deficiency anemia, thalassemia, and lead poisoning. Iron deficiency is suggested by microcytic anemia with low reticulocyte count. Thalassemia is suggested by microcytic anemia (and history of ethnic background). Lead poisoning is suggested by microcytic anemia (and history of lead exposure).

50-1 D. *Learning objective:* **Identify laboratory tests to evaluate microcytic anemia.**
Iron deficiency: Serum iron, total iron binding capacity, and ferritin. A trial of therapeutic iron (3 to 5 mg/kg/day) should produce a prompt increase in the reticulocyte count if the anemia is caused by iron deficiency.
Thalassemia: Hemoglobin electrophoresis
Lead poisoning: Blood lead level > 25 g/dl causes the anemia seen in lead poisoning.

50-2 A. *Learning objective:* **Identify the key issues to evaluate an infant with a positive newborn screen for sickle cell anemia.** You should inquire about the maternal and paternal sickle cell status and the family history of others with sickling disorders. In addition, it is important to ask whether the child had any problems since birth, especially unexplained infections, fevers, or pain. The initial newborn screen test should be repeated to document the diagnosis.

50-2 B. *Learning objective:* **Discuss the specific management of sickle cell anemia that reduces morbidity and mortality.** Individuals with sickle cell anemia are functionally asplenic in infancy (even though they develop splenomegaly) and have splenic infarction later in life. They are thus highly susceptible to systemic infection with encapsulated organisms. Penicillin must be given twice daily to reduce the likelihood of life-threatening infection. Immunization with conjugated 7 valent pneumococcal vaccine in infancy and 23 valent pneumococcal vaccine at the age of 2 years will further decrease the incidence of bacteremia and sepsis in these children. Prompt evaluation for any fever and early institution of parenteral antibiotic therapy is essential to reduce morbidity and mortality resulting from sepsis in patients with sickling disorders.

50-2 C. *Learning objective:* **Be able to counsel families about the basics of sickle cell anemia, its ongoing management, and its prognosis.** You should be able to discuss the genetics of sickle cell disease (method of inheritance). You should be able to counsel parents so that they understand (1) the need for penicillin to prevent morbidity, (2) the need for routine immunizations, including pneumococcal vaccination, (3) the need for immediate evaluation if the child develops a temperature higher than 38.5° C (101° F), and (4) the need for a comprehensive evaluation. You should also provide information about potential problems, including the possibility of infection, pain (hand-foot syndrome), jaundice, and pallor. Teach the parents to palpate for enlarging spleen.

BIBLIOGRAPHY

Behrman RE, Kliegman RM, Jenson, HB, editors: *Nelson's textbook of pediatrics*, ed 17, Philadelphia, 2004, WB Saunders.

Hoekelman RA et al, editors: *Primary pediatric care*, ed 4, St Louis, 2001, Mosby-Year Book.

Lanzkowsky P, editor: *Manual of pediatric hematology and oncology*, ed 4, New York, 2005, Elsevier.

Nathan DG et al, editors: *Nathan and Oski's hematology of infancy and childhood*, ed 6, Philadelphia, 2003, WB Saunders.

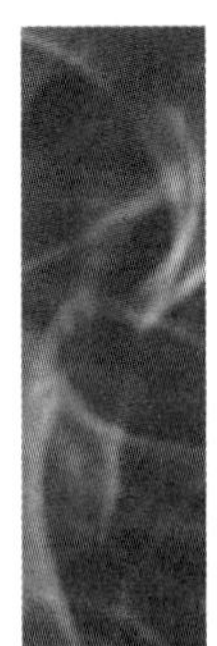

51

Elevated or Depressed White Blood Cell Count

ROGER BERKOW

The white blood cell (WBC) count is often obtained to screen for infection or in response to a wide variety of clinical problems. Interpretation of results depends on knowledge of the changes that occur from birth to adolescence. It also demands an appreciation of how the WBC count varies in different disease states.

ETIOLOGY

How Do White Blood Cells Vary with Age?

At birth, an infant's WBC count is high and the differential shows a predominance of neutrophils. This neutrophilic predominance is brief, and by 1 month of age the lymphocytes predominate. The WBC count and differential pattern become similar to that of an adult during early adolescence (Table 51-1). Both leukocytosis and leukopenia can indicate infectious, immunologic, or malignant processes (see Chapter 63 for leukemia).

What Causes an Elevated White Blood Cell Count?

Elevated WBC or leukocytosis is most commonly associated with bacterial infection when there is also predominance of neutrophils and immature (band) forms. A WBC count of 15,000/mm^3 or higher, with an immature or "band" neutrophil count of 1500/mm^3 or higher, is especially concerning when accompanied by clinical signs of "toxicity." Leukocytosis also accompanies hemorrhage and hemolysis as a result of increased bone marrow activity. Leukocytosis with mature forms occurs after exercise, from the release of marginated neutrophils. Metabolic disorders, leukemia, myeloproliferative disorders, and treatment with steroids, epinephrine, and cytokines also cause leukocytosis. Lymphocytosis with mature lymphocytes is associated with viral illness, notably mononucleosis. If a marked lymphocytosis is seen, pertussis must be considered. Eosinophilia is associated with allergies, eczema, parasitic infections, neoplasm, asthma, and collagen vascular disease.

Table 51-1

WBC and Differential Leukocyte Count by Age

Age	Leukocytes ($\times 10^3$)	Neutrophils (%)	Lymphocytes (%)	Monocytes (%)	Eosinophils (%)
Birth	18	61	31	6	2
1 week	12.2	45	41	9	4
1 mo	10.8	35	56	7	3
6 mo	11.9	32	61	5	3
1 yr	11.4	31	61	5	3
4 yr	9.1	42	50	5	3
10 yr	8.1	54	38	4	2
16 yr	7.8	57	35	4	3

WBC, White blood cell.

What Causes a Depressed White Blood Cell Count?

A depressed WBC or leukopenia count usually occurs in response to viral illnesses, drug exposure, or malignancy, and manifests as either lymphopenia or neutropenia. *Lymphopenia* is associated with an increased risk of opportunistic infections in congenital immune deficiency syndromes and human immunodeficiency virus (HIV) infection. *Neutropenia* is defined as an absolute neutrophil count (ANC) of less than 2500/mm^3 in the newborn and less than 1500/mm^3 in children and adults. The chances of bacterial infection increase dramatically as ANC decreases. Fever in a patient with a neutrophil count less than 500/mm^3 represents a medical emergency and calls for a complete investigation for bacterial infection and the early institution of broad-spectrum antibiotic therapy.

What Causes Neutropenia?

Neutropenia results from decreased production or increased destruction of neutrophils. Transient neutropenia occurs most commonly during a febrile viral illness from temporary marrow suppression, with decreased production of neutrophils. The neutrophil count typically returns to baseline as the viral illness resolves, but if the count is less than 500/mm^3, blood cultures and the institution of broad-spectrum antibiotics should be considered. Malignancy, especially leukemia, causes neutropenia, as do aplastic anemia and a number of rare syndromes. Cyclic neutropenia is manifested by oscillations in the neutrophil count, with the nadir occurring approximately every 21 days, associated with fever and oral ulcerations; within days, the neutrophil count cycles back up, and the child improves. Immune-mediated neutrophil destruction can also occur as an isoimmune phenomenon, as a result of viral infections, in autoimmune disorders, or as an idiopathic phenomenon called *chronic benign neutropenia.* Hypersplenism destroys WBCs (and red blood cells [RBCs]) in the sinusoids of the spleen. Pseudoneutropenia reflects increased margination of neutrophils in the vasculature; stress usually results in a prompt release of neutrophils into the circulation. Neutropenia can be seen at or shortly after birth in severe congenital neutropenia (Kostmann's neutropenia), as the first finding in congenital bone marrow failure syndromes (Fanconi's anemia), and in idiopathic aplastic anemia. A complete medication history is essential in evaluating the causes of neutropenia.

EVALUATION

When Should I Order a White Blood Cell Count?

Recognition of characteristic clinical syndromes should prompt assessment of the WBC and differential leukocyte count. Fever, the appearance of "toxicity," and other findings of infection warrant this workup, particularly if an infant or young child is incompletely immunized. Additional tests, including blood and cerebrospinal fluid (CSF) cultures, urine culture, radiographs, and bone marrow aspirate and biopsy, depend on the clinical scenario and the differential diagnosis. Evaluation of leukemia is discussed in Chapter 63.

TREATMENT

How Do I Manage a Febrile Child with Leukocytosis?

The risk of serious bacterial infection increases when a child younger than 2 years has a temperature of 40° C or higher, appears toxic, has a WBC count of 15,000/mm^3 or higher, and has an immature or "band" neutrophil count of 1500/mm^3 or higher. Risk is especially high if immunization against *Haemophilus influenzae* type B and *Streptococcus pneumoniae* are incomplete. If a specific source for the fever, such as UTI, cannot be identified, it is appropriate to treat a toxic-appearing child empirically with a broad-spectrum antibiotic, usually a third-generation cephalosporin, while awaiting results of blood, urine, and other cultures (see Chapter 33).

Is Treatment Needed for Nonmalignant Neutropenia?

Infection is the major risk of neutropenia, and broad-spectrum antibiotic therapy is warranted if the ANC is below 500/mm^3 and the patient appears toxic with fever, pain, or respiratory distress. In addition, patients with known HIV infection must be continuously monitored for opportunistic infections and treated promptly.

KEY POINTS

- The WBC and differential leukocyte count change as the child ages.
- Both infection and leukemia may produce elevated or decreased WBC counts.

Case 51-1

A 24-month-old boy is brought for a routine health supervision visit. He has had frequent otitis media and has been on prophylactic antibiotic therapy with trimethoprim-sulfamethoxazole since 18 months of age. He has been free of ear infections during this time. Examination today is unremarkable, including tympanic membranes. As a routine screening test you order a complete blood count (CBC) and differential, which reveals the following:

WBC 2500/mm^3
Hemoglobin 12.0 g/dl
Hematocrit 36%
MCV 76 fl
Neutrophils 5%
Lymphocytes 88%
Monocytes 4%
Eosinophils 3%

A. What component(s) of the CBC is/are an area for concern? What is the ANC?
B. What is the most likely cause of the neutropenia? What is the mechanism?
C. What is the appropriate management of this child?
D. How would management change if the child develops a fever of 101° F tonight?
E. What if the neutrophil count persists after the causative agent is discontinued?

Case Answers

51-1 A. *Learning objective:* **Interpret a CBC and differential; identify neutropenia.** The total WBC is 2500/mm^3 (low) and demonstrates neutropenia (neutrophils are only 5% of the total WBC). The absolute neutrophil count is 125/mm^3 (5% × 2500/mm^3).

51-1 B. *Learning objective:* **Identify the cause of neutropenia from the history.** Trimethoprim-sulfamethoxazole causes neutropenia by suppression of bone marrow.

51-1 C. *Learning objective:* **Discuss the management of neutropenia, recognizing its possible complications.** Stop the trimethoprim-sulfamethoxazole and repeat CBC weekly to monitor the expected rise in absolute neutrophil count. While the child is neutropenic, the parents must be aware of the risks of bacterial infection and of the need to notify you if fever develops.

51-1 D. *Learning objective:* **Discuss the management of fever in a neutropenic child.** Because of the high risk of invasive bacterial infection in neutropenia, you should culture the blood, urine, and throat. You should also obtain a chest radiograph and begin broad-spectrum antibiotics.

51-1 E. *Learning objective:* **Discuss the causes of persistent neutropenia.** Malignancy or aplastic anemia can cause persistent neutropenia. You should obtain a bone marrow aspirate for further evaluation.

BIBLIOGRAPHY

Lanzkowsky P, editor: *Manual of pediatric hematology and oncology,* ed 4, New York, 2005, Elsevier.

Nathan DG et al, editors: *Nathan and Oski's hematology of infancy and childhood,* ed 6, Philadelphia, 2003, WB Saunders.

Pizzo PA, Poplack DG, editors: *Principles and practice of pediatric oncology,* ed 4, Philadelphia, 2002, Lippincott-Raven.

Ries LAG et al, editors: *Cancer incidence and survival among children and adolescents: United States SEER Program, 1975-1995* (NIH Publication No. 99-4649), Bethesda, MD, 1999, National Cancer Institute, SEER Program.

52

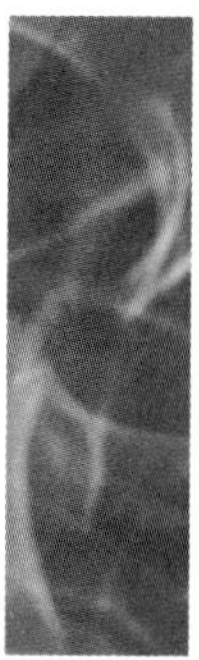

Hematuria

LAVJAY BUTANI and BRUCE Z. MORGENSTERN

ETIOLOGY

Does the Urine Dipstick Detect Blood Reliably?

Urine dipsticks are sensitive and will detect even small numbers of red blood cells (RBCs), especially if the specimen is concentrated. Blood is often identified by dipstick on a routine urinalysis for a totally asymptomatic child. When the dipstick test is "trace," it reflects < 5 RBCs per high-power field on microscopic examination and is physiologic. Occasionally, the presence of substances other than RBCs, such as hemoglobin and myoglobin, can also cause discoloration of the urine dipstick.

How Is Hematuria Defined?

Microscopic hematuria is defined as more than 5 RBCs per high-power field on a centrifuged urine specimen, and is found on one occasion in as many as 4% of all urine specimens in American school children. It is generally benign when present without proteinuria. When the dipstick reading is "moderate" or "large," and especially when associated with proteinuria, the hematuria may reflect underlying renal disease. *Persistent microscopic hematuria* occurs in fewer than 1% of children. *Gross hematuria* means that urine contains visible blood and occurs in < 0.1% of children.

What Causes Hematuria?

A list of the common causes of hematuria is found in Table 52-1.

EVALUATION

How Do I Evaluate Isolated Microscopic Hematuria?

An otherwise healthy child with isolated microscopic hematuria needs only a repeat urine specimen while you review the child's growth, development, and blood pressure. The urine should be sent for urinalysis

Table 52-1

Causes of Hematuria in Children

Parenchymal Source	Urinary Tract Source
Glomerulonephritis	Stones, hypercalciuria
Pyelonephritis	Hemorrhagic cystitis (usually viral), urethritis
Less common	
Trauma	Exercise (bladder trauma)
Arteriovenous malformations	Tumors
Anatomic malformations (polycystic kidney disease or ureteropelvic junction obstruction)	Coagulation disorder (von Willebrand's disease, etc.)

with microscopic evaluation for RBCs. Isolated microscopic hematuria will resolve spontaneously in most cases and no further workup is needed. Presence of white blood cells (WBCs), crystals, or casts would suggest a diagnosis other than isolated microscopic hematuria.

How Do I Evaluate Persistent Microscopic Hematuria?

Most patients who have asymptomatic persistent microscopic hematuria have no history of gross hematuria and have age-appropriate growth, development, blood pressure, and renal function. Proteinuria is not present on urinalysis. Such patients have, at most, mild renal disorders, which have little chance of progressing to renal failure. Treatment does not alter the management or natural history. A *limited workup* is appropriate for these patients, including random urine calcium-to-creatinine ratio, and screening for microscopic hematuria in family members to detect familial glomerulonephritis (Chapter 65). A *complete workup*, as outlined later for gross hematuria, would be necessary if the physician or family wishes to rule out all significant renal diseases or if the patient has microscopic hematuria *plus* other associated signs or symptoms.

How Do I Evaluate Gross Hematuria?

If your patient has visible blood in the urine a complete workup is needed. A thorough history, physical examination, and urinalysis can usually determine whether the hematuria originates in the renal parenchyma or the collecting system (Table 52-2). If the source is identified, perform the pertinent workup, as discussed later. If you cannot determine the source of hematuria with any reasonable degree of accuracy, do further testing as dictated by the patient's condition. Referral to a nephrologist or urologist is justified.

How Do I Determine the Source of Hematuria?

The history and initial urinalysis will give the first clues. Isolated hematuria is unlikely as a sign of urinary tract infection (UTI); much more

Table 52-2

Clinical Findings in Hematuria Based on Source of Bleeding

	Source of Bleeding	
Clinical Finding	**Parenchyma (Intrarenal)**	**Collecting System Ureter, Bladder (Extrarenal)**
Appearance of urine	"Tea colored"	Bright red or blood clots
Urinary symptoms	Painless hematuria	Dysuria, urgency, frequency
Associated symptoms	Sore throat Hypertension, edema	Fever and colicky pain
Family history	Deafness, renal failure	Renal stones, UTI
Proteinuria	> 2+ on dipstick Urine protein-to-creatinine ratio > 1	Trace to 1+ on dipstick
Other	RBC casts (high specificity but low sensitivity)	Crystals in urine

RBC, Red blood cell; UTI, urinary tract infection.

commonly, UTI would be identified in a patient with fever, dysuria, and cloudy urine, plus hematuria, positive leukocyte esterase and nitrite tests, and microscopic evidence of pyuria and bacteriuria. Urine culture would be needed to identify the organism. If the hematuria occurs in a patient with signs of glomerulonephritis, a workup as discussed in Chapter 65 is necessary. When colicky abdominal pain accompanies microscopic or gross hematuria, consider renal stones or hypercalciuria. Kidney-ureter-bladder (KUB) x-ray and possibly a computed tomography (CT) scan may detect renal stones, and a random urine for calcium-to-creatinine ratio will identify hypercalciuria. Other tests might include renal ultrasound or CT to assess for polycystic kidney disease or renal masses and a sickle cell screen when appropriate. A bleeding disorder may rarely present with hematuria.

TREATMENT

How Is Hematuria Managed?

Management is directed toward the identified underlying disease process. The evaluation often does not yield a diagnosis in cases of isolated microscopic hematuria; management consists of patient education and ongoing monitoring for any change in the clinical presentation and for development of hypertension or proteinuria.

KEY POINTS

- Microhematuria is common and usually benign in otherwise healthy children.
- History, physical examination, and urinalysis usually identify the source of the bleeding in children with gross hematuria.
- Close follow-up of children with hematuria allows early detection of a change in renal status.

Case 52-1

A 5-year-old girl is found to have microscopic hematuria without proteinuria at the time of a routine well-child visit. She has also had recent dysuria. Her physical examination is unremarkable.

A. What are the possible explanations for her symptoms?
B. What further historical information may be of help in evaluating your patient?
C. What further laboratory testing would you consider?

Case 52-2

A 17-year-old girl is brought to the emergency department for evaluation of a 5-day history of grossly bloody (brownish-colored) urine. She is in no pain but has had a 10-pound weight loss and low-grade recurrent fevers for the past month. Blood pressure is 140/90 mm Hg. Physical examination finds a faint erythematous rash on both cheeks and generalized edema. The urine dipstick shows 4+ blood and 4+ protein.

A. What is the most likely source of the patient's hematuria, and why?
B. What are the possible causes of the hematuria?
C. What further tests would you order?

Case Answers

52-1 A. *Learning objective:* **List the differential diagnosis for microscopic hematuria in a child or adolescent.** Differential diagnosis of hematuria associated with dysuria includes UTI, trauma, and hypercalciuria. Nephrolithiasis can also cause microscopic hematuria but is usually accompanied by abdominal or groin pain.

52-1 B. *Learning objective:* **Use the history to obtain the information needed to narrow the differential diagnosis of hematuria.** Ask about voiding frequency and the pattern of urination, including hesitancy, urgency, and incontinence. Be sure to ask about abdominal pain. In an infant, crying with urination suggests dysuria, and a foul odor in the diaper should suggest possible infection. Ask also about the past history of UTIs, the use of bubble baths, and details of perineal hygiene, especially wiping after bowel movements. Constipation is a common finding in girls with UTI. Additional questions should address any perineal or abdominal trauma. Inquire about the family history of hematuria, UTI, renal disease, and kidney stones.

52-1 C. *Learning objective:* **Select laboratory tests to evaluate hematuria.** The initial laboratory tests include urinalysis with microscopic examination, urine culture, and determination of the calcium-to-creatinine ratio. Further tests depend on the findings on the initial screen.

52-2 A. *Learning objective:* **Use the history, physical examination, and laboratory tests to identify the origin of blood in the urine.** This patient's hematuria originates in the upper urinary tract or from renal parenchymal source because (1) the hematuria is painless, (2) the patient is hypertensive and has edema, and (3) significant proteinuria accompanies the hematuria.

52-2 B. *Learning objective:* **List the differential diagnosis for gross hematuria.** Acute or chronic glomerulonephritis is the most likely cause of this teenager's findings. Trauma is unlikely without a history and physical findings to support it. Nephrolithiasis can cause gross hematuria but is associated with prominent abdominal pain. A renal tumor can cause either gross or microscopic hematuria, but a mass would be identified in the abdomen and the hematuria would not likely be accompanied by heavy proteinuria.

52-2 C. *Learning objective:* **Select laboratory tests to evaluate gross hematuria.** The initial laboratory test should be the urinalysis with microscopic examination to look for red blood cell casts. Patients with suspected glomerulonephritis (see Chapter 65) should also have serum creatinine and blood urea nitrogen studies to assess renal function, and serum C3 and C4 complement levels. A teenage girl with hematuria, proteinuria, fever, and facial rash should be investigated for systemic lupus erythematosus (Chapter 70).

BIBLIOGRAPHY

Bergstein J, Leiser J, Andreoli S: The clinical significance of asymptomatic gross and microscopic hematuria in children, *Arch Pediatr Adolesc Med* 159:353, 2005.

Diven SC, Travis LB: A practical primary care approach to hematuria in children, *Pediatr Nephrol* 14:65, 2000.

Feld LG et al: Limited evaluation of microscopic hematuria in pediatrics, *Pediatrics* 102(4):e42, 1998.
Matos V et al: Urinary phosphate/creatinine, calcium/creatinine, and magnesium/creatinine ratios in a healthy pediatric population, *J Pediatr* 131:252, 1997.
Roy S et al: Hematuria preceding renal calculus formation in children with hypercalciuria, *J Pediatr* 99:712, 1981.

53

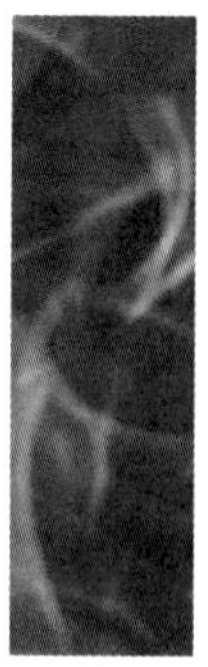

Proteinuria

LAVJAY BUTANI and BRUCE Z. MORGENSTERN

ETIOLOGY

Is Proteinuria a Sign of Kidney Disease?

Protein in the urine is a nonspecific finding and does not necessarily indicate an underlying kidney disorder. *Physiologic proteinuria* occurs commonly in children and adults from leakage of small amounts of albumin and low-molecular-weight proteins into the urine and may be exaggerated after standing *(orthostatic proteinuria)*. Physiologic urine protein concentration is typically < 4 mg/m^2/hr in children and reaches 150 mg/24 hr in adults (Table 53-1). *Pathologic proteinuria* is usually far in excess of physiologic values. Acute febrile illnesses or vigorous physical activity can cause transient elevations of protein excretion above physiologic levels.

What Causes Persistent Pathologic Proteinuria?

When pathologic proteinuria is persistent, it is usually a sign of an underlying kidney disease. In addition, when children are known to have kidney disease, the presence and the magnitude of proteinuria are independent factors that predict a poor outcome. A patient with both blood and protein in the urine has a high likelihood of having glomerulonephritis (Chapter 65). Persistent proteinuria *without* blood occurs in two situations: *Glomerular proteinuria* occurs in disorders that cause increased permeability of the glomerular basement membrane that allows leakage of large-molecular-weight proteins such as albumin. Examples include nephrotic syndrome, glomerulopathies such as focal segmental glomerulosclerosis, and reflux nephropathy/renal scarring from acute pyelonephritis (Chapter 65). *Tubular proteinuria* results from defective tubular resorption of low-molecular-weight proteins such as beta$_2$-microglobulin and occurs in Fanconi's syndrome, tubulointerstitial nephritis, acute tubular necrosis, reflux nephropathy, and a variety of hereditary diseases.

Table 53-1

Quantifying Proteinuria

Protein in a 24-Hour Urine Collection		
mg/m^2/hr (Child)	**mg/24 hr (Adult)**	**Random Urine Protein-to-Creatinine Ratio**
< 4	< 150	< 0.5 (< 2 yr) < 0.2 (> 2 yr)
Pathologic		
4–40	150–3500	0.2–2.5
> 40	> 3500	> 2.5

What Is Orthostatic Proteinuria?

Orthostatic proteinuria accounts for 70% to 80% of all cases of proteinuria in adolescents. Its pathogenesis is not entirely clear but is thought to be mediated by hemodynamic mechanisms during prolonged standing. Children and adolescents with orthostatic proteinuria usually have protein excretion < 1 g/24 hr. They have a benign long-term course and minimal risk of developing renal insufficiency. Establishing the diagnosis is straightforward (see later). Therapy is not needed, but careful explanation and reassurance about the benign nature of this phenomenon are important. Annual follow-up to monitor blood pressure and growth and to perform urinalysis is recommended because orthostatic proteinuria has not been optimally studied.

EVALUATION

When Is Proteinuria Likely to Be Detected?

Proteinuria is most commonly identified when a "routine" dipstick urinalysis is performed on an asymptomatic patient at a well-child visit or sports physical examination. Occasionally, findings such as edema, a purpuric rash, hypertension, or gross hematuria will prompt urinalysis that detects proteinuria. The urine dipstick is highly sensitive and specific for albumin. False-positive tests occur when the urine has high specific gravity or is highly alkaline; false-negative tests occur when the urine has low specific gravity or when only non-albumin proteins such as immunoglobulin light chains are present.

What Findings from History Are Important?

Whether a child has symptomatic or asymptomatic persistent proteinuria, you should inquire specifically about fever, recent viral or bacterial illnesses, gross hematuria, swelling of eyes and legs, and abdominal distention. Heavy physical exertion shortly before the office visit may cause proteinuria. Past history of previous urinary tract infections, arthritis, rash, or other underlying disorders may help with diagnosis. A detailed medication history, especially for chronic use of nonsteroidal antiinflammatory drugs, may identify a cause of proteinuria.

What Should I Look for on Physical Examination?

On physical examination, look for signs of growth failure or recent weight gain, and measure the blood pressure. Check for edema in the periorbital area, the extremities, and the sacral area. Examine the abdomen for ascites. Specific diseases that cause proteinuria, such as glomerulonephritis, may have characteristic findings, including arthritis or rashes (Chapter 65).

How Should I Begin the Evaluation of Proteinuria?

Your goal is to differentiate benign from pathologic proteinuria and to detect persistent proteinuria. If your patient is truly asymptomatic and has no other findings suggestive of an underlying disease, a practical approach is to repeat the urine dipstick on two separate random urine specimens, preferably on first-voided morning samples. Also, send the two urine samples to the laboratory for urinalysis and for determination of the urine protein-to-urine creatinine ratio (Up/c = Urine protein in mg/dl ÷ urine creatinine in mg/dl). This ratio correlates well with the 24-hour urine protein excretion. Table 53-1 defines physiologic and pathologic proteinuria using both methods. If the Up/c of the first-voided morning urine sample is less than 0.2, the patient either has transient or orthostatic proteinuria; no further workup is needed. If the first morning Up/c is persistently higher than 0.2, your patient has pathologic proteinuria and needs further workup to rule out kidney disease. What other tests help identify the cause of proteinuria?

If the cause of proteinuria is unclear, consider the following additional tests:

- Serum creatinine to assess renal function
- Serum total protein, albumin, and cholesterol to look for nephrotic syndrome
- Quantitation of proteinuria by timed urine collection
- Renal ultrasonography as a crude screen for renal parenchymal abnormalities
- Second-line tests should be considered on a case-by-case basis:
  - Dimercaptosuccinic acid (DMSA) renal scan to look for the scarring seen in reflux nephropathy
  - Renal biopsy, especially if your patient has an elevated serum creatinine level or is hypertensive

TREATMENT

How Do I Treat Proteinuria?

Treatment of a child with proteinuria depends entirely on the etiology. Nephrotic syndrome, focal segmental glomerulosclerosis, and glomerulonephritis are discussed in Chapter 65. For children with tubular proteinuria, treat the underlying disease or condition if possible. Persistent proteinuria itself may be harmful to the kidneys over an extended period; angiotensin-converting enzyme inhibitors and angiotensin-receptor blockers have a renoprotective effect and should be considered in such a setting.

KEY POINTS

- Proteinuria is a common and often benign finding in children.
- Orthostatic proteinuria is the most common cause of proteinuria in older children and adolescents and is benign.
- Persistent proteinuria may be a sign of an underlying kidney disease.

Case 53-1

An 18-year-old athlete is found to have 2+ protein on a urine dipstick at a routine sports physical, which took place after practice at school. He is asymptomatic. His blood pressure is 110/70 mm Hg, and the physical examination is unremarkable.

A. What is the most likely explanation for your patient's proteinuria?
B. What should be your next step in evaluating your patient's problem?

Case 53-2

A 3-year-old African-American boy is noted to have 3+ protein on a urine dipstick at a health supervision visit. The family has not noted any change in his appearance or well-being. Height and weight are at the 50th percentile for age and blood pressure (BP) is 113/67 mm Hg (>95th percentile for age and height). His physical examination is unremarkable. The urine dipstick and first morning urinalysis are repeated twice and each time show 3+ protein but no blood. The first morning Up/c = 3 from both samples.

A. What is the likely source of this boy's proteinuria?
B. How would you begin his evaluation?

Case Answers

53–1 A. *Learning objective:* **Interpret a positive test for urine protein.** This patient's age, the negative history and physical examination, and the absence of blood in the urine make orthostatic proteinuria the most likely diagnosis.

53–1 B. *Learning objective:* **Use history, physical examination, and selected laboratory tests to evaluate proteinuria.** A detailed history and physical examination must be done to look for signs and symptoms of an underlying disease. Repeat the urine dipstick on a first morning urine specimen on two separate occasions and send the urine to the laboratory to determine the urinary protein-to-creatinine (Up/c) ratio.

53–2 A. *Learning objective:* **Interpret Up/c from a first morning urine specimen.** The Up/c of 3 on both first voided samples indicates that this child has persistent proteinuria that is not orthostatic and is in the nephrotic range. This points to the presence of a glomerular disease. Differential diagnoses include all the conditions that can cause nephrotic syndrome or glomerulopathies or less likely (because of young age and gender) reflux nephropathy/renal scarring.

53–2 B. *Learning objective:* **Select laboratory testing to investigate persistent proteinuria.** Obtain serum levels of creatinine, albumin, and cholesterol to determine if your patient has nephrotic syndrome. Further testing will depend on the results of your initial tests and is likely to include a detailed workup for glomerular diseases (Chapter 65). Renal ultrasound or a DMSA scan may be needed to look for reflux nephropathy/renal scarring.

BIBLIOGRAPHY

Bergstein JM: A practical approach to proteinuria, *Pediatr Nephrol* 13:697, 1999.

Houser M: Assessment of proteinuria using random urine samples, *J Pediatr* 104:845, 1984.

Morgenstern BZ et al: Validity of protein-osmolality versus protein-creatinine ratios in the estimation of quantitative proteinuria from random samples of urine in children, *Am J Kidney Dis* 41:760, 2003.

Rytand DA, Spreiter S: Prognosis in postural (orthostatic) proteinuria: forty- to fifty-year follow-up of six patients after diagnosis by Thomas Addis, *N Engl J Med* 305:618, 1981.

Schieppati A, Remuzzi G: The June 2003 Barry M. Brenner Comgan lecture. The future of renoprotection: frustration and promises, *Kidney Int* 64:1947, 2003.

Thompson AL, Durrett RR, Robinson R: Fixed and reproducible orthostatic proteinuria. VI. Results of a 10-year follow-up evaluation, *Ann Intern Med* 73:235, 1970.

Section

5

Patients Presenting with Known Conditions

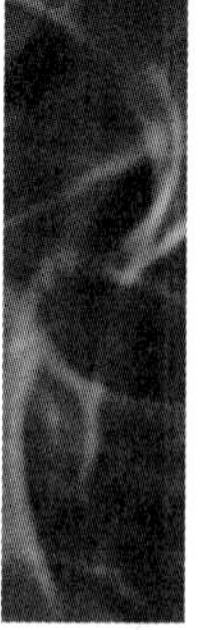

54 Adolescents with Known Conditions

KEN CHEYNE and MICHAEL R. LAWLESS

ACNE

ETIOLOGY

What Causes Acne?

Adolescent acne is caused by obstruction of the sebaceous follicles located primarily on the face and trunk. This process is activated by androgens and aggravated by *Propionibacterium acnes*. Acne can begin as early as age 8 years and affects as many as 85% of individuals between the ages of 12 and 25 years. Acne can be aggravated or induced by friction, oil-based cosmetics, and drugs that elevate plasma testosterone levels.

EVALUATION

How Does Acne Appear Clinically?

Depending on the interaction of the causative processes and the host response, acne may appear as open comedones ("blackheads"), closed comedones ("whiteheads"), or inflammatory papules, pustules, or cysts. Severity is determined by the extensiveness of the affected skin and by the types of lesions, with pustular and cystic lesions representing more serious involvement.

TREATMENT

What Are Treatment Choices for Acne?

Topical retinoids are the first choice for acne treatment. They relieve follicular obstruction and reduce inflammation. Retinoids can be combined with topical antimicrobial agents (e.g., benzoyl peroxide, erythromycin, or clindamycin). Systemic antibiotics such as erythromycin, tetracycline, doxycycline, and minocycline may also be needed in more severe inflammatory acne. Oral contraceptives with an estrogenic effect and a weak androgenic effect may also be useful in the treatment of acne in adolescent girls.

Isotretinoin (Accutane) should be *used only under the direction of a dermatologist.* It is an oral retinoid that is effective for severe cystic acne. Food and Drug Administration (FDA) regulations mandate that all adolescents who are candidates for isotretinoin treatment *must* be counseled about the teratogenic effects of the drug and monitored for possible psychiatric effects. Girls *must* use effective oral and barrier methods of contraception, and *must* be followed regularly with pregnancy tests (see *www.fda.gov/cder/drug/infopage/accutane/default.htm*).

EATING DISORDERS

ETIOLOGY

How Common Are Eating Disorders?

Approximately 0.5% to 1% of adolescent girls develop anorexia nervosa, which makes this disorder the third most common chronic condition among adolescent girls after obesity and asthma. Up to 5% of older adolescents and young adult women develop bulimia nervosa. Prevalence rates for bulimia nervosa among high school students are generally lower than those among college-age women. Although their behaviors do not meet the *Diagnostic and Statistical Manual of Mental Disorders, Fourth Edition* (DSM-IV) criteria for bulimia nervosa, as many as 10% to 50% of adolescent women report occasional self-induced vomiting or binge eating.

Can Boys Develop Eating Disorders?

Recent studies suggest that up to one in six individuals with an eating disorder are male. In general, adolescent boys are shape-oriented, tend to be dissatisfied about their appearance from the waist up, and almost always diet for specific personal reasons. Males commonly diet to improve athletic performance, avoid being teased for being fat, avoid developing medical diseases associated with men in the family, or improve a gay relationship.

What Causes Eating Disorders?

Eating disorders are characterized by the misuse of eating in an attempt to solve other life problems. The etiologies of anorexia nervosa and bulimia nervosa are complex and multifactorial. A combination of biologic, psychologic, and societal factors contributes to the predisposition and perpetuation of eating disorders. Difficulty with the developmental transition from childhood to adulthood has been associated with eating disorders. Depression and sexual trauma are two psychological factors that have been associated with bulimia nervosa.

EVALUATION

What Are the DSM-IV Criteria for Eating Disorders?

- *Anorexia nervosa* diagnostic criteria include persistent and severe restriction of energy intake, often combined with compulsive exercise in the pursuit of thinness. This drive for thinness is relentless. Patients who have anorexia nervosa may be subdivided into a restrictive type or a binge eating–purging type.

- *Bulimia nervosa* criteria include binge eating followed by some compensatory behavior to rid the body of ingested calories. The most common type of purging behavior in adolescents is self-induced vomiting. Adolescents with bulimia nervosa are usually of average to above average weight for height. They often engage in impulsive behaviors such as substance abuse, self-mutilation, self-harm, or sexual promiscuity.

What Are the Signs and Symptoms of Eating Disorders?

Eating disorders may present with any of the following:

- Disturbed body image leading to an irrational interpretation of appearance
- Dieting with vehemence
- Visible weight loss
- Disorganized eating patterns such as skipping meals on various pretenses, unusual or extreme food preferences (especially carbohydrate avoidance), hoarding of food, cooking for others, playing with food at meals, eating alone, refusing to eat with family or to eat a meal out, and feeling extreme bloating after eating
- Changes in menstrual cycle or amenorrhea
- Excessive and/or ritualistic exercise, especially sit-ups
- Abuse of laxatives, diet pills, diuretics, sugar-free gum (sorbitol), caffeine, and/or syrup of ipecac
- Binge eating, especially of sweets, breads, and salty snack foods, secretive postprandial vomiting, stealing of food or money for food
- Hair loss, cold hands and feet, syncopal episodes, constipation, calluses on dorsum of the fingers, parotid gland swelling, or dental enamel erosion
- Inability to recognize feelings or basic needs such as hunger or fatigue
- Withdrawal from family and friends (for some adolescents, involvement in structured interactions, such as school organizations, may continue, although in a driven way)
- Slowing of normative psychosocial development
- Rigid adherence to a highly prescribed set of values, with a relative lack of curiosity and questioning
- Compulsive neatness and orderliness
- Change in mood such as increased irritability, increased anxiety, depression
- Changes in school and/or work performance, especially regarding simultaneous striving for perfection while verbalizing a sense of ineffectiveness

Are Laboratory Tests Helpful?

The diagnosis of an eating disorder is clinical; there are no confirmatory laboratory tests. Information from the history and physical examination will help you choose laboratory tests to detect abnormalities that arise from weight control habits used by the adolescent and from malnutrition. Routine laboratory tests may include a complete blood count, erythrocyte sedimentation rate, and biochemical profile.

TREATMENT

How Are Eating Disorders Treated?

The successful treatment of eating disorders requires an interdisciplinary team. Medical monitoring, nutritional counseling, and individual and family counseling are the backbone of treatment. Family involvement is essential from the beginning. Establishment of a trusting relationship and the early restoration of the adolescent's nutritional and physiologic state are the initial goals of treatment. Comorbidities such as depression also need to be treated. The successful treatment of an adolescent with an eating disorder may take months to years.

What Are the Complications of Eating Disorders?

Eating disorders are classified as psychiatric disorders, but they are associated with significant medical complications that must be treated to reduce likelihood of morbidity and mortality. Adolescents with eating disorders are at risk for significant growth retardation, pubertal delay, and reduction in bone mass. Medical complications generally reflect the weight control behavior used by the adolescent.

- Caloric restriction causes decreased metabolic rate, easy fatigability, hypothermia, cold intolerance, and irregular menstrual cycles or amenorrhea. Patients may exhibit lanugo-type hair growth. Cardiovascular complications may include bradycardia and other dysrhythmias, orthostatic hypotension, and syncope.
- Self-induced vomiting may result in dehydration, alkalosis, hypokalemia, esophagitis, salivary gland enlargement, dental enamel erosion, and subconjunctival hemorrhages.
- Laxative use may lead to dehydration, malabsorption, and abdominal cramping.
- Diuretic use may lead to dehydration and hypokalemia.

What Is the Prognosis for Eating Disorders?

Recent data indicate that 75% to 85% of adolescents with anorexia nervosa recover completely. Of those with bulimia nervosa, approximately 60% achieve a good outcome, with approximately 30% having an intermediate outcome.

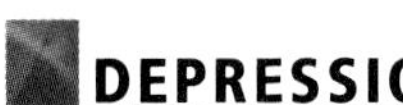

DEPRESSION

ETIOLOGY

How Common Is Depression in Adolescents?

In the Centers for Disease Control and Prevention's 2005 Youth Risk Behavior Survey, 28.5% of high school students reported feeling sad or hopeless, and 16.9% seriously considered attempting suicide, 13.0% made a suicide plan, and 8.4% had made a suicide attempt. Five percent to 9% of adolescents meet the DSM-IV criteria for major depressive disorder, and 3% to 8% meet the criteria for dysthymic disorder. Depressive disorders are diagnosed twice as often in adolescent women as in adolescent men.

EVALUATION

What Are the Diagnostic Criteria for Depression?

The DSM-IV outlines the diagnostic criteria for major depressive disorder and dysthymia. Major depressive disorder is usually associated with discrete episodes of more severe depression, which can be distinguished from the person's usual level of functioning. Dysthymic disorder is primarily a chronic disturbance of mood, involving a depressed or irritable mood for most days for at least 1 year in adolescents.

What Are the Signs and Symptoms of Depression?

The signs and symptoms of depressive disorders in adolescents are variable. Depressed adolescents often have physical complaints such as persistent fatigue, headaches, or abdominal pain. Useful screening questions for depression are "How are you sleeping?" and "How is your concentration?" If answers to these questions suggest problems, you should evaluate the adolescent for the possibility of depression.

Adolescents may present with any of the following symptoms and signs of depression:

- Feelings of being sad, blue, or "down in the dumps"
- Strong feelings of guilt, boredom, inadequacy, or hopelessness
- Loss of pleasure in daily activities
- Withdrawal from social activities at school or with friends
- Increase or decrease in activity level (depressed adolescent boys often engage in more frequent acting-out behavior such as fighting)
- Difficulty concentrating with reading or study, increased school absenteeism or truancy, poor or declining academic performance
- Use of alcohol or other drugs
- Somatic complaints
- Change in sleep or eating patterns
- Accident proneness

How Can I Evaluate for Depression?

A useful mnemonic to evaluate for depression is SIGECAPS:

*S*leep—initial/middle/terminal insomnia or hypersomnia
*I*nterests—decreased interest in usual activities
*G*uilt—feelings of guilt, dysphoria, irritability, or excessive moodiness
*E*nergy—decreased energy level
*C*oncentration—decreased ability to concentrate
*A*ppetite—decreased or increased appetite with associated weight loss or gain
*P*sychomotor retardation
*S*uicide—suicidal ideation

When Are Laboratory Tests Needed?

Laboratory tests are *not* routinely indicated in the evaluation of depression. If the adolescent has associated symptoms of hypothyroidism, such as weight gain, constipation, or temperature intolerance, a thyroid-stimulating hormone level may be indicated.

TREATMENT

How Do I Treat Depression?

The treatment of depression in an adolescent consists of education, counseling, and often medication. Families should be educated about the biologic basis and familial transmission of depressive disorders. They should be made aware of the signs and symptoms of depression. Counseling, although primarily directed toward the depressed adolescent, should involve the parents to ensure treatment success. Antidepressant drugs, such as selective serotonin reuptake inhibitors (SSRIs), are also often indicated. The use of medication is dictated by the severity of the presenting symptoms, the adolescent's willingness to take medication, and the parent's acceptance of the use of medication. Successful pharmacologic treatment should be maintained for at least 6 months and then be reassessed. Currently the FDA has a "black box" warning on the use of SSRIs in persons less than 18 years of age *(www.fda.gov/cder/drug/antidepressants/)*. The FDA recommends close follow-up of adolescents started on SSRIs because of a potential increased risk of suicidal thoughts with the initiation of SSRIs. The recurrence rate for depression in adolescents is 50% after the first episode, 70% after the second, and 90% after the third.

SUBSTANCE ABUSE

ETIOLOGY

What Drugs Do Adolescents Use Most Commonly?

Alcohol, tobacco, and marijuana are the three drugs most commonly used by adolescents. They are often referred to as "gateway drugs" because it is unusual for an adolescent to use other drugs without having used one of the gateway drugs first. Alcohol and tobacco use is legal for adults, making these two drugs readily available to adolescents.

How Do We Know What Drugs Adolescents Use?

Monitoring the Future, the long-term, ongoing study of the behaviors, attitudes, and values of American adolescents conducted by the University of Michigan's Institute for Social Research, reported in 2005 that 50% of adolescents have used an illicit drug by the time they leave high school. The proportion of high school seniors who have used any drug other than marijuana in their lifetime is 27%. Seventy-five percent of 12th graders, 63% of 10th graders, and 41% of 8th graders have used alcohol at least once. Fifty-eight percent of 12th graders, 42% of 10th graders, and 20% of 8th graders have been drunk at least once. Binge drinking, defined in this study as five or more drinks in one sitting within the past 2 weeks, is a pattern of alcohol consumption that is associated with adverse health outcomes. In 2005, 28% of 12th graders, 21% of 10th graders, and 10% of 8th graders admitted to binge drinking. With respect to cigarettes, 23% of 12th graders, 15% of 10th graders, and 9% of 8th graders admit to use within the past month. Forty-five percent of 12th graders, 34% of 10th graders, and 16% of 8th graders in 2005 had used marijuana at least once.

Do Adolescents Use Other Drugs?

Many other drugs used less frequently by adolescents are still of concern. "Club drugs" such as Ecstasy (3,4-methylenedioxymethamphetamine [MDMA]), gamma hydroxybutyrate (GHB), ketamine, and flunitrazepam (Rohypnol) are popular at nightclubs and all-night dance parties called "raves." Anabolic steroids are also a concern, especially among adolescent boys involved in bodybuilding, football, and wrestling. Methylphenidate has also become a drug of abuse. Adolescents crush the tablets and "snort" the powder. Most recently, there has been a rise in the use of prescription pain relievers such as OxyContin and Vicodin by adolescents. Clearly the problems of substance abuse remain widespread among American adolescents.

EVALUATION

How Does Substance Abuse by Adolescents Present?

Adolescents generally try to hide their use of alcohol and other drugs. Substance abuse by adolescents is suggested by the following:

- Poor school performance/attendance
- More pronounced mood swings than usual
- Recent change in friends, especially to older ones
- Increased interest in the drug culture
- Sloppy dress, poor grooming, and poor hygiene
- Rebellious or paranoid flavor to interpersonal relationships
- Symptoms of acute and/or chronic depression

- Unexplained or recurrent accidents and/or fights
- Runaway behavior
- Active lying
- Preoccupation with social activities at which alcohol and drugs might be present
- Overt episodes of intoxication and/or overdose
- Legal system involvement

How Can I Screen for Substance Abuse?

The CRAFFT questionnaire developed by Knight and associates (1999) is a quick screen for substance abuse in adolescents. It does not ask adolescents to reveal the quantity or frequency of their drug use but instead looks at the consequences of their drug use. *Two or more positive responses indicate a significant substance abuse problem,* and further evaluation is required.

C—Have you ever ridden in a *C*AR driven by someone (including yourself) who was "high" or had been using alcohol or drugs?
R—Do you ever use alcohol or drugs to *R*ELAX, feel better about yourself, or fit in?
A—Do you ever use alcohol or drugs while you are by yourself, ALONE?
F—Do you ever *F*ORGET things you did while using alcohol or drugs?
F—Does your family or do your *F*RIENDS ever tell you that you should cut down on your drinking or drug use?
T—Have you ever gotten into *T*ROUBLE while you were using alcohol or drugs?

When Should I Order a Drug Screen?

Drug testing for substances of abuse can be performed on blood, urine, or hair specimens. Urine is the most commonly used specimen. Each drug is detectable for a unique period of time in the urine. False-negative and false-positive drug screens do occur. Positive screening tests should be confirmed by a more specific test such as gas chromatography–mass spectrometry. It is important to remember that a positive test does not determine the extent of drug use. Similarly, a negative drug screen does not ensure that the adolescent is not using drugs. Drug testing is not a substitute for an assessment by a substance abuse professional.

Can I Obtain a Drug Screen without Consent?

The American Academy of Pediatrics Committee on Substance Abuse issued a policy statement titled "Testing for Drugs of Abuse in Children and Adolescents" in 1996. This policy states that involuntary testing is *not* appropriate in adolescents with decisional capacity, even with parental consent. A drug screen may be performed without the consent of the adolescent *only if there are strong medical or legal reasons.* Such reasons may include an adolescent with altered mental status presenting to the emergency department, an adolescent who is involved in the juvenile justice system, or an adolescent who is participating in a substance abuse treatment program.

TREATMENT

Can Substance Abuse Be Treated?

Treatment options available to the adolescent with substance abuse problems range from individual counseling for the adolescent who may have just begun experimenting with drugs to inpatient or residential treatment for the addicted adolescent. The spectrum of treatment options (from least to most restrictive) includes individual counseling, after-school or evening programming, day treatment, inpatient treatment, and residential treatment. Ongoing participation in an after-care program or a support group such as Alcoholics Anonymous or Narcotics Anonymous is essential for the maintenance of abstinence.

KEY POINTS

- Acne can be managed effectively for most adolescents without referral to a dermatologist.
- Eating disorders occur most commonly in adolescent women, but adolescent men also develop them.
- School failure, withdrawal from usual activities, disordered sleep, and vague physical complaints all may indicate depression.
- The "gateway drugs" used by adolescents are alcohol, tobacco, and marijuana.
- Drug testing should be performed only if the adolescent consents to it unless there are strong medical or legal reasons for testing.

Case 54-1

A 14-year-old boy expresses concerns about "zits" at a preparticipation sports examination. You note that he has moderate comedonal acne on his face, with a few inflamed nodules on his chest and shoulders.

A. What will you tell him and his parents about the cause of acne?
B. Describe a practical approach to acne management for this patient.
C. What would make you consider prescribing isotretinoin? If the patient were a girl, would you need to take any special precautions?

Case 54-2

A 14-year-old girl presents to the clinic with a 15-pound weight loss over the past 2 months. Her menstrual periods have become irregular, and she complains of frequent dizziness. Her mother states that she religiously does 100 sit-ups each day. She no longer eats meals with the rest of her family.

A. What is your differential diagnosis for this girl's weight loss?
B. What other behaviors that are related to weight control do you need to evaluate for this patient?

Case 54-3

Parents of a 16-year-old boy call for advice. Their son has had a decline in school performance during the second semester of his sophomore year in high school. He has become increasingly moody and complains of frequent headaches. He has missed nearly 1 month of school because of headaches and fatigue. He has also dropped out of soccer and has quit his music lessons.

A. What conditions could be the cause of his symptoms?
B. How can you distinguish depression from a physical disorder?
C. If you diagnose depression in an adolescent, what treatment options can you offer?

Case 54-4

A 17-year-old boy is brought to the emergency department by his parents after he came home late for his curfew with slurred speech and behaviors that were inappropriate. According to his parents, he could not answer questions appropriately. They discovered some drug paraphernalia in his coat pocket.

A. What questions would you ask the parents to identify possible signs and symptoms of substance abuse?
B. What drugs are the adolescent most likely to have used?
C. Is a drug screen indicated in this adolescent boy?
D. Do you need the adolescent's consent to perform the drug screen?

Case Answers

54-1 A. *Learning objective:* **Discuss the pathophysiology and clinical findings of acne.** Acne is caused by the obstruction of sebaceous follicles. It is aggravated by hormones produced at the time of puberty, as well as by the presence of skin bacteria. It can be aggravated by friction and by the use of oil-based cosmetics. Skin lesions can be inflammatory lesions, whiteheads, or blackheads.

54-1 B. *Learning objective:* **List major treatment methods for acne.** The initial approach is to use topical retinoids. Benzoyl peroxide and/or topical antibiotics, such as erythromycin, are added if the initial management does not provide adequate control. If acne worsens, a systemic antibiotic such as doxycycline could be added. Remember that all of these treatments increase sensitivity to sun, so remind the patient about regular use of sunblock.

54-1 C. *Learning objective:* **Recognize cystic acne, discuss its management, and recognize that adolescent girls must provide informed consent and use effective contraception if isotretinoin is prescribed.** Isotretinoin is indicated for the treatment of cystic acne or severe acne that is recalcitrant to other forms of treatment. Mandatory informed consent is now required for females who are treated with isotretinoin. They must have two negative pregnancy tests before starting the drug, must use two effective methods of contraception, and must have regular pregnancy tests during therapy. A dermatologist may be the best clinician to direct this treatment, but primary-care physicians must be aware of isotretinoin use and its potential impacts.

54-2 A. *Learning objective:* **Recognize eating disorders as a possible cause of weight loss in adolescents.** An eating disorder such as anorexia nervosa seems to be most likely, because the adolescent is engaged in ritualistic exercise and is avoiding eating meals with the rest of the family. The adolescent should be asked screening questions to rule out inflammatory bowel disease, diabetes mellitus, an unrecognized malignancy, or hyperthyroidism.

54-2 B. *Learning objective:* **Describe the signs and symptoms of eating disorders in adolescents.** Developmental issues, including the adolescent's drive for thinness and the importance of peer pressure and conformity should be considered as you evaluate the patient. Ask about use of diuretics, laxatives, emetics (such as syrup of ipecac), or diet pills. Inquire about binge eating and self-induced vomiting. Also remember to ask about mental health issues, including depression and anxiety.

54-3 A. *Learning objective:* **Identify depression as a cause of behavioral and physical symptoms in adolescents.** Depression, substance abuse, and infectious mononucleosis all can cause this constellation of findings.

54-3 B. *Learning objective:* **List the key findings that characterize depression in an adolescent.** A detailed history should be done to identify whether the patient feels sad or blue, has lost pleasure in daily activities, has developed a sleep disturbance (either excessive sleepiness or altered sleep patterns), has withdrawn from school or social activities, has difficulty concentrating or has had declining academic performance, or has vague but intrusive somatic complaints (such as headache, abdominal pain, joint aches). Irritability and worsening parent/adolescent relations can also be a clue to depression. It is crucial to identify suicidal ideation and to ask about any suicide attempts or gestures, now and in the past. Family history of depression is a key component of the evaluation.

54-3 C. *Learning objective:* **Discuss key management issues for the treatment of depression in adolescents.** Recognize the need for psychiatric referral. The key components in the treatment of adolescent depression include education of the patient and family, counseling to assist the individual and parents to cope with the behaviors, and medication (such as the selective serotonin reuptake inhibitors). Psychiatric referral may be needed.

54-4 A. *Learning objective:* **List the signs and symptoms of adolescent substance abuse.** Findings that suggest substance abuse include changes in appearance or friends, poor/declining academic performance, mood swings, unexplained/recurrent fights or accidents, and decreased compliance with rules at home. Parents may be able to provide answers to the CRAFFT questionnaire that is discussed in the chapter.

54-4 B. *Learning objective:* **Identify the three drugs most commonly used by adolescents.** Alcohol, tobacco, and marijuana are the three drugs most commonly used by adolescents.

54-4 C. *Learning objective:* **Identify the indications for performing a drug screen on an adolescent.** Yes, a drug screen is indicated because the adolescent is intoxicated and the substance is not known for certain.

54-4 D. *Learning objective:* **Discuss the legal and ethical issues related to drug testing in adolescents.** Permission/consent from the adolescent is not needed because at this time the patient lacks the capacity to make an informed decision. If the adolescent were not intoxicated, and there were no medical or legal imperatives to identify a substance, you should not perform a drug screen without the adolescent's consent, even if the parents request the test.

BIBLIOGRAPHY

American Academy of Pediatrics Committee on Substance Abuse: Testing for drugs of abuse in children and adolescents, *Pediatrics* 98:305, 1996.

American Psychiatric Association: *Diagnostic and statistical manual of medical disorders (revised)*, ed 4, Washington, DC, 1994, American Psychiatric Association.

Monitoring the Future. *www.monitoringthefuture.org.*

Knight JR et al: A new brief screen for adolescent substance abuse, *Arch Pediatr Adolesc Med* 153:591, 1999.

Zaenglin AL, Thiboutout DM: Expert committee recommendations for acne management. *Pediatrics* 118:1188, 2006.

55

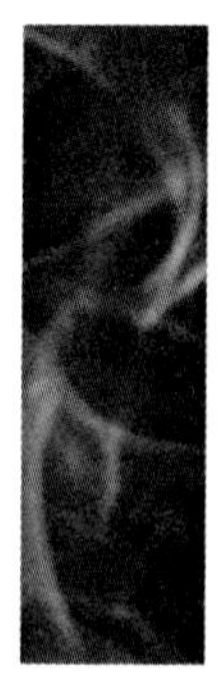

Behavior and Learning Disorders

STACEY McCONKEY and LINDA J. COOPER-BROWN

An individual who demonstrates a frequent, severe, persistent, and characteristic pattern of behavior that causes significant impairment of function is said to have a behavior disorder. Specific disorders discussed in this chapter include attention deficit hyperactivity disorder (ADHD), conduct disorder, and learning disorder. Attention deficit hyperactivity disorder is the most commonly diagnosed behavior disorder. Conduct disorder and learning disorders must be recognized in the primary-care office. Learning disorder is also discussed because it is commonly misidentified or overlooked. The diagnosis of behavioral, emotional, and learning disorders is discussed in detail in *The Classification of Child and Adolescent Mental Diagnoses in Primary Care: Diagnostic and Statistical Manual for Primary Care (DSM-PC)*.

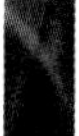

ATTENTION DEFICIT HYPERACTIVITY DISORDER

ETIOLOGY

What Is Attention Deficit Hyperactivity Disorder?

ADHD is a neurobehavioral disorder that occurs in 3% to 7% of school-aged children. The disorder is often suspected by parents, teachers, and other adults who work with children because of concerns about hyperactivity, inattentiveness, impulsivity, and poor progress in school. Behaviors such as anger and aggressiveness may also prompt concern, but these are not part of the ADHD spectrum. The physician's role is to ensure that the proper diagnosis has been made and that any other comorbid conditions are addressed. In addition, it is critical to monitor the child's response to treatment and tolerance of medical therapy, if that is prescribed.

EVALUATION

How Is Attention Deficit Hyperactivity Disorder Classified?

ADHD has three categories in the DSM-PC:

- **Inattentive-only type (ADHD IA)**—These children are primarily inattentive and tend to be noticed less often than children with overactive behavior. This form is often underdiagnosed, although it is the most common subtype in girls.
- **Hyperactive/impulsive (ADHD H/I)**—These children tend to be overactive and have problems with impulsivity but are able to focus on tasks. This is the least common form.
- **Combined type ADHD**—This is the most common form and demonstrates symptoms of hyperactivity, impulsivity, and inattentiveness.

How Do I Diagnosis Attention Deficit Hyperactivity Disorder?

In general, the diagnosis of ADHD should only be made in children after age 7 years, even when symptoms occur earlier. Age-appropriate development of young children often includes impulsive, inattentive, and highly energetic behaviors. A child suspected of having ADHD must demonstrate the behaviors listed in the DSM-IV criteria for one of the subtypes (Table 55-1). The concerning behaviors also must meet the following criteria:

- Occur to a greater degree than appropriate for age, gender, and cognitive ability

Table 55-1

DSM-IV Classification of Attention Deficit Hyperactivity Disorder (ADHD)

Inattentive Type ADHD IA Behaviors
Lack of attention
Rapidly shifting attention
Does not finish things
Shifts from one activity to another
Easily distracted
Very short attention span
Hyperactive/Impulsive Type ADHD H/I Behaviors
Can't sit still
Restless and fidgety
Talks constantly
Interrupts
Acts without thinking
Combined Type ADHD Behaviors
Combination of inattention, hyperactivity, and impulsiveness

Adapted from Wolraich M, editor: *Classification of child and adolescent mental diagnoses in primary care: diagnosis and statistical manual for primary care (DSM-PC)—child and adolescent version,* Elk Grove Village, IL, 1996, American Academy of Pediatrics, pp. 93-110.

- Have onset before age seven and persist
- Occur on a regular basis for more than 6 months
- Cannot be explained by another diagnosis

Of primary importance is that the symptoms must cause significant functional impairment that does not allow the child to perform up to full potential in *two different environments*. For most children, these environments are home and school. You should consider alternative diagnoses if symptoms are only present in one environment.

How Are Behaviors Identified and Documented?

Parent and teacher behavioral rating scales (such as the Vanderbilt or Connors scales) are very useful for collecting information. These scales ask the parent and teacher to identify a child's behaviors, including those commonly associated with ADHD. The frequency of behaviors can then be compared with age- and gender-specific norms to ascertain whether the child meets criteria for the various types of ADHD in all settings. Parents should make observations at home of daily activities, common family situations, and anything that seems to trigger a concerning behavior. The teacher who spends the most time with the child in school should fill out the forms. Often, school psychologists may have been consulted by teachers and can provide additional information.

What Other Problems Occur with Attention Deficit Hyperactivity Disorder?

ADHD occurs in approximately 50% of patients with conduct disorder. Children with learning disorders may be misdiagnosed as having ADHD. Children with ADHD occasionally manifest a variety of tics, and Tourette disorder may coexist with ADHD. A number of serious mental health problems, including substance abuse, autism, and major depression, may cause behaviors that resemble those of ADHD.

What Is the Medical Evaluation of Attention Deficit Hyperactivity Disorder?

The concerns identified by parents and teachers must be taken seriously and evaluated carefully. History must be comprehensive and must focus on the behavior, its patterns, triggers, and reinforcers. In addition, the environments in which problem behaviors occur must be identified (see Chapter 22). Growth, development, behavior, and the family, school, and social environments must be evaluated. Detailed past medical history and a thorough review of systems are also needed. The physical examination must focus on observed behaviors plus the details of all organ systems, especially neurologic findings. Laboratory testing, if any is needed, will be based on clinical suspicions. This approach should identify problems that mimic ADHD, including hyperthyroidism, absence seizures, hearing loss, and learning disorders.

Syndromes that are associated with increased frequency of ADHD, such as fragile X or fetal alcohol syndrome, must also be identified. You will use the information gathered from parents, teachers, and the medical evaluation to decide if one of the ADHD subtypes is a possible diagnosis and if referral to a psychologist is needed for further psychometric evaluation. If the diagnosis is clear from the evaluation, you will then decide whether medication is appropriate. Comorbid problems such as depression or tics may also be identified and require management.

TREATMENT

What Treatment Options Are Available for Attention Deficit Hyperactivity Disorder?

The goal of treatment is to improve a child's ability to function in the multiple environments in which learning occurs. Successful treatment includes the combination of behavioral management, family and teacher education, and selective use of medication. Behavioral management helps children improve their social skills and learning strategies both at home and at school. Parent and teacher education will ensure that a consistent approach will be taken in the home and school and will also counter the misinformation that abounds in public media and on the Internet. Medication should be viewed as an adjunct to behavioral and environmental management, not as a panacea. In addition, it is important that medical professionals serve as advocates for children with behavioral and other mental health problems in schools, communities, and society at large.

What Medications Are Used to Treat Attention Deficit Hyperactivity Disorder?

Stimulant medications such as methylphenidate (Ritalin, Concerta, Metadate) or dextroamphetamine (Dexedrine, Adderall) promptly improve attention, reduce impulsivity, and decrease activity level, all of which should improve performance during learning activities. These medications are available in short-, intermediate-, and long-acting forms, with duration of action ranging from 4 to 12 hours. Side effects such as appetite suppression, headaches, and sleep problems are usually related to medication dose and timing. Other nonstimulant medications such as atomoxetine (Strattera) and clonidine have been used with mixed success for ADHD and are not the first choice for treatment.

How Is Medication Therapy Managed?

Medication dose will generally be started at the low end of the dosing range, with adjustment upward made as school performance is monitored over time. Another approach used commonly when diagnosis and management are shared between a physician and a psychologist is to base the initial dose on results of psychometric testing done after a test dose of medication. It is important that ongoing monitoring uses parent and teacher observations, school grade reports, and objective measures of the ADHD characteristics, such as performance on psychometric tests and behavior rating forms. Frequent office visits will be needed to evaluate response to the medication, make adjustments to the dose, or even change the dosage form. Children with ADHD must be followed long-term to monitor growth, blood pressure, medication side effects, and school performance. This will increase the likelihood that medical and behavioral management will be effective.

CONDUCT DISORDER

ETIOLOGY

What Is Conduct Disorder?

Conduct disorder refers to severe antisocial behavior and is generally considered to have genetic, social, and environmental antecedents. Conduct disorder may occur as early as age 5 but usually is first identified in school-aged or adolescent children. Children with oppositional defiant disorder demonstrate less serious behaviors and have a better outcome than those with conduct disorder.

EVALUATION

What Behaviors Identify Conduct Disorder?

A child with conduct disorder demonstrates persistent *antisocial behavior* and often shows little concern for others. Behaviors that suggest conduct disorder include

- Aggressive behavior that harms or threatens to harm people or animals
- Destructive behavior that damages or destroys property
- Habitual lying
- Theft
- Skipping school or other serious violations of rules
- Deviant sexual behavior
- Substance abuse
- Habitual involvement with the legal system

The diagnosis must be made cautiously, especially in early childhood, because many behaviors that resemble conduct disorder reflect lack of supervision or lack of involvement by responsible adults in the lives of children and adolescents. For example, a 3-year-old child who starts a fire with a cigarette lighter that was left on the living room sofa by a parent does *not* have conduct disorder. Lack of supervision and parental irresponsibility led to the unfortunate outcome. Conversely, a 10-year-old child who repeatedly acts out in aggressive, impulsive, and destructive ways and who shows little remorse for his actions may have conduct disorder. Other problems that coexist in patients with conduct disorder include ADHD, anxiety, depression, academic difficulties, and problems with peer relationships.

TREATMENT

Can Conduct Disorder Be Treated?

Treatment must be directed at the specific behaviors and at any associated (comorbid) problems. The majority of children with conduct disorder have learning and reading problems and ADHD coexists in 50%. Such patients benefit from treatment with the stimulant medications that are used to treat ADHD. Special education programs in behavior disorder classes may be needed, along with behavior management plans for school and home. Some children may require medication to manage aggressive outbursts, but careful consideration should be given to possible medication side effects and long-term consequences. Every family will need services to help them with the multiple needs associated with conduct disorder and to prevent child abuse, which often occurs in families challenged by a child with conduct disorder. The range of services includes parent training, family therapy, training in problem-solving skills, and community-based services. Early intervention, adequate child-care services, and family treatment may prevent many cases of conduct disorder. Screening for domestic violence is also appropriate.

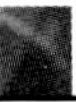

LEARNING DISORDER

ETIOLOGY

What Is a Learning Disorder?

Learning disorder reflects a discrepancy between achievement and ability and may be identified in 5% to 15% of school-aged children. A learning disorder should be suspected when achievement on an individually administered standardized test of reading, mathematics, or written expression is substantially below the level expected for age, gender, schooling, and level of intelligence. Learning disorders must be differentiated from the expected variations in academic achievement among otherwise developmentally appropriate children. In addition, academic difficulties unrelated to a learning disorder may result from lack of opportunity to learn, a mismatch between educational strategy and the child's learning style, and cultural factors. Children with delayed language development, those who were born prematurely, and those who have had head injury are at increased risk for learning disorders. Isolated problems with visual acuity, astigmatism, and hearing loss do *not* cause learning disorders. Children who have a variety of underlying emotional and behavioral problems or disorders may have problems with learning that do not represent learning disorders. Chronic illness may have a negative impact on learning that is not a learning disorder. Sudden deterioration in school performance may be caused by substance abuse or depression. Disorders that are occasionally comorbid with learning disorders include ADHD, depression, conduct/oppositional defiant disorder, mental retardation, and others.

EVALUATION

What Are the Signs and Symptoms of Learning Disorders?

Learning disorders manifest in many ways and are often misdiagnosed. A child with a learning disorder may have problems in specific academic subjects but may also appear to be inattentive, impulsive, and/or hyperactive, behaviors that are the hallmarks of ADHD. Conversely, a child with an emotional or behavioral disorder may have learning problems as the initial or even the most prominent manifestation of the underlying problem. Without careful assessment, the wrong diagnosis may be made and inappropriate treatment started. Learning disorders are thought to be related to underlying deficits in memory, language, and/or visual-spatial abilities. Children with memory deficits may have reading or math difficulties because they forget numbers, words, letters, or facts. Children with language deficits often have problems understanding directions or expressing themselves in written work. Children with visual-spatial deficits often are "clumsy," have poor handwriting, or messy homework, and they may have reading or writing problems related to letter or word reversals.

How Is a Learning Disorder Diagnosed?

The first concern about learning usually comes up during a health supervision visit when a child's progress in school is reviewed with parents. If school progress is not at expected levels for age, formal assessment should be recommended, either through the school system or with referral to a child psychologist experienced in learning issues. Physical examination must pay careful attention to the special senses, particularly vision and hearing, but a child with hearing loss or impaired vision should not be diagnosed with a learning disorder unless the learning difficulties exceed those expected with the deficit. Observation of the interaction between parent(s) and child; assessment of affect, mental status, and behavior; and a careful neurologic examination are also crucial components of the evaluation. You need to identify any underlying medical or emotional condition that causes or contributes to the achievement problems. Cognitive and neuropsychological testing by specialists will often identify the specific deficits and recommendations for treatment.

TREATMENT

How Is a Learning Disorder Treated?

Treatment must be based on the results of a comprehensive evaluation of the child's cognitive skills and deficits. Federal law mandates that public schools provide children with support services in the form of an "individualized learning plan" to address the learning problems. This generally includes specialized educational instruction and psychoemotional support services. Medications have no place in management of learning disorder, but comorbid conditions may require treatment. Correction of visual acuity problems and hearing deficits will enhance optimal learning but will not improve a learning disorder.

KEY POINTS

- Behavior disorders reflect the interaction among an individual child, genetic factors, and the social and physical environment.
- A child with ADHD demonstrates the characteristic behaviors in multiple environments.
- Conduct disorder must be diagnosed with care because behaviors may be caused by lack of supervision or involvement by responsible adults.
- Learning disorders may be mistaken for ADHD unless careful evaluation is performed.

Case 55-1

William is a 7-year-old boy in second grade. His mother is concerned because at school and in organized out-of-school activities William must often be reminded to pay attention, be quiet, and wait his turn. At school he will blurt out answers and has trouble sitting still. The teacher has suggested that William have an evaluation for ADHD. She states that he does not really have any problems at home.

A. What questions will you ask to evaluate the mother's concerns?
B. How can you determine if developmental or learning delays are causing his behaviors?
C. How should you proceed with an evaluation for William?

Case 55-2

Justin is a 12-year-old sixth grader who has been suspended from school. He has been removed from the bus for fighting on several occasions this school year, and yesterday he injured another child on the playground. His father says that Justin started a fire at home last month and has to be carefully supervised.

A. What further information do you need to make the diagnosis of conduct disorder?
B. What recommendations will you make for management of Justin's behavior?

Case Answers

55-1 A. *Learning objective:* **Use the history to identify possible attention deficit hyperactivity disorder (ADHD); recognize the genetic characteristics of ADHD.** You should ask how old William was when these problems were first noted. Details of the behaviors should be sought from observers, including parents, teachers, and coaches. A behavior checklist may identify behaviors at home that are being overlooked by parents but that suggest ADHD. Family history can also help, so ask if parents, siblings, or other relatives have had similar problems.

55-1 B. *Learning objective:* **Identify developmental, congenital, and mental health conditions that have a high risk of ADHD.** Physical examination will detect many congenital abnormalities that are associated with mental retardation and will also detect neurologic deficits. Ask for evidence to document performance in school and other activities, such as report cards or results of any testing done at school. You would anticipate that a child with ADHD would be easily distracted, would have difficulty with impulse control, and would have excessive physical activity. Teacher reports can identify such behaviors and can also inform you whether the child is keeping up with school work.

55-1 C. *Learning objective:* **Discuss the evaluation of a child suspected of ADHD.** Gather more information from the teacher, including structured questionnaires such as the Connor Rating Scale. Recommend that the school psychologist or other educational specialist evaluate William at his school. If this evaluation cannot be done, referral to a pediatric psychologist knowledgeable in diagnosis of ADHD is indicated.

55-2 A. *Learning objective:* **Describe the features of conduct disorder and distinguish it from other common behavior disorders.** You must determine whether Justin has any other problems with behavior or learning, including comorbid conditions such as ADHD and oppositional defiant disorder (noncompliant and uncooperative). Find out about other behaviors including theft, abuse of animals, and destruction of property. You also must determine if Justin ever had been arrested, intoxicated, or uses tobacco or other substances. Identify the make-up of his peer group. Inquire about the family: Are there financial or other stressors? Is the family intact? Has anyone had trouble with the law? Is substance abuse a concern? Who supervises Justin when he comes home from school? Ask specifically about behaviors of siblings and parents.

55-2 B. *Learning objective:* **Discuss management of a patient with conduct disorder.** Referral to a child psychologist or psychiatrist will be beneficial in this case. Comorbid conditions such as ADHD should be treated, which may improve overall behavior. The family will need support and counseling, but you must also recognize the possibility that the family may be a major factor in causing the patient's behavior. The school has an important role in providing an educational program directed at the patient's abilities. Behavior management plans will be beneficial both in school and in the home. Ensuring adequate supervision is important. Legal authorities may already be involved, and foster care may be needed.

BIBLIOGRAPHY

American Academy of Pediatrics: *Caring for children with ADHD: A resource toolkit for clinicians*, 2002, Elk Grove Village, IL, AAP.

American Academy of Pediatrics, Committee on Psychosocial Aspects of Child and Family Health: The new morbidity revisited: a renewed commitment to the psychosocial aspects of pediatric care, *Pediatrics* 108:1227, 2001.

Fact Sheet: Caring for every child's mental health, Washington, DC, CMHS National Mental Health Knowledge Exchange Network, 2000. Available at: *www.mentalhealth.org/child/*. Individual fact sheets include the following: (1) Mental, Emotional, and Behavior Disorders in Children and Adolescents; (2) Attention Deficit/Hyperactivity Disorder in Children and Adolescents; (3) Conduct Disorder; (4) Major Depression in Children and Adolescents; (5) Autism in Children and Adolescents.

Reiff MI, editor: *ADHD: a complete and authoritative guide*, 2004, AAP.

Wolraich M, editor: *Classification of child and adolescent mental diagnoses in primary care: diagnosis and statistical manual for primary care (DSM-PC)—child and adolescent version*, Elk Grove Village, IL, 1996, American Academy of Pediatrics.

56

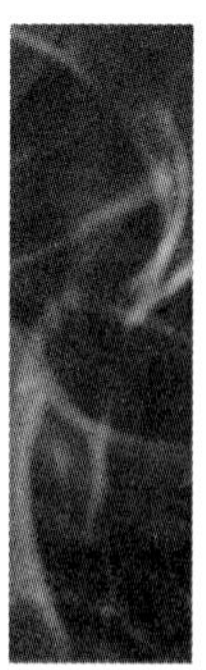

Cardiology

NORMAN B. BERMAN

VENTRICULAR SEPTAL DEFECT

ETIOLOGY

What Is a Ventricular Septal Defect?

Ventricular septal defect (VSD) is the most common congenital heart defect. Most VSDs are small, do not cause any cardiac symptoms, and eventually close spontaneously. Large VSDs are clinically more problematic, however, because the high-volume left-to-right shunt causes increased pulmonary blood flow, increased pulmonary venous return, and left ventricular volume overload. The volume overload causes congestive heart failure (CHF), which presents in infants with increased respiratory rate and effort, diaphoresis, difficulty feeding, and poor weight gain (failure to thrive). If a large VSD is untreated, the chronically increased pulmonary artery pressures eventually cause increased pulmonary vascular resistance and progressive cyanosis (Eisenmenger's syndrome).

EVALUATION

What Do I Need to Look for in an Infant with a Ventricular Septal Defect?

Always look for signs of CHF. Ask about the specifics of feeding: how much the infant takes, how long each feeding takes, if respiratory distress occurs during feeding, or if other feeding difficulties occur. An infant with a VSD should not be cyanotic, but this is still a good issue to ask about. The growth chart should be carefully plotted, with particular attention to the weight curve, because poor feeding may manifest as a falloff in weight gain. On physical examination, it is most important to observe the infant's work of breathing: respiratory rate, chest wall excursion, use of accessory muscles, and retractions. Hepatomegaly is common in infants with CHF, with the liver edge usually more than 2 cm below the right costal margin. Crackles (rales) are not commonly heard on auscultation of the lungs in infants with CHF. Jugular venous distention and peripheral edema, common signs of CHF in adults, are rarely seen in infants with CHF. A large VSD will typically cause a loud, harsh, holosystolic murmur, but the intensity of the murmur does not correlate well with the size of the VSD or the presence of CHF.

What Studies Are Needed to Diagnose Ventricular Septal Defect?

The most important problems to assess are growth and signs of CHF—no diagnostic studies are needed to make this assessment. CHF is a clinical diagnosis; it cannot be diagnosed by electrocardiogram (ECG), chest radiograph, or echocardiogram. The chest radiograph may be helpful to assess heart size, pulmonary blood flow, or the presence of pneumonia in a child with respiratory symptoms that are not clearly CHF. The ECG may demonstrate left or right ventricular hypertrophy, and this may help in the overall assessment of the infant's hemodynamic state. Echocardiography is essential for the initial diagnosis of the VSD but does not really aid day-to-day management.

TREATMENT

What Treatment Is Needed for an Infant with Ventricular Septal Defect?

Small VSDs almost all close spontaneously and thus require no specific therapy. Larger VSDs that cause CHF can be managed medically, and many of these defects will become smaller with time as well. Medical management consists primarily of digoxin and diuretics (furosemide). If CHF and failure to thrive do not improve with medical management, open-heart surgery to close the VSD will be required. Large VSDs resulting in pulmonary hypertension also require surgical closure. Overall, the prognosis of infants with a VSD is excellent, even if surgical closure is needed. Antibiotic prophylaxis to prevent subacute bacterial endocarditis (SEB) is no longer recommended for a VSD.

ATRIAL SEPTAL DEFECT

ETIOLOGY

What Is an Atrial Septal Defect?

Atrial septal defect (ASD) is common, with isolated ASDs accounting for approximately 5% of all congenital heart defects. An ASD can also be present in association with more complex heart defects. Most ASDs are located in the region of the foramen ovale (secundum ASD). Less commonly, ASDs can be close to the atrioventricular valves (primum ASD) or the superior vena cava (sinus venosus ASD). All types of ASD cause left-to-right shunting from left atrium to right atrium, increased pulmonary blood flow, and right ventricular volume overload. Isolated ASDs rarely cause symptoms in children but will often result in symptomatic right heart failure in adults if not corrected.

EVALUATION

What Do I Need to Look for in a Child with an Atrial Septal Defect?

A child with an ASD typically presents at a few years of age with an asymptomatic heart murmur that may not have been noticed previously. Symptoms, if present, are caused by the increased pulmonary blood flow and will most likely manifest as shortness of breath with exertion or as respiratory infections that are more frequent or more severe than expected. Symptomatic infants typically have failure to thrive.

What Findings Should Make Me Suspect an Atrial Septal Defect?

The murmur in a child with an ASD is caused by the increased pulmonary blood flow. This pulmonary flow murmur can be very subtle and unimpressive, or it may be obvious. Wide, fixed splitting of the second heart sound is the pathognomonic finding of an ASD but may be difficult to appreciate. Wide, fixed splitting occurs because increased pulmonary blood flow causes delayed pulmonic valve closure.

What ECG Findings Are Characteristic of Atrial Septal Defect?

The ECG is almost always abnormal in children with a significant ASD, making this a valuable tool for assessing any asymptomatic heart murmur. ECG findings of an ASD include right axis deviation, right atrial enlargement, and right ventricular hypertrophy with a right ventricular volume overload pattern (rsR′ in V_1).

Are Other Diagnostic Studies Needed?

The diagnosis of an ASD can be strongly suspected based on physical examination and ECG. When ASD is suspected it should be confirmed by echocardiography.

TREATMENT

What Treatment Is Required for an Atrial Septal Defect?

A clinically apparent ASD is likely large enough to cause significant right ventricular volume overload and thus to require closure. Surgery is typically delayed until 3 to 5 years of age because some ASDs will spontaneously diminish in size and thus may not require closure. Although most ASDs often require open-heart surgery, some can be closed by a device delivered via catheterization. In either case the long-term prognosis is excellent. Antibiotic prophylaxis to prevent SEB is *not* recommended for ASDs.

TETRALOGY OF FALLOT

ETIOLOGY

What Is Tetralogy of Fallot?

Tetralogy of Fallot (TOF) is the most common *cyanotic* congenital heart defect. The four components of the tetralogy are VSD, aortic override, pulmonic stenosis, and right ventricular hypertrophy. Cyanosis is the most important clinical finding and develops when the VSD and right ventricular outflow obstruction combine to cause right-to-left shunting through the VSD.

EVALUATION

What Do I Need to Look for in an Infant with Tetralogy of Fallot?

Infants with TOF may have cyanosis at birth but may also be acyanotic and develop cyanosis weeks to months later. Look for presence and/or degree of cyanosis on physical examination. Pulse oximetry will detect oxygen desaturation, which, when mild, can be subtle or even impossible to detect by physical examination alone. An infant with oxygen saturation above 85% may appear acyanotic, particularly to an untrained observer. Essentially all infants with TOF have a heart murmur caused by the right ventricular outflow tract obstruction, but the murmur is not a reliable indicator of the severity of the obstruction.

What Complications Occur in an Infant with Tetralogy of Fallot?

Hypercyanotic spells, also called "tet spells," can occur in infants with TOF before surgical correction. Classically, the infant's crying triggers these spells because crying causes increased systemic venous return to the right ventricle, which has a fixed outflow obstruction. This increased volume cannot get past the right ventricular obstruction, so the deoxygenated blood shunts from right to left through the VSD and into the systemic arterial circulation, causing increased cyanosis. Tet spells can be life threatening and thus require emergency treatment. Other complications of TOF, rarely seen now with early surgical correction, include polycythemia, stroke, and brain abscess.

What Diagnostic Studies Are Needed?

Oxygen saturation obtained by pulse oximetry is the most important information for an infant with TOF. An ECG will show evidence of right ventricular hypertrophy, but this is not particularly helpful in management. A chest radiograph may show the characteristic boot-shaped heart but does not really aid in managing the infant. Echocardiography is essential in the diagnosis of TOF but is not part of the routine management performed by the pediatrician.

TREATMENT

What Treatment Is Required for an Infant with Tetralogy of Fallot?

Infants with TOF undergo surgical correction of the defect by 6 months of age in most centers, sooner if the infant becomes progressively cyanotic. The repair includes patch closure of the VSD and resection of the right ventricular outflow tract obstruction that causes right-to-left shunting and cyanosis. The prognosis for infants with TOF is excellent, despite the need for surgical intervention. Antibiotic prophylaxis to prevent SEB is recommended TOF before repair and may be needed after repair.

COARCTATION OF THE AORTA

ETIOLOGY

What Is Coarctation of the Aorta?

Coarctation of the aorta is a narrowing in the proximal descending aorta just distal to the origin of the left subclavian artery. The obstruction limits descending aortic flow and causes elevated blood pressure proximal to the obstruction. This can lead to systemic hypertension in the upper body and decreased perfusion in the lower body. Coarctation of the aorta may present in very different ways, depending on the age of the child and the severity of the obstruction. Newborns with severe coarctation may develop CHF or shock because of inadequate cardiac output to the lower body and kidneys. Milder coarctation may go undetected for many years, and older children with coarctation may develop systemic hypertension as a result. Girls with Turner's syndrome have a high incidence of coarctation.

EVALUATION

What Findings Suggest Coarctation in a Newborn?

It is important to assess for any discrepancy between the upper and lower extremity pulses in children at any age and especially in newborns. Diminished femoral pulses strongly suggest the presence of a coarctation. In newborns, coarctation of the aorta can be difficult to detect clinically in the presence of a patent ductus arteriosus: flow through the ductus arteriosus can bypass the obstruction and can make the coarctation clinically inapparent. When the ductus arteriosus closes, a severe coarctation will present as congestive heart failure or shock. A mild coarctation may not cause an appreciable decrease in femoral pulses, and the only finding may be a murmur noted predominantly in the back.

What Findings Suggest Coarctation in an Older Child?

Coarctation is unlikely to cause symptoms beyond infancy and can easily escape detection if blood pressures and pulses are not assessed.

Blood pressure measurements are difficult in infants but should be part of routine health supervision starting at 3 years of age. The presence of systemic hypertension in a child should raise suspicion of a coarctation and should prompt careful auscultation for the presence of a heart murmur and careful examination of the femoral pulses.

TREATMENT

How Is Coarctation of the Aorta Treated?

Coarctation of the aorta requires intervention to relieve the obstruction if it is severe enough to cause clinical symptoms or if systemic hypertension develops. In most centers, coarctation is still repaired surgically by resecting the coarctation and reanastomosing the aorta end to end. Some centers perform balloon dilation of the coarctation using interventional catheterization techniques. It is important to monitor the femoral pulses and blood pressure regularly in children with known coarctation. After surgical repair, a recurrent coarctation may develop, manifested by a return of decreased femoral pulses, systemic hypertension, or a discrepancy between upper and lower extremity blood pressures. Antibiotic prophylaxis to prevent SEB is no longer recommended for children with coarctation of the aorta.

How Is Coarctation-Associated Hypertension Treated?

Hypertension results from obstruction of the descending aorta, so it must be treated by removal of the obstruction. It is not appropriate to treat the upper extremity systemic hypertension caused by an unrepaired coarctation with antihypertensive medications. This will lower the blood pressure both proximal and distal to the coarctation and can result in hypoperfusion of the kidneys and renal failure. The prognosis for children with repaired coarctation is generally excellent unless coarctation is diagnosed late and systemic hypertension has already been present for many years. In such a scenario, the child may be left with chronic systemic hypertension despite adequate surgical relief of the coarctation. Antihypertensive medications will be needed.

POSTOPERATIVE CARDIAC PATIENTS

ETIOLOGY

What Surgical Procedures Might I Encounter?

The most common procedures you may encounter include surgical repair of ASD, VSD, coarctation of the aorta, and TOF. Other complex defects are less common, but collectively they account for a significant percentage of children having surgery for congenital heart disease. The Fontan operation is performed for several different types of complex heart defects. The Blalock-Taussig shunt is less commonly done now than it was 10 to 20 years ago, but it remains an important operation for specific cyanotic heart defects.

What Is the Fontan Operation?

The Fontan operation is a complex palliative procedure used for patients with a variety of congenital heart defects that have only a single ventricle (tricuspid atresia, hypoplastic left heart syndrome, and others). The operation has been modified many times over the last 30 years and is performed in different ways in different centers. Ultimately, the Fontan operation directs systemic venous return to the pulmonary arteries without using a ventricle to pump blood to the pulmonary circuit. Despite the complexity of the resulting hemodynamics, the Fontan operation is generally successful and most patients do well for many years. There is, however, a significant long-term risk for atrial arrhythmias. Exercise tolerance is generally good but less than that of the child's peers.

What Is a Blalock-Taussig Shunt?

The Blalock-Taussig shunt is a connection from the systemic arterial system to the pulmonary artery, most commonly from the right subclavian artery to the right pulmonary artery. The operation is performed to increase pulmonary blood flow in patients with cyanotic heart defects that cause decreased pulmonary blood flow, such as TOF and tricuspid atresia. Originally, this was a direct anastomosis of the right subclavian artery to the right pulmonary artery, but now this connection is performed with a Gore-Tex tube. The Blalock-Taussig shunt was the first operation performed to palliate patients with cyanotic heart defects, and its development led to the growth of the field of pediatric cardiology. The Blalock-Taussig shunt is performed less because many defects are frequently more completely repaired earlier in life in ways that do not require a shunt.

EVALUATION

What Do I Look for if a Child Has Had Heart Surgery?

First, you must find out the nature of the congenital defect for which surgical repair was performed and whether the surgery was recent. In the 2 to 3 weeks after surgery, operative complications are an important concern. Post-pericardiotomy syndrome is more common in older children after surgery and leads to a large pericardial effusion. This can present as vomiting or respiratory symptoms, usually with low-grade fever. Knowing the natural history of the repaired congenital heart defects will assist you to anticipate problems. A general assessment of the child's health is always important. Most children with repaired congenital heart defects are expected to be as healthy and active as their peers; some, however, may have persistent heart murmurs, cyanosis, or limitations to activity. Exercise tolerance is important to assess because decreased exercise tolerance, shortness of breath with exertion, and syncope are the most common symptoms of ongoing hemodynamic abnormalities.

Do Heart Murmurs Persist after Surgical Repair?

Many children will continue to have heart murmurs after successful repair of their heart defects. It is important to try to assess the murmur for any changes over time. The presence of a diastolic murmur that was not noted previously can be significant and suggests new valvular regurgitation.

Does Cyanosis Persist?

Most patients with repaired cyanotic defects should be acyanotic after repair, with oxygen saturation greater than 95%. Persistent cyanosis or low oxygen saturation may be an indicator of a problem with the repair.

How Common Are Arrhythmias after Repair?

Significant arrhythmias occur in approximately 5% of patients who have had open-heart surgery, and most occur many years after surgery. Most congenital heart defects are repaired through an atrial incision, and thus these patients are at risk for developing atrial arrhythmias. Atrial tachycardia, atrial flutter, and atrial fibrillation all can occur following heart surgery. Any ventricular incision adds to the risk of ventricular arrhythmias, such as premature ventricular contractions and ventricular tachycardia.

TREATMENT

How Is a Child Managed after Surgical Repair?

The pediatrician will manage general health and the pediatric cardiologist will manage heart-related problems.

- *Antibiotic prophylaxis* to prevent SEB. Evidence shows that prophylaxis before dental or surgical procedures does *not* prevent SBE reliably. New (2007) guidelines recommend SBE prophylaxis *only* for patients with cyanotic cardiac defects, during the six-month period after surgical repair, and when a residual defect persists at the site of prosthetic material after surgical repair.
- *Physical activity.* Most children with repaired congenital heart defects can participate in sports or other activities without restriction. Activity restrictions may be recommended if a defect places the child at risk for ischemia or sudden death.

KEY POINTS

- ◆ The murmur of a VSD may be harsh or blowing, but the intensity of the murmur does not correlate with the size of the defect.
- ◆ Congestive heart failure is a common presentation of VSD in infancy.

- Listen carefully to the second heart sound: a wide, fixed split S_2 signifies ASD.
- Hypercyanotic spells in infants with tetralogy of Fallot can be life-threatening.
- Absent femoral pulses or unexplained hypertension may indicate coarctation of the aorta.

Case 56-1

A 2-week-old infant presents with a history of feeding difficulties and mild respiratory distress. On physical examination, the infant is tachypneic with increased work of breathing and has a loud systolic murmur that was not noted in the newborn nursery. The liver edge is palpated 3 cm below the right costal margin.

A. What is the most likely cause of this infant's clinical findings?
B. Why was a murmur not heard at birth or in early infancy?

Case 56-2

At a routine health supervision visit for a 3-year-old child, you detect a systolic murmur that you had not heard previously. In addition, the cardiac examination demonstrates a right ventricular impulse in the precordium and a widely split second heart sound. An electrocardiogram demonstrates right ventricular hypertrophy.

A. What is the likely cause of the infant's murmur?
B. Why does an ASD cause a systolic heart murmur?

Case 56-3

Parents of a 2-month-old infant bring him for evaluation because he appears blue when he cries. His color at other times is fine, and he is feeding and growing well. He has had a heart murmur since he was a newborn.

A. What is the most likely cause of this infant's cyanosis?
B. What causes the cyanosis in TOF?

Case 56-4

A 5-year-old child is noted to be hypertensive at a routine health supervision visit. Blood pressure in the right arm is 124/78 mm Hg, which is above the 95th percentile for age and size. In retrospect, blood pressures were above the 90th percentile for age at the previous two health supervision visits. In addition, you hear a heart murmur that is most prominent in the back. The femoral pulses are diminished compared with the brachial pulses.

A. What is the most likely cause of this patient's findings?
B. What are the most important physical examination findings in coarctation of the aorta?

Case 56-5

An 8-year-old girl had surgical repair of an atrial septal defect 10 days ago, and the mother calls to report that the child has a fever to 101° F, vomited 3 times in the last hour, and is having difficulty breathing.

A. What is the likely cause of the child's symptoms?

Case Answers

56-1 A. *Learning objective:* **Identify ventricular septal defect in infancy.** This is a typical presentation of an infant with congestive heart failure from a ventricular septal defect. History identifies poor feeding and rapid, labored breathing. Examination finds poor weight gain, a loud, harsh systolic murmur, and hepatomegaly.

56-1 B. *Learning objective:* **Discuss the pathophysiology of ventricular septal defect.** The murmur was not noted initially because newborn infants have elevated pulmonary vascular resistance. There is, therefore, little left-to-right shunting in a newborn with a ventricular septal defect. The shunt increases and the murmur appears as pulmonary vascular resistance decreases during the first few weeks after birth.

56-2 A. *Learning objective:* **Identify the clinical features of atrial septal defect.** This is the classic presentation of an atrial septal defect. Findings include a systolic murmur with a fixed, widely split second heart sound and evidence of right ventricular overload (right ventricular impulse and electrocardiographic changes).

56-2 B. *Learning objective:* **Discuss the cause of the murmur in atrial septal defect.** The murmur is caused by increased blood flow in the pulmonary outflow tract that results from the left-to-right shunt. The murmur is not caused by blood flow across the atrial septal defect.

56-3 A. *Learning objective:* **List the common heart diseases that produce cyanosis in infancy.** TOF is the most common cyanotic congenital heart defect. Cyanosis may not be present at birth but often develops in the first month or two of life. This presentation is not specific to TOF. The other common cyanotic heart defects are transposition of the great arteries, tricuspid atresia, truncus arteriosus, and total anomalous pulmonary venous return (note that these defects all begin the letter "T" and are often referred to as the 5 T's of cyanotic heart disease). It is very important to know that mild cyanosis can be difficult to recognize on examination, so pulse oximetry is critical whenever there is a question about possible cyanosis.

56-3 B. *Learning objective:* **Discuss the pathophysiology of cyanosis in congenital heart disease.** Cyanosis occurs in TOF because the large ventricular septal defect, in combination with right ventricular outflow tract obstruction, leads to right-to-left shunting through the defect. The desaturated blood that enters the arterial circulation causes the cyanosis.

56-4 A. *Learning objective:* **Identify hypertension in children and list common cardiac causes.** Hypertension in a child should prompt an evaluation for coarctation of the aorta, which is usually asymptomatic.

56-4 B. *Learning objective:* **Identify the physical findings that are commonly found in patients with coarctation of the aorta.** Diminished or absent femoral pulses, a systolic heart murmur, and blood pressure elevation in the upper extremities are the common findings in coarctation of the aorta. In addition, the prominence of the murmur in the back further supports the diagnosis of coarctation.

56-5 A. *Learning objective:* **Identify the presenting signs of post-pericardiotomy syndrome.** Post-pericardiotomy syndrome typically presents 10 to 14 days after open-heart surgery as vomiting or respiratory symptoms, usually with low-grade fever.

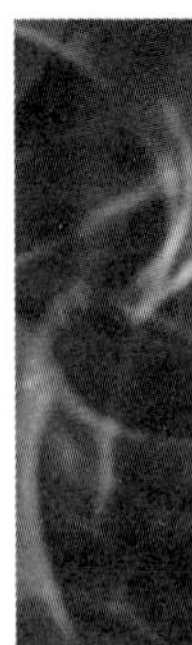

57 Dermatology

DANIEL P. KROWCHUK

Skin conditions are common in pediatrics. This chapter presents an introductory discussion of dermatitis, diaper rashes, cutaneous infections, infestations, papulosquamous disorders, and childhood exanthems. A discussion of acne and its treatment is included in Chapter 54. Clinical photographs are available in electronic atlases (e.g., the Johns Hopkins University Dermatlas, *http://dermatlas.med.jhmi.edu/derm/index.cfm*) or standard textbooks (see References at the end of this chapter).

DERMATITIS

ATOPIC DERMATITIS

ETIOLOGY

What Is Atopic Dermatitis?

Atopic dermatitis is the most common chronic pediatric skin disorder. It generally begins during infancy or childhood; 90% of affected patients present before 5 years of age. The diagnosis is made clinically, based on the presence of three or more of the following: typical morphology and distribution of lesions, pruritus, chronic relapsing course, and a family or personal history of atopic disorders.

EVALUATION

How Do I Recognize Atopic Dermatitis?

The appearance of lesions varies with age and racial background. Infants and toddlers, for example, often have involvement of the face, trunk, and extremities. During childhood, lesions are concentrated in flexural areas, such as the antecubital and popliteal fossae, wrists, and ankles. Adolescents exhibit flexural involvement but often develop lesions on the hands, face, and neck. In light-colored skin, lesions are erythematous, somewhat scaly or crusted papules, patches, or thin plaques. In contrast, in skin of color, erythema is less obvious, and lesions may appear gray. In addition, the eruption is more papular, and postinflammatory hypopigmentation or hyperpigmentation may be present.

TREATMENT

How Is Atopic Dermatitis Treated?

Although there is no cure, most patients can be managed effectively with the measures outlined in Boxes 57-1 and 57-2.

BOX 57-1

DAILY MEASURES TO CONTROL ATOPIC DERMATITIS

Control Pruritus

- Apply an emollient as needed. Lotions work well, but ointments are the best moisturizers (often not well tolerated because of greasy feel).
- Use a mild, unscented soap or soap substitute for bathing.
- Use an additive-free detergent for laundering clothes.
- To the extent possible, wear cotton clothing next to the skin.
- Avoid bathing in very hot water.

Hydrate the Skin

- Apply an emollient as needed, especially after bathing.
- Limit the frequency of bathing.

BOX 57-2

WHEN ATOPIC DERMATITIS FLARES

Reduce Inflammation

- Apply a topical corticosteroid twice daily as needed.
  - Face (any age): low-potency (e.g., hydrocortisone cream 1% or 2.5%).
  - Infants (except the face): low-potency (as above).
  - Children (except the face): low-potency (as above) or, if needed, mid-potency (e.g., triamcinolone cream 0.025%).
  - Adolescents (except the face): mid-potency (e.g., triamcinolone cream 0.1%).
- Apply a topical calcineurin inhibitor (e.g., pimecrolimus, tacrolimus) if there is no response to topical corticosteroids.

Control Pruritus

- Use antihistamine at bedtime (e.g., hydroxyzine, 1 mg/kg/dose).

Control Infection

- If there is crusting or oozing, consider an oral antistaphylococcal antibiotic (e.g., cephalexin).

CONTACT DERMATITIS

ETIOLOGY

What Is Contact Dermatitis?

Contact dermatitis occurs when an antigen penetrates the epidermis and sensitizes T lymphocytes. On reexposure to the antigen, sensitized T lymphocytes release cytokines that produce an inflammatory response, usually within 12 to 24 hours. Most often, contact dermatitis in pediatric patients results from exposure to plant allergens. Other allergens include nickel (present in jewelry, belt buckles, and clothing snaps), potassium dichromate (present in some shoes), neomycin, thimerosal, or formaldehyde (used in topical medications) or balsam of Peru or other fragrances (used in perfumes or soaps).

EVALUATION

What Are the Signs of Contact Dermatitis?

Potent antigens, such as urushiol (present in poison ivy, oak, or sumac), typically cause an acute dermatitis that consists of vesicles, bullae, erythematous papules, and edema. New lesions continue to appear for several days. If untreated, the dermatitis may persist for 3 to 4 weeks. Weaker antigens (e.g., nickel) produce a subacute dermatitis characterized by erythema, scaling, and lichenification. The key to recognizing contact dermatitis is the observation that the eruption is limited to certain areas. Linear vesicles or bullae on exposed surfaces suggest exposure to plant allergens. Nickel dermatitis occurs at sites of contact with jewelry or below the umbilicus where there is contact with a belt buckle or clothing snap. An eruption on the dorsa of the feet raises suspicion of shoe dermatitis.

TREATMENT

How Is Contact Dermatitis Treated?

For a patient with localized dermatitis involving areas other than the face, a mid-potency topical corticosteroid (e.g., triamcinolone acetonide 0.1% or fluocinolone acetonide 0.01%) may be applied twice daily; low-potency preparations (e.g., hydrocortisone 1%) are ineffective. However, when more than 10% to 15% of the body surface is involved, as may occur in plant dermatitis, oral prednisone may be required. An initial dose of 1 mg/kg may be administered once daily, then tapered by

20% to 25% every 3 days to complete a 12- to 21-day course. Discontinuing therapy earlier may result in a return of symptoms. Other treatments also may be beneficial. When vesicles rupture, drying can be promoted by taking tepid baths or applying cool compresses or shake lotions (e.g., calamine). An oral antihistamine provides sedation that offers relief from itching. Topical anesthetics containing benzocaine and topical antihistamines (e.g., diphenhydramine) are best avoided because they may induce a contact dermatitis.

How Is Contact Dermatitis Prevented?

Prevention of further episodes is important. Those who have experienced plant dermatitis should learn to recognize and avoid poison ivy, sumac, and oak. When exposure may be unavoidable (e.g., during hikes or camping trips), wearing protective clothing or applying a barrier preparation, such as Ivy Block, may be useful. For those with nickel allergy, avoiding jewelry containing the metal is important. Patients who wear earrings, for example, are advised to use varieties with solid gold or surgical stainless-steel posts. Clothing snaps may be painted with clear nail polish or covered with cloth tape.

SEBORRHEIC DERMATITIS

ETIOLOGY

What Is Seborrheic Dermatitis?

Seborrheic dermatitis is an inflammatory disorder of the skin that involves areas of the body where sebaceous glands are concentrated. The cause is unknown, but the inflammatory response is dependent on the presence of the yeast *Pityrosporum ovale.* It occurs at times when sebaceous glands are most active (e.g., in infants until age 9 to 12 months and during adolescence).

EVALUATION

How Do I Recognize Seborrheic Dermatitis?

In infants, seborrheic dermatitis causes scaling of the scalp ("cradle cap") or salmon-pink scaling patches concentrated in skin folds (e.g., retroauricular and axillary) and the diaper area. Adolescents and adults experience scaling of the scalp ("dandruff") or erythematous, scaling patches in the eyebrows, behind the ears, and in the nasolabial folds.

TREATMENT

How Is Seborrheic Dermatitis Treated?

The site involved determines the type of treatment. In infants with cradle cap, shampooing, during which the scalp is scrubbed with a soft brush to physically remove scale, may be sufficient. If scaling persists, an antiseborrheic shampoo (e.g., one containing zinc pyrithione or selenium sulfide) may be substituted. Adolescents with scalp involvement may be treated with an antiseborrheic shampoo or one containing ketoconazole; if inflammation is present, an appropriate topical corticosteroid (e.g., a mid-potency lotion or solution) may be applied at bedtime or, if needed, twice daily. Lesions elsewhere on the body (e.g., the face) are treated with a low-potency topical corticosteroid (e.g., hydrocortisone cream 1% twice daily) or, in adolescents, with a topical antiyeast preparation (e.g., ketoconazole cream twice daily).

DIAPER RASHES

What Are the Most Common Forms of Diaper Rash and How Are They Treated?

Diaper rashes are a common problem in infants. The most prevalent forms are irritant (because of excessive wetness that reduces the skin's ability to withstand frictional forces and enzymes in stool that act as irritants), candidal, and seborrheic. The clinical features and treatment of these forms of diaper rashes are summarized in Table 57-1.

Table 57-1

Manifestations and Management of Common Diaper Dermatitis

Type	Clinical Manifestations	Treatment
Irritant	Convexities involved Erythema, superficial erosions	Change diaper frequently Apply barrier preparation (e.g., zinc oxide paste) If inflammation severe, apply hydrocortisone cream 1% bid
Candidal	Convexities and creases involved Erythema, scaling, satellite papules or pustules	Apply topical antiyeast preparation (e.g., nystatin, miconazole nitrate)
Seborrheic	Convexities and creases involved Salmon-pink erythema, greasy scale Involvement of other areas (e.g., scalp, retroauricular folds, neck folds, axillae)	Diaper area: apply hydrocortisone cream 1% bid Scalp: shampoo hair and brush scalp to remove scale (if ineffective, use keratolytic shampoo) Skin: apply hydrocortisone cream 1% bid

bid, Twice daily.

BACTERIAL INFECTION (IMPETIGO)

ETIOLOGY

What Is Impetigo and What Causes It?

Impetigo is a bacterial infection of the skin. It occurs in two forms: crusted (or nonbullous) and bullous. The crusted form accounts for more than 70% of cases and is particularly prevalent in warm, humid climates. It results from infection with *Staphylococcus aureus* and, possibly, group A beta-hemolytic streptococci (GABHS). Bullous impetigo is caused by strains of *S. aureus* that produce an epidermolytic toxin, which damages intercellular adherence, causing a cleft high in the epidermis and the formation of fragile blisters that rupture rapidly.

EVALUATION

How Do I Recognize Impetigo?

Children with crusted (nonbullous) impetigo have erosions covered with a yellow or honey-colored crust that typically are located around the nares. In contrast, bullous impetigo is characterized by flaccid bullae and round, erythematous, superficial erosions surrounded by a rim of scale, the remnant of the bulla roof.

TREATMENT

How Is Impetigo Treated?

Children with impetigo are treated with an antibiotic active against both *S. aureus* and GABHS. If the infection is widespread or multifocal, an oral agent such as a first-generation cephalosporin (e.g., cephalexin) or dicloxacillin is prescribed for 7 to 10 days. If infection is localized, a topical antibiotic (e.g., mupirocin) is sufficient. For those with bullous impetigo, oral therapy with a first-generation cephalosporin or dicloxacillin is indicated.

FUNGAL INFECTIONS

TINEA CORPORIS

ETIOLOGY

What Is Tinea Corporis?

Tinea corporis (ringworm) is an infection of the skin with one of a group of fungi known as dermatophytes, organisms that infect keratinized structures such as the skin, hair, and nails.

EVALUATION

How do I recognize tinea corporis? Tinea corporis is characterized by one or a few expanding erythematous, scaling annuli (rings) or thin plaques. The border is well defined and often more elevated and inflamed than the center. Central clearing is often but not always present. In some children, small pustules are present at the border or throughout the lesion. Although these clinical features generally permit a diagnosis, if uncertainty exists, a potassium hydroxide preparation will demonstrate the branching hyphae.

TREATMENT

How Is Tinea Corporis Treated?

For children with one or a few lesions, a topical imidazole (e.g., miconazole nitrate) or other suitable topical antifungal agent may be applied twice daily until the lesion resolves, typically within 2 to 4 weeks. In the occasional patient with numerous or very large lesions, an oral antifungal agent such as griseofulvin is required.

TINEA CAPITIS

ETIOLOGY

What Is Tinea Capitis?

Tinea capitis is a dermatophyte infection of the scalp. In the United States, the organism most often responsible is *Trichophyton tonsurans*. Infection is spread from person to person and, for reasons unknown, predominantly affects African-American children. Tinea capitis also may be caused by infection with *Microsporum canis*, an organism usually acquired from cats or dogs.

EVALUATION

What Are the Signs of Tinea Capitis?

In the most prevalent form of tinea capitis, the patient has one or more patches of hair loss (i.e., alopecia) within which are seen "black dots," the remnants of infected hairs within follicles that have broken at the scalp line. Other presentations include diffuse scaling of the scalp (the seborrheic form), an inflammatory form characterized by scattered pustules and papules, and a tender, boggy mass (kerion). Tinea capitis resulting from *M. canis* causes patches of alopecia within which are scale and short hairs. Because hairs do not break at the scalp line, black dots are not observed. A potassium hydroxide preparation or fungal culture will confirm the diagnosis of tinea capitis.

TREATMENT

How Is Tinea Capitis Treated?

Tinea capitis requires treatment with an oral antifungal agent, usually griseofulvin, at a dose of 15 to 20 mg/kg (of the microsize form) daily for 6 to 8 weeks. Adjunctive therapy with selenium sulfide 1% or 2.5%, used as a shampoo, eradicates surface fungal elements and may reduce the likelihood of spread.

OTHER FUNGAL INFECTIONS

Other fungal infections that are particularly prevalent among adolescents include the following:

Tinea cruris: This infection produces erythematous scaling patches located on the medial proximal thighs and in the crural folds. It is treated with a topical imidazole or other antifungal agent.

Tinea pedis: In most patients, tinea pedis causes fissuring, scaling, and pruritus between the toes. Like tinea cruris, it is treated with a topical imidazole or other antifungal.

Tinea versicolor: Infection with the yeast *P. ovale* causes this condition. The chest, back, neck, and upper arms most often are involved. Lesions are hypopigmented or hyperpigmented macules that may coalesce into large patches; often they possess a fine, powdery scale. Treatment is with selenium sulfide lotion 2.5% applied from the neck to the waist for 10 minutes daily for 7 days. To prevent recurrences, patients are advised to apply the medication for 8 to 12 hours once every 1 to 2 months for a total of 6 months.

VIRAL INFECTIONS

WARTS

ETIOLOGY

What Causes Warts?

Warts are the result of infection with various types of human papillomavirus (HPV). Infection is spread primarily by direct contact, but fomites (i.e., objects that can transmit infection) also have been implicated.

EVALUATION

What Are the Types of Warts?

Common warts (verruca vulgaris) are skin-colored papules with a rough surface that range in size from a few millimeters to a centimeter or more; most often they occur on the hands and knees.

Plantar warts are often painful papules or nodules located on the sole of the foot. Multiple small lesions may coalesce to form a large "mosaic" wart. The presence of black specks on their surfaces (thrombosed capillaries) and an absence of normal epidermal ridges distinguish plantar warts from calluses.

Flat warts appear as multiple small (measuring a few millimeters in diameter), smooth, flesh-colored, thin plaques or papules typically located on the face or extremities.

Condylomata acuminata, or genital warts, are round or flat-topped papules located in the perineum, introitus, and perianal area or on the penis. The finding of genital warts in children should raise concern about possible sexual abuse, although benign forms of transmission are possible.

TREATMENT

What Treatments Are Available for Warts?

The response of individual warts to any modality is variable. In view of this and the natural history of lesions to resolve spontaneously, it is prudent to discuss with the patient, when appropriate, and parents whether any form of treatment should be initiated. Therapies commonly employed in the treatment of warts are summarized in Table 57-2. Immunization with the HPV vaccine was approved by the Food and Drug Administration (FDA) in May 2006 but had not been recommended for routine use at the time of this revision. The vaccine prevents cancer and skin lesions caused by four strains of the virus.

MOLLUSCUM CONTAGIOSUM

ETIOLOGY

What Is Molluscum Contagiosum?

Molluscum contagiosum is caused by infection with the molluscipox virus. Infection is spread by direct contact, including sexual activity, although the role of fomites cannot be excluded. Individual lesions tend to resolve within several weeks, but new lesions may appear for 12 to 18 months or longer.

Table 57-2

Commonly Used Treatments for Warts

Type of Wart	Treatment	How Used	Efficacy	Comments
Common or plantar	Keratolytic Common warts: start with product containing 15% to 17% salicylic acid Plantar warts: may use higher concentration of salicylic acid	Apply daily and cover with tape or Band-Aid In 24 hours, soak wart in warm water, dry, and débride with emery board Repeat daily	58% to 84% effective	Safe Requires prolonged treatment (1 to 2 months)
	Cryotherapy (e.g., with liquid nitrogen or other cryogen)	Applied by provider (treat wart and 1 to 5 mm margin of normal skin until it turns white; white color should remain for 10 seconds)	80% of patients cured in 12 weeks after 2 to 4 treatments	Painful Bullae may form following treatment (when bulla ruptures, wound care required to prevent secondary bacterial infection)
	Cantharidin (chemical extract that causes formation of a blister in the epidermis)	Applied by provider Using a toothpick or stick end of a cotton-tipped applicator, apply a small amount to the wart and allow to dry Wash area in 4 hours	Anecdotally effective	Bullae may form following treatment (see above, cryotherapy) A ring of warts occasionally forms around the site of treatment

(continued)

Table 57-2

Commonly Used Treatments for Warts (Continued)

Type of Wart	Treatment	How Used	Efficacy	Comments
Flat	Keratolytic (use product containing 15% to 17% salicylic acid)	See above	See above	See above
	Imiquimod	Apply daily to warts	Anecdotally effective	Expensive May cause skin irritation
	Cryotherapy	See above; less intense freeze is required	See above	See above
Genital	Podophyllin 25%	Applied by provider every 1 to 3 weeks; washed off in 4 to 6 hours	32% to 79% effective	May cause skin irritation Contraindicated in pregnancy
	Podofilox	Applied by patient bid for 3 days each week for 4 weeks	68% to 86% effective	May cause skin irritation Contraindicated in pregnancy
	Imiquimod	Applied for 6 to 10 hours, 3 times weekly for 16 weeks	Effectiveness: 72% females, 33% males	May cause skin irritation
	Cryotherapy	See above	See above	See above

bid, Twice daily.

EVALUATION

How Do I Recognize Molluscum Contagiosum?

Molluscum contagiosum appears as one or more translucent or white papules that may resemble vesicles or pustules. Lesions typically measure one to a few millimeters in diameter but occasionally grow to a centimeter or more. A central "dimple" or umbilication is a hallmark of molluscum lesions, although it may be absent in very small papules. Often, there is an area of erythema and mild scaling surrounding lesions. Patients may have one or many lesions, but the presence of very numerous lesions (e.g., hundreds) should suggest the possibility of underlying immunodeficiency. Molluscum contagiosum on or near the genitalia of children almost always is the result of autoinoculation from other areas of the body. However, the observation of lesions limited to this area should raise concern about possible sexual abuse.

TREATMENT

How Should Molluscum Contagiosum Be Treated?

The approach to the treatment of molluscum contagiosum is similar, in many respects, to that of warts. Because the infection eventually resolves spontaneously, no intervention is a reasonable option for an otherwise healthy, immunocompetent individual. If a decision is made to treat, parents should be advised that available therapies eradicate individual lesions but not the underlying infection. Thus, new lesions may continue to appear for several months. Options for treatment include cryotherapy, physical removal by curettage, and the application of cantharidin or other keratolytic, imiquimod, or tretinoin (Table 57-2).

INFESTATIONS

SCABIES

ETIOLOGY

What Is Scabies?

Scabies is a pruritic eruption caused by infestation with the mite *Sarcoptes scabiei*. It usually is acquired through close contact, although transmission by fomites such as clothing or bedding is possible.

EVALUATION

How Do I Recognize Scabies?

In infants, scabies produces erythematous papules, vesicles, or pustules that are distributed in a generalized fashion on the trunk and extremities. Older children, adolescents, and adults exhibit erythematous papules, nodules, or burrows in the interdigital webs, in the flexural areas of the wrists and elbows, in the axillae, at the belt line, on the areolae, or beneath the breasts in women and on the penis in men.

TREATMENT

How Is Scabies Treated?

The treatment of choice, particularly for infants and toddlers, is permethrin cream 5%. It is applied to the entire body surface of infants, including the head and face, and under the nails for 8 to 14 hours. Toddlers and older patients are treated from the neck to toes. Although a single treatment is 90% effective, a second treatment 7 days later is advised. Lindane 1% also may be effective but is considered a second-line therapy. Concerns about potential neurotoxicity, usually caused by excessive application or inadvertent ingestion, preclude its use in infants or young children. When scabies is diagnosed, all asymptomatic close contacts and family members should be treated once. Following treatment, all clothing and bedding should be washed in hot water. Clothing that cannot be laundered may be dry-cleaned or stored in a plastic bag for 2 weeks. Families should be counseled that itching might persist for several weeks after effective treatment.

HEAD LICE (PEDICULOSIS CAPITIS)

ETIOLOGY

What Are Head Lice?

Lice are small insects (2 to 3 mm in length) that feed on blood. There are three forms that infest humans (head, body, and pubic or crab lice). Infestation with head lice, the most common form, is spread primarily by direct contact, although shared combs, brushes, or hats may serve as fomites.

EVALUATION

How Do I Recognize a Child with Head Lice?

Children with head lice often complain of pruritus or a sense of something crawling in the scalp. Parents or teachers may observe live lice or their eggs (nits) attached to hairs.

TREATMENT

How Is an Infestation Treated?

The preferred initial treatment is with permethrin 1% (e.g., Nix) or a pyrethrin (e.g., RID, A-200). In the event of a treatment failure, alternative agents may be used, such malathion 0.5%, permethrin 5%, occlusive agents (e.g., petrolatum), or trimethoprim-sulfamethoxazole. Although lindane was widely used in the past, potential resistance, slow killing time, and concerns about potential toxicity (if used inappropriately or inadvertently ingested) limit its use. An important adjunct to treatment is careful combing with a nit comb. Family members who share a bed with the index case should be treated. Combs, hairbrushes, clothing, and bed linens should be washed, soaked, or dried at a temperature above 130° F. Those items that cannot be washed may be placed in a plastic bag for 2 weeks. Furniture, carpeting, and car seats should be vacuumed.

PAPULOSQUAMOUS DISORDERS

What Are Papulosquamous Disorders?

Papulosquamous disorders are those conditions characterized by elevated lesions (e.g., papules or plaques) that have scale. Among the most common papulosquamous disorders are chronic atopic or contact dermatitis, seborrheic dermatitis, and tinea corporis (discussed previously). Other papulosquamous disorders that may be encountered are pityriasis rosea, psoriasis, dermatomyositis, and lupus erythematosus. The clinical features of these four diseases are summarized in Table 57-3.

Table 57-3

Clinical Features and Treatment of Selected Papulosquamous Disorders

Disease	Clinical Features	Treatment
Pityriasis rosea	In 60% of patients, the initial lesion is a herald patch, a scaling patch that precedes the generalized eruption by 2–3 weeks Small, thin, oval, scaling plaques with long axes parallel to lines of skin stress Lesions are concentrated on the trunk and spare the face and extremities	There is no specific therapy and spontaneous resolution occurs in 6–8 weeks For patients with pruritus, an oral antihistamine or emollient containing menthol, phenol, or pramoxine may be prescribed

(continued)

Table 57-3

Clinical Features and Treatment of Selected Papulosquamous Disorders (Continued)

Disease	Clinical Features	Treatment
	In persons of color, an "inverse" distribution may occur, with involvement of the extremities and relative sparing of the trunk	
Psoriasis	Erythematous scaling papules and plaques that have a predilection for the elbows, knees, eyebrows, umbilicus, and gluteal cleft Most children and adolescents have scaling of the scalp Lesions often occur in areas of trauma (Koebner phenomenon)	Treatment may include a topical corticosteroid, calcipotriene, or tar preparation
Dermatomyositis	Violaceous discoloration of the bridge of the nose, face, hands, and knees Erythematous scaling papules over the interphalangeal joints, nail fold telangiectasias Muscle weakness often present	If evidence of muscle involvement, a systemic steroid (e.g., prednisone) is employed The rash may be prevented by the regular use of sunscreen
Lupus	An erythematous macular or papular eruption involving the malar area is the most common manifestation; scaling plaques may occur elsewhere Systemic involvement (e.g., renal, gastrointestinal, cardiovascular, central nervous system) may be present	Cutaneous lesions are managed with a topical corticosteroid, sunscreen, and, if necessary, hydroxychloroquine

CHILDHOOD EXANTHEMS

What Are Childhood Exanthems?

A number of systemic infections in children are accompanied by fever and a rash; these are termed exanthems or exanthematous diseases. The most common of these diseases are summarized in Table 57-4.

Table 57-4

Guide To Common Childhood Exanthems

Disease	Etiologic Agent	Clinical Features
Erythema infectiosum	Parvovirus B19	The rash begins as confluent erythema of the cheeks followed by a lacy, reticulated pink erythema of the extremities or trunk. The eruption fades after 3 to 5 days but may return for up to 4 months following exercise, overheating, or sun exposure.
Hand, foot, and mouth	Coxsackievirus A16, other coxsackieviruses, echoviruses, enteroviruses	Typically occurs during the summer or fall. Shallow ulcers appear on the soft palate, uvula, tonsillar pillars, and tongue. Cutaneous lesions are erythematous papules or oval vesicles concentrated on the palms, soles, and digits. The thighs and buttocks may be involved. The eruption resolves within 1 week.
Measles	Measles virus	Measles is characterized by fever, cough, coryza, conjunctivitis, and an exanthem composed of erythematous macules and papules. The rash first appears on the lateral aspects of the neck and behind the ears. It then progresses to involve the face, trunk, and extremities. By the time the rash reaches the feet, the face is clearing. Koplik spots may be observed on the buccal mucosa.
Roseola (exanthem subitum)	Human herpesvirus 6 or echovirus 16	Typically occurs in children younger than 3 years. Characterized by high fever for 2 to 3 days. As the fever resolves, erythematous pink macules appear on the trunk and extremities. The rash fades in 24 hours.
Rubella	Rubella virus	Erythematous macules first appear on the face and then spread to the trunk and extremities. As the rash appears on the distal extremities, it resolves on the face and trunk. Patients may have associated fever, posterior cervical lymphadenopathy, or arthritis.
Scarlet fever	Group A β-hemolytic streptococci	Pharyngeal infection with group A β-hemolytic streptococci that is associated with fever and a rash. The rash is composed of fine erythematous papules that have a rough or sandpaper feel.

(continued)

Table 57-4

Guide To Common Childhood Exanthems (Continued)

Disease	Etiologic Agent	Clinical Features
		Initially, the eruption is concentrated in skin flexures (e.g., axillae or groin). Linear petechiae in skin flexures (Pastia's lines) may be observed. Patients often have erythema of the face, with perioral pallor and a strawberry tongue.
Varicella	Varicella-zoster virus	The lesions of varicella are erythematous macules or papules that rapidly develop a central vesicle. Vesicles then rupture, forming a crust. Crops of new lesions appear for 3 to 4 days; they usually begin on the trunk and subsequently spread to the extremities and head. Vesicles that rapidly rupture to form ulcers may occur on mucosal surfaces.

KEY POINTS

- Atopic dermatitis usually has its onset before age 5 years, has a chronic relapsing course, and is accompanied by pruritus and a characteristic distribution of lesions.
- Contact dermatitis is a T-cell mediated allergic reaction. The best "treatment" is prevention by avoidance of known sensitizers such as poison ivy or nickel.
- Seborrhea commonly occurs on the scalp and in skin folds.
- A diaper rash that does not respond to barrier creams and hygiene may be caused by a *Candida* infection.
- Extensive impetigo, especially involving the nasal mucosa, requires systemic antibiotic treatment.
- Tinea infection of scalp and nails requires systemic antifungal treatment.
- Common warts and molluscum contagiosum are viral infections.
- When a child has scabies or head lice, the entire family should be treated.

Case 57-1

A 5-year-old African-American child presents for evaluation of hair loss of 2 weeks' duration. Physical examination reveals a 3-cm patch of alopecia in the occipital region within which are hairs broken at the level of the scalp and scale.

A. What is the most likely diagnosis?
B. What other conditions might you consider in the differential diagnosis?
C. How would you confirm the diagnosis?
D. What treatment is required?

Case 57-2

A 6-month-old infant presents for evaluation of a recurring pruritic rash. The family history is remarkable for allergic rhinitis in the mother and asthma in an older sibling. On physical examination, you observe erythematous, chapped-appearing patches on the cheeks and erythematous minimally scaling patches on the trunk and extensor surfaces of the extremities.

A. What is the most likely diagnosis?
B. Outline a plan for management.

Case 57-3

A 6-year-old presents for evaluation of a rash of 2 days' duration. She has been well without fever or other symptoms and is taking no medications. Her past medical history is unremarkable; specifically, she has no history of skin disease. Physical examination reveals a temperature of 37°C, red cheeks, and a lacy, reticulated erythema of the extremities.

A. What is the most likely diagnosis?
B. What is the etiology of her eruption?

Case 57-4

A 9-month-old infant has had a rash for 2 weeks. He has been fussier than usual but has had no fever or other symptoms. Physical examination reveals erythematous papules, many of which are eroded and crusted, distributed widely over the trunk and extremities. Papules and pustules are present on the palms and soles. No other family members are similarly affected.

A. What is the most likely diagnosis? What other disorders should be considered in the differential diagnosis?
B. What treatment is indicated?

Case 57-5

A 2-month-old infant has a diaper rash. On physical examination you find erythematous patches and superficial erosions involving the proximal thighs and suprapubic area; the inguinal folds are spared, but not the creases, in the diaper area.

A. What is the most likely cause of this infant's diaper rash?
B. What are the other common causes of diaper rash?
C. Outline a plan for management.

Case Answers

57-1 A. *Learning objective:* **Identify tinea capitis.** The presence of an acquired patch of alopecia, within which are scale and hairs broken at the scalp (i.e., "black dot" hairs), suggests tinea capitis resulting from *Trichophyton tonsurans.*

57-1 B. *Learning objective:* **Review the causes of localized alopecia in children.** Common causes of localized alopecia without scarring of the scalp include traction alopecia, friction alopecia, alopecia areata, and trichotillomania. None of these disorders, however, are associated with scaling or "black dot" hairs as manifested by the child described in the case.

57-1 C. *Learning objective:* **Discuss the diagnosis of tinea capitis.** To confirm the diagnosis of tinea capitis, one may perform a potassium hydroxide preparation of "black dot" hairs and scale obtained from the scalp. Alternately, a fungal culture (e.g., using dermatophyte test medium or other suitable medium) can be performed using scale or "black dot" hairs obtained from the scalp.

57-1 D. *Learning objective:* **Discuss the treatment of tinea capitis.** Griseofulvin orally for 6 to 8 weeks is the preferred treatment for tinea capitis; selenium sulfide 1% or 2.5% used adjunctively as a shampoo eradicates surface fungal elements and may reduce the spread of infection.

57-2 A. *Learning objective:* **Recognize atopic dermatitis.** A recurring pruritic eruption, coupled with the physical findings exhibited by the infant presented in the case, suggests a diagnosis of atopic dermatitis.

57-2 B. *Learning objective:* **Discuss the management of atopic dermatitis.** During flares of atopic dermatitis in an infant, hydrocortisone 1% or 2.5% may be applied twice daily to affected areas. A bedtime dose of a sedating antihistamine improves sleep and reduces scratching. Aspects of daily management might include limiting bathing, using a mild soap or soap substitute for bathing, using an additive-free laundry detergent, wearing cotton clothing, and, during colder months, the regular application of an emollient and the use of a vaporizer or humidifier in the infant's room.

57-3 A. *Learning objective:* **Recognize erythema infectiosum.** The girl presented has a "slapped cheek" appearance and a reticulated flat rash on the extremities. These are features of erythema infectiosum (Fifth disease).

57-3 B. *Learning objective:* **Identify the causative agent of erythema infectiosum.** Erythema infectiosum (Fifth disease) is caused by infection with human parvovirus B19.

57-4 A. *Learning objective:* **Identify scabies infestation.** In an infant, the onset of a generalized, pruritic papular eruption that involves the palms and soles suggests a diagnosis of scabies.

57-4 B. *Learning objective:* **Review the differential diagnosis of scabies.** Atopic dermatitis is the disorder most likely to mimic scabies. Unlike scabies, however, it is a recurring eruption characterized by erythematous patches and small papules that typically do not involve the palms and soles. Less common disorders to be considered in the differential diagnosis include lichen planus and dermatitis herpetiformis.

57-4 C. *Learning objective:* **Discuss the treatment of scabies.** Permethrin 5%, applied topically, is the agent preferred for the treatment of infants with scabies and all close contacts. In infants, the medication should be applied to the entire body surface, including the head. Bedding and clothing must be laundered.

57-5 A. *Learning objective:* **Recognize irritant diaper dermatitis.** The infant presented in the case has findings (e.g., erythematous patches that involve the convexities, not the creases) consistent with the diagnosis of irritant diaper dermatitis.

57-5 B. *Learning objective:* **Review common causes of diaper dermatitis.** Common causes of diaper rash, aside from irritant dermatitis, include candidiasis and seborrheic dermatitis. Unlike irritant diaper dermatitis, both of these conditions involve the creases as well as the convexities. In addition, infants with candidiasis exhibit satellite lesions, while those with seborrheic dermatitis often have concomitant involvement of the scalp or other skin flexures (e.g., the axillae or neck folds).

57-5 C. *Learning objective:* **Discuss the management of irritant diaper dermatitis.** Management of irritant diaper dermatitis includes frequent diaper changes, the application of a barrier preparation (e.g., Desitin or zinc oxide paste) and, possibly, the application of a low-potency topical corticosteroid (e.g., hydrocortisone 1%).

BIBLIOGRAPHY

Textbooks

Cohen BA: *Pediatric dermatology,* ed 3, Philadelphia, 2005, Elsevier Mosby.

Paller AS, Mancini AJ: *Hurwitz clinical pediatric dermatology,* ed 3, Philadelphia, 2005, Saunders Elsevier.

Weston WL, Lane AT, Morelli JG: *Color textbook of pediatric dermatology,* ed 3, St Louis, 2007, Mosby.

Electronic Textbooks

Habif TP: *Clinical dermatology,* ed 4, Philadelphia, 2004, Mosby. Available via MD Consult.

Electronic Atlases

http://dermatlas.med.jhmi.edu/derm/index.cfm. Johns Hopkins University Dermatlas. It contains more than 7900 images of pediatric dermatologic disorders. Each image is accompanied by a brief case history. One may search by diagnosis, disease category, or body site involved. There is a quiz to test your knowledge. This is a highly useful resource.

http://tray.dermatology.uiowa.edu/DermImag.htm. Atlas of general dermatology maintained by the Department of Dermatology, University of Iowa. Images of conditions are listed alphabetically.

www.dermis.net/pedoia/en/home/index.htm. Dermatologic Online Image Atlas maintained by the University of Erlangen, Germany. It contains more than 4500 images of adult and pediatric dermatologic disorders. Conditions may be searched alphabetically or by body area. There is a quiz to test your knowledge.

58

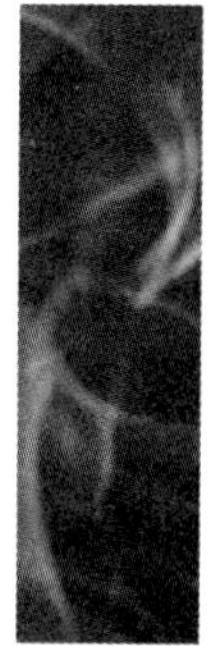

Developmental Disabilities

DIANNE M. McBRIEN

INTRODUCTION

What Is a Developmental Disability?

Approximately 17% of Americans younger than 18 years have been diagnosed with a developmental disability. The 2000 reauthorization of the Developmental Disabilities Act defines developmental disability as a "severe, chronic disability in an individual five years of age or older that is attributable to a mental or physical impairment or a combination of mental and physical impairments." The developmental disability must manifest before 22 years of age, continue indefinitely, and result in substantial functional limitation in multiple areas of life. Children with developmental disabilities often have complex health care needs and may receive care from multiple subspecialists. Such patients are also identified as having special health care needs, which is discussed in Chapter 16.

What Developmental Disabilities Am I Likely to See?

A review of every developmental disability is beyond the scope of this chapter. The focus is on autistic disorder, cerebral palsy, and Down syndrome because they are common and because management principles may be applied to other developmental diagnoses. Diagnosis and management of common associated health issues will be reviewed. Where appropriate, information about incidence and genetic factors will be provided. Finally, you will be referred to text and electronic resources for more developmental disability-related information.

Who Is at Risk for Developmental Disability?

Developmental disabilities occur in every race and socioeconomic group. As outlined in Chapter 27, genetic, prenatal, and perinatal factors contribute to the genesis of certain developmental disorders. Children with these predisposing factors may be at higher risk of disability. Many affected children, however, have unremarkable family, prenatal and birth histories.

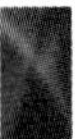

AUTISM/PERVASIVE DEVELOPMENTAL DISORDER

ETIOLOGY

What Is Autism?

Autism, or autistic disorder (AD), was first described by Leo Kanner in 1943. Decades ago, the medical community believed that AD was caused by cold and rejecting mothers. Most investigators today agree on a neurobiologic cause, although a specific lesion has not been identified. AD is one of five *autism spectrum disorders* that are classified under the category of pervasive developmental disorders (PDDs) in the *Diagnostic and Statistical Manual* (DSM-IV). The diagnosis of AD requires symptoms in three areas:

- Qualitative impairments in verbal and nonverbal communication
- Deficits in social interaction
- Restricted or repetitive behaviors and/or interests

What Are the Other Autistic Spectrum Disorders?

The other autistic spectrum disorders have various combinations of the AD clinical features. Children with *Asperger's disorder* have problems with social interaction, pragmatic language, and restricted interests but show normal cognitive abilities and language development. *Rett syndrome* is an X-linked condition affecting girls that typically has onset before age 4 years. Patients with Rett syndrome have deceleration of head growth plus loss of social skills, expressive language, and both gross motor and purposeful hand skills. *Childhood disintegrative disorder* is diagnosed in children who demonstrated normal development for at least 2 years then began to regress in more than one developmental area. *Pervasive developmental disorder not otherwise specified* (PDD-NOS) describes children who display some autistic symptoms but do not meet the criteria for the other four spectrum disorders.

How Common Is Autistic Disorder?

Autistic spectrum disorder develops in 60 out of 10,000 children. Boys have more than three times higher risk than girls. Autism in girls, however, is much more likely to be accompanied by significant mental retardation. AD coexists with some degree of mental retardation in 70% of cases. Often, AD can be correlated with a specific genetic, metabolic, or structural cause of mental retardation, including fragile X syndrome, tuberous sclerosis, Angelman syndrome, Down syndrome, phenylketonuria, neurofibromatosis, Rett syndrome, or congenital brain malformation.

What Causes Autism?

There is no unifying hypothesis about the etiology of autism. Neuroanatomic, neurochemical, neuroelectrical, and genetic factors have all been implicated. Various brain anomalies are commonly seen on imaging studies, and seizure disorders occur in 11% to 42% of individuals with AD. Neurochemical studies suggest abnormal neurotransmitter activity in some autistic individuals, although the significance of this finding is not clear. The evidence for a genetic basis is striking: AD has a 60% concordance in monozygotic twins. Siblings of autistic individuals have up to 25 to 50 times higher risk of AD than the general population. First-degree relatives of individuals with AD have higher than average rates of personality traits such as anxiety, rigidity, and social awkwardness, a group of traits known as the *broader autism phenotype* (BAP). BAP implies that the spectrum of autistic traits may be much wider than originally thought. A single gene has not been identified, but studies to date point to three locations: the long arm of chromosome 7 (7q), a region on the long arm of chromosome 15, and a region on chromosome 13.

EVALUATION

What History Is Needed to Diagnose Autism?

Family members or teachers are very likely to express concern about a child's language, social development, or behavior. Your task is to obtain a detailed history with particular attention to communication, social skills, and behaviors. Table 58-1 shows a general list of associated signs and symptoms. Screening tools such as the Checklist for Autism in Toddlers (CHAT) help focus your questions during primary care visits. The five key items from the CHAT can be found in Table 58-2. Children who fail *all* these items have a high risk of developing autism.

How Should I Assess Communication?

You must assess for speech and language delay because most children with AD acquire these skills much more slowly than motor skills. Ask family members if the child communicates with words and sentences,

Table 58-1

Impairments Common to Autistic Syndromes
Impairments in social skills
Limitations in the use of interactive language
Sensorimotor deficiencies
Echolalia
Deficiencies in symbolic thinking
Stereotypic behaviors
Self-injury behaviors
Mental retardation
Seizure disorders

Information from the American Psychiatric Association: *Diagnostic and statistical manual of mental disorders, ed 4,* Washington, DC, 1994, American Psychiatric Association, pp 65–78. Copyright 1994.

Table 58-2

5 Key Items in the CHAT (Failure of All 5 Means High Risk for Autism)

Ask the parent:
Does your child ever PRETEND, for example, to make a cup of tea using a toy cup and teapot, or pretend other things?
Does your child ever use his/her finger to point, to indicate INTEREST in something?
Examiner observation:
Get child's attention, then point across the room at an interesting object and say, "Oh look! There's a (name of toy)!" Watch child's face. Does the child look across to see what you are pointing at?
Get the child's attention. Then give child a baby doll and toy bottle, and say, "Can you feed the baby?" Does the child pretend to give the doll the bottle, rock the doll, etc.?
Say to the child, "Where's the light?" or "Show me the light." Does the child point with his/her index finger at the light?

CHAT, Checklist for autism in toddlers.

by pointing, use of hand signs, or jargoning. If the child speaks, inquire about vocabulary size and complexity of utterances. Next, ask about unusual features of speech. Does the child often *echo* what he or she hears? *Immediate echolalia* occurs when a child promptly repeats the final fragments of sentences or songs; *delayed echolalia* occurs when the child repeats past information out of context. A child with AD/PDD commonly demonstrates delayed echolalia by habitually reciting portions of movies or television programs. In addition, a child may also misuse pronouns, speak in a pedantic tone of voice, or fail to respond to his or her own name. Hearing loss, language disorders, and some learning disabilities can mimic AD/PDD symptoms. Evaluation by an interdisciplinary team should include audiometry, psychometric testing, and speech and language assessment, in addition to cognitive testing and a medical evaluation.

How Does a Child with Autistic Disorder Interact with Others?

Social skills are delayed relative to developmental age in AD/PDD. Examples of social deficits include poor eye contact, incongruent facial expressions, inappropriate volume or rate of speech, and resistance to being touched. A good screening question is "Does your child point out things for you to look at?" A normally developing young child usually draws the attention of a parent or other adult to an object of interest by pointing, reciprocal eye contact, verbalizations, and body language. These *joint attention behaviors* demonstrate the child's growing awareness that others may share their experiences. Young children with AD/PDD perform far fewer joint attention behaviors than do typical children. They are occasionally described by parents as less interested in cuddling than their siblings, although this may vary markedly. Ask if the child seeks comfort from parents when hurt, and if he initiates hugs and kisses.

What Are Restricted Activities?

A child may "ignore" surroundings and people, yet show unusual interest in a single object such as a ceiling fan or running water. Pretend play is reduced in children with AD/PDD, so it is appropriate to inquire about favorite toys and activities, and about the nature of play. If the child likes to play with toy cars, does he set up races and crashes, make appropriate noises, and put toy figures inside the cars? Or does he play with them by lining them up or banging them together? Ask about play that is imitative of adult activity such as cooking on a toy stove or pretending to drive a toy vehicle. Also inquire if the child has a transitional object, such as a teddy bear. A child with AD/PDD tends not to have such objects or may choose an unusual item, such as a wooden spoon.

What Repetitive Activities Characterize Autistic Disorder?

Repetitive activities in AD/PDD may take many forms, including hand flapping, finger posturing, rocking, and spinning. Children may play for hours looping a particular piece of string or pouring water from one cup into another. The propensity for repetition may be demonstrated by a rigid insistence on routine, with severe behavioral outbursts greeting even a minor alteration in routine.

What Developmental Findings Suggest Autism?

It is especially important to consider the child's overall developmental status before concluding that a particular symptom is indicative of AD/PDD. For example, a 5-year-old boy with known mental retardation may have a developmental age of 18 months. He may prefer to play alongside, but not with, other children, may flap his hands when excited, and speak only in 2-word phrases. His behaviors are consistent with his delayed development and do not by themselves support a diagnosis of AD/PDD.

What Should I Look for on Physical Examination?

The examination is an opportunity to *observe the child's interactions* with family members and with you. Note how the child responds to his or her name and to instructions. You should look carefully for dysmorphic features, including microcephaly and neurocutaneous disorders.

What Workup Is Indicated for Autistic Disorder/Pervasive Developmental Disorder?

The diagnosis is based entirely on clinical findings and the DSM-IV criteria. Laboratory tests are indicated mainly to evaluate clinical suspicions of an associated acquired or congenital disorder. Consider blood lead level if the lead screening history is positive. Molecular genetic studies are needed if findings suggest fragile X syndrome. MECP2 mutation study is appropriate in a girl with slow head growth and suspected Rett syndrome. Electroencephalogram (EEG) may be indicated if the history suggests seizure activity. Head imaging may be helpful for a child with cranial abnormalities or suspicion of neurocutaneous disease. A child with dysmorphic features or findings suggestive of neurocutaneous disorder may benefit from referral to a medical geneticist for further evaluation.

TREATMENT

How Is Autism Treated?

At this writing, autism and its spectrum disorders cannot be cured. Most treatment plans emphasize intensive academic and behavioral intervention beginning as soon as possible after the diagnosis is made. Classroom environments must be highly structured, heavily reliant on visual aids, and provide frequent positive reinforcement to the child. Behavioral techniques are used to teach social skills and activities of daily living. Parents need to be trained in these techniques to teach their children at home.

Are Medications Ever Useful?

Psychotropic medications may provide isolated benefits to some children with severe behavioral challenges. Atypical antipsychotic agents, including risperidone and quetiapine, have been shown to reduce aggressive behaviors in autistic children and are generally well tolerated. Selective serotonin reuptake inhibitors may alleviate the rigidity and perseveration of some autistic symptoms. Drug therapy is not indicated for or useful in treatment of social or language deficits associated with AD/PDD.

Do "Alternative" Treatments Help?

Although it is critical that you listen to parental concerns and beliefs, you also must provide appropriate, reliable, valid information to counter the misinformation that abounds in popular media and on the Internet. Elimination diets, vitamin and herb supplements, heavy metal chelation, and avoidance of immunizations all are examples of practices favored by many parents of children with AD/PDD. None of these measures has been demonstrated to be safe or effective and none can be recommended. Immunizations have no identified relationship to any of the autistic spectrum disorders, and referral to reliable Web sites such as those of the Centers for Disease Control and Prevention and the American Academy of Pediatrics may be helpful to families. Avoidance of immunizations puts a child at risk for preventable infections.

CEREBRAL PALSY

ETIOLOGY

What Is Cerebral Palsy?

Cerebral palsy describes a group of static, nonprogressive disorders of the developing brain. Although it may manifest in many different ways, cerebral palsy is consistently characterized by abnormalities in muscle tone and posture and by some degree of permanent motor impairment.

The incidence of cerebral palsy is between 2 and 3 per 1000 births, a figure that has not changed for the past two decades.

How Is Cerebral Palsy Classified?

Individual cases are classified by subtype and by distribution of neurologic impairment. Approximately 80% of patients have one of the three subtypes of cerebral palsy; the remaining 20% demonstrate either a mix of subtypes or muscle rigidity throughout range of motion.

What Are the Subtypes of Cerebral Palsy?

1. *Spastic* cerebral palsy accounts for more than 60% of cases. Marked by spasticity and hyperreflexia, it is associated with motor cortex and corticospinal tract injury. Primitive reflexes are persistent.
2. *Dyskinetic* cerebral palsy affects 20% of people with the disorder and is associated with basal ganglia injury. Athetoid and dystonic movements are seen in this subtype.
3. *Ataxic* cerebral palsy is associated with cerebellar damage and is seen in 1% of cases. Tremor and broad-based, lurching gait are seen.

Which Regions of the Body Are Affected?

Cerebral palsy of the spastic subtype is further classified by the distribution of neurologic impairment. *Diplegia* refers to impairment of trunk and extremities, with the lower extremities usually most severely affected. *Hemiplegia* describes impairment of function of only one side of the body. *Quadriplegia* affects all extremities, plus truncal, head, and neck musculature. *Paraplegia,* involvement of the lower extremities alone, is rare, as are *monoplegia* and *triplegia.*

What Causes Cerebral Palsy?

Any agent that damages the immature brain is capable of causing cerebral palsy. A list of potential etiologic factors is provided in Table 58-3. Note that causative factors in preterm and term infants differ somewhat. Also bear in mind that many children with cerebral palsy may not have histories indicative of any of these etiologies. Maternal infection, neonatal infection, and coagulopathy have emerged as important etiologic agents in the past decade, while birth asphyxia is now thought to

Table 58-3

Factors Associated With Development of Cerebral Palsy

Preterm Birth	Term Birth
Maternal infection	Hypoxic/ischemic injury
Multiple gestation, including vanishing twin syndrome	Maternal autoimmune disorder
Periventricular leukomalacia	Maternal coagulopathy
	Maternal infection

account for a minority of cases. Extreme prematurity and multiple gestations are also increasingly significant etiologic factors.

EVALUATION

What History Should I Obtain?

The mother's history should be reviewed for evidence of thrombosis, collagen vascular disease, recurrent fetal loss, and treatment with antibiotics just before or immediately following delivery. Prenatal information, if available, should be reviewed carefully for evidence suggestive of intrauterine growth retardation, bleeding, or twin loss. Labor and delivery records will provide information about resuscitation, if it was needed. Go over any neonatal medical problems, being alert for asphyxia-related problems including seizures and anuria. If the child underwent head imaging, review the films or their interpretations. Note the results of any hearing or vision assessments, including acoustic brainstem response and evaluation for retinopathy of prematurity. See Chapter 27 for an approach to suspected developmental delay.

What Family History Is Important?

Because some cerebral palsy has an X-linked genetic component, family history should inquire about relatives with motor impairments or other disabilities. Bear in mind that families may not recognize that an affected relative has cerebral palsy. You are more likely to find out relevant information if you ask *"Does anyone related by blood to you have trouble walking or moving?"* Social history should include lead screening questions.

How Should I Assess Developmental Progress?

If a young child has a delay in gross motor development, you should first identify developmental achievements in all areas (see Chapters 9 and 27). Quantify the degree of motor delay by asking about and observing the child's abilities. To help exclude progressive neurologic disease, *always* ask whether development seems to be regressing in any area. Then, ask questions about muscle tone: stiffness or floppiness. Do the child's arms and legs feel stiff and difficult to move? Some parents will not articulate this but will comment that this child is unusually difficult to dress or diaper. Bear in mind that affected children may actually be hypotonic as infants and develop spasticity and increased tone as myelinization continues around the injured area in the brain. Inquire about abnormalities in posture and persistence of primitive reflexes. Does the child often arch when held or when placed in his car seat? Is one hand held fisted much of the time? Is there a strong and persistent hand preference prior to age 1 year, which may suggest a paresis of the contralateral hand? Are writhing or posturing motions seen? Does the child automatically "stand" when suspended on a flat surface, even if the rest of his motor development has not advanced even close to the standing milestone? Does the child "startle" easily and seemingly spontaneously, especially after 4 months of age?

What Medical Problems Occur in Cerebral Palsy?

Problems commonly encountered in patients with cerebral palsy are listed in Table 58-4. Some of the more frequently identified problems include poor feeding and growth, respiratory illness related to aspiration or the residual lung disease of prematurity, seizures, constipation, sleep disturbance, vision and hearing loss, and multiple orthopedic disorders such as contractures and foot deformities.

What Should I Look for on Physical Examination?

First, *observe* the child while you speak with other family members. Does behavior seem age-appropriate? Is the infant or child alert, interactive, vocal, and sociable? Are spontaneous movements reduced in number? Note movement quality: is it easy and fluid, or do you observe jerks, tremors, or twisting? When you start the physical examination, proceed slowly, with warm hands and a warm stethoscope. This preparation will help to keep the child as relaxed as possible and enable you to perform a reliable neuromuscular examination. You will find the physical examination detailed in Chapter 27 helpful as a guide. During the general examination, look for evidence of neurologic impairment. Gently, then more briskly, move the joints through as much range of motion as is possible, noting if you feel resistance suddenly "give way." Known as the *clasp-knife reflex,* this finding is a hallmark of spasticity. Evaluate antigravity muscle tone by holding the child under the arms and in midair. Hypotonic children will "slip" through your hands (see Chapter 42), whereas those with spasticity typically exhibit "scissoring" by extending their limbs and adducting at the hips (Figure 58-1). As you test reflexes, look for briskness (3 to 4+/4+) and persistent clonus. Remember that 1 to 2 beats of clonus can be elicited in healthy young infants. Persistence of primitive reflexes is a concerning finding.

Table 58-4

Medical Problems in Patients with Cerebral Palsy
Visual problems, including strabismus, cortical blindness, and refractive errors
Sensorineural hearing loss
Drooling
Seizures
Mental retardation, learning disabilities, and ADHD
Gastrointestinal disorders, including aspiration, reflux, and constipation
Feeding and growth problems
Sleep disorders
Orthopedic consequences of spasticity: Contractures and pain. Hip dislocation and scoliosis common
Skin breakdown ("pressure sores" on dependent areas)

ADHD, Attention deficit hyperactivity disorder.

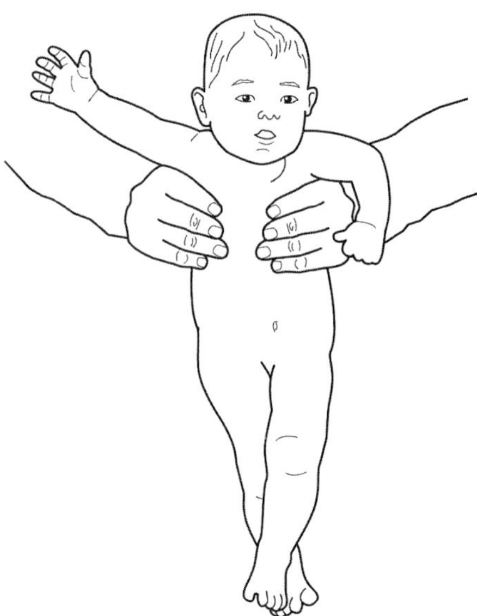

FIGURE 58-1 Scissoring.

How Do I Test for Persistent Primitive Reflexes?

Primitive reflexes should have completely disappeared by age 6 months, and they are abnormal if obligatory at any age. Persistence of the *Moro reflex* and *palmar grasp* are two examples of primitive reflexes that should be looked for during the evaluation of a child with suspected cerebral palsy. The *asymmetric tonic neck reflex* is elicited by gently turning the infant's head to the side for 15 seconds. A positive response consists of extension of the extremities on the side to which the face is turned, with flexion of those on the contralateral side (Figure 58-2). Try to assess postural tone by eliciting reactions such as the *positive supporting reflex*. Perform this reaction by suspending the child over the examination table so that the soles of the feet just touch the surface and the toes are slightly flexed (Figure 58-3). A positive response consists of extension of the legs that resembles a standing attempt.

What Other Physical Findings Should I Look for?

Complete your neuromuscular examination by looking for *skeletal deformities* caused by muscle use imbalance, including scoliosis, contractures, foot deformities, and limitations in hip range of motion. Also assess extraocular movements, listen to lung sounds, palpate the abdomen for stool masses, and do a complete skin check for pressure sores.

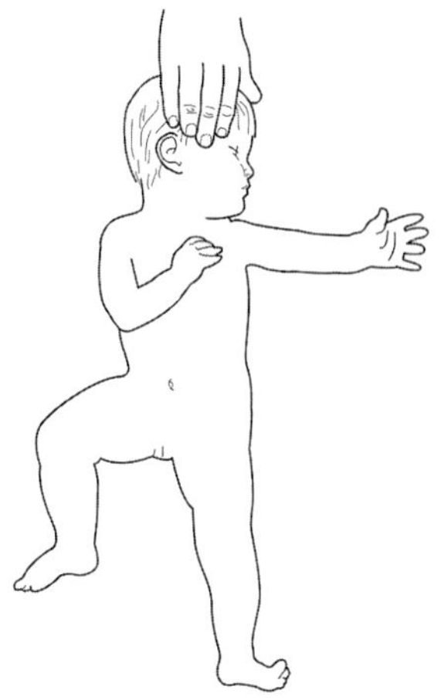

FIGURE 58-2 Asymmetrical tonic neck reflex.

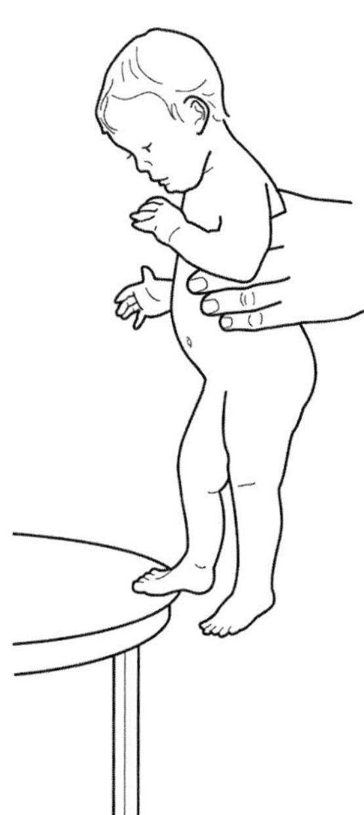

FIGURE 58-3 Positive supporting reflex.

Are Laboratory and Imaging Studies Needed?

The diagnosis of cerebral palsy is made on clinical grounds. Laboratory and radiographic studies mainly help to clarify the diagnosis, identify the cause of the impairment, and manage complications. Chapter 27 provides general recommendations for the laboratory evaluation of the developmentally delayed child. Head magnetic resonance imaging (MRI) may yield information about congenital malformations, atrophy, posterior fossa anomalies, or white matter abnormalities. Head computed tomography (CT) is more appropriate for the detection of calcifications and assessment of ventricular size. Serum creatine kinase measurement should be ordered on floppy or weak children. If a child is found to have developmental regression, deceleration in head growth, failure to thrive, seizures, organomegaly, cataracts, or muscle fasciculation or atrophy, further evaluation by a developmental specialist is warranted. A patient with clear risk factors, such as an affected child who is the product of a 27-week twin pregnancy, will not need an extensive workup.

TREATMENT

How Are Children with Cerebral Palsy Treated?

Treatments for children with cerebral palsy are designed to optimize function, prevent secondary disability, such as contractures and muscle atrophy, and manage related complications, such as seizures and strabismus. Physical, occupational, and speech therapies should be started as soon as possible after diagnosis. Orthoses, including hand splints and ankle/foot braces, will maintain spastic joints in functional position and prevent contractures. For infants and young children, adaptive car seats and feeding chairs that help reduce extensor tone are available. Wheelchair seating is needed for older children with quadriplegia and usually must be custom designed.

When Would Surgery Be Needed?

Orthopedic surgery is often needed by children with cerebral palsy to lengthen or transfer tendons and release contractures. Adolescents and young adults often need spinal fusion for scoliosis and reduction of dislocated hips. *Neurosurgical* treatments include botulinum toxin injections in selected muscle groups and the intrathecal baclofen pump, which may be an option for children with severe spasticity. Selective dorsal rhizotomy, in which intraoperative electromyogram (EMG) is used to identify overactive spinal nerve rootlets before they are severed, may be an option for selected patients.

What Medications Are Documented to Help?

Diazepam and baclofen decrease spasticity, although their potential benefits must be weighed against adverse effects such as drowsiness and constipation. Other medications may be needed to manage coexisting medical problems: anticonvulsants, bronchodilators, H2 blockers, and stool softeners. Excessive secretions can be controlled with anticholinergic therapy.

What Nutritional Support Is Needed?

Increased energy requirements, oral motor difficulties, gastroesophageal reflux, and aspiration all place children with cerebral palsy at high risk of poor nutrition. Height, weight and body mass index (BMI) should be checked at each office visit. Arm span reflects growth in height and should be measured for children with severe scoliosis. Pediatric texture swallow study should be performed if symptoms suggest aspiration or reflux. Supplements may be needed to boost calories. Gastrostomy placement is beneficial for selected children.

How Can a Multidisciplinary Team Help Management?

Children with cerebral palsy often require the coordinated care of multiple subspecialists, including gastroenterology, neurology, ophthalmology, orthopedics, and otolaryngology services. Because more than half of affected children have mental retardation, special education services and support are also needed in the majority of cases. Periodic interdisciplinary developmental evaluation, including cognitive, academic, visual, auditory, gross, and fine motor assessments, is recommended.

DOWN SYNDROME

What Is Down Syndrome?

Down syndrome is the most common identifiable cause of mental retardation and has an incidence of 1 in 750 to 900 live births. Ninety percent of Down syndrome cases result from pure trisomy 21; the rest are related to translocation or mosaicism.

What Causes Down Syndrome?

Down syndrome risk is directly correlated to maternal age. A 25-year-old woman's risk is estimated at 1 in 1300, a 35-year-old woman's risk jumps to 1 in 365, and a 45-year-old woman's risk is 1 in 30. It is hypothesized that advanced maternal age lengthens the meiosis I period, which increases the time for potential nondisjunction errors. Advanced paternal age may occasionally cause nondisjunction errors in spermatocytes. Researchers are exploring the contribution of oral contraceptives and periconceptional tobacco smoking to risk of Down syndrome.

What Information Should I Obtain?

A child with Down syndrome may have learning and behavior problems in addition to the multiple medical problems associated with the genetic lesion. Because Down syndrome can affect every organ system, the history and physical examination should be comprehensive. The *Down Syndrome Health Care Guidelines* (Table 58-5) are helpful for preventive health and chronic illness care. Growth measurements should be plotted on growth charts specific for children with Down syndrome.

What Organ System Problems Might I Anticipate?

Cardiac

Congenital cardiac malformations are seen in 40% to 50% of neonates with Down syndrome; half of these babies will need surgical repair.

Table 58-5

Down Syndrome: A Preventive Medical Checklist

Infancy (birth–12 months)

Karyotype confirmation and genetic counseling—newborn period
Cardiac evaluation and echocardiogram—newborn period
SBE prophylaxis in susceptible children
Check newborn thyroid screen
Consider flu vaccine
Monitor: cardiac, gastrointestinal, and neurodevelopmental function
Audiology (hearing) evaluation—by 6 months
Compile a medical information log
Appointment at a Down syndrome clinic

Childhood (1–12 years)

Recheck thyroid function tests—yearly
Continue SBE prophylaxis in susceptible children
Consider flu vaccine—yearly
Monitor: ENT, cardiac, gastrointestinal, behavioral, and neurodevelopmental function
Consider antibiotic prophylaxis, allergies, ventilation tubes, and ENT consultation
Recheck hearing—at least annually
Ophthalmology (vision) evaluation—at 1 year
Cervical spine x-ray—once between 3 and 5 years; repeat only if clinically warranted
  Lateral neck (neutral, flexion, and extension views); measure ADI and neural canal width
Dental evaluation—at 3 years, then twice yearly
Twice-daily teeth brushing
Regular physical exercise and recreational programs
Continue mental information log
Appointment at a Down syndrome clinic—yearly

Adolescence (12–18 years)

Continue SBE prophylaxis in susceptible individuals
Consider flu vaccine—yearly
Monitor: behavior and mental health; recheck thyroid function tests—yearly
Recheck hearing—at least every 2 years
Recheck vision—every 2 to 3 years
Cervical spine x-ray—only if clinically warranted
Females: gynecology evaluation (pelvic examination and Pap smear)
Dental evaluation twice yearly
Twice-daily teeth brushing
Regular physical exercise and recreational program

ADI, Atlanto-Dens interval; ENT, ear, nose, throat; SBE, subacute bacterial endocarditis.
From Cohen W et al: Down Syndrome Preventive Medical Checklist. Report of The Down Syndrome Medical Interest Group, *Down Syndrome Quarterly,* Volume 1(2), Down Syndrome Medical Interest Group, 1996.

Inquire about energy level, color, feeding difficulties, growth problems, or breathing difficulties. Review the medical record for cardiac echo results, history of cardiac surgeries, plans for cardiac and surgical follow-up, and diuretics or other medications for congestive heart failure.

Ear, Nose, and Throat

The midfacial hypoplasia associated with Down syndrome makes ear, nose, and throat (ENT) problems pervasive in this population. Ask about hearing loss, results of hearing tests, use of hearing aids, and discharge or bleeding from the ears or nose. Review the history of surgeries such as myringotomy tubes or tonsillectomy. To screen for sleep apnea, ask about daytime drowsiness, loud snoring, choking, and breathing pauses during sleep.

Metabolic

The lifetime risk of thyroid dysfunction is estimated to be as high as 17% in Down syndrome. Most children will have acquired lymphocytic thyroiditis, but congenital hypothyroidism and Graves' disease occur as well. Children with Down syndrome are also at increased risk of type I diabetes. Ask about appetite, temperature intolerance, dry skin, sweating, bowel function, abdominal pain, vomiting, lethargy, excessive sleeping, or hyperactive, aggressive behavior.

Gastrointestinal

Approximately 12% of newborns with Down syndrome have a congenital gastrointestinal anomaly. Duodenal atresia is the most common lesion, identified by the "double-bubble sign" on abdominal plain film. Tracheoesophageal fistula, Meckel's diverticulum, annular pancreas, and imperforate anus are also associated with Down syndrome, as is Hirschsprung's disease. Celiac disease may occur in 3% to 17% of newborns with Down syndrome. Low abdominal muscle tone contributes to constipation. Inquire about surgery, feeding difficulties, and the child's stooling pattern.

Hematology and Oncology

Individuals with Down syndrome have 10 to 20 times greater lifetime likelihood of developing leukemia than the general population. Acute lymphocytic leukemia (ALL) is most common in children and adults; in infants, acute myelocytic leukemia (AML) is most prevalent. Newborns with Down syndrome may develop a transient myeloproliferative disorder with striking leukocytosis. Although these infants undergo spontaneous remission, they have a 30% risk of future AML. Ask about fever, pallor, weight loss, rash, unexplained bruising, or bleeding. Ask if the child is limping or is refusing to walk, because leukemia may present with bone pain.

Neurology and Psychiatry

All children with Down syndrome have hypotonia early in life, but tone improves somewhat with time. Incidence of seizures is increased compared with the general population. Individuals with Down syndrome generally have mental retardation, but the majority can learn self-care and basic literacy skills, and many live semi-independently. Autistic disorder and more severe retardation occur in 10% to 15% of Down syndrome patients.

Other

Children with Down syndrome have a high incidence of refractive error, astigmatism, and cataract, so you should ask about squinting, headaches, and visual concerns. Ensure that immunizations are up to date, and review the history for frequent respiratory and skin infections, as this population has a number of immune system deficits. Ask about joint dislocations, sprains, and pain that might result from hypermobile joints that are prone to injury from chronic excessive range of motion. Question the family about itching or rashes because very dry skin and eczema are common. Review questions about puberty.

What Should I Look for on Physical Examination?

First, look for the characteristic midfacial hypoplasia (Figure 58-4). Note epicanthal folds, oblique palpebral fissures, flattened nasal bridge, and small nares. Examine the eyes for *Brushfield spots,* a ring of white spots around the iris, and look carefully for strabismus and nystagmus. The ears are small and low-set and tympanic membranes may be difficult to visualize. The head has characteristic *brachycephaly.* The tongue may protrude slightly because the oral cavity is small. Examine the pharynx to identify a notched or bifid uvula or soft palate defects. Teeth may be congenitally absent, abnormally shaped, or delayed in eruption. The thyroid may be enlarged. Identify any cervical adenopathy. Examine the heart carefully to identify any murmurs. Palpate the abdomen for any stool masses or splenomegaly. Assess sexual maturity with Tanner staging. Examine the skin for bruising, rashes, or dryness. Examine joints for swelling, pain, or erythema. Check for palmar creases and for clinodactyly. Check for a noticeable space ("sandal gap") between the first and second toes. Assess large joints for hypermobility. Perform a neurologic examination to evaluate for hypotonia. Plot height, weight, and head circumference on charts standardized for boys and girls with Down syndrome.

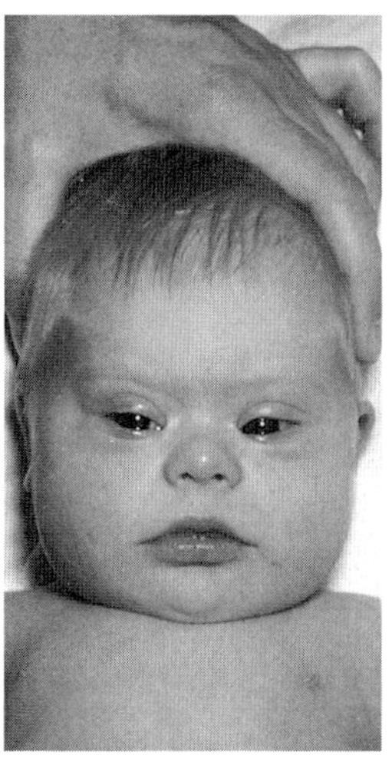

FIGURE 58-4 Down syndrome mid-facial hypoplasia. (From Zitelli B, Davis H: *Atlas of physical diagnosis,* ed 4, St Louis, 2002, Mosby, p 10.)

What Workup Is Appropriate?

A karyotype confirms the diagnosis and defines the specific chromosomal defect (trisomy 21, translocation, or mosaicism), which then guides genetic counseling. The Down Syndrome Health Care Guidelines describe the timing of various screening tests. As a general rule, workup of organic illness or sensory loss should *always* be considered first if a child with Down syndrome demonstrates behavioral problems.

TREATMENT

What Treatments Are Available?

Although Down syndrome cannot be cured at this time, improved medical management and early interventions have brightened the outlook for this population. Infants should be referred for early intervention services as soon as possible. Children should undergo periodic evaluation of speech, cognitive, and motor function so that school programming can be optimized. Primary health care providers should be aware of potential acute and chronic health issues in this population, as well as necessary preventive health care.

Case 58-1

The mother of an 18-month-old-girl is concerned because the child has not yet started to walk. She cannot sit independently, even for a brief period. She recently rolled from front to back but cannot roll back to front. She reaches for toys with her left hand with a "batting" motion. She makes vowel sounds and vocalizes mainly in response to familiar faces. She coughs when drinking and has a small hard stool every other day. She was born at 26 weeks' gestation and had a complicated, prolonged stay in the neonatal intensive care unit. Intraventricular hemorrhage was identified with subsequent cystic changes in periventricular white matter seen on head ultrasound. She was discharged 5 months after birth on nasal-canula oxygen and a high-calorie formula. Physical examination shows length at 5th percentile, weight below 5th percentile and head circumference (HC) 10th to 25th percentile. Head is long and narrow (dolichocephalic). When suspended under the arms, she internally rotates and adducts her hips, appearing to "scissor" her legs in midair. She also demonstrates a persistent asymmetric tonic neck reflex and a stepping reflex. She holds her right hand fisted during the examination. Gentle range of motion of the extremities encounters resistance until the end of the arc, when the resistance suddenly gives way. The resistance feels greatest on the right side. Deep tendon reflexes are globally hyperactive, with three beats of clonus at the right ankle.

A. How should gestational age be considered when evaluating the development of a child who was born prematurely?
B. What is the significance of the head ultrasound findings?

C. What contributes to this child's poor weight gain?
D. How will you answer the mother's questions about whether the child will ever walk?

Case 58-2

The mother of a 4-year-old boy brings a letter from the preschool teacher that expresses concerns about the boy's delayed language and behavior problems and asks whether he has autism. The boy communicates with two- and three-word phrases, with grunts, and by pointing at desired objects. He can undress himself but cannot dress or brush his own teeth. He plays alongside his peers but cries and bites if a child attempts to join in his solitary play. He has good eye contact with his parents; eye contact with teachers is intermittent and improves in quiet situations. His favorite activity is building with blocks. Birth history was unremarkable. He sat unsupported at 9 months and walked at 18 months. He first used words at 2 years and combined words at 3 years. He has not demonstrated any regression in development. His mother has no family history of developmental disorders; his father is adopted. The boy cries when he sees you and runs to his mother, with whom he cuddles for comfort. He displays minimal eye contact with you until you have chatted for several minutes with the family. He allows you to examine him on his mother's lap. The physical examination itself is unremarkable. Height and weight are at the 25th percentile; head circumference is 25th to 50th percentile. At one point you wind up a mechanical toy bear. As it moves across the floor, the boy laughs and says to his parents, "Look, teddy!" He then grabs a toy stethoscope and tries to "examine" the bear. Cognitive assessment by the clinic psychologist estimates developmental age at 24 months, with some scatter into 30 months. Speech and language tests reveal receptive language abilities at 28 months and expressive language abilities between 20 and 24 months. Hearing is tested as normal.

A. Why would the teacher be concerned about autism?
B. What information indicates that autism is not the problem?
C. How helpful is family history in evaluating a child with possible autism?

Case 58-3

A 15-year-old girl with Down syndrome is brought by her parents to clinic because she is not listening in class and is refusing to follow instructions. A note from the teacher's aide wonders if she must be treated for attention deficit hyperactivity disorder (ADHD). Parents note that she has become less cooperative with them at home, often staring blankly when they ask her to do things. History identifies loud snoring, choking and pauses during sleep, difficulty awakening, and falling asleep in school. Aside from a patent ductus arteriosus that closed spontaneously in infancy and two sets of myringotomy tubes as a toddler, her past medical history is unremarkable. On examination, she is an obese, pleasant girl with characteristic findings of Down syndrome, who appears considerably fatigued. She nods off several times as you are talking with her parents. Oropharynx has no obvious lesions and tonsils are not hypertrophied. Her right tympanic membrane has a large central perforation, and her left tympanic membrane has air-fluid levels. Heart and lung examination is noncontributory.

A. What information from the history can explain the problems noted at school and at home?
B. What further evaluation would be helpful?

Case Answers

58-1 A. *Learning objective:* **Discuss the impact of gestational age on development.** The length of time by which the child was premature is typically subtracted from the child's chronologic age to arrive at the corrected developmental age. In this case, the child was born approximately 3 months prematurely. When this time is subtracted from her chronologic age of 18 months, we would say that she has a *corrected gestational age* of 15 months. She should have achieved the developmental milestones common to most 15 month olds, such as saying single words and walking independently.

58-1 B. *Learning objective:* **Identify neurologic consequences of prematurity.** Severe intraventricular hemorrhage occurs commonly in premature infants and increases the risk for future developmental problems. Cystic changes in the periventricular white matter *(periventricular leukomalacia)* are strongly and specifically predictive for the later development of cerebral palsy.

58-1 C. *Learning objective:* **Discuss the nutritional problems experienced by infants and young children with cerebral palsy.** Feeding and growth problems are common in children with cerebral palsy and are typically multifactorial in origin. Because bulbopharyngeal musculature is often affected by the disorder, oral motor problems are common and cause abnormal swallowing. People with cerebral palsy are also prone to gastroesophageal reflux and to chronic aspiration. Children with spastic cerebral palsy also have increased caloric needs relative to children with normal tone. Weight gain must be monitored carefully.

58-1 D. *Learning objective:* **Demonstrate ability to counsel parents about cerebral palsy.** Try to avoid having to prognosticate if at all possible. Children present continual surprises to their families and their doctors whether they have or do not have disabilities. The best approach is to provide support and let the child develop to the extent possible. Encourage the family to maximize the child's potential and to accept the child as a unique individual. If the family insists that you give an impression of what the future may hold, it is reasonable to say that the prognosis for walking is poor if a child demonstrates persistent primitive reflexes at 2 years of age or is not sitting independently by this time.

58-2 A. *Learning objective:* **Identify the characteristic findings in autism.** Language and social deficits are characteristic of autism spectrum disorders but are also common in overall developmental delay. In comparison with his classmates, this boy has delayed language and social skills. His parallel play and inconsistent eye contact are behaviors typical of a much younger child, as are his outbursts of crying and biting. Further evaluation identified delayed development as the likely cause of the observed behaviors.

58-2 B. *Learning objective:* **Discuss the evaluation of a child in whom autism is suspected.** This child cuddles when he needs comforting. Although children with autism are often very loving with family members, they may not seek comfort or cuddle. Instead, many autistic children flap hands, spin, or scream in stressful situations. In addition, he pointed out the toy bear to his parents, which reflects the emergence of joint attention behavior, a milestone in social reciprocity that is absent or markedly reduced in children with autism. When he attempted to examine the bear with the stethoscope he demonstrated imaginative play, which is also greatly reduced or even absent in autism. This boy's skills are at the level appropriate for his delayed development. He does not have autism.

58-2 C. *Learning objective:* **Discuss the heredity of autism.** This boy's maternal history has no risk factors; the father's history cannot be assessed. A strong maternal family history of autism, anxiety, ADHD, academic failure, or conduct problems in males should prompt a workup for fragile X in a boy being evaluated for autism. Characteristic dysmorphic features may be subtle or absent on examination, especially early in life. Information about more subtle familial personality traits may also be helpful in the evaluation because first-degree family members of individuals with autism may have higher rates of timidity, aloofness, inflexibility, and difficulty with social language use. A sensitively collected family history may reveal high degrees of social awkwardness and rigidity for several generations.

58-3 A. *Learning objective:* **Discuss the approach to behavioral problems in a child with Down syndrome.** Whenever a child with Down syndrome presents with behavioral changes, *medical problems must always be ruled out.* This teenager with Down syndrome has inattention and defiance. Her parents report loud snoring and daytime sleepiness. On examination, you find obesity and bilateral middle ear pathology. Individuals with Down syndrome are at high risk for sleep apnea because of the predisposing narrow airway and the hypotonia of the musculature supporting the airway. Sleep deficits can manifest themselves as attentional and behavioral problems. In addition, the characteristic craniofacial hypoplasia in this population predisposes them to chronic ENT infection, obstruction, and hearing loss.

58-3 B. *Learning objective:* **Discuss the appropriate workup for children with Down syndrome who have behavioral or medical problems.** Given the history and physical examination, it would be reasonable to order an overnight sleep study to determine if she has sleep apnea. She should also be referred to an otolaryngologist experienced in treating children with Down syndrome. Then, she will need audiometry. It is also prudent to obtain thyroid functions on any individual with Down syndrome who presents with a behavioral change.

BIBLIOGRAPHY

Autism

Bauman ML, Kemper TL: *The neurobiology of autism*, ed 2, 2005, Baltimore, MD, The Johns Hopkins University Press. This comprehensive review of current autism-based research theories and clinical applications discusses recommendations for the initial workup.

Volkmar FR: *Handbook of autism and pervasive developmental disorders*, ed 3, 2005, Hoboken, NJ, John Wiley & Sons.

www.autism-resources.com/. Information-rich site containing numerous helpful links, book reviews, a FAQ page, parent commentaries, and much more.

Cerebral Palsy

Capute A, Accardo P: *Developmental disabilities in infancy and childhood, Vol II: The spectrum of developmental disabilities*, Baltimore, 1996, Paul Brookes. The second of a two-volume book, a detailed exploration of cerebral palsy and other disabilities and their manifestations from infancy to young adulthood. Recommendations for assessment and treatment.

Miller F: *Cerebral palsy*, Cambridge, 2005, Springer. Informative review of orthopedic issues in this population, including seating and physical therapy.

United Cerebral Palsy Association Web site: *www.ucpa.org/*. Links to topics in research, advocacy, education, employment, housing, and public policy.

Down Syndrome

The National Down Syndrome Society Web site: *www.ndss.org*. Comprehensive portal site offering not only up-to-date medical information but also links to research and advocacy resources.

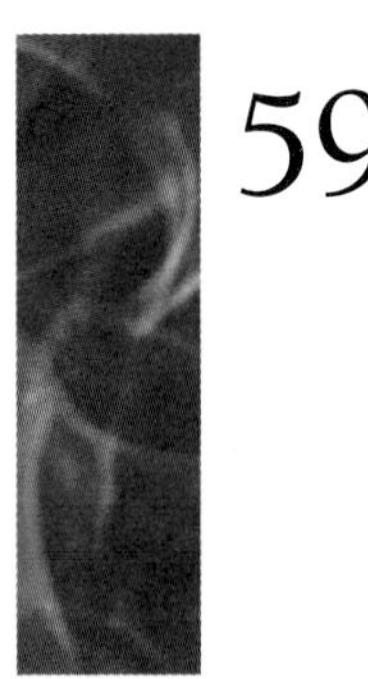

59

Emergencies

CHARLES A. JENNISSEN and STEVEN Z. MILLER[†]

SEIZURES

ETIOLOGY

What Causes Seizures?

Identification of the specific cause of a seizure (Table 59-1) usually comes only after the patient is stable but may be very important in initiating appropriate treatment. Any time a patient has the new onset of seizures, you must first think of the dangerous and reversible causes. Chapter 37 discusses seizures in greater detail.

What Causes Seizure in a Child Who Has a Fever?

A "simple" febrile seizure is the most likely type of generalized tonic-clonic seizure in a febrile child between 6 months and 6 years of age (Table 37–1). Other seizures that occur with fever include "complex" febrile seizure, underlying epilepsy or metabolic disease with seizure triggered by fever, and seizure associated with central nervous system infection (Chapter 37).

EVALUATION

How Do I Determine the Cause of a Seizure?

Your immediate reaction to a seizing patient should be to perform the ABCs (see Chapter 31) and to stabilize the patient. It is important to test for hypoglycemia and to identify hypoxemia with oximetry. Poisoning may have a characteristic toxidrome, which is a unique pattern of signs and symptoms affecting the heart rate, blood pressure, pupil size, and body temperature (Table 59-2). Electrolyte abnormalities and inborn errors of metabolism may be identified by blood chemistry tests. Central nervous system (CNS) infection usually has characteristic signs and will be detected with lumbar puncture and cultures. Concern about possible intracranial hemorrhage or tumor will prompt imaging studies.

[†]Deceased.

Table 59-1

Causes of Seizures

Category	Specific Cause
Insufficient substrate to the brain	Hypoxemia Shock Increased intracranial pressure Hypoglycemia
Poisonings	Amphetamines, opioids, anticonvulsants, cocaine, ethanol, lead (and many more)
Electrolyte abnormalities	Calcium or magnesium abnormalities Sodium abnormalities
Serious conditions that need to be diagnosed quickly	Meningitis/encephalitis Central nervous system hemorrhage Tumor Inborn errors of metabolism
Diagnoses of exclusion	Febrile seizure Idiopathic epilepsy

Table 59-2

Toxidromes (Selected List)

Toxidrome	Cause
Tachycardia, hypertension, large, briskly reactive pupils	Sympathomimetics
Tachycardia, hypertension, large, sluggish pupils	Anticholinergics
Bradycardia, tachypnea, small pupils	Cholinergics (organophosphates or nerve gas)
Bradycardia, decreased respirations, pinpoint pupils	Opioids (and clonidine)

A seizing infant may be the victim of physical abuse (see Chapter 24 and the sections on altered level of consciousness and head trauma in this chapter). Finally, idiopathic epilepsy and febrile seizure are diagnoses of exclusion.

Do All Febrile Patients Who Have Seizures Need Lumbar Puncture?

Patients with a simple febrile seizure rarely require a lumbar puncture. If the patient is awake and alert after the seizure, you can rule out meningitis clinically with history and physical examination. On the other hand, a lumbar puncture *must* be done if the febrile child appears "toxic" or if there is obvious meningeal irritation (stiff neck, Kernig's and/or Brudzinski's sign). If the patient is sleepy after the seizure but seems to be slowly waking up, you can observe for a period of time. If the patient is not awake and alert after about 30 minutes, a lumbar puncture should be considered. Also, if the child is younger than 6 months, most authorities recommend a spinal tap after a seizure with fever.

TREATMENT

What Should I Do If a Patient Is Seizing?

The key is to take a limited number of actions in a specific sequence that will keep you task-oriented (see Chapter 31):

- Start with the ABCs.
- Provide oxygen and establish vascular access (give intravenous fluids if necessary).
- Assess the response to your interventions.
- Obtain a finger-stick glucose level.
- Consider sending blood samples for electrolyte levels.
- Consider possible poisonings and administer the antidote for any specific poison identified.

After you have stabilized your patient and considered the dangerous and reversible causes of seizures, you should administer a medication to stop the seizure. Once the seizure has stopped, identify other seizure causes with a thorough history and physical examination and selected diagnostic and imaging tests.

When Should I Give an Anticonvulsant to a Patient Who Is Having a Seizure?

Anticonvulsants should only be administered after the steps discussed previously. If the seizure has gone on 5 minutes or more, you should consider anticonvulsant administration.

What Anticonvulsant Should I Use to Stop a Seizure?

The benzodiazepines (lorazepam, diazepam, midazolam) are usually used first because they have a short onset of action and are relatively safe. These may be given intravenously, intraosseously, or by rectal administration. Lorazepam is often considered the drug of choice for persistent seizures because of its longer duration of action. If these fail, an intravenous loading dose of phenobarbital or phenytoin is the next choice.

RESPIRATORY DISTRESS

ETIOLOGY

What Causes a Child to Have Difficulty Breathing?

Some important causes of respiratory distress that affect children include the following:

- Asthma
- Bronchiolitis (usually caused by respiratory syncytial virus [RSV])

- Croup
- Bacterial pneumonia
- Congestive heart failure
- Foreign body aspiration
- Chronic lung disease (such as cystic fibrosis or bronchopulmonary dysplasia)

EVALUATION

What Findings Help Me Identify Respiratory Distress?

Evaluation of the following will identify patients with ventilation problems and difficulty breathing:

- General responsiveness: Hypoxemic children are often agitated and those with CO_2 retention may be drowsy.
- Respiratory rate: Count the respirations yourself. Remember that the upper limit for respiratory rate in healthy young infants is approximately 50 breaths/min; respiratory rate decreases to about 30 breaths/min by 1 year of age.
- Chest wall movement: Intercostal or supraclavicular retractions are signs of increased work of breathing.
- Abdominal breathing: Infants will have "see-saw" breathing when in distress—the chest pulls in when the abdomen moves out, and vice versa—because of the compliance of the infant chest.
- Head bobbing: Infants will often rock their heads (as if nodding "yes") when in respiratory distress.
- Skin color: Cyanosis is a sign of hypoxemia.
- Pulse oximetry: Oxygen saturation below 91% is concerning because this is at the beginning of the steep part of the O_2 saturation curve.
- Decreased breath sounds and air flow: Auscultate carefully!
- Abnormal sounds: *Wheezing* indicates bronchiolar obstruction, but you may not hear wheeze if there is very poor air flow. *Crackles* reflect alveolar collapse, fluid, or pneumonia.
- Pulsus paradoxus: This very concerning finding is identified by a marked change in the systolic blood pressure between the end of inspiration and the end of expiration. Blood pressure normally drops slightly during inspiration, but the gap should not be greater than 10 mm Hg. You measure pulsus paradoxus by taking the blood pressure and identifying the gap between the pressure of the first heart beat that you hear when deflating the cuff and the pressure at which you begin to hear every beat. Pulsus paradoxus greater than 20 mm Hg in an asthmatic patient reflects impending respiratory collapse.

TREATMENT

How Do I Treat an Infant Who Is Wheezing?

A wheezing infant younger than 1 year most likely has bronchiolitis, especially during the winter months. This is usually caused by RSV

(Chapter 69). Most infants require only supportive treatment, but some may need more aggressive management. *Hypoxia* is a common complication of bronchiolitis and pulse oximetry is an important test. Administration of oxygen should be considered when the oxygen saturation is below 94%. *Apnea* is another potential complication of RSV bronchiolitis, especially in young infants, and will necessitate hospitalization when present. Because wheezing is a prominent clinical finding, many physicians empirically treat bronchiolitis with inhaled bronchodilators (nebulized albuterol or racemic epinephrine). Anecdotal evidence suggests that bronchodilator therapy results in short-term improvement of bronchiolitis, but systematic reviews of the literature have not provided evidence that bronchodilator treatment reduces rates of admission to hospital, improves oxygen saturation, or affects long-term outcome. Use of oral corticosteroids is not recommended for bronchiolitis. Wheezing is discussed further in Chapters 25 and 69.

Is Management Different for an Older Child with Wheezing?

Symmetrical, diffuse, polyphonic wheezing in a child older than 1 year or with recurrent wheezing is much more likely to be asthma (Chapter 69) than bronchiolitis. Bronchodilators and corticosteroids have documented efficacy, both acutely and long-term. Oxygen may be needed for severe asthma attacks, so pulse oximetry should be used for all patients. If asymmetrical, monophonic wheezing is detected, foreign-body aspiration must be considered. Imaging studies and bronchoscopy may be needed for diagnosis and management.

ALTERED LEVEL OF CONSCIOUSNESS

ETIOLOGY

What Diagnoses Should I Consider When I See a Child Who Is Difficult to Arouse?

Altered level of consciousness and seizures have similar causes. Think about a cluster of causes that are prioritized by seriousness.

First, consider urgent, life-threatening problems:

- Hypoxemia
- Hypoglycemia
- Shock (septic, cardiogenic, hypovolemic, neurogenic, anaphylactic shock; in addition, congenital adrenal hyperplasia and diabetic ketoacidosis can present as shock.

Next, identify dangerous yet reversible causes:

- Poisoning (especially carbon monoxide, opioid, anticholinergic, cholinergic, cyclic antidepressant, and cardiotoxic drugs)
- Electrolyte abnormalities (calcium/magnesium, sodium, potassium)
- Status epilepticus in a patient with partial complex seizures

Then, consider serious causes that require aggressive evaluation and management:

- CNS hemorrhage (consider child abuse, such as shaken baby syndrome in an infant)
- Meningitis/encephalitis
- Tumor

Finally, think about intussusception. The diagnosis is counterintuitive because it seems to have nothing to do with the CNS directly, but this gastrointestinal obstruction can present as lethargy without obvious gastrointestinal symptoms in a young child (usually between 3 months and 3 years of age, with a peak at 11 months). An experienced pediatrician will often think of this diagnosis and perform a rectal examination to look for blood in the stool. A child who presents late with intussusception may have enough injury to the bowel to present with "currant jelly stool," a grossly bloody stool classic for this problem.

EVALUATION

How Do I Make Sure That I Do Not Overlook a Serious Cause of Lethargy?

Remember, a limited number of actions will identify the life-threatening cause of lethargy:

- Start with the ABCs (to assess for hypoxemia, shock, and brain herniation).
- Give oxygen and obtain access (administer intravascular fluids if necessary).
- Assess the response to your interventions (do not forget this important step).
- Obtain finger-stick glucose level. Assess serum electrolytes and consider poisonings.
- Consider status epilepticus with complex partial epilepsy. Look for mouth twitching and other subtle signs of seizure activity.
- Consider intracranial causes, such as hemorrhage, tumor, or meningitis. Use clinical findings first and perform computed tomography (CT) scan and spinal tap as necessary.
- Consider inborn errors of metabolism in infants and young children. Blood levels of CO_2, ammonia, and lactate are a good starting point.
- Consider intussusception. Perform a rectal examination and obtain abdominal radiographs to identify bowel obstruction. A contrast enema is the "gold standard" for diagnosis and treatment.

TREATMENT

What Treatment Is Needed for a Patient with an Altered Level of Consciousness?

Treatment depends entirely on the cause. Initial management is supportive and stabilizes the patient. You should review the specific management options for the most likely disorders that cause altered level of consciousness.

POISONING

ETIOLOGY

Who Is Most Likely to Be a Poisoning Victim?

Poisoning occurs most commonly in toddlers, between 12 months and 3 years of age, and adolescents. *Toddlers* have a high risk for *unintentional* poisoning because of their curiosity and the developmental drive to explore. The most common ingestions include acetaminophen, cough and cold preparations, cleaning substances, cosmetics, and plants. Toddlers occasionally ingest medications prescribed for other family members. *Adolescents* usually are victims of self-inflicted, *intentional* poisoning, most of which involves pharmaceuticals such as acetaminophen, barbiturates, stimulants, and antidepressants. Alcohol is a common "unintentional" poison in this age group.

EVALUATION

What Is the Initial Approach to an Overdose?

As always, start with the ABCs and stabilize the patient. You may want to add another "A" for antidotes and another "D" for decontaminate in your primary survey. These are discussed in the treatment section. Check the pupils, heart rate, respiratory rate, and blood pressure to identify a toxidrome so that the antidote for a specific toxin may be administered.

How Do I Determine the Cause of an Overdose?

Often, no obvious toxidrome is present on examination. Ask about the details of the ingestion, especially timing, ingested substance(s), and reports from any observers. Identify all medications that are in the home and assume that they were *all* taken until proven otherwise. Ask a family member to go home and bring back all the medications that are in the home, including all empty containers. Remember, patients and families often do not consider birth control pills, vitamins, acetaminophen, aspirin, other over-the-counter preparations, and complementary, alternative, and herbal preparations as medications. These should be brought from home, too.

What Tests Should I Consider for a Poisoned Patient?

Screening tests include:

- Electrocardiogram with a rhythm strip may be the *most important* test. It allows you to identify the effects of cardiotoxic drugs, which are among the most dangerous poisonings. Keep the patient on a cardiac monitor.
- Acetaminophen level is critical. The patient may be asymptomatic and may not report the ingestion or consider acetaminophen to be a medication. Hepatic toxicity begins approximately 48 hours after the overdose, but the window of opportunity to treat with the antidote is within 24 hours and best results are obtained if treatment is started within 8 hours.

- Complete blood count, serum chemistries, and liver function tests as a baseline.
- Osmolar gap will identify unknown alcohol ingestion. The osmolar gap is the difference between serum osmols measured directly and osmols calculated from a chemistry panel.
- Salicylate blood levels are done routinely at some centers.
- Toxicology screens and alcohol levels are usually sent, especially for adolescents.
- Abdominal radiographs are not routine but may identify radiopaque pills, such as iron tablets.

TREATMENT

How Would I Decontaminate an Overdose Patient?

Decontamination is a mainstay of poisoning treatment but must be initiated as soon as possible to be effective. *Activated charcoal* is the most effective decontaminant and is best used within 1 hour of the ingestion. Use after this time period may still be helpful for overdose with slow-release medications, and some specific poisonings are treated with repetitive activated charcoal dosing (details are available from Poison Control Centers). *Syrup of ipecac has virtually no role in the management of poisonings.* Its use will make it more difficult to use activated charcoal. *Gastric lavage is rarely useful* except in comatose patients within 30 minutes of a lethal overdose, and it is effective only if done with a large tube (if the tube fits in the nose, it is too small). The airway must be protected during lavage. None of these treatments should be used for caustic or hydrocarbon ingestions.

How Do I Treat Specific Ingestions?

Many medications or ingested substances have a particular antidote. Table 59-3 includes antidotes for common and dangerous ingestions.

Table 59-3

Antidotes for Common Ingestions

Toxic Ingestion	Antidote
Acetaminophen	*N*-acetyl cysteine
Anticholinergics	Physostigmine
Cholinergics	Atropine (and sometimes pralidoxime)
Beta-blockers	Glucagon
Digitalis	Fab antibodies (Digibind)
Iron	Deferoxamine
Isoniazid	Pyridoxine
Opioids (and possibly clonidine)	Naloxone
Phenothiazines	Diphenhydramine or benztropine
Cyclic antidepressants	Sodium bicarbonate

How Do I Use Blood Levels to Make Treatment Decisions?

Blood levels can be measured for many medications, including acetaminophen, salicylates, theophylline, and anticonvulsants. Nomograms are readily available in emergency departments to compare the blood levels of acetaminophen and salicylates with the expected outcome.

How Do I Treat a Toxic Acetaminophen Ingestion?

Treatment of an acetaminophen overdose with *N*-acetyl-cysteine (Mucomyst) is based on the blood level 4 hours after the ingestion. Treatment can be delayed until the blood level comes back, but because the antidote is most effective when administered within 8 hours of the ingestion, treatment should be started if you anticipate any delay in obtaining the blood level beyond this point. The *nomogram absolutely does not apply to sustained-release forms of acetaminophen,* so all patients who overdose with a sustained-release product must be treated with *N*-acetyl-cysteine and monitored closely for hepatic toxicity. The combination of acetaminophen overdose and acute or chronic alcohol ingestion may put the patient at increased risk of hepatic toxicity.

HEAD TRAUMA

ETIOLOGY

What Diagnoses Should I Consider for a Patient with Traumatic Loss of Consciousness?

Your most important task is to determine whether the loss of consciousness occurred *before* or *after* the head trauma. When loss of consciousness occurs before head trauma, consider the diagnoses discussed in the sections on seizures and altered loss of consciousness in this chapter. When trauma *causes* loss of consciousness, you must be prepared to manage one or more of the following:

- Diffuse axonal injury: This is usually associated with a violent mechanism, such as a motor vehicle crash, and almost always causes persistent symptoms and prolonged loss of consciousness.
- CNS hemorrhage: *Epidural hemorrhage* is arterial in origin and can occur from relatively minor trauma, especially to the temporoparietal region of the head through which the middle meningeal artery traverses. Patients who have epidural hemorrhage may be totally lucid for a period of time after the head trauma, then abruptly lose consciousness. *Subdural hemorrhage* is usually venous in origin, and symptoms may develop only after several days.
- Contusion: Transient symptoms such as amnesia after head trauma may indicate a contusion. A brain contusion is a parenchymal bruise (hemorrhage and edema) on the surface of the brain resulting from

primary neuronal and vascular injury from trauma. The bleeding may extend into the white matter and subdural/subarachnoid spaces. There may be long-term and sometimes subtle consequences to this injury.

- Concussion: This results from trauma that causes altered mental status but no radiographic evidence of CNS injury. Loss of consciousness is not necessary for the diagnosis of concussion. Grading schemes are based on the duration and severity of the symptoms. Concussion may be relatively benign or may result in significant sequelae such as recurrent headache, dizziness, or intolerance of exercise.
- Abusive head injury: This sad but prevalent occurrence must be considered for any infant who presents with altered level of consciousness. Any of the brain injuries discussed above may be present.

EVALUATION

How Do I Determine If a Head Injury Is the Result of Abuse?

Although medical students are not yet mandatory reporters, you should learn the "red flags" (Table 24–2) that make the diagnosis of abuse more likely. A history of trauma that is not consistent with the injury and the child's development should raise concern about the possibility of intentional trauma/abuse. You should notify your attending of the concern. A physician who *suspects* abuse in a case of head trauma must file a report to child protective services. Definite diagnosis of abuse and identification of the abuser are *not* the responsibility of the reporting physician. A detailed discussion of child abuse can be found in Chapter 24.

Should I Order a Skull X-Ray or Computed Tomography Scan?

Imaging in the evaluation of head trauma continues to be controversial. For infants up to 1 year of age, a moderate-sized hematoma is an indication for a *skull x-ray* to screen for an underlying fracture. If a linear fracture is identified, a *CT scan* would be warranted. This is particularly true for infants younger than 3 months of age and in any case where abuse is suspected. Signs or symptoms that are considered indications for CT scan include:

- Loss of consciousness for more than a brief period
- Amnesia for the event and/or for preceding or subsequent events
- Persistent vomiting
- Seizure
- Drowsiness
- Persistent, high-pitched crying
- Significant skull fracture on physical examination
- Altered level of consciousness
- Neurologic deficit on examination
- Abnormal behavior
- Coagulopathy

TREATMENT

If a Head-Injured Patient Appears to Be Herniating, What Can I Do?

Brain herniation is a life-threatening consequence of head injury. Management of impending herniation includes the following:

- Raise the head of the bed 30 degrees (unless the cervical spine is unstable).
- Sedate patient if combative or agitated.
- Infuse mannitol.

Hyperventilate the patient using a bag-valve-mask (BVM) or through an endotracheal tube until the signs of herniation are reversed. (Excessive hyperventilation must be avoided in patients with increased intracranial pressure who are not herniating. Hyperventilation may cause reduced CNS arteriolar blood flow because of vasoconstriction. Subsequent decreased delivery of oxygen and other needed substrates may cause additional brain injury.)

KEY POINTS

- Start with the ABCs for all emergencies.
- Assess response to your initial stabilization efforts.
- Problem-specific management begins only after the patient is stable.
- A seizing child may be hypoglycemic.
- Check oxygen saturation when a child has respiratory distress or altered level of consciousness.
- Look for toxidromes when evaluating a poisoned child.
- Head trauma may be accidental or inflicted: Be sure that the injury is consistent with the history.

Case 59-1

A 2-year-old boy is rushed into the emergency department by his parents. You observe generalized tonic-clonic seizure activity.

A. What should you do first?
B. Does this child need urgent anticonvulsant treatment?
C. Does this child need long-term therapy?

Case 59-2

A 16-year-old boy presents to the emergency department agitated and in respiratory distress. His respiratory rate is 28 breaths/min, heart rate is 130 beats/min, and his oxygen saturation is 90%. His parents tell you that he has had asthma since early childhood. He has been using an albuterol inhaler five or six times daily for the past several days. Someone recommends treating the boy with lorazepam because he is agitated. In addition, the concern is expressed that albuterol might further increase his heart rate, leading to cardiac ischemia.

A. What is this boy's diagnosis?
B. How would you treat this patient?
C. Does albuterol pose a risk to this patient?

Case 59-3

A 6-month-old boy is brought to the emergency department by his mother, who says that he has been acting "out of it." She tells you that earlier today her son would not wake for a feeding. A similar episode happened 1 month ago. When you examine the infant, you find that he is alert and interactive and has an unremarkable physical examination.

A. Why does this history concern you?
B. What three major diagnoses might you consider?

Case 59-4

A 16-year-old boy presents to the emergency department in a lethargic state. He has pinpoint pupils, a pulse of 80 beats/min, respirations of 16 breaths/min, and blood pressure of 122/76 mm Hg. Because of the presumption of an opioid overdose, you give a single dose of naloxone. The patient does not respond to this treatment and remains lethargic.

A. Does this patient really have an opioid overdose?
B. Why did he not respond to naloxone?
C. What characteristic of naloxone requires special attention when managing an opioid overdose?

Case 59-5

A 16-year-old boy was hit on the head with a baseball bat 8 hours earlier. He has no memory of the event. Witnesses state that he had momentary loss of consciousness at the time of the injury but was lucid and coherent once he awoke. Aside from pain and swelling at the site of the injury, he felt well until approximately 2 hours ago when vomiting developed. The vomiting has been persistent since then. His physical examination demonstrates an alert but uncomfortable boy who is complaining of headache. He has a hematoma over the right temporal region. He vomited twice during the examination.

A. What concerns you about this patient?
B. What diagnostic workup will you pursue?
C. What findings are commonly associated with intracranial injury?

Case Answers

59-1 A. *Learning objective:* **Describe the initial approach to an actively seizing patient.** Generally speaking, seizures of short duration do not cause significant damage as long as you maintain adequate delivery of oxygen and glucose to the brain. Therefore, the steps in management of this child would include the following:

- Position the airway and administer oxygen. Monitor effectiveness of this management by measuring the oxygen saturation.
- Check perfusion and give fluids if patient is in shock.
- Check blood glucose level and administer intravenous glucose if low.

59-1 B. *Learning objective:* **Discuss the indications for treating a seizing patient with anticonvulsants.** Once you have stabilized the patient and have addressed the potentially reversible causes of seizures, you can consider administration of a medication to stop the seizure. One of the benzodiazepines should be administered if a generalized, tonic-clonic seizure does not stop spontaneously after 5 minutes or after administration of intravenous glucose if the sugar level was low.

59-1 C. *Learning objective:* **Discuss the prognosis of a generalized seizure, based on its cause, and the need for long-term treatment.** The need for long-term management with anticonvulsants depends on the cause of the seizure. Neither a simple febrile seizure nor the first generalized seizure of epilepsy requires anticonvulsant therapy.

59-2 A. *Learning objective:* **Use the history and physical examination to identify status asthmaticus and recognize agitation as a sign of hypoxia.** This patient is in status asthmaticus. The history of long-standing asthma, his excessive use of inhaled albuterol, and his respiratory distress all point to this diagnosis. For any patient who is agitated, you must rule out lack of oxygen as the cause. In this case, an oxygen saturation of 90% tells you that he needs oxygen, not lorazepam.

59-2 B. *Learning objective:* **Describe how to treat a patient with status asthmaticus.** This patient needs oxygen, beta agonist therapy, and systemic corticosteroids. He will also need to be hospitalized in a monitored unit.

59-2 C. *Learning objective:* **Discuss the therapeutic effects and the side effects of common medications used to treat asthma.** Beta agonists such as albuterol are safe for children and adolescents even if they have tachycardia. Cardiac ischemia is essentially not a concern in the pediatric age range. The tachycardia is most likely related to the hypoxemia and respiratory distress.

59-3 A. *Learning objective:* **Discuss the major reasons that lethargy in an infant should cause concern.** Lethargy in an infant suggests the possibility of a number of serious disorders. You must consider anything that affects the substrates available for central nervous system function. Other causes include poisonings, seizures, trauma, and intussusception. An infant with lethargy or altered consciousness may have been subjected to abusive head trauma. The history of the event must be obtained with care. The physical examination also must look for signs of physical abuse, although findings such as bruises or long bone fractures may be absent.

59-3 B. *Learning objective:* **Discuss the causes of recurring lethargy in an infant.** Based on this infant's presentation, the following diagnoses need to be considered:

- *Shaken baby syndrome:* Infants subjected to trauma by shaking often recover from their injuries and often have no visible injuries. They may be intermittently lethargic and irritable, depending on the frequency and severity of shaking episodes. Unexplained, recurrent visits for lethargy, even in well-appearing infants, warrant a meticulous history to determine the details of the illness and to ensure that the history is consistent with the physical findings. The physical examination should search for signs of trauma, increased intracranial pressure, and neurologic dysfunction. An ophthalmologic examination should be done to look for retinal hemorrhages and a CT scan of the head may be indicated to identify subdural hemorrhage.
- *Inborn errors of metabolism,* including congenital adrenal hyperplasia: Partial defects in the enzyme system can lead to recurrent episodes of lethargy that resolve with appropriate hydration. Although this is typically detected with the neonatal screen, some infants are not tested. Physical examination may demonstrate ambiguous genitalia in girls, but boys may be difficult to identify. Abnormalities of serum electrolytes, including hyponatremia in combination with hyperkalemia, can be a clue to this diagnosis.

- *Intussusception:* This can manifest as intermittent episodes of irritability or lethargy. The waxing and waning symptoms might be labeled as recurrent. An abdominal mass and currant jelly stools are physical findings that support this diagnosis, although they may be absent early in the disease.

59-4 A. *Learning objective:* **Recognize opioid overdose using clinical findings.** Pinpoint pupils and lethargy are the hallmarks of opioid overdose, so the presumptive diagnosis is reasonable.

59-4 B. *Learning objective:* **Describe the treatment of suspected opioid overdose.** Naloxone is the treatment of choice, but the initial dose may not have been adequate. Certain opioids need a large dose of naloxone to reverse the drug effects. Repeat doses of naloxone may be needed every 2 minutes, for five total doses (10 mg total).

59-4 C. *Learning objective:* **Discuss the practical aspects of naloxone pharmacokinetics.** Naloxone has a duration of action of approximately 20 minutes. Thus, effective reversal of opioid toxicity may require repeat doses or even use of a naloxone drip. Monitor the patient's level of consciousness and pupil responses closely.

59-5 A. *Learning objective:* **Identify the information from the history that points to intracranial injury caused by head trauma.** Head trauma with loss of consciousness and later development of persistent vomiting indicate the need to evaluate the patient for possible intracranial bleeding. In particular, the site of the injury and the period between trauma and development of other symptoms suggest a possible epidural hemorrhage.

59-5 B. *Learning objective:* **Discuss the evaluation for possible intracranial injury.** This boy should have a head CT scan to look for intracranial bleeding. During the imaging study, you must monitor the patient and be prepared to intervene in the event that increased intracranial pressure develops and causes life-threatening problems.

59-5 C. *Learning objective:* **Discuss the risk factors that suggest intracranial injury.** "Red flags" that raise concern about intracranial injury include the following:

- Mechanism of the injury suggests severe trauma (e.g., a direct blow to the head with a hard object or a fall from an extreme height). The mechanism must be considered carefully despite initial absence of signs and symptoms of intracranial injury.
- Amnesia
- Persistent vomiting
- Injury to the temporoparietal region (because of the potential involvement of the middle meningeal artery)
- Glasgow Coma Scale score < 15 (especially if this persists)
- Abnormal neurologic examination

60

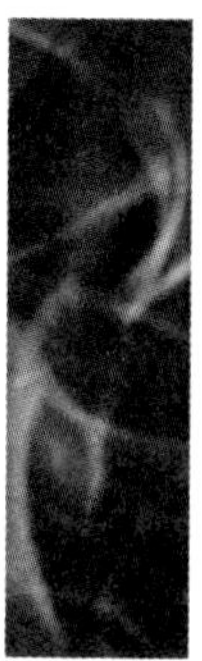

Endocrinology

NICHOLAS JOSPE

DIABETES MELLITUS

ETIOLOGY

What Causes Diabetes?

Type 1 diabetes mellitus results from autoimmune destruction of the insulin-producing β cells in the pancreatic islets. Numerous genes play a role in type 1 diabetes, although their exact function is still unclear. Environmental factors, such as viral infections and stress, may also contribute to the development of the disease. *In type 2 diabetes mellitus,* the initial insulin resistance and subsequent relative insulin deficiency result in abnormal glucose metabolism and its consequences. Obese individuals in particular are thought to have insulin resistance before development of relative insulin deficiency. Symptoms of diabetes occur in type 2 diabetes when insulin secretion is inadequate to overcome insulin resistance. Type 2 diabetes is emerging as an important pediatric problem, reflecting the epidemic of obesity in the industrialized world. In the United States, 10% to 40% of children with newly diagnosed diabetes have type 2 disease, with regional variation based on the prevalence of obesity and other risk factors, including race.

EVALUATION

How Do Type 1 and Type 2 Diabetes Differ?

Distinguishing type 1 diabetes from type 2 diabetes is important and may present a diagnostic dilemma in children. Although there is a genetic component to type 1 diabetes, a family history of diabetes is positive in only 1 of 10 patients. By contrast, the family history in type 2 diabetes is usually more prominent. Both type 1 and type 2 diabetes cause polyuria and polydipsia. Type 1 diabetes has mainly nonspecific physical findings, including dehydration, weight loss, and, rarely, growth failure. Type 2 diabetes is strongly associated with obesity as a component of the metabolic syndrome and may have additional

Table 60-1

Characteristics of Type 1 and Type 2 Diabetes Mellitus

Characteristics	Type 1 Diabetes	Type 2 Diabetes
Age at diagnosis	All ages	Puberty
Gender	Male = female	Female > male
Highest prevalence	Caucasians	African-Americans, Latinos, Native Americans
Symptom onset	Rapid	Progressive
Diagnosis on routine physical examination	Uncommon	Common
Hx of polyuria, polydipsia, weight loss	Common	Less common
FHx of diabetes	Infrequent	Frequent
FHx of autoimmune disease, such as hypothyroidism or hyperthyroidism	More frequent	Less frequent
Obesity	Less common	Very common
Acanthosis nigricans	Rare	Common
DKA at onset	Common	Rare
Ketones in urine	Common	Rare to absent
Islet cell autoantibodies	Present	Absent

DKA, Diabetic ketoacidosis; FHx, family history; Hx, history.

findings, including acanthosis nigricans, hypertension, hyperlipidemia, and, in females, polycystic ovary syndrome. Table 60-1 lists the features of both types of diabetes.

How Is Blood Glucose Used to Diagnose Diabetes?

The following blood glucose findings are diagnostic of diabetes:

- Casual blood glucose greater than 200 mg/dl along with symptoms of diabetes ("casual" = random, without regard to time since last meal)
- Fasting glucose above 126 mg/dl
- Blood glucose greater than 200 mg/dl, 2 hours after a glucose load during an oral glucose tolerance test

Impaired fasting glucose or impaired glucose tolerance implies a significant risk of developing diabetes. *Impaired fasting glucose* is defined as glucose levels of 100 to 125 mg/dl in fasting patients. *Impaired glucose tolerance* is defined as 2-hour glucose levels of 140 to 199 mg/dl on the 75-g oral glucose tolerance test. The oral glucose tolerance test is not recommended for routine clinical use to screen for the diagnosis.

How Is Type 1 Diabetes Diagnosed?

Type 1 diabetes becomes clinically apparent when excessive thirst and urination develop, along with increased appetite, enuresis, weight loss, and fatigue. If symptoms are not recognized, the child may become markedly dehydrated and progress to diabetic ketoacidosis (DKA). Rarely, an asymptomatic patient will be identified because of glucosuria on a routine urinalysis. Diagnosis of diabetes is based on hyperglycemia. Glucosuria, with or without ketonuria, also is diagnostic.

How Is Type 2 Diabetes Diagnosed in Children?

Type 2 diabetes is increasing in prevalence among obese children and adolescents. Risk factors include a family history of type 2 diabetes, a body mass index above the 95th percentile for age, physical inactivity, hypertension, and low levels of high-density lipoprotein cholesterol. Populations at high risk include African-Americans, Latinos, Native Americans, and Asian-Pacific Islanders. The typical patient with type 2 diabetes is an obese adolescent with acanthosis nigricans who may be asymptomatic or may have polyuria, polydipsia, and sometimes dehydration. Evaluation of such a patient should include inquiry into the family history and a screening test for blood glucose level. Referral of obese patients to pediatric endocrinologists for evaluation, diagnosis, and treatment of type 2 diabetes has increased markedly.

TREATMENT

How Is Diabetes Managed?

The goal in diabetes management is to delay or prevent complications by maintaining the best possible degree of blood glucose control. Most newly diagnosed diabetic children have type 1 diabetes and thus require insulin. Blood glucose levels must be monitored closely at home to allow adjustments of insulin dosages. Management must include discussion of nutrition, physical activity, psychobehavioral issues, and the continuous changes of childhood and adolescence. For type 2 diabetes, the initial treatment may include insulin, but this can usually be replaced with oral hypoglycemic agents and dietary control, with additional management similar to that for the type 1 diabetic. Efforts to improve lifestyle, eating behavior, and activity may be appropriate.

What Are the Guidelines for Blood Glucose Control?

The principal goal of home blood glucose monitoring is to maintain blood glucose within the age-specific target range. In practice, tight blood glucose control is difficult, and most patients have frequent excursions both below and above the target range (Table 60-2).

Table 60-2

Target Ranges for Blood Glucose Control

Age	Blood Glucose (mg/dl)
Infants and preschool children	100-200
School-aged children and adolescents	70-150

Effectiveness of the treatment regimen and adherence by the patient are assessed by regular blood glucose determinations. All blood test results should be recorded in a log that is reviewed at each clinic visit so that insulin or oral medication doses may be adjusted. Approximately every 3 months, glycosylated hemoglobin (HbA_{1c}) should be measured to assess chronic blood glucose control.

How Is Insulin Used to Treat Type 1 Diabetes?

Treatment depends on whether the patient has type 1 diabetes or type 2 diabetes. On occasion, the distinction cannot be made and it is usually safest to begin treatment with insulin. Type 1 diabetes is always treated with insulin. Short-acting and long-acting insulins are typically injected alone or in combinations three or more times daily. You must be aware of the speed of onset and the duration of action of each commonly used type of insulin (Table 60-3). Increasing numbers of adolescents and young children are now using external insulin pumps for continuous subcutaneous insulin infusion. The pump delivers short-acting insulin at a basal rate during the day and night and as a bolus whenever needed to correspond to a meal. Patients learn to match the amount of insulin to the carbohydrate content of the food they are about to eat.

What Medications Are Used for Type 2 Diabetes?

Type 2 diabetes is treated with oral medications and sometimes with insulin. Commonly used oral hypoglycemic agents and their mechanisms of action are listed in Table 60-4.

Table 60-3

Insulin and Its Actions

Insulin Type	Onset (hr)	Peak (hr)	Duration (hr)
Short-acting regular	0.5	2-3	4-6
Short-acting: Lispro, Aspart, glulysine	< 0.5	1-2	2-3
Intermediate-acting: NPH, Lente	2-4	4-8	12-18
Long-acting: Glargine, Detemir	6-10	Flat	18-24+

Table 60-4

Oral Hypoglycemic Agents

Mechanism of Action	Examples
Insulin secretogogues	Sulfonylureas, meglitinide
Insulin sensitizers	Metformin, thiazolidinediones
Alpha-glucosidase inhibitors	Acarbose, miglitol

What Are the Consequences of Poor Diabetic Control?

Retinopathy, nephropathy, and both peripheral and autonomic neuropathy result from chronic poor control. Beginning approximately 5 years after the diagnosis of diabetes, all patients should have ophthalmologic evaluations yearly. Ongoing assessment of growth and blood pressure are important. In addition, a yearly urinalysis should be done to detect the presence of microalbuminuria. Recognition that complications may occur is important if they are to be detected early. It is also important to remember that intensive treatment of hyperglycemia with insulin or oral hypoglycemic agents prevents or delays all of these complications. Nutritional management and attention to emotional and behavioral issues are crucial.

When Does Diabetic Ketoacidosis Occur in Diabetes?

Diabetic ketoacidosis (DKA) is the most dangerous acute complication and may occur during an acute illness because of relative insulin deficiency or insulin resistance. Profound hyperglycemia, metabolic anion gap acidosis, and severe dehydration may lead to life-threatening shock. Patients and their parents need to know about signs and symptoms of DKA. Fever, upper respiratory infection, headache, abdominal pain, diarrhea, nausea, vomiting, and increased rate of breathing should raise the concern of DKA. In adolescence, DKA commonly results from omission of insulin in a setting of psychobehavioral conflict.

Does Hypoglycemia Have Adverse Consequences?

Maintenance of blood glucose levels within the target range for age is important to prevent hypoglycemia, which is the most common acute complication of diabetes. Hypoglycemia occurs frequently at all ages and much more often in type 1 than type 2 diabetes. It is usually mild and manifests as hunger, shakiness, sweatiness, rapid heart rate, pallor, and behavioral changes. A single acute episode of hypoglycemia causes a transient reduction in mental efficiency but does not cause long-term cognitive problems. Recurrent, severe hypoglycemia places children younger than 5 years at an increased risk of neurocognitive impairment but does not typically have cognitive effects in older children and adolescents.

What Behavioral and Emotional Problems Occur?

Low self-esteem and depression are common with diabetes and may be associated with an increased risk for complications. Poor control of diabetes in children and adolescents is often associated with stress in the family, home, school, or peer group. Adherence to the demanding therapeutic regimen limits an individual's perceived freedom and independence, issues that are central to adolescence. Denial, anger, sadness, and stress all can contribute to nonadherence, which leads to deterioration of diabetes care and development of DKA. Counseling may help.

When Is Hospitalization Needed?

Children with new-onset diabetes are hospitalized at most institutions, more often for type 1 than type 2 diabetes. The hospitalization is designed to manage any acute symptoms such as dehydration, initiate glucose control and provide the patient and the family with the education needed to manage diabetes at home. After hospitalization, all patients with diabetes will need close follow-up in the primary care office, in partnership with the pediatric endocrinologist and the diabetes team. Typically, patients visit the endocrinologist quarterly and maintain regular telephone contact with the diabetes care team. Hospitalization is rarely needed after initial diagnosis except to manage acute complications such as DKA.

THYROID DISEASE

ETIOLOGY

What Causes Thyroid Disease?

Thyroid disease may be congenital or acquired. Congenital hypothyroidism most often results from abnormal embryologic development of the thyroid gland. Diagnosis is now part of the newborn screening programs in all states in the United States and allows the early treatment needed to prevent the severe consequences of inadequate thyroid hormone on the developing brain. Autoimmune thyroid disease is the most common cause of acquired thyroid dysfunction in childhood and adolescence. Autoimmunity against thyroid tissue may either lead to destruction of the gland causing hypothyroidism or Hashimoto's disease or to excess stimulation of the gland with resultant hyperthyroidism or Graves' disease.

What Findings Suggest Thyroid Disease?

Signs and symptoms of congenital hypothyroidism are nonspecific in the newborn, so the disease *must be detected by screening*. Once diagnosed, treatment will be started promptly, and these infants will display no abnormal clinical features. Congenital hypothyroidism should no longer have the disastrous neurodevelopmental consequences of cretinism. Children and adolescents with acquired hypothyroidism will have the classical clinical findings of hypothyroidism plus delayed skeletal maturation, delayed puberty, or menstrual disorders. Table 60-5 lists the characteristic findings of hypothyroidism and hyperthyroidism.

How Do I Identify Abnormal Thyroid Function?

Abnormalities of thyroid function are established at all ages by measuring free thyroxine (free T_4) and thyroid-stimulating hormone (TSH) levels. Antithyroid antibody levels may provide information about the cause of thyroid disease. Congenital hypothyroidism is identified by an abnormal newborn thyroid screen and confirmed with free T_4 and TSH levels. Values of free T_4 and TSH are age-dependent, so pediatric references should be consulted; do not rely on the hospital laboratory reports unless reference values are listed by age. Regular measurement of free T_4 and TSH levels is necessary as children grow to assess adequacy of treatment and to adjust thyroid replacement therapy.

Table 60-5

Clinical Findings of Thyroid Disease

Finding	Hypothyroidism	Hyperthyroidism
Temperament	Placid, "dull" in school	Emotional lability, hyperactive, nervous
Temperature tolerance	Cold intolerance	Heat intolerance
Bowel habits	Constipation	Diarrhea
Sleep habits	Sleepiness, low energy	Trouble sleeping
Weight	Weight gain	Weight loss
Statural growth	Slowed ("flat curve")	Accelerated
Pulse	Slow	Fast
Skin	Cool, dry, coarse	Warm, smooth, diaphoretic
Eye	No eye findings	Exophthalmos
Neurologic	Slow deep tendon reflexes	Increased deep tendon reflexes
Muscle strength	No muscle changes	Decreased proximal muscle strength

TREATMENT

What is the Treatment of Hypothyroidism?

Hypothyroid children are treated with hormone replacement, consisting of l-thyroxine. Each child will have adjustments made in thyroid hormone replacement based on measurement of thyroid function tests at regular intervals, but further follow-up of thyroid antibodies is no longer needed after the diagnosis is established.

How is Hyperthyroidism Treated?

Children with hyperthyroidism are treated with antithyroid medications, and sometimes with ablation with radioactive iodine or surgery. Antithyroid medication reduces excessive thyroid hormone secretion and is usually continued for 12 to 24 months, followed by a trial off medication with close follow-up. Most patients remain euthyroid, some become spontaneously hypothyroid, and others relapse into hyperthyroidism. Treatment of recurring hyperthyroidism with radioablative iodine typically results in permanent hypothyroidism, requiring lifelong therapy with l-thyroxine. Careful monitoring of thyroid function is essential with all therapies. In addition, you must assess for side effects from antithyroid medication and for evolution of eye disease.

ADRENAL DISEASE

ETIOLOGY

What Causes Adrenal Disease?

Cushing's syndrome is the result of glucocorticoid excess. The most common cause of glucocorticoid excess and Cushing's syndrome in children and adolescents is chronic therapy with corticosteroid medication. Cushing's disease is hyperadrenalism and results when pituitary or other tumors produce adrenocorticotropic hormone (ACTH) that stimulates excessive secretion of glucocorticoid by the adrenal gland, which also results in Cushing's syndrome. Hypoadrenalism may occur congenitally or from an autoimmune disorder. Most frequently, the diagnosis is made in patients with hypopituitarism caused by radiation therapy to the central nervous system as part of therapy for cancer or in children with congenital central nervous system (CNS) anomalies, such as Arnold-Chiari malformation or hydrocephalus.

EVALUATION

What Findings Suggest Hyperadrenalism?

The evaluation of a child with suspected hyperadrenalism requires a careful history to identify the use of glucocorticoid medications. Cushing's disease is quite rare in childhood and is suspected clinically when a child is markedly *overweight and short.* Cushing's syndrome caused by treatment with corticosteroids is more common, and history of steroid use for a variety of disorders should be sought. Signs of Cushing's syndrome include overweight, slowed statural growth, plus thin skin, purple stretch marks, muscle weakness, easy bruising, increased body hair, acne, and psychological disturbances. Children and adolescents with exogenous obesity are often thought to have a "hormonal" problem, but their age-appropriate height (or even tall stature) makes an endocrine disorder highly unlikely. Identification of pituitary and adrenal tumors is made with imaging studies and blood and urine tests for measurement of cortisol and its metabolites.

What Findings Occur in Hypoadrenalism?

Adrenocortical deficiency or hypofunction rarely occurs but may be suspected from the history. Signs and symptoms include weakness, anorexia, fatigue, nausea, abdominal pain, weight loss, hyperpigmentation, and low blood pressure. These are so readily confused with other clinical diseases that a pediatrician will rarely refer a child for evaluation of this specific entity. Blood and urine studies of cortisol levels will be needed to document hypoadrenalism. As mentioned earlier, children who have a high risk of pituitary dysfunction, whether acquired or congenital, should be monitored for symptoms and signs of hypoadrenalism.

TREATMENT

How Are Hyperadrenal Disorders Managed?

Chronic glucocorticoid therapy may be necessary for treatment of many illnesses, and Cushing's syndrome is an unavoidable consequence. If glucocorticoids can be reduced in dose or changed to alternate-day dosing, signs of Cushing's syndrome may abate. Treatment of specific diseases that cause stimulation of excess glucocorticoid production will result in resolution of the physical findings and return of cortisol levels toward physiologic ranges.

What Is the Treatment for Hypoadrenal Function?

Replacement of glucocorticoids is the mainstay of therapy. It is important to adjust therapy to maintain adequate physical growth. Overtreatment with glucocorticoid will result in a fall in height velocity accompanied by weight gain, perhaps along with acne and lanugo. Undertreatment may decrease overall level of energy and result in fluctuations of weight as well as appetite. It is important to inquire whether the patient has salt craving, which may indicate the need for mineralocorticoid replacement.

KEY POINTS

- Type 1 diabetes should be suspected in the child with increased thirst and urination. Weight loss, dehydration, and diabetic ketoacidosis develop if the diagnosis is made late.
- Obesity is associated with type 2 diabetes in adolescents.
- Hypothyroid children have prominent slowing of statural growth.
- Prolonged corticosteroid treatment is the most common cause of Cushing's syndrome.

Case 60-1

A 13-year-old girl is brought to the emergency department by her parents because they think she has been "acting strangely" and "breathing too fast" for the past several days. She has not been "herself" recently and has complained of fatigue, abdominal pain, and increased thirst. Parents think that she is acting out, because she is upset about being prevented from attending the junior high dance. The emergency department physician thinks that it is appropriate to rule out diabetes.

A. What questions should the physician ask to clarify the diagnosis and plan an evaluation?
B. What findings on physical examination are consistent with DKA?

C. Why does the emergency department physician suspect DKA in this patient?
D. What laboratory tests should be ordered for this patient?
E. How will the physician differentiate type 1 diabetes from type 2 diabetes?

Case 60-2

A mother brings her 14-year-old son to you because he is concerned that he is too short. You note that he is also quite overweight, but neither the boy nor his mother is concerned about this because everyone else in the family is also overweight.

A. What history and examination features would make you consider hypothyroidism?
B. What laboratory studies do you wish to obtain? What results do you expect if he has hypothyroidism?
C. How will you distinguish exogenous obesity from obesity caused by an endocrine disorder?

Case 60-3

A 14-year-old, overweight adolescent girl comes to your clinic. Her chief complaint is that she has irregular periods. Her mother is concerned that the girl has a "gland problem."

A. What features on physical examination might make you concerned about type 2 diabetes mellitus or Cushing's syndrome?
B. What laboratory studies do you wish to obtain?
C. What series of interventions may be warranted?

Case Answers

60-1 A. *Learning objective:* **Use the medical history to identify the clinical features of diabetes mellitus.** The physician should ask about the presence of polyuria, polydipsia, recent weight loss, changes in appetite (especially polyphagia, which often precedes symptoms of diabetes), and a family history of diabetes or other autoimmune disease.

60-1 B. *Learning objective:* **Identify the physical examination findings in diabetic ketoacidosis.** Recent weight loss and dehydration are two key findings. If available, a growth chart can provide a pre-illness weight to document any acute weight loss. Vital signs may indicate a shock, with hypotension and tachycardia. Signs of dehydration include sunken eyes, dry lips and mucous membranes, cool extremities, and delayed capillary refill (> 4 seconds). A characteristic finding in diabetic ketoacidosis is breath that smells fruity or like acetone.

60-1 C. *Learning objective:* **Discuss the pathophysiology of diabetic ketoacidosis, and relate it to the physical findings.** Lack of insulin results in the inability to metabolize glucose, with consequent glucosuria, metabolic acidosis, dehydration, and weight loss. The tachypnea reflects respiratory alkalosis to compensate for the metabolic acidosis. Diabetic ketoacidosis is high in the differential diagnosis for a young adolescent with the sudden onset of behavioral changes, thirst, tachypnea, and dehydration.

60-1 D. *Learning objective:* **Select laboratory tests to diagnose diabetes mellitus; comment on the test results that would be found in diabetic ketoacidosis.** The tests that the physician might order in the emergency department include blood glucose, urinalysis, serum electrolytes, and venous blood gas. You would anticipate that this patient would have markedly elevated blood glucose, metabolic acidosis, ketonuria, and glucosuria.

60-1 E. *Learning objective:* **Discuss the differences between type 1 and type 2 diabetes in adolescence.** Although both types of diabetes may present as diabetic ketoacidosis, this complication occurs more commonly with type 1 disease. In addition, type 2 diabetes is most common in obese, often hypertensive, adolescents, especially when the family history is positive.

60-2 A. *Learning objective:* **Identify the history and physical examination features of hypothyroidism in a child or adolescent.** The clinical findings that suggest hypothyroidism include growth stunting and obesity. You should review the growth chart to identify a flattening of the curve for growth in height. Ask about cold intolerance, constipation, low energy, increased tiredness, mood changes, skin changes, and poor appetite despite weight gain. Physical examination may identify coarse, dry skin that feels cool to touch and may be slightly sallow. A slow pulse rate and delayed deep tendon reflexes are other findings.

60-2 B. *Learning objective:* **Select laboratory tests to identify hypothyroidism and interpret the results.** Thyroid function tests include free T_4, which would be low, and TSH, which would be elevated. A bone age radiograph (left hand and left wrist) will allow you to evaluate skeletal maturation, which is usually markedly delayed in hypothyroidism.

60-2 C. *Learning objective:* **Distinguish exogenous obesity from the obesity of an endocrine disorder such as hypothyroidism.** Long-standing hypothyroidism causes growth stunting, whereas exogenous obesity tends to be associated with tall stature in childhood. In very longstanding, untreated hypothyroidism, ultimate adult stature may be reduced, whereas children with exogenous obesity reach their predicted genetic height potential early. Unlike children with hypothyroidism, who tend to have delayed bone age, children with exogenous obesity tend to have slightly advanced bone age.

60-3 A. *Learning objective:* **Use the physical examination to identify obesity caused by endocrinopathy.** Obesity is a feature of both type 2 diabetes and Cushing's syndrome. Acanthosis nigricans is commonly identified in adolescents with type 2 diabetes. Hirsutism in adolescent girls results from elevated circulating androgens in polycystic ovary syndrome, which is linked to insulin resistance. In Cushing's syndrome, obesity is accompanied by short stature because the endocrinopathy interferes with statural growth. The obesity has a characteristic central pattern, with "moon face" and a "buffalo hump." Striae, weakness, and thin skin are also found.

60-3 B. *Learning objective:* **Select laboratory tests to evaluate obesity. The selection of laboratory tests should be based on the findings.** If obesity is accompanied by short stature, then thyroid studies and blood and urine levels of cortisol and its metabolites should be done. Further evaluation to determine the cause of hyperadrenalism will be needed. If the patient has appropriate or tall stature, then exogenous obesity is likely, and the evaluation should be directed to identification of possible type 2 diabetes mellitus: serum glucose, serum electrolytes, serum lipids, and urinalysis.

60-3 C. *Learning objective:* **Discuss management issues for the obese adolescent.** Management depends on the diagnosis. The rare adolescent with Cushing's disease will require treatment for the cause of the hyperadrenalism. Treatment of Cushing's syndrome caused by corticosteroid medication depends on the ability to reduce the dose or switch to "steroid-sparing" alternative medications to manage the underlying disease. The obesity of hypothyroidism responds gradually to thyroid replacement therapy. The much more common case of exogenous obesity, often with the metabolic syndrome or even type 2 diabetes mellitus, will necessitate management that focuses on lifestyle changes. This includes a weight reduction program with dietary counseling, exercise, peer support, family involvement, and other social and psychological services. The goal should be slowed weight gain rather than weight loss. Moderate dietary restrictions have been shown to be safe in children and do not have adverse effects on linear growth.

BIBLIOGRAPHY

Diabetes Mellitus

Atkinson MA, Eisenbarth GS: Type 1 diabetes: new perspectives on disease pathogenesis and treatment, *Lancet* 358:221, 2001.

Kaufman FR: Diabetes mellitus, *Pediatr Rev* 18:382, 1997.

Nature insight review articles, in *Nature* 414:781, 2001.

Thyroid Disease

Cooper DS: Antithyroid drugs, *N Engl J Med* 352:905, 2005.

Fisher DA: Hypothyroidism, *Pediatr Rev* 15:227, 1994.

LaFranchi S: Congenital hypothyroidism: etiologies, diagnosis, and management, *Thyroid* 9:735, 1999.

Adrenal Disease

Leinung MC, Zimmerman D: Cushing's disease in children, *Endocrinol Metab Clin North Am* 23:629, 1994.

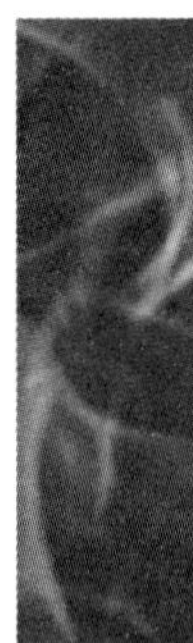

61 Gastroenterology

WARREN P. BISHOP and DINESH S. PASHANKAR

GASTROINTESTINAL BLEEDING

ETIOLOGY

What Causes Gastrointestinal (GI) Bleeding?

Blood in the stool or vomitus is typically of great concern to parents and physicians. Massive bleeding can be life threatening and must be treated rapidly to replenish the vascular compartment and stop the hemorrhage. In many other cases the quantity of blood lost is not so large as to be immediately dangerous. Table 61-1 lists the common causes of bleeding by age. Congenital lesions cause problems early in life, but some types of bleeding can occur at any age.

EVALUATION

What Questions Help Assess GI Bleeding?

Is it blood? Foods with intense red coloring such as candy, soft drinks, and beets can produce red-colored stool. If a parent shows you a cherry-red diaper, you should consider that the color may be from something other than blood. A simple test for occult blood should be performed.

How much blood has been lost? Ask how much blood has been seen. Streaks of blood on the surface of a hard stool, bloody mucus mixed in stool, teaspoon-sized clots, or a larger amount of bloody material? If the child passed blood into the toilet, ask about the color of the water in the toilet bowl: Light pink is of less concern than opaque red. You must also consider that there may be a larger quantity of blood in the intestinal lumen that has not yet shown itself. Evaluating the child for signs of shock, tachycardia, and systolic hypotension is therefore critical.

Where is the bleeding coming from? Not all blood in the toilet, diaper, or vomitus comes from the digestive system. Your history and examination must seek evidence of bleeding from surrounding structures.

Table 61-1

Causes of Gastrointestinal Bleeding by Age

Age	Hematemesis*	Rectal Bleeding
Neonatal period (birth-6 weeks)	Ingested maternal blood—first days of life	Anal fissure
	Peptic disease	Allergic colitis
	Coagulopathy	NEC
	Arteriovenous malformation	Hirschsprung's disease
	Duplication cyst	Volvulus
Infancy to 2 years	Peptic disease	Allergic colitis
	Varices	Intussusception
	Foreign body	Meckel's diverticulum
	NSAIDs	Bacterial colitis
	Arteriovenous malformation	
	Coagulopathy	
Children older than 2 years	Peptic disease	Juvenile polyp
	Esophageal varices	Meckel's diverticulum
	Mallory-Weiss tear	Bacterial colitis
	NSAIDs	Nodular lymphoid hyperplasia
	Foreign body	
	Arteriovenous malformation	HSP, HUS
	Coagulopathy	IBD
Any age	Peptic disease	Bacterial/amebic dysentery
	Arteriovenous malformation	

*Any cause of hematemesis can also present as rectal bleeding.
HSP, Henoch-Schönlein purpura; HUS, hemolytic uremic syndrome; IBD, inflammatory bowel disease; NEC, necrotizing enterocolitis; NSAIDs, nonsteroidal antiinflammatory drugs.

Vomited blood may have originated in the lungs, mouth, or nasopharynx. Blood coming from below may have a vaginal or urinary tract source. When no other source seems likely, think about where in the gut the bleeding may be coming from. *Vomited blood* is nearly always from the esophagus, stomach, or duodenum. *Rectal bleeding* may come from anywhere within the gut. Melena (black, sticky, tarry, sickly sweet–smelling stools) typically indicates a very high source of bleeding, whereas bright red blood suggests very distal bleeding. Dark red blood mixed with stool suggests bleeding higher in the colon. When blood is only on the surface of the stool, a much more distal source is likely. With large volumes of rectal bleeding, the degree of redness becomes less reliable, because of rapid transit of the blood through the gut. In this case, passing a nasogastric tube to sample gastric contents helps rule out a proximal source.

What is the cause of the hemorrhage? To answer to this question you must have information about the symptoms that preceded and accompanied bleeding, the age of the patient, the medical history, the medication history, and the amount and source of bleeding. Refer to Table 61-1 for causes of bleeding by age and Table 61-2 for causes of bleeding by clinical presentation.

What Should I Look for on Physical Examination?

First, remember the ABCs (Chapter 31): Determine the hemodynamic status. Is the child pink, blue, or pale? Is there increased work of breathing? Are blood pressure and pulse rate appropriate for age, high, or low? Are pulses palpable and strong? Is capillary refill < 2 seconds or prolonged? Look for bruising and petechiae, which indicate possible coagulopathy. Signs of liver disease include hepatosplenomegaly, jaundice, and prominent abdominal veins. Evaluate the abdomen carefully for tenderness, distention, bowel sounds, and mass lesions. Location of tenderness may help identify the source of bleeding. For example, epigastric tenderness suggests peptic disease, whereas a tender mass in the right lower quadrant may indicate Crohn's disease. Bowel obstruction such as volvulus or intussusception causes hyperactive,

Table 61-2

Causes of Gastrointestinal Bleeding by Clinical Presentation

Presentation	Suspected Condition	Imaging Test(s)
Bowel obstruction symptoms (colicky pain, vomiting) accompanying bleeding	Volvulus Intussusception	Flat and upright plain films of abdomen Abdominal ultrasonogram Upper GI series (volvulus) Barium enema (intussusception)
Epigastric pain, hematemesis	Peptic ulcer	Upper GI series (low sensitivity, endoscopy preferred)
Massive, painless hematemesis	Esophageal varices Peptic ulcer	None. Upper endoscopy indicated to diagnose and treat bleeding
Massive, painless rectal bleeding	Meckel's diverticulum	Meckel's scan
	AV malformation	Arteriogram, labeled RBC scan
Bloody diarrhea	Inflammatory bowel disease	Barium enema (colonoscopy preferred)
Formed stool with streaks of blood	Allergic colitis (infant) Rectal fissure Juvenile polyps	None. Consider sigmoidoscopy or colonoscopy instead

AV, Arteriovenous; GI, gastrointestinal; RBC, red blood cell.

high-pitched "pinging" bowel sounds; distention; bilious emesis; and colicky pain. *Always perform a rectal examination and test stool for blood,* regardless of stool color.

What Laboratory Tests Should I Perform?

Table 61-3 lists suggested laboratory studies for children with GI bleeding. Remember that acute bleeding will not immediately cause a drop in the hemoglobin or hematocrit. You must select tests to rule out coagulopathy, identify liver disease, and assess hydration status, renal function, and electrolytes. When there is evidence of massive bleeding, send a specimen to the blood bank immediately!

What Imaging Studies Should I Order?

Your clinical judgment is important at this point. Do not order every test available—focus on those studies that will best test your diagnostic hypothesis. In many cases, endoscopy is preferred to any other test. Table 61-2 lists imaging studies for the evaluation of different clinical presentations.

TREATMENT

How Should I Begin Management of Gastrointestinal Bleeding?

Your initial evaluation determines possible sources of bleeding and the patient's hemodynamic status. If the child has normal vital signs and a history of only minor blood loss, such as a few streaks of bright red blood in the stool, proceed directly to appropriate diagnostic tests. If bleeding is more severe, you must stabilize the patient and stop the bleeding. Figure 61-1 gives a suggested approach to management.

When Should a Gastroenterologist Be Consulted?

Consulting a pediatric gastroenterologist is a high priority in all cases of significant GI bleeding, especially when you suspect a condition that

Table 61-3

Laboratory Investigation of Gastrointestinal Bleeding
CBC with WBC differential, platelet count
PT, PTT
AST, ALT, alkaline phosphatase, GGT
Electrolytes, BUN, creatinine
Stool for WBC, culture (bloody diarrhea)
Type and crossmatch
Hemoccult or similar test for suspected blood in stool and vomitus

ALT, Alanine aminotransferase; AST, aspartate aminotransferase; BUN, blood urea nitrogen; CBC, complete blood count; GGT, γ-glutamyltransferase; PT, prothrombin time; PTT, partial thromboplastin time; WBC, white blood cell.

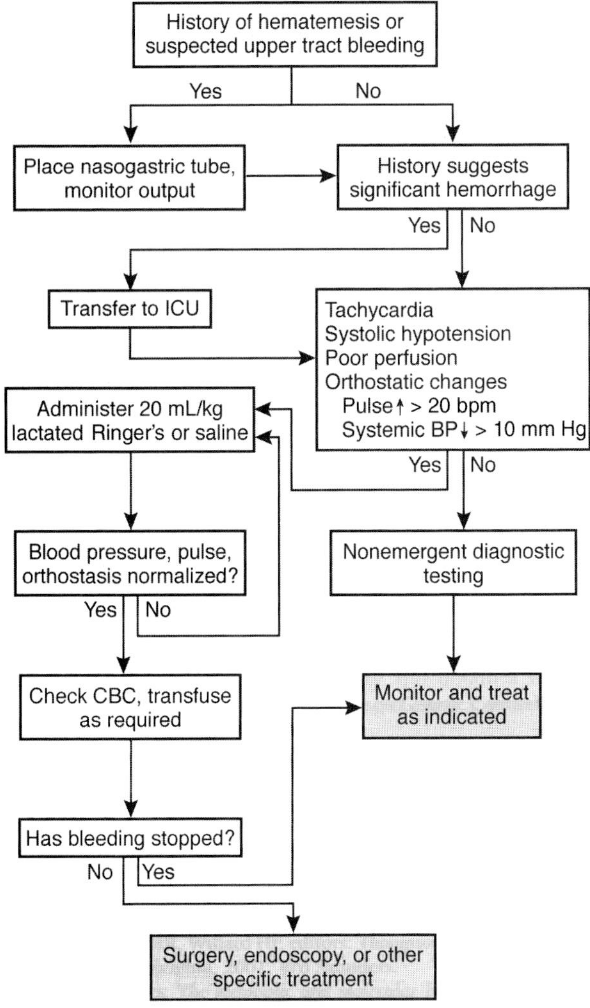

FIGURE 61-1 Initial therapy for gastrointestinal bleeding. BP, Blood pressure; bpm, beats per minute; CBC, complete blood count; ICU, intensive care unit.

can be treated directly through the endoscope, or when an accurate diagnosis is most likely to be achieved by direct visualization or biopsy. A gastroenterologist can usually stop the bleeding from esophageal varices, peptic ulcers, and arteriovenous malformations if they are within reach of the endoscope. Endoscopic biopsy can diagnose inflammatory bowel disease and other conditions, such as allergic colitis of infancy.

INFLAMMATORY BOWEL DISEASE

ETIOLOGY

What Is Inflammatory Bowel Disease?

Inflammatory bowel disease (IBD) refers to disorders that cause chronic inflammation of the GI tract. *Ulcerative colitis (UC)* is characterized by continuous, chronic mucosal inflammation *only in the colon,* starting from the anus and extending proximally to a variable extent. *Crohn's disease (CD),* on the other hand, is a chronic inflammatory disorder that may involve any part of the GI tract, from the mouth to the anus. UC and CD usually can be differentiated by the clinical features listed in Table 61-4.

What Are the Causes and Risk Factors for Inflammatory Bowel Disease?

The cause of IBD remains unknown. Genetic susceptibility and environmental influences both have a role in pathogenesis. The most important risk factor is family history: When close relatives are affected, risk of IBD in a symptomatic patient is in the range of 7% to 22%.

What Is the Differential Diagnosis of Inflammatory Bowel Disease?

Because IBD has a wide spectrum of clinical presentations, the differential diagnosis can be quite wide. Bacterial infections and parasitic infestations can mimic UC and Crohn's colitis. Chronicity of symptoms and negative stool culture results favor IBD as opposed to infection. Abdominal pain has a very broad list of potential causes (see Chapter 17). Celiac disease can present with growth failure, anemia, abdominal pain, and nonbloody diarrhea.

Table 61-4

Differentiating Features of Ulcerative Colitis and Crohn's Disease

	Ulcerative Colitis	Crohn's Disease
Distribution	Colon only	Any part of gastrointestinal tract
Involvement	Mucosal only Continuous	Transmural Discontinuous ("skip areas")
Clinical features		
Rectal bleeding	Usual	Sometimes
Abdominal mass	Absent	Sometimes
Perianal disease	Absent	Sometimes
Histology		
Intestinal fistulas	Absent	Sometimes
Granuloma	Absent	Sometimes

EVALUATION

In Which Patients Should I Suspect Inflammatory Bowel Disease?

IBD most often occurs in adolescents, but should be suspected in children with anemia, chronic abdominal pain, or failure to thrive, as well as those with more obvious symptoms such as bloody diarrhea and perianal fistulae. Symptoms of CD can be quite subtle, including short stature and delayed puberty in adolescents.

How Does Inflammatory Bowel Disease Typically Present?

IBD, particularly CD, has a wide variety of presentations, including extraintestinal manifestations (Table 61-5). These features may appear before, with, or after the onset of the GI symptoms. Growth failure is a prominent extraintestinal manifestation of CD.

Ulcerative colitis: Children with UC have frequent loose, watery stools that contain blood and mucus. They also have colicky abdominal pain, urgency, tenesmus (sensation of incomplete emptying), and often wake up at night for bowel movements.

Crohn's disease: The clinical presentation of CD varies, depending on the involved region of the GI tract. The ileocecal region is the most common site affected, and patients typically have crampy abdominal pain and diarrhea, with or without visible blood. Patients with extensive CD in the colon have symptoms similar to UC. CD localized to the small bowel is often relatively silent, except when inflammation and scarring lead to obstructive symptoms such as vomiting, abdominal pain, and distention. More commonly, these children have poor weight gain, decreased energy, and anemia. Adolescents with CD may have delayed puberty. Patients with gastric or duodenal involvement complain of epigastric pain and vomiting.

What Should I Look for on Physical Examination?

Vital signs and hydration status should be assessed. Assessment of growth is essential: Children with small bowel CD often appear

Table 61-5

Extraintestinal Manifestations of Inflammatory Bowel Disease

Site	Manifestations
Extremities	Arthralgia, arthritis, clubbing
Skin	Erythema nodosum, pyoderma gangrenosum
Liver	Sclerosing cholangitis, autoimmune hepatitis
Eye	Uveitis, episcleritis
Bone	Osteopenia
Renal	Urolithiasis, enterovesical fistulas
General	Fever, growth failure, pubertal delay

chronically ill because of growth failure, malnutrition, and anemia. Also assess the sexual maturity of adolescents. Look for abdominal tenderness, guarding, and masses. In most cases of CD and UC, abdominal tenderness is minimal, but a tender right lower quadrant mass resulting from inflamed, thickened bowel may be found in CD. Severe abdominal tenderness with distention and guarding is an ominous sign indicating toxic megacolon or bowel perforation. The presence of oral ulcers or perianal skin tags, abscesses, or fistulas are typical of CD. Do not forget to look for the extraintestinal manifestations listed in Table 61-5.

What Studies Should I Order for Suspected Inflammatory Bowel Disease?

Start with a complete blood count (CBC), erythrocyte sedimentation rate (ESR), and C-reactive protein. Serum albumin and liver function tests should also be determined. Low serum albumin indicates chronic GI loss of protein and poor nutritional status. Elevation of liver enzymes may suggest accompanying sclerosing cholangitis or autoimmune hepatitis. Patients who appear acutely ill should have serum electrolytes, blood urea nitrogen (BUN), and creatinine measured. Patients with diarrhea should have stool sent for culture and *Clostridium difficile* toxin assay. Always test stool for blood.

When Are Endoscopy and Imaging Studies Useful?

Upper endoscopy and colonoscopy with biopsy are the most important diagnostic tests for IBD. UC is characterized by continuous inflammation of the colon that may extend from the anus to the cecum. The proximal GI tract and small bowel are never involved. CD can involve the entire gut and is characterized by "skip areas" of normal bowel between areas of chronic inflammation. On biopsy, the presence of granulomas strongly suggests CD, but these are not present in all cases. Because the entire gut cannot be visualized by the usual instruments, evaluation of the small bowel is best performed by barium upper GI series. A new device, the capsule endoscope, is of use in difficult-to-diagnose cases of small bowel CD.

TREATMENT

How Do I Treat the Patient with Inflammatory Bowel Disease?

The goals of treatment are to decrease bowel inflammation, alleviate symptoms, address complications, and promote optimal growth. Table 61-6 lists medications with indications and complications. Patients with severe colitis require hospitalization, fluid resuscitation, and intravenous steroids.

- *Steroids* are highly effective for acute exacerbation, but long-term use is to be avoided because of serious adverse effects. Taper steroids as soon as possible after the treatment of an acute attack.
- *Immunomodulators* such as 6-mercaptopurine and azathioprine are increasingly used for both UC and CD because of their therapeutic

Table 61-6

Medications Used for Inflammatory Bowel Disease

Medications	Indications	Comments
Aminosalicylates		
Mesalamine or sulfasalazine	Mild to moderate UC and CD	Well tolerated Complications—rash, headache, rare worsening of colitis
Corticosteroids		
Prednisone: oral/ intravenous	Acute colitis; moderate to severe UC and CD	Rapid action; many side effects of long-term steroid therapy
Immunomodulators		
6-Mercaptopurine or azathioprine	Moderate to severe chronic UC and CD; steroid dependency	Steroid sparing Complications of azathioprine—pancreatitis, bone marrow suppression
Infliximab	Severe Crohn's colitis and fistula	Complication—hypersensitivity
Enemas		
Mesalamine or steroid	Distal colonic disease of UC and CD	
Antibiotics		
Metronidazole	Perianal fistulas, abscess	Complications—nausea, neuropathy
Ciprofloxacin	Mild colitis	Complication—nausea

CD, Crohn's disease, UC, ulcerative colitis.

efficacy and steroid-sparing action. Recently, infliximab (antitumor necrosis factor alpha antibody) has been used with remarkable success when CD or UC is unresponsive to other management.

- *Nutrition* and *psychosocial support* are important for optimal management of IBD. For children with significant growth failure because of CD, nasogastric tube feeding or parenteral nutrition is sometimes required.

What Is the Role of Surgery in Inflammatory Bowel Disease?

Urgent surgical intervention may be needed for acute problems such as uncontrolled GI bleeding, bowel perforation, and bowel obstruction. Elective surgery may be indicated for severe disease unresponsive to medical therapy or for suspicion of malignancy. In UC, colectomy with ileoanal anastomosis is curative. The role of surgery is limited in CD because recurrence of disease is typical. Therefore, bowel resection in CD is kept to a minimum.

What Is the Prognosis of Inflammatory Bowel Disease in Children?

IBD is a chronic disease characterized by exacerbations and remission. Spectrum of severity ranges from mild disease that requires minimal medications to severe disease that requires frequent hospitalizations and surgery. IBD has a high morbidity but low mortality. There is a risk of colon cancer in long-standing UC. Therefore, these patients need colonoscopic surveillance, beginning around 8 to 10 years after diagnosis. Colectomy is curative for patients with UC and eliminates the risk of cancer.

LIVER DISEASE IN CHILDHOOD

ETIOLOGY

How Does Liver Disease Affect Children?

The differential diagnosis of liver disease in infants and children differs significantly from that of adults because alcoholic liver disease and symptomatic hepatitis C are uncommon. Liver disease in the newborn is a special category that includes congenital disorders unique to this age group. Liver disease in infancy and childhood varies from mild to severe, and even infants sometimes require liver transplantation.

What Liver Diseases Are Commonly Found in the Newborn Period?

Table 61-7 lists the causes of liver disease in the newborn period. ***Italics*** highlight the most common disorders. Diagnoses that have a specific treatment are *underlined*.

What Liver Diseases Are Commonly Seen beyond the Newborn Period?

Congenital lesions that present in the newborn period may linger as chronic disease throughout childhood. New onset of liver disease beyond the newborn period generally results from conditions such as acute viral (and rarely bacterial) hepatitis, autoimmune hepatitis, primary sclerosing cholangitis, toxic hepatitis, and late-onset metabolic diseases, such as Wilson's disease (Table 61-8).

What Are the Consequences of Liver Disease in Children?

Liver functions include synthesis, excretion, and metabolism, all of which may be affected by disease, either together or separately. Severe liver disease causes *jaundice, prolonged clotting time, hypoalbuminemia, hypoglycemia, hyperammonemia, abnormal amino acid profile, impaired drug clearance,* and *hepatic encephalopathy*. Hepatic excretory function is primarily affected when a stone, mass lesion, or duct injury blocks the biliary system. Inborn errors of metabolism can have narrow or broad effects on liver function. Any liver injury, if persistent, will

Table 61-7

Differential Diagnosis of Neonatal Liver Disease[†]

Obstructed bile flow
- *Biliary atresia**
- *Alagille's syndrome*
- *Choledochal cyst**
- *Gallstone, sludge**
- Mass lesion
- Caroli's disease
- Congenital hepatic fibrosis

Metabolic
- *α_1-Antitrypsin deficiency*
- *Galactosemia**
- *Tyrosinemia**
- Hereditary fructose intolerance*
- *Cystic fibrosis*
- Neonatal hemochromatosis
- Zellweger's syndrome
- Progressive familial intrahepatic cholestasis (several types)
- Bile acid synthesis disorders
- Wolman's disease

Infectious
- *Cytomegalovirus*
- *Urinary tract infection**
- *Sepsis**
- Toxoplasmosis
- Herpesvirus
- Enterovirus
- Parvovirus
- Hepatitis B
- Listeria
- Syphilis

Toxic
- *Parenteral nutrition*
- Drug reaction*

Other
- Neonatal hepatitis (giant cell hepatitis)
- Ischemic injury (shock, asphyxia, congenital heart disease)

[†]The most common conditions causing neonatal cholestasis are shown in italics. Conditions for which specific treatment is available are marked by an asterisk (*).

eventually lead to more global impairment of liver function. An example is biliary atresia, in which blockage of bile flow initially causes jaundice, with later development of nutritional problems, hepatic inflammation, fibrosis, cirrhosis, portal hypertension, and synthetic dysfunction leading to death or liver transplantation.

Table 61-8

Etiology of Liver Disease beyond the Neonatal Period

Infectious hepatitis
Hepatitis A, B, and C
Epstein-Barr virus
Adenovirus, echovirus, parvovirus
Listeria, brucella, tularemia, leptospirosis
Cat scratch disease
Rocky Mountain spotted fever
Q fever

Metabolic diseases
Wilson's disease
α_1-Antitrypsin deficiency
Cystic fibrosis
Glycogen storage diseases
Cholesterol ester disease
Defects of fatty acid oxidation
Navajo neurohepatopathy
Zellweger's syndrome
Adrenoleukodystrophy

Toxic
Acetaminophen
Iron
Valproic acid
Parenteral nutrition
Other drug reaction

Miscellaneous
Nonalcoholic steatohepatitis

Neoplastic
Hepatoblastoma
Hepatocellular carcinoma
Hemangioendothelioma

Autoimmune
Autoimmune hepatitis
Primary sclerosing cholangitis

What Is Portal Hypertension?

The portal vein flows into the liver, carrying blood from the intestine and spleen. It branches into smaller and smaller tributaries, finally filtering through the sinusoids before draining into the hepatic vein. When portal blood flow is blocked by cirrhosis, the pressure in the portal vein rises. Symptoms of portal hypertension include *enlarged abdominal veins, splenomegaly,* and *GI bleeding.*

EVALUATION

How Do I Test Liver Function?

- *Excretory function tests:* total and direct bilirubin, serum bile acids, and cholesterol
- *Synthetic function tests:* prothrombin time, partial thromboplastin time, albumin, and specific clotting factor levels
- *Metabolic function tests:* ammonia and glucose levels
- *Hepatic injury markers*: alkaline phosphatase, gamma-glutamyltransferase (GGT) and transaminases. Hepatocellular injury, such as that seen with viral hepatitis, causes elevated aspartate aminotransferase (AST) and alanine aminotransferase (ALT). GGT is a microsomal enzyme found in biliary epithelium and in several other tissues. Increased GGT in the setting of liver disease suggests biliary injury. The GGT activity may also be elevated by microsomal enzyme-inducing agents such as phenobarbital, warfarin, and phenytoin and may be up to six times the normal adult level during the first weeks of life.

How Do I Investigate Neonatal Liver Disease?

Biliary atresia, neonatal hepatitis, and alpha$_1$-antitrypsin deficiency are the three most common causes of neonatal liver disease. Of these, only biliary atresia is treatable, and only when it is diagnosed before 8 to 12 weeks of age. Therefore, considerable urgency exists to identify this and other obstructive lesions to allow surgical relief before irreversible liver injury occurs. Other treatable conditions, such as some infections and metabolic disorders, must also be found quickly so that prompt therapy may be given.

How Do I Identify Neonatal Cholestasis?

Most newborn infants with liver disease present with cholestasis, the result of reduced bile flow. This is characterized by an elevation of direct bilirubin (> 2 mg/dl and > 10% of the total bilirubin). *Infants with cholestasis differ from babies with physiologic jaundice, in whom the direct bilirubin is not increased.* The diagnostic approach to neonatal cholestasis starts with noninvasive tests, then progresses to more invasive and specialized investigations as required. Table 61-9 lists suggested initial and secondary laboratory and imaging studies. Figure 61-2 presents the sequence of subsequent testing. Remember that the primary goal of your evaluation is to identify treatable disorders quickly.

How Do I Evaluate Liver Disease in Older Patients?

Table 61-10 lists a suggested evaluation of liver disease with onset after the newborn period. Infectious, metabolic, autoimmune, and obstructive disorders must be identified so that proper treatment and supportive care may be provided. Some conditions must be urgently identified and treated to minimize further hepatic injury, especially autoimmune hepatitis, biliary obstruction, bacterial infections, and Wilson's disease.

Table 61-9

Diagnostic Studies in Neonatal Cholestasis

Initial tests	*Secondary tests*
Total and direct bilirubin	Urine CMV culture
AST, ALT, GGT	Serum amino acids
RBC galactose 1-phosphate uridyltransferase	Urine organic acids
α_1-Antitrypsin level and phenotype	Hepatobiliary scintigraphy
Blood culture	Percutaneous liver biopsy
Urinalysis and urine culture	
Abdominal ultrasound	

ALT, Alanine aminotransferase; AST, aspartate aminotransferase; CMV, cytomegalovirus; GGT, γ-glutamyltransferase; RBC, red blood cell.

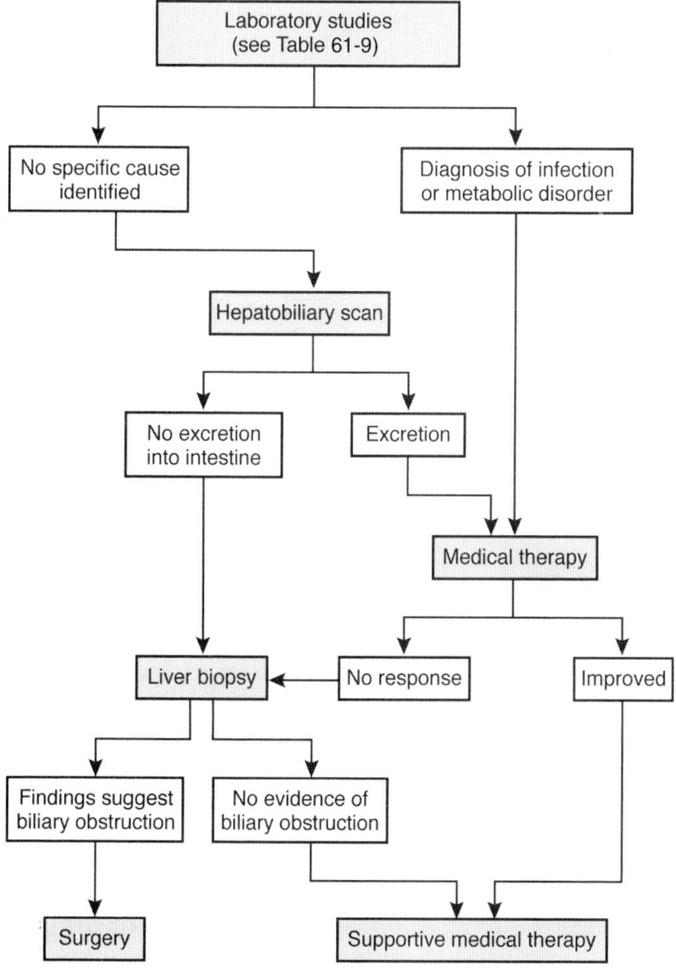

FIGURE 61-2 Diagnostic approach to neonatal cholestasis.

Table 61-10

Laboratory Evaluation of Liver Disease beyond the Neonatal Period

Initial Studies	Secondary Studies
Etiology	***Etiology and prognosis***
Hepatitis B	Liver biopsy
Surface antigen and antibody, IgG and IgM core antibodies, e antigen	Endoscopic retrograde cholangiopancreatography
Hepatitis A antibody	Metabolic studies
Epstein-Barr virus serology	CT scan
Autoantibodies	Surgical exploration and biopsy
Antinuclear antigen	
Antismooth muscle	
Anti–liver-kidney microsomal antigen	
Antineutrophil cytoplasmic antibody	
Antimitochondrial antibody	
Wilson's disease studies	
Serum ceruloplasmin	
24-hr urine copper excretion	
Slit lamp examination of iris	
Amylase and lipase	
Ultrasound imaging of liver and bile ducts	
Blood and urine culture	
Urinalysis	
Liver injury and function	
AST, ALT, GGT, alkaline phosphatase	
PT, PTT, INR	
Total protein and albumin	
CBC with WBC differential and platelets	

ALT, Alanine aminotransferase; AST, aspartate aminotransferase; CBC, complete blood count; CT, computed tomography; GGT, γ-glutamyltransferase; INR, international normalized ratio; PT, prothrombin time; PTT, partial thromboplastin time; WBC, white blood cell.

TREATMENT

How Is Biliary Atresia Treated?

Untreated biliary atresia is uniformly fatal. When diagnosed before irreversible liver injury occurs, biliary atresia can potentially be treated surgically by the Kasai procedure. This operation uses an intestinal conduit to replace the obliterated extrahepatic bile duct. The success rate of this procedure varies, but many children achieve at least some degree of palliation. Despite timely surgery, the majority will eventually require liver transplantation.

How Is Viral Hepatitis Treated?

There is no specific therapy available for hepatitis A. Fortunately, the vast majority of children infected with this virus will recover fully. Vaccination against hepatitis A and B are making these infections a rarity in the developed world. Therapies are available for chronic hepatitis B and for hepatitis C. The specifics are beyond the scope of this chapter, especially as recommendations are changing rapidly. Children with these disorders should be referred to a pediatric gastroenterologist.

How Is Chronic Liver Disease Treated?

Specific therapy is available for some chronic liver diseases. Wilson's disease is treated with a low-copper diet and copper-chelating agents. Autoimmune hepatitis is treated with immunosuppressants. Biliary conditions such as primary sclerosing cholangitis may respond to surgery or endoscopic intervention. Table 61-11 lists supportive therapies commonly used in patients with liver conditions.

Table 61-11

Supportive Care for Chronic Liver Disease
Cholestasis
Fat-soluble vitamins (A, D, E, K)
Formula enriched with MCT oil
Ursodiol
Autoimmune hepatitis
Steroids
Immunosuppressives
Hepatitis B
Lamivudine
Interferon
Adefovir
Hepatitis C
Interferon, ribavirin
Ascites
Low-sodium diet
Diuretics
Therapeutic paracentesis
Portal hypertension
Nonselective beta-blocker
Nitrates
Portosystemic shunts
Surgical
TIPSS
Encephalopathy
Lactulose
Oral antibiotic (neomycin, others)

MCT, Medium chain triglyceride; TIPSS, transjugular intrahepatic portosystemic shunt.

KEY POINTS

- Blood in the toilet, the diaper, or in vomitus may have its source outside of the GI tract.
- Inflammatory bowel disease often presents with bloody diarrhea in an adolescent who has delayed puberty and slow growth.
- Liver disease in infancy often manifests as prolonged jaundice with elevated direct bilirubin.

Case 61-1

A 6-month-old infant is brought to the emergency department with a 6-hour history of nonstop crying and has just passed a frankly bloody stool. Temperature is 37.8° C, pulse is 120 beats/min, and respiratory rate is 22 breaths/min. Your examination reveals an ill-appearing, somewhat obtunded infant with a distended abdomen. A soft abdominal mass is palpable.

A. What is the most likely diagnosis for this patient?
B. What diagnostic tests will you order?

Case 61-2

A 5-year-old boy presents to the emergency department with a 1-hour history of passing four large stools consisting mostly of dark red blood and clots. Physical examination demonstrates a resting pulse of 140 beats/min, poor capillary refill (10 seconds), and an orthostatic systolic blood pressure decrease of 20 mm Hg.

A. What diagnoses do you suspect?
B. How will you rule out a massive upper tract hemorrhage?
C. What diagnostic studies will you order?

Case 61-3

A 13-year-old girl has had diarrhea and abdominal pain for 1 week. She has loose, watery stools up to five times a day. She also has low-grade fever. On examination she looks well hydrated and her abdominal examination is benign.

A. What is the differential diagnosis?
B. What investigations would you like to do for the initial evaluation?
C. At the initial visit, this patient had a negative stool culture and negative *C. difficile* toxin, but the occult blood test was positive. Consequently, you

scheduled her for a follow-up visit in 1 week to monitor her progress. At her return visit, she reports worsening pain and diarrhea and recent bright red blood and mucus in her stools. On further inquiry, she also admits to having had abdominal pain and loose stools off and on for the last 3 months. What additional investigations would you order in view of this new information?

Case 61-4

A 15-year-old boy presents with a 20-pound weight loss over the last 3 months. He has one loose stool per day without any visible blood or mucus. He has abdominal pain that occurs only once or twice a week. On examination he is afebrile and appears pale and quite thin. His abdominal examination demonstrates no tenderness or masses.

A. What is the differential diagnosis?
B. What important family history would you like to ask about?
C. How would you investigate his weight loss?

Case 61-5

A 3-week-old infant girl is brought to your office because of jaundice. The child was born at term, weighing 3300 g, and is being breast-fed. She has been thriving and now weighs 3500 g. She had mild jaundice on the second day of life, but the jaundice has been worsening for the past week. Today, total bilirubin is 13.2 mg/dl with direct bilirubin of 5.6 mg/dl.

A. What is your initial differential diagnosis?
B. What additional diagnostic tests should you order?
C. If this infant is diagnosed with biliary atresia, what information can you give to the parents?

Case Answers

61-1 A. *Learning objective:* **Discuss the differential diagnosis of gastrointestinal bleeding in an infant.** The history of irritability followed by bloody stools and lethargy in an infant points to intussusception. The abdominal mass adds to the suspicion. Other causes of gastrointestinal bleeding would be less common. A younger infant with milk protein allergy might have bloody stools and irritability but would not have an abdominal mass. Bacterial gastroenteritis would not likely cause an abdominal mass.

61-1 B. *Learning objective:* **Select diagnostic tests for an infant with gastrointestinal bleeding and abdominal mass.** A contrast barium enema is the diagnostic test of choice. It would also likely be the treatment of choice to reduce the intussusception. The frankly bloody stool does not need laboratory confirmation. If the child had irritability and lethargy, but did not (yet) have frankly bloody stool, a test for occult blood might be positive.

61-2 A. *Learning objective:* **Identify the causes of gastrointestinal bleeding in children.** Meckel's diverticulum and an arteriovenous malformation are the most common causes of massive, painless rectal bleeding. Other causes of bleeding in children older than 2 years include juvenile polyp, bacterial colitis, nodular lymphoid hyperplasia, Henoch-Schönlein purpura, hemolytic uremic syndrome, and inflammatory bowel disease. Each would have symptoms and signs that aid in diagnosis.

61-2 B. *Learning objective:* **Identify the source of gastrointestinal bleeding from history, physical examination, and diagnostic interventions.** The best way to identify upper gastrointestinal bleeding is to insert a nasogastric tube to detect blood in the stomach. In addition, history will confirm the onset and time course of the bleeding. Physical examination will not reveal major changes in blood pressure early in the process. It is difficult to pinpoint the source of massive bleeding based on the color of the blood in the stool. Prolonged capillary refill and tachycardia indicate blood loss. You should assess the quality of the pulses and look for evidence of abdominal tenderness. Also, look for ecchymoses and petechiae, which suggest a coagulation disorder.

61-2 C. *Learning objective:* **Select diagnostic studies to evaluate gastrointestinal bleeding.** Order a CBC, but remember that massive bleeding will not immediately cause a drop in the hemoglobin or hematocrit until circulating volume is restored. You must also rule out coagulopathy, look for liver disease, and assess the patient's hydration status, renal function, and electrolytes. Send a sample of blood to the blood bank for possible transfusion.

61-3 A. *Learning objective:* **List common causes of acute diarrhea with abdominal pain.** The differential diagnosis at this stage would include acute gastroenteritis or early inflammatory bowel disease.

61-3 B. *Learning objective:* **Select laboratory tests to evaluate a febrile patient with diarrhea and abdominal pain.** Stool cultures and an assay for *Clostridium difficile* toxin should be ordered to look for infection. Because inflammatory bowel disease is a consideration, a stool test for occult blood should be done.

61-3 C. *Learning objective:* **Discuss the progression of inflammatory bowel disease and the diagnostic testing that will identify it.** Because teenagers often tend to underreport unpleasant symptoms, you reviewed the history and discovered information that was not identified at the first visit. Inflammatory bowel disease is now a likely possibility because infection was not identified on the earlier evaluation and symptoms have worsened. In view of the new information about chronic diarrhea and pain, plus the progression of symptoms, you should order CBC, white blood cell (WBC) differential, ESR, and/or C-reactive protein and should refer her to a gastroenterologist for colonoscopy with biopsies.

61-4 A. *Learning objective:* **Discuss the differential diagnosis of an adolescent with weight loss and gastrointestinal symptoms.** Significant weight loss with diarrhea and abdominal pain should raise suspicion of a chronic GI condition such as Crohn's disease or celiac disease.

61-4 B. *Learning objective:* **Recognize the genetic/familial nature of chronic bowel disorders.** Positive history of IBD in any family members, especially in a close relative, is an important risk factor for IBD in your patient. Celiac disease also has a high familial incidence.

61-4 C. *Learning objective:* **Select diagnostic studies to confirm the diagnosis of chronic bowel disease.** Upper GI endoscopy and colonoscopy with biopsies should be performed. Crohn's disease is characterized by granulomatous chronic inflammation, whereas celiac disease is diagnosed by villous atrophy in small bowel mucosa. If celiac disease is suspected, you should also assay antiendomysial antibody, tissue transglutaminase, and IgA levels.

61-5 A. *Learning objective:* **Identify the common congenital, infectious, and toxic causes of liver disease in childhood.** This child has cholestatic jaundice. Causes include biliary atresia, neonatal hepatitis, and α_1-antitrypsin disease.

61-5 B. *Learning objective:* **Select tests for the initial evaluation of an infant with cholestatic jaundice.** Initial tests include abdominal ultrasound, tests of liver function (aspartate transaminase, alanine transaminase, gamma-glutamyltransferase), blood culture, urinalysis, α_1-antitrypsin level, and a repeat of the neonatal screen. Additional tests are listed in Table 61-9.

61-5 C. *Learning objective:* **Discuss the management of biliary atresia.** This is the only cause of neonatal cholestasis that can be treated. Prompt diagnosis leads to surgical intervention with the Kasai procedure. Liver transplantation may eventually be necessary.

BIBLIOGRAPHY

Gastrointestinal Bleeding

Arain Z, Rossi TM: Gastrointestinal bleeding in children: an overview of conditions requiring nonoperative management, *Semin Pediatr Surg* 8:172, 1999.

Fox VL: Gastrointestinal bleeding in infancy and childhood, *Gastroenterol Clin North Am* 29:37, 2000.

Irish MS: Bleeding in children caused by gastrointestinal vascular lesions, *Semin Pediatr Surg* 8:210, 1999.

Silber G: Lower gastrointestinal bleeding, *Pediatr Rev* 12:85, 1990.

Inflammatory Bowel Disease

Griffiths AM et al: Growth and clinical course of children with Crohn's disease, *Gut* 34:939, 1993.

Hyams JS: Inflammatory bowel disease, *Pediatr Rev* 21:291, 2000.

Kirschner BS: Ulcerative colitis, *Pediatr Clin North Am* 43:235, 1996.

Liver Disease in Childhood

Chang MH: Chronic hepatitis virus infection in children, *J Gastroenterol Hepatol* 13:541, 1998.

D'Agata ID, Balistreri WF: Evaluation of liver disease in the pediatric patient, *Pediatr Rev* 20:376, 1999.

Moseley RH: Evaluation of abnormal liver function tests, *Med Clin North Am* 80:887, 1996.

Pashankar D, Schreiber RA: Neonatal cholestasis: a red alert for the jaundiced newborn, *Can J Gastroenterol* 14 (suppl D), 67D, 2000.

62

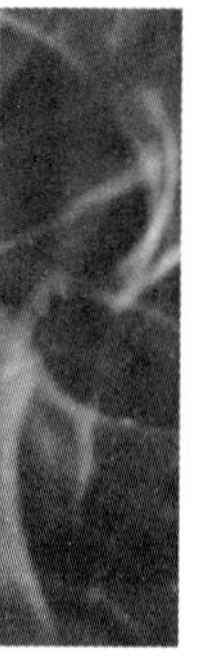

Genetics

KIM M. KEPPLER-NOREUIL and ADAM B. KANIS

Our understanding of human genes and of the genetic basis of disease has grown dramatically, especially with the completion of mapping of the Human Genome Project. Molecular technology for identifying human genes has allowed for the diagnosis and understanding of the mechanisms of human diseases. Medical genetics involves not only the diagnosis, treatment, and management of individuals with multiple congenital anomalies, developmental disabilities, and hereditary diseases, but it also involves human disorders having complex inheritance, such as diabetes, many types of cancer, and heart disease (e.g., cardiomyopathy). Knowledge of medical genetics is relevant to all medical practice, particularly pediatrics.

What Are the Reasons for a Genetic Consultation?

Children and their families are most commonly referred for clinical genetics evaluation because of birth defects or a known or suspected genetic disorder. Examples include the following:

- Multiple birth defects
- Growth problems, including short stature, failure to thrive, or overgrowth
- Neurodevelopmental problems, such as mental retardation, developmental regression, seizures, ataxia, or behavioral problems
- Premature or delayed puberty or ambiguous genitalia
- Prenatal exposure to alcohol, drugs, or other teratogens
- Recurrent miscarriages or advanced maternal age
- Family history of a known disorder, such as cystic fibrosis or fragile X syndrome
- Metabolic acidosis or hyperammonemia

BIRTH DEFECTS

ETIOLOGY

How Common Are Birth Defects?

A birth defect that interferes with normal function of the affected tissue or organ is identified in approximately 3% of all children within the first year of life and in 5% by adolescence. Several studies have indicated that congenital abnormalities account for about 17% to 27% of all hospitalizations for pediatric patients.

What Causes Birth Defects?

Birth defects and genetic disorders may be caused by (1) single-gene mutations, (2) chromosome abnormalities, (3) multifactorial factors, the interaction between genes and environment, and (4) teratogens.

- *Single-gene disorders* may have autosomal dominant, autosomal recessive, X-linked recessive, or X-linked dominant inheritance. There are now more than 5000 such disorders recognized. It is estimated that single-gene disorders affect 2% of the general population over a lifetime and 6% to 8% of hospitalized children.
- *Chromosome disorders* affect almost 1% of live-born children and account for approximately 50% of spontaneous abortions. These involve both numerical and structural chromosome defects.
- *Multifactorial inheritance* may account for up to 60% of disease in the entire population in a lifetime. Common disorders in adults and isolated congenital anomalies in children result from the combined effects of genetic mutation and environmental factors.
- *Teratogens* cause morphologic and/or functional abnormalities in a fetus. They include infectious agents, physical agents, drug and chemical agents, and maternal metabolic and genetic factors. The effects of teratogens are preventable in the absence of the offending factor.

What Mechanisms Can Cause Birth Defects?

The mechanisms that cause birth defects include deformation, disruption, dysplasia, and malformation. Each has specific implications for clinical presentation and prognosis (Table 62-1).

EVALUATION

How Do I Evaluate a Child with Multiple Birth Defects?

The history for a child with multiple congenital anomalies should specifically emphasize prenatal events. These include (1) maternal factors such as diabetes, hypertension, exposures to prescription and other drugs, uterine abnormalities, and others and (2) fetal factors including abnormal fetal movements, ultrasound findings in the fetus, and amniotic fluid analyses. Ask about development, behavior, growth patterns, and presence of impaired hearing or vision. The family history should include information

Table 62-1

Types of Pathogenetic Mechanisms Causing Birth Defects

Types	Description	Prognosis	Recurrence	Example(s)
Deformation	Abnormal shape or form caused by extrinsic mechanical forces (twinning, uterine defects, oligohydramnios); usually occur in last trimester of pregnancy	Good	Low recurrence risk	Plagiocephaly; metatarsus adductus; tibial bowing
Disruption	Abnormalities from extrinsic breakdown or interference with normal developmental process; adjacent structures often unaffected	Good	Low recurrence risk	Amniotic bands
Dysplasia	Defects resulting from abnormal cellular organization or function that affect one general tissue type; often not evident at birth	Depends on particular disorder, but may worsen with age		Cutis laxa; ectodermal dysplasias; achondroplasia
Malformation	Defect resulting from an intrinsic abnormality of development of a body structure during prenatal life; may involve multiple tissue types	Often require surgery or medical treatments	Risk of recurrence of an isolated malformation is in the range of 2%-5% (multifactorial)	Cleft lip and palate; congenital heart defects

on ethnic origin, consanguinity, similar abnormalities in other family members, and recurrent miscarriages or stillbirths. Parental age is also important because advanced maternal age is associated with risk of chromosomal abnormalities in the fetus, and advanced paternal age is associated with risk of new autosomal dominant mutations.

How Do I Develop a Family Pedigree?

A family pedigree is essential to help determine whether an identifiable mode of inheritance can explain the presenting problem: autosomal dominant, autosomal recessive, X-linked, or chromosome translocation. The family history is recorded in a pedigree with symbols representing individuals and their symptoms or disorders. *At least three generations* are needed to establish inheritance patterns. If the pedigree shows male-to-male transmission, an equal number of males and females affected, and affected individuals in each successive generation, this confirms *autosomal dominant inheritance.* If males are predominantly affected on the maternal side of the family and vertical transmission is demonstrated, then *X-linked inheritance* is likely. Horizontal patterns of affected individuals or siblings, or consanguinity (relatedness), suggest *autosomal recessive inheritance.* The family history is recorded in a pedigree with symbols representing individuals and their symptoms or disorders (Figure 62-1).

How Do I Recognize a Birth Defect?

An anomaly can be either a minor or a major structural abnormality. *Minor anomalies* have no serious medical or cosmetic effects. They serve as clues to the diagnosis of a specific pattern of malformation. Examples of minor anomalies include preauricular ear pits, fifth finger clinodactyly, single palmar crease, and epicanthal folds. The presence of two

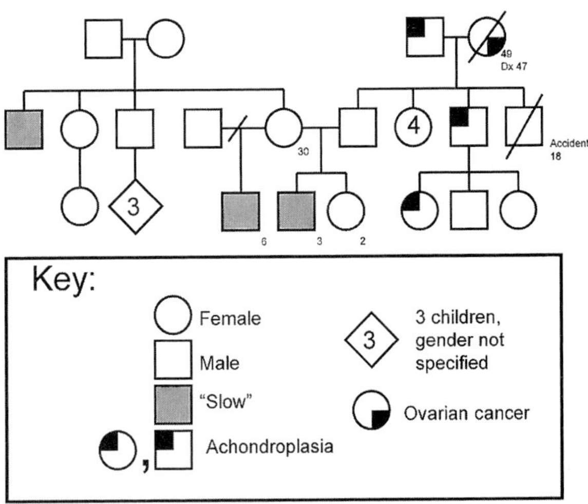

FIGURE 62-1 Example pedigree and legend of symbols.

or more minor malformations should "raise a red flag" and warrants a search for an underlying major malformation. *Major malformations* usually require surgical or medical intervention and can reduce life expectancy if not corrected. Examples of major anomalies include microphthalmia, hydrocephalus, gastroschisis, and clubfeet.

What Is Important on Physical Examination?

The physical examination must look for minor and major structural anomalies and specifically note the physical growth of various parts of the body such as upper and lower segment measurements or size of the ears. This requires careful measurements to provide quantitative assessment and comparison with established norms. There are published graphs of these measures (Hall et al., 1995).

Is Testing Needed for an Isolated Anomaly?

An isolated birth defect or major anomaly is most likely caused by multifactorial inheritance but could be familial with autosomal dominant inheritance. In most cases, further testing *cannot* confirm this mode of inheritance. Parents should be counseled that the risk of recurrence of the anomaly in future offspring is approximately 2% to 5%. In some cases, gene mutations may have been identified as the cause of a particular malformation. An example is coronal craniosynostosis, in which mutations in the fibroblast growth factor receptor 3 *(FGFR3)* gene may be causative. Because many of the major malformations have associated minor anomalies, it may be warranted to obtain routine chromosome analysis when evaluating such a child.

Do Multiple Birth Defects Have Recognizable Patterns?

Multiple major and minor structural anomalies can have recognizable patterns: *syndrome, sequence, association,* and *complex.* Table 62-2 defines and gives examples of each pattern. Each of these patterns has implications for etiology, natural history, and prognosis. The *patterns of malformation* must be considered when a child has multiple major and minor anomalies, especially if accompanied by growth, developmental, or behavioral abnormalities. Each pattern may have different modes of inheritance: single gene, chromosome abnormality, or multifactorial causes.

What Is the Evaluation for Multiple Birth Defects?

The child with two or more minor anomalies should undergo an evaluation for underlying major anomalies, because many are occult. A meticulous physical examination and selected imaging studies and laboratory tests can help identify associated birth defects or medical problems. For instance, a child who has preauricular pits or protruding ears (minor anomalies) should undergo hearing testing and renal ultrasound studies to search for the hearing loss and renal malformations found in the branchio-oto-renal (BOR) syndrome. Complications associated with suspected disorders should also be sought using imaging and/or laboratory studies. For example, a child suspected of having Williams syndrome (caused by microdeletion of chromosome 7q11) is at risk for hypercalcemia, renal artery stenoses and/or calculi, supravalvular

Table 62-2

Patterns of Birth Defects

Pattern	Definition	Cause(s)	Example(s)
Syndrome	Recognizable pattern of structural defects often with a predictable natural history	Single-gene inheritance (AR, AD, XLR, XLD); chromosome defects; teratogens	Down syndrome (trisomy 21); Fragile X syndrome; Cornelia de Lange syndrome
Sequence	Single identifiable event/ abnormality in development that triggers a cascade of other developmental defects	Often unknown	Pierre-Robin sequence (initial mandibular hypoplasia → displacement of tongue → interruption of palatal closure → cleft palate, micrognathia, glossoptosis → respiratory and feeding problems)
Association	Grouping of certain birth defects resulting from interruption of development at a particular embryonic period	Often unknown	VATER or VACTERL association (*v*ertebral defects, *a*nal atresia, *c*ardiac defects, *t*racheo-*e*sophageal defects, *r*enal or *r*adial limb defects)
Complex	Pattern of birth defects derived from different structures that all lie together in the same local body region during embryologic development (known as *developmental field*)	Unknown	OEIS complex (omphalocele, exstrophy of the bladder, imperforate anus, spinal defects)

AD, Autosomal dominant; AR, autosomal recessive; XLD, X-linked dominant; XLR, X-linked recessive.

aortic stenosis, and pulmonic stenosis. Surveillance testing with total and ionized serum calcium levels, electrolytes, blood urea nitrogen (BUN) and creatinine, urinalysis, renal ultrasound, and echocardiogram may identify abnormalities. Other birth defects may justify chromosome analysis, fluorescence in situ hybridization (FISH) analysis, and DNA testing.

When Should Chromosome Analysis Be Done?

Chromosome analysis is recommended for the child with multiple congenital anomalies, developmental delay, and/or growth abnormalities, as well as for couples with multiple pregnancy losses. A normal karyotype or chromosome analysis consists of 23 pairs of chromosomes, including 22 pairs of autosomes and 1 pair of sex chromosomes (46,XX in females, and 46,XY in males). Microdeletions and microduplications are detected by chromosomal microarray analysis, which targets telomeres, centromeres, and known microdeletion/microduplication syndromes.

What Is the Fluorescence In Situ Hybridization Test?

Very small deletions or duplications detected by chromosome microarray analysis are confirmed by FISH. This study is useful to identify conditions caused by "microdeletions," such as DiGeorge/velocardiofacial syndromes (chromosome 22q11 deletion) and Williams syndrome (chromosome 7q11.2 deletion).

What Must I Do before Requesting DNA or Molecular Tests?

You must make a precise and correct clinical diagnosis for a patient with multiple birth defects, mental retardation, or metabolic abnormality before considering DNA or molecular testing. These tests can be used only if there is a known gene mutation. In addition, there must be a clinical and/or research laboratory available to perform the tests. Most genetic disorders do not have an identified gene mutation, so DNA testing is not available.

What Is DNA Testing?

DNA testing detects gene mutations or changes in the DNA sequence as small as a single nucleotide or as large as thousands of base pairs. These are too small to be detected by chromosome or FISH analysis. Molecular techniques can detect gene mutations for many different genetic disorders.

TREATMENT

What Treatment Is Possible for Birth Defects?

Treatment is possible at several levels for patients with birth defects or genetic disorders. The structural abnormalities of many sporadic birth defects or genetic disorders, such as congenital heart disease, are often amenable to surgical or medical therapies.

METABOLIC DISORDERS

ETIOLOGY

What Metabolic Diseases Might I Encounter?

Several single-gene disorders affect biochemical pathways involved in protein, carbohydrate, or lipid metabolism. These "inborn errors of metabolism" have importance beyond their prevalence because they are *treatable*. They generally cause damage by preventing synthesis of crucial compounds, by blocking degradation or removal of toxic compounds, or by a combination of both mechanisms. For example, in phenylketonuria (PKU), accumulated phenylalanine is toxic, whereas in Smith-Lemli-Opitz syndrome the inability to make cholesterol is responsible for many problems. Most metabolic disorders have autosomal recessive inheritance, but some have X-linked recessive or mitochondrial inheritance.

EVALUATION

How Does Metabolic Disease Present Clinically?

The diagnostic clues that lead to the suspicion of a metabolic disease depend on the specific disorder. Children with metabolic disease often have *delayed growth and impaired brain function*. Therefore, metabolic disease should be considered when a child is physically small as well as developmentally delayed. Developmental *regression* usually signals the presence of an accumulating toxic metabolite and should bring metabolic disease to mind. Some patients, however, may have appropriate growth or even be overgrown and may have normal brain function. Structural abnormalities can be seen occasionally, but they are not as common in metabolic diseases as in chromosome or other single-gene disorders.

What Laboratory Tests Detect Metabolic Diseases?

The metabolic diseases are dependent on laboratory testing for diagnosis. When metabolic disease is suspected, initial testing should focus on carbohydrate, fatty acid, and amino acid metabolism. Initial blood tests usually include measurement of serum electrolytes, blood glucose, lactate, ammonia, amino acids, and the acyl-carnitine profile. Urine tests that are sometimes helpful include determinations of amino acids, organic acids, and ketones. Sample collection, fasting state, concomitant medications, sample preparation, and even the particular laboratory chosen all may affect results and their interpretation. These tests usually do not give a final diagnosis but rather are a broad screen to determine if further testing is warranted. On occasion, the presence of metabolic disease may be identified from testing done for other reasons. For example, metabolic disorders will be suspected when electrolyte studies show low total serum CO_2, when magnetic resonance imaging demonstrates abnormal myelination, or when an ophthalmologic examination identifies a "cherry-red spot." DNA and other molecular diagnostic tests make diagnosis of metabolic diseases simpler, faster, more precise, and often cheaper—but only for a limited number of disorders at this time. Expanded newborn screening, in which all newborns are screened for larger numbers of metabolic disorders, is also rapidly changing the diagnosis of metabolic diseases.

TREATMENT

Can Metabolic Diseases Be Treated?

Treatment reflects the pathogenesis of the inborn errors of metabolism, and either *replaces* a biologic product that the patient is unable to produce or *reduces or removes* a dietary component that the patient is unable to metabolize. PKU is the prototype for successful therapy of genetic disease. Patients with PKU cannot metabolize phenylalanine, which accumulates and is toxic to the brain. Careful control of dietary phenylalanine provides enough of this essential amino acid for growth and no more. Good dietary control allows these patients to be developmentally normal instead of mentally retarded, which would be the outcome in untreated PKU. "Gene therapy" for the treatment of human genetic disorders is still in its infancy.

Can Abnormal Gene Products Be Replaced?

Enzymes and other proteins can be produced in the laboratory and given to a patient (as in Gaucher's disease). Liver and bone marrow transplants give the recipient "normal" genes, along with the cells and tissues to produce the normal gene products. Several storage disorders are currently being treated by this method. The treatment commonly called *gene therapy* refers to giving donor genes to a patient to correct a defect. At the time of this writing (2006), gene therapy was undergoing limited clinical trials and will likely become a mainstream treatment modality for several disorders in the next decade.

CANCER

ETIOLOGY

Is There a Genetic Predisposition to Cancer?

Although 33% to 50% of all individuals will have some type of cancer during their life spans, the great majority of cancer occurs sporadically and is not related to a genetic predisposition. Certain features of a pedigree suggest that a cancer risk gene is segregating in the family, including *cancer at an age younger than commonly seen for that cancer type, bilateral or multifocal tumors, multiple individuals with the same cancer type, and occurrence of cancers that are known to be associated with each other (e.g., breast and ovarian cancer)*. Additionally, certain uncommon cancers such as medullary carcinoma of the thyroid have a high likelihood of genetic predisposition. The family "oral history" is often inaccurate concerning a relative's cancer, especially for cancer occurrences before the latter part of the 20th century. Careful review of the pathology records of family members who have had cancer will clarify the family cancer history. Physical examination is also crucial because some familial cancer syndromes have characteristic features. Once the details have been gathered, the patient can then be provided with a preliminary risk assessment and given the option of further evaluation, including genetic testing if available. If the patient being evaluated is presymptomatic (i.e., has not actually had cancer), then choosing the appropriate family member to test demands careful consideration.

What Cancer Syndromes Affect Children?

Familial cancer syndromes primarily have their impact in adulthood, but several syndromes affect children, including Von Hippel-Lindau syndrome (VHL), multiple endocrine neoplasia (MEN) syndromes, and familial adenomatous polyposis (FAP). The large majority of familial cancer predisposition syndromes are transmitted as autosomal dominant disorders, and therefore cancer in a parent would mean a 50% risk for the child. Organ systems at risk include the endocrine (VHL and MEN), gastrointestinal (FAP), and ophthalmologic (VHL, FAP).

EVALUATION

What Testing Is Available for Cancer Syndromes?

Family history is the essential "test" in familial cancer syndromes. Failure to identify the family history of cancer and to act on the history could have disastrous consequences for a child, even if presymptomatic. A genetics consultation can determine the need for surveillance or screening in familial cancer syndromes. Screening may be either DNA diagnostics to determine if the patient in question did indeed inherit the disorder or a combination of physical examination, biochemical analysis, and imaging studies to evaluate for the actual development of tumors.

TREATMENT

Is Treatment Available for Cancer Syndromes?

In general, the malignancies that result from a familial cancer predisposition are treated similarly to those that occur sporadically. Surveillance may allow early diagnosis so that treatment can begin at earlier stages. Additionally, in certain syndromes with extremely high risk of malignancy, surgeries can be performed prophylactically in presymptomatic individuals.

GENETIC COUNSELING

What Is Genetic Counseling?

Much of the treatment for patients and their families involves genetic counseling. The content and timing of counseling sessions vary depending on the concerns of each individual family. The information provided about the diagnosis, the options available, and the risk of recurrence must be presented in a compassionate, unbiased, nondirective, nonjudgmental way. It is important that such information be presented in person, not over the telephone, and with as many family members present as possible. The American Society of Human Genetics (1975) provides a definition of genetic counseling that emphasizes communication to help an individual or family

1. Comprehend the medical facts, including the diagnosis, probable course of the disorder, and the available management.
2. Appreciate the way heredity contributes to the disorder and the risk of recurrence in specified relatives.
3. Understand the options for dealing with the risk of recurrence.
4. Choose the course of action that seems appropriate to them in view of their risk and their family goals and act in accordance with that decision.
5. Make the best possible adjustment to the disorder in an affected family member.

Where Can I Learn More about Genetic Disorders?

Numerous textbooks describe known syndromes, associations, and sequences caused by chromosome and single-gene abnormalities. A few of the valuable ones are included in the bibliography. The *On-line Mendelian Inheritance in Man* (OMIM) database contains all known human diseases with single gene etiologies *(www.ncbi.nlm.nih.gov [click on OMIM])*; GeneReviews *(www.genereviews.org/)* is also a very useful resource

How Do I Provide Health Supervision for Children with Genetic Disorders?

The American Society of Human Genetics and the American Academy of Pediatrics (AAP) have jointly developed a series of health supervision guidelines for children with genetic disorders. These statements can be found on the AAP Web site at *http://aappolicy.aappublications.org/policy_statement/index.dtl#H*. They provide information about specific disorders and make recommendations for anticipatory guidance and routine screening. These guidelines are available for most of the common genetic conditions, including Down syndrome, achondroplasia, neurofibromatosis (type I), fragile X syndrome, Marfan syndrome, sickle cell disease, and Turner syndrome, to name a few. Also refer to Chapter 16, Special Healthcare Needs. Table 62-3 lists other Internet resources that are useful for professionals, patients, and families.

Table 62-3

Selected Genetic Internet Resources

Group	Site
Alliance of Genetic Support Groups	*www.geneticalliance.org*
GeneClinics/GeneTests	*www.geneclinics.org*
Public Health Genomics	*www.cdc.gov/genomics*
National Organization for Rare Disorders	*www.rarediseases.org* ("Index of Rare Diseases")
OMIM (Online Mendelian Inheritance in Man)	*www.ncbi.nlm.nih.gov* (click on OMIM)
Organization of Teratology Information Specialists	*www.otispregnancy.org* (click on "Fact Sheets")
Teratology Society	*www.teratology.org*

KEY POINTS

- The family pedigree is an important tool in the evaluation of possible genetic disorders.
- Careful physical examination and measurement of affected body parts aids in the assessment of the child with congenital anomalies.

(continued)

- Counseling and support are key components of genetic evaluation.
- Neonatal screening is one of the most effective diagnostic tools for identification of genetic disorders.

Case 62-1

A family brings a 5-year-old boy to the office with concerns about behavior and development. They want to know if he is "normal," if his problems will resolve, and if his condition is inherited. Various people have told the parents that their child must have a genetic problem because he is "retarded," has "ADHD," and is "autistic." He was born at term, after an uneventful pregnancy. His medical history includes only viral illnesses, but his development has always been slower than expected by the parents. His language and social skills are especially problematic. He was enrolled in a preschool at age 4 years but was withdrawn from school because of his disruptive behavior and because he "could not learn." Your physical examination demonstrates a child who appears afraid of contact, makes sounds but no recognizable words, behaves at a level much below his chronologic age, and has no physical findings consistent with any specific syndrome. Family history reveals two maternal uncles with moderate mental retardation and a maternal great uncle who was institutionalized.

A. What historical information will help you better understand this child's problem?
B. How can the family pedigree assist with diagnosis?
C. If this child is ultimately diagnosed with fragile X syndrome, what will you discuss with the family about prognosis and management?

Case 62-2

A 5-pound, 3-ounce male infant was just born in a small community hospital to a 24-year-old woman after an uncomplicated, full-term pregnancy. You are concerned because the infant has bilateral cleft lip and palate, small eyes, a loud heart murmur, undescended testicles, and clubfeet. The infant is also small for gestational age. The infant's problems were a surprise, because this is the mother's first pregnancy and she had no history of abortions or miscarriages.

A. What information do you need to obtain to evaluate this patient?
B. Draw the pedigree for the following family history: The baby's mother has two healthy brothers, ages 21 and 28 years. Her older brother has a 3-year-old son and a 1-year-old daughter, both healthy. Her mother is 56 years old and her father is 58 years old, and both are also healthy. The baby's father is 25 years old and healthy. He has four sisters, each of whom has two children, all healthy. His father died at age 55 years of a heart attack. His mother is healthy at age 57 years.

C. Based on the pedigree and the infant's findings, what is the most likely cause?
D. How would you evaluate this infant? What do you need to discuss with the family?

Case 62-3

A male infant with achondroplasia is born to a G2P2A0 28-year-old mother and a 40-year-old father. Neither parent has achondroplasia. Their other child, a 3-year-old boy, has grown appropriately. Family history shows that the mother is adopted and knows nothing of her biologic family. The father has three brothers: the youngest, age 16 years, has cystic fibrosis; the older brothers are healthy and each have two children, all of normal stature. Paternal grandparents are both in their sixties and healthy.

A. Draw the family pedigree and interpret the inheritance pattern.
B. How can an infant have an autosomal dominant disorder if there is no evidence of the disease in prior generations?
C. What is the risk that this patient's father is a carrier for cystic fibrosis?
D. What will you tell the parents about their risk for future children with achondroplasia? Is their other son likely to have achondroplasia or to transmit it to his offspring?

Case Answers

62-1 A. *Learning objective:* **Discuss the general approach to assessment of a possible genetic disorder.** The history should emphasize details of the problem from the perspective of the family. A pedigree should be drawn, based on a thorough family history with information from at least three generations on both sides of the family. Growth records, developmental milestones, school records, and behavioral concerns all should be examined. A careful physical examination that includes additional measurements beyond height, weight, and head circumference might identify subtle findings that point to a syndrome. If any diagnostic testing has been done, the results should be reviewed. Think about the relationship between the history and the physical examination and develop a differential diagnosis that includes conditions that can explain the combination of findings identified. Diagnostic tests should be selected to clarify hypotheses generated during the history and physical examination.

62-1 B. *Learning objective:* **Use a pedigree to identify the mode of inheritance of a hereditary disorder.** The pedigree allows a visual representation of hereditary traits and disorders. It may identify a specific pattern of inheritance, including autosomal dominant, autosomal recessive, and X-linked traits. Look for these patterns of transmission for the trait in question: Is every generation affected? Is there a pattern of male-to-male transmission, indicating autosomal dominant inheritance? Does the family have evidence of consanguinity, suggesting autosomal recessive inheritance? Are males more involved than females, on the maternal side of the family, suggesting X-linked inheritance? A new mutation may be identified if the trait appears without prior clinical manifestation. The family's pedigree is shown in the figure.

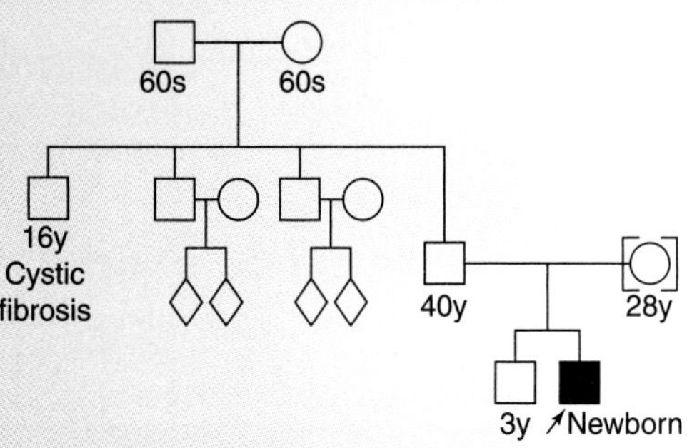

62-1 C. *Learning objective:* **Discuss the characteristic features of fragile X syndrome, and outline broad management issues.** Fragile X syndrome is an X-linked trait that manifests as mental retardation, hyperactivity, and behaviors that may resemble those expressed by autistic children. Physical features often, but not always, found include large testicles, long jaw, long ears, and hyperextensible joints. Family history may be positive for mental retardation among male offspring. Families must be counseled about the need for developmental assistance, individualized education plans, and assistance with activities of daily living.

62-2 A. *Learning objective:* **Discuss the information that should be obtained from the history to evaluate a newborn with congenital anomalies.** First, do a careful review of this pregnancy, including maternal fever, other illnesses, bleeding, diabetes, hypertension, and rashes. Ask about alcohol, tobacco, and prescription or over-the-counter drug use (including herbs). Review the mother's reproductive history, especially previous fetal loss by miscarriage, abortion, or stillbirth. Ask whether prenatal studies were done, including ultrasound, amniocentesis, and triple screen. Obtain a detailed family history.

62-2 B. *Learning objective:* **Use a pedigree to assess the possibility of familial transmission of a trait and to determine the mode of inheritance.** The pedigree shows no familial transmission of the problem.

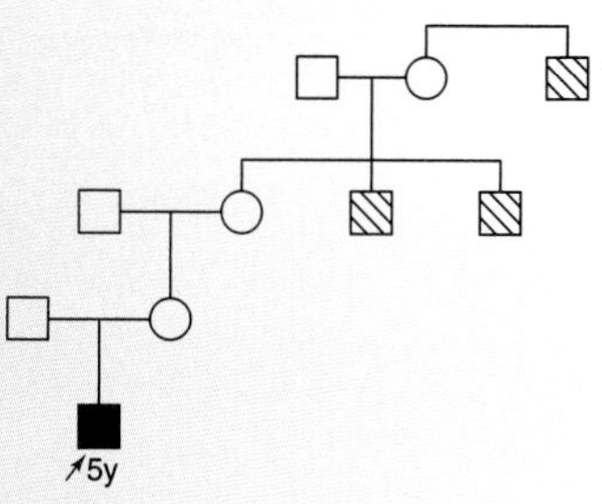

62-2 C. *Learning objective:* **Recognize that an infant with in utero growth retardation and multiple congenital anomalies most likely has a chromosomal abnormality.** An infant with multiple congenital anomalies and in utero growth retardation whose family pedigree does not demonstrate familial transmission of the problem most likely has a chromosomal abnormality. Examples of such anomalies include trisomies, deletions, and duplications.

62-2 D. *Learning objective:* **Develop an evaluation and management plan, including diagnostic tests to evaluate a suspected chromosomal anomaly, and use results to counsel the family.** Consultation with a geneticist will allow identification of a recognizable syndrome. Chromosomal analysis (karyotype) is the most important laboratory test. Other laboratory tests may be indicated depending on the nature of the anomalies and the ease with which a syndrome or pattern can be identified. Studies such as head ultrasound, other central nervous system imaging tests, or echocardiogram should be performed. When a child has two or more obvious anomalies (in this case, in utero growth retardation, bilateral cleft lip and palate, heart defects, and eye and skeletal anomalies), a search for other occult anomalies is warranted. Consultation with a cardiologist or an ophthalmologist may also aid the diagnosis. The family must know the results of the diagnostic evaluation and must be given detailed information about prognosis and the risks of recurrence (if known). The infant in this case has trisomy 13, a condition with a high likelihood of death in the newborn period.

62-3 A. *Learning objective:* **Interpret a pedigree.** There is no evidence of achondroplasia in this family.

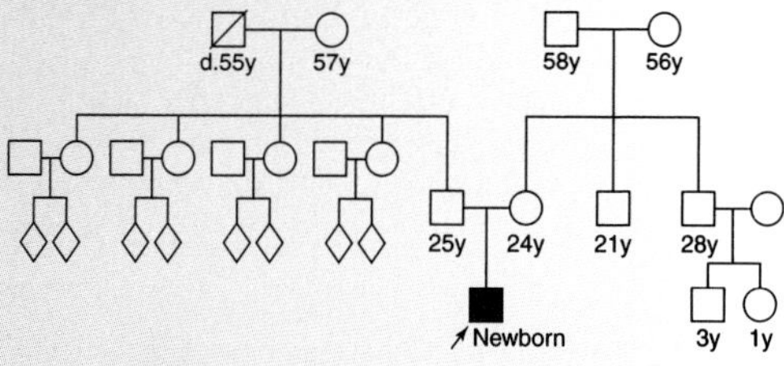

62-3 B. *Learning objective:* **Discuss the common modes of inheritance: autosomal recessive, autosomal dominant, X-linked.** This infant most likely has a new mutation in the fibroblast growth factor receptor 3 *(FGFR3)* gene. Approximately 80% of cases of achondroplasia are caused by a new mutation. Advanced paternal age is a risk factor for new autosomal dominant mutations, especially in achondroplasia. When the infant reaches reproductive age, he will have a 50% risk of passing the anomaly to his offspring.

62-3 C. *Learning objective:* **Discuss the concept of the "carrier state" for common genetic conditions.** Because the patient's uncle (father's brother) has cystic fibrosis, a disease that is inherited as an autosomal recessive trait, the father has a 2/3 likelihood of being a carrier for the CF gene. Both paternal grandparents are obligatory carriers, because they have an affected son.

62-3 D. *Learning objective:* **Discuss the importance of family counseling when a child is diagnosed with a hereditary disorder.** Because neither parent has achondroplasia, the disorder was not transmitted in the usual autosomal dominant mode. The risk of another spontaneous mutation in the FGFR3 gene is low. The family's other child has no risk of manifesting achondroplasia or of transmitting it to his future offspring.

BIBLIOGRAPHY

American Society of Human Genetics, Committee on Genetic Counseling, Genetic counseling, *Am J Hum Genet* 27:240, 1975.

Borgaonkar DS et al: *Chromosomal variation in man,* ed 8, New York, 1997, Wiley-Liss.

Gorlin RS, Cohen MM Jr, Hennekam RCM: *Syndromes of the head and neck,* ed 4, Oxford, 2001, Oxford University Press.

Hall JG, Froster-Iskenius UG, Allanson JE: *Handbook of normal physical measurements,* Oxford, 1995, Oxford University Press, .

Jones KL: *Smith's recognizable patterns of human malformation,* ed 6, Philadelphia, 2006, Elsevier-Saunders.

Nussbaum RL, McInne RR, Willard HF, editors: *Thompson & Thompson genetics in medicine,* ed 7, Philadelphia, 2007, WB Saunders.

Scriver CR et al, editors: *The metabolic and molecular bases of inherited disease,* ed 8, New York, 2001, McGraw-Hill.

Stevenson RE, Hall JG, Goodman RM, editors: *Human malformations and related anomalies,* Oxford, 1993, Oxford University Press.

63

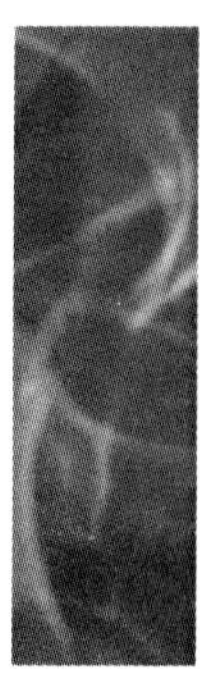

Hematology

ROGER BERKOW

 IRON DEFICIENCY ANEMIA

ETIOLOGY

What Causes Iron Deficiency in Children?

Iron deficiency most often develops from poor gastrointestinal absorption of iron and poor bioavailability of iron from food, combined with microscopic gastrointestinal (GI) blood loss. Human milk has low iron content (0.5 to 1 mg/L) but high iron bioavailability (~50% absorption) and provides breast-fed infants with adequate iron for the first 6 months of life, after which iron-containing foods should be introduced. Infant formula contains 12 mg/L of iron, of which ~10% is absorbed. Unmodified cow's milk has low iron content (0.5 mg/L), has poor iron bioavailability (3% to 5% absorption), and also irritates the infant gut mucosa, leading to chronic blood loss. Switching from breast milk or formula to unmodified cow's milk before age 12 months is the leading cause of iron deficiency in the developed nations. In the developing world, parasitic infection is the leading cause of iron deficiency. Adolescent females may develop iron deficiency from heavy menstrual blood loss. Iron deficiency in children outside of infancy should lead to a search for blood loss and consideration of bowel pathology (polyps or Meckel's diverticulum).

EVALUATION

How Should I Evaluate Suspected Iron Deficiency Anemia?

An anemic infant or child commonly has a history of pallor and of being switched to cow's milk before age 12 months. Milk is usually the primary source of calories, but the child may eat other foods. No obvious blood loss is reported in most cases. The physical examination shows a pale child without bruising, petechiae, lymphadenopathy, or hepatosplenomegaly. A cardiac "flow" murmur may be heard. Complete blood count (CBC) shows anemia, microcytosis (low mean corpuscular volume [MCV]), and hypochromia (low mean corpuscular hemoglobin

[MCH]). Reticulocyte count is low (see Table 50-1). The white blood cell (WBC) count and differential should be normal, but the platelet count is often elevated. If the tests are done, serum iron level will be low, total iron-binding capacity will be elevated, and iron saturation (iron ÷ total iron-binding capacity) and serum ferritin will be very low. The test for stool occult blood is often positive.

TREATMENT

How Is Iron Deficiency Anemia Treated?

Iron dose is 6 mg/kg/day of *elemental iron*. Ferrous sulfate, the most common form of iron used for children, has 20% elemental iron. The iron should be given separately from food to increase absorption. Response to treatment is marked by a rise in the reticulocyte count within 3 or 4 days and an increase in hemoglobin within 1 to 2 weeks. Treatment must be given for several months to replenish iron stores, and dietary iron supplementation is important after successful treatment. If a child remains anemic with microcytic red blood cells (RBCs) despite iron therapy, consider thalassemia, lead exposure, or copper deficiency (seen occasionally in severe nutritional deficiency).

HEMOLYSIS

ETIOLOGY

What Causes Hemolysis?

Hemolysis results from disorders that affect the RBC membrane, the cytoplasm, or the hemoglobin. Careful consideration of these RBC components must be a part of the evaluation. *Extrinsic* factors act on the membrane to cause hemolysis and *intrinsic* defects cause cell breakdown (Table 63-1).

Table 63-1

Red Blood Cell (RBC) Defects That Result in Hemolysis

Extrinsic Factors	Intrinsic Factors
Antibody formation: autoimmune hemolysis, isoimmune hemolysis Microangiopathic hemolysis: HUS, DIC, artificial heart valves	Genetic defects of membrane structural proteins: spherocytosis and elliptocytosis Genetic defect of the lipid layers, vitamin E deficiency Enzyme defects: pyruvate kinase, G-6-PD

DIC, Disseminated intravascular coagulation; G-6-PD, glucose-6-phosphate dehydrogenase; HUS, hemolytic uremic syndrome.

How Do Autoantibodies Cause Hemolysis?

The RBC membrane contains more than 200 different glycoprotein antigens. Autoantibodies directed against RBC antigens, other than the A, B, and Rh blood groups, shorten the life of the RBCs through a process known as *autoimmune hemolytic anemia* (AIHA). Part of the RBC membrane is removed as the antibody-coated RBC traverses the sinusoids of the spleen, leading to the formation of spherocytes that undergo hemolysis. Occasionally, intravascular hemolysis occurs in the presence of a strong complement-fixing antibody. In either case, rapid destruction of RBCs can lead to a potentially life-threatening anemia. The formation of "autoantibodies" can be an early sign of a more generalized autoimmune disorder.

What Are Isohemagglutinins and When Do They Cause Hemolysis?

The A and B antigens on RBCs are similar to naturally occurring proteins and cause the formation of isohemagglutinins: anti-A antibodies in type O and B individuals and anti-B antibodies in type O and A individuals. These antibodies are *not* the same as the autoantibodies discussed earlier. When a mother with blood type O has a baby with blood type A (known as an "ABO setup"), isohemagglutinins can cross the placenta and induce hemolysis, causing isoimmune hemolytic anemia of the newborn. Anti-A and anti-B antibodies can also cause hemolysis after transfusion if blood is not carefully cross-matched or if clerical errors lead to mismatched transfusion.

What Is Rh Incompatibility?

The Rh blood group does not mimic naturally occurring antigens, so prior exposure to Rh-positive RBCs must occur for antibodies to form. This most often occurs when an Rh-negative mother gives birth to an Rh-positive infant. The baby's RBCs enter the mother's circulation and trigger anti-Rh antibody production. The Rh-negative mother must be given anti-Rh globulin to destroy any fetal or infant cells to which she is exposed. If this does not occur, or if anti-Rh antibodies form despite attempts to remove Rh-positive RBCs, the mother is said to be "Rh sensitized." Any subsequent pregnancy in which the fetus is Rh positive will be at risk, because the anti-Rh antibodies cross the placenta and cause hemolysis in the fetus.

What Causes Mechanical Red Blood Cell Damage?

The hemolysis that occurs in hemolytic uremic syndrome (HUS), in disseminated intravascular hemolysis, and in the presence of giant hemangiomas (Kasabach-Merritt syndrome) results from damage to the RBCs during passage through fibrin-coated microvasculature. This process is called *microangiopathic hemolytic anemia* and produces fragments of RBCs called *schistocytes*. Extrinsic damage to RBCs can also occur as the cells pass through an artificial heart valve or an enlarged spleen and from extremes of temperatures, as can be seen in burn victims.

Do Red Blood Cell Membrane Abnormalities Cause Hemolysis?

The RBC membrane is a lipid bilayer into which glycoprotein antigens and channels for the transport of electrolytes are inserted. Underlying and attached to the membrane are structural proteins that help support the shape and flexibility of the RBC. Disorders that affect the structural protein layer or the lipid bilayer will cause hemolysis. The defects may be within the membrane itself or may be caused by damage from enzyme or cofactor deficiencies.

What Structural Protein Abnormalities Cause Hemolysis?

Hereditary spherocytosis (HS) and hereditary elliptocytosis (HE) are the most common disorders resulting from intrinsic abnormalities of the RBC membrane. They are inherited as autosomal dominant traits, although 20% to 25% of patients have no family history and most likely have new mutations in structural proteins, such as spectrin, actin, ankyrin, and others. The severity of hemolysis in HS or HE varies greatly: Some children require repeated transfusion therapy, whereas others are identified only by a routine screening CBC.

How Do Hemoglobin Abnormalities Cause Hemolysis?

The predominant abnormalities of hemoglobin that lead to hemolysis are the sickling disorders: hemoglobin SS, SC, and S-β thalassemia. Sickle cell disease (Hb SS) results from the substitution of valine for glutamine at the sixth amino acid position on the β chain of hemoglobin. This autosomal recessive disorder is characterized by polymerization of the hemoglobin molecule in conditions of low oxygen. These polymers induce changes in the RBCs that lead to hemolysis. The RBCs also take on a sickle shape, which leads to occlusion of blood flow through small blood vessels and leads to pain, splenic infarction, stroke, pulmonary infarction, and priapism. The progressive splenic infarction places affected children at high risk for life-threatening infection from encapsulated bacteria (*Streptococcus pneumoniae, Neisseria meningitidis, Haemophilus influenzae* type b, and *Salmonella* species).

Do Red Blood Cell Enzyme Abnormalities Cause Hemolysis?

The cytosol contains the key enzymes that provide the energy to maintain cellular activities and membrane transport (glycolytic pathway). Cytosol also contains the antioxidants that protect the hemoglobin from oxidative damage (pentose phosphate pathway). Deficiencies in any of the components of these pathways result in hemolysis.

What Is Pyruvate Kinase Deficiency?

Pyruvate kinase deficiency is an autosomal recessive trait and usually produces a mild hemolytic anemia. It is the most common abnormality of the glycolytic pathway, which metabolizes glucose to lactate and produces adenosine triphosphate (ATP). A different enzyme controls each step in this pathway. Deficiency or abnormal function of any of these enzymes can decrease production of ATP, alter the ionic environment of the RBC, and shorten RBC survival. In general, deficiency of enzymes early in the pathway produces more severe and global abnormalities, as compared with enzymes in the more distal parts of this pathway.

How Does Glucose-6-Phosphate Dehydrogenase Deficiency Cause Hemolysis?

Hemoglobin is protected from oxidant damage by NADPH. Glucose-6-phosphate dehydrogenase (G-6-PD) is the enzyme primarily responsible for the production of NADPH, and its activity decreases as the RBC ages. Several isoforms of this enzyme exist. Pathologic forms of G-6-PD degrade more rapidly, inducing oxidant stress within the RBC as the cell ages. Males are usually affected, because the gene is inherited as an X-linked recessive disorder. The rate of decrease of the enzyme activity defines the different forms of G-6-PD deficiency. The enzyme isoforms with more rapid rates of decrease are common in people of Mediterranean and Middle Eastern descent. In the Mediterranean variety, rapid rate of enzyme loss leads to a baseline oxidant stress and hemolysis that increases dramatically on exposure to medications or foods that increase the oxidant stress. The African variety is usually mild, with hemolysis only occurring with exposure to foods (fava beans) or medications (sulfonamides, acetaminophen).

EVALUATION

What Is the First Step in the Evaluation of Hemolysis?

If the anemia is the first sign of a problem, the CBC will direct the diagnostic evaluation (see Chapter 50). If the underlying disorder is identified first, then the risk of hemolysis must be recognized and the patient evaluated. In general, hemolysis results in normocytic anemia with an increased reticulocyte count and decreased haptoglobin concentration. The serum indirect bilirubin may be elevated and there may be nonspecific evidence of hemolysis, such as an increase in lactate dehydrogenase. Findings on the blood smear may be specific to the cause of hemolysis.

How Do I Identify Antibody-Mediated Hemolysis?

The major initial information comes from the Coombs' test. The direct Coombs' test will be positive when antibody is bound to the RBC, and the indirect Coombs' test will be positive in the presence of circulating antibody. Tests to identify the specific antibody responsible for hemolysis will make the final diagnosis.

What Is Found in Microangiopathic Hemolysis?

The finding of RBC fragments (schistocytes) on the blood smear is specific to a microangiopathic process. Schistocytes are bizarrely shaped RBCs, sometimes called *helmet cells*. Sometimes the underlying disorder, such as HUS, is identified first, which leads to a search for hemolysis.

How Is an Intrinsic Red Blood Cell Membrane Defect Identified?

A typical patient with hereditary spherocytosis is a 1- to 2-year-old child with mild to moderate anemia at routine screening. Past history reveals prolonged jaundice at birth. The family history reveals that a parent and grandparent on the same side of the family both had anemia in childhood that resolved after removal of the spleen. Physical examination shows mild pallor, minimal or no scleral icterus, and a spleen that is palpable ~2 cm below the left costal margin. A corrected reticulocyte count is elevated. Review of the peripheral blood smear identifies numerous spherocytes. The Coombs' test is negative. The osmotic fragility test will help confirm the diagnosis. After diagnosis of HS, long-term follow-up is important to detect increased hemolysis or a rapid drop in hematocrit at times of intercurrent illnesses. Infection with parvovirus B19 commonly triggers hemolysis and inhibits erythrocyte production. As hemolysis continues without replacement of RBCs by the marrow, life-threatening anemia may occur.

How Are Hemoglobinopathies Identified?

Newborn screening to detect hemoglobinopathies is routine in almost all states. This screening primarily serves to detect sickle cell anemia, but any hemoglobinopathy may be identified. An older child who was not screened at birth may present with anemia or with signs and symptoms consistent with a hemoglobinopathy. In addition to the basic workup, hemoglobin electrophoresis should be obtained.

How Are Red Blood Cell Enzyme Defects Identified?

Hemolysis that cannot be related to a microangiopathic process, effects of antibody formation, a membrane defect, or a hemoglobinopathy must be evaluated for defects in RBC enzymes. Staining of the RBCs to detect Heinz bodies (denatured hemoglobin precipitates) or review of the peripheral blood smear for the presence of "bite" cells will help support a diagnosis of G-6-PD deficiency. Specific enzyme analyses identify deficiencies of G-6-PD, pyruvate kinase, or other enzymes in the glycolytic pathway.

TREATMENT

Can Antibody-Mediated Hemolysis Be Treated?

Transfusion is the primary immediate treatment, but it is often extremely difficult to find "compatible" blood because of the presence of antibodies in the child's serum. In autoimmune hemolytic anemia (AIHA) it is often impossible to find compatible blood. Corticosteroids and intravenous immunoglobulin (IVIG) are useful adjuncts to the treatment of AIHA. For newborns with isoimmune hemolytic anemia it is most appropriate to use the mother's blood to cross-match for a compatible unit of blood if transfusion is needed. Exchange transfusion may be indicated to decrease the bilirubin level and to lower antibody levels.

How Are Other Hemolytic Anemias Treated?

Transfusion may be needed, but the major management is support of the patient against the disease that produces the hemolysis. Avoidance of medications and foods that cause oxidative stress is key in the presence of G-6-PD deficiency.

What Are the Treatment Options for Sickle Cell Anemia?

Early diagnosis and penicillin prophylaxis are crucial to prevent death from infection. Penicillin must be started as soon as a sickling disorder is identified, usually within the first month or two of life. Immunization against *S. pneumoniae* and *H. influenzae* type b must be done. This aggressive treatment has significantly decreased the incidence of life-threatening bacteremia. However, any child with a sickling disorder who has an elevated temperature requires immediate evaluation, blood cultures, and treatment with parenteral antibiotics. If a child with hemoglobin SS has a new onset of acute neurologic changes, the possibility of stroke should be considered. Stroke is a devastating complication that occurs in about 10% of children with SS genotype. Treatment includes administration of oxygen and an exchange transfusion to reduce rapidly the amount of sickle hemoglobin. This treatment often prevents progression of the stroke and allows the correction of some of the neurologic deficit. To prevent recurrent stroke, chronic transfusion with RBCs is essential.

LEUKEMIA

ETIOLOGY

Which Malignancies Cause Disorders of Leukocytes?

Acute lymphoid leukemia accounts for 75% of all childhood leukemia, with *acute myelogenous leukemia* accounting for approximately 20% of cases. Five percent of childhood leukemia is chronic in nature. Acute leukemia can present with a normal, low, or elevated WBC count. Malignant transformation of developing leukocytes leads to replacement of the bone marrow components, causing neutropenia, anemia, and thrombocytopenia. Malignant cells can also infiltrate lymph nodes, thymus, liver, spleen, and kidneys.

What Are the Complications of Leukemia?

Initial concerns on diagnosis and initial treatment of leukemia include the possibility of infection, immune dysfunction, anemia, and bleeding. Breakdown of leukemic cells, with the release of potassium, phosphate, and nucleic acids, can cause *tumor lysis syndrome* and acute renal failure. Marked leukocytosis (> 100,000/mm^3) in some patients with leukemia can be associated with confusion, respiratory distress, and a greater likelihood of tumor lysis syndrome.

What Is the Prognosis of Leukemia?

More than 70% of acute lymphocytic leukemia can be cured. Favorable prognostic factors at diagnosis include ages between 2 and 10 years, female sex, low WBC count, absence of organomegaly and central nervous system (CNS) disease, and the presence of certain chromosomal and molecular markers. Acute myelogenous leukemia can be cured in 40% to 50% of cases.

EVALUATION

How Is Leukemia Diagnosed?

Diagnosis is made by the presence of anemia, thrombocytopenia, and neutropenia, accompanied by increased, decreased, or normal numbers of leukocytes. Leukemia can present with or without lymphadenopathy and hepatosplenomegaly. Bruising, petechiae, and abnormal bleeding often occur. The appearance of abnormal cells in the peripheral blood and bone marrow confirms the presence of leukemia. Analysis for immature cell antigens using immune markers is an adjunct to diagnosis and classifies the type of leukemia. Accurate diagnosis is essential because treatment differs markedly for acute lymphocytic leukemia and acute myelogenous leukemia.

TREATMENT

How Is Leukemia Treated?

Treatment for acute lymphocytic leukemia involves chemotherapy and sometimes radiation therapy. Most children participate in standardized therapies designed to advance leukemia treatment. Remission occurs when leukemic cells are no longer present in the bone marrow and the peripheral blood count normalizes. Intrathecal chemotherapy or CNS radiation therapy is needed to prevent the development of CNS leukemia. After remission, intensive therapy is continued for 6 to 12 months and then maintenance chemotherapy continues for 2 to 2.5 years. Once chemotherapy is completed, the potential for recurrent disease and the long-term effects of the disease and its treatment become the focus of follow-up.

KEY POINTS

- Iron deficiency is the most common cause of microcytic anemia in childhood.
- Hemolysis may result from RBC membrane defects, autoimmune damage to RBCs, or mechanical disruption of RBCs.
- Sickle cell anemia predisposes the child to life-threatening infections.
- Leukemia may produce elevated or decreased WBC counts.

Case 63-1

A 15-month-old African-American boy comes for evaluation of yellow eyes. He was well until 2 weeks ago when he developed an upper respiratory infection. Since that time the mother states that his eyes have been somewhat yellow. He is active and playful and has had no fever at home. He was born at term to a G1P0 mother who had no complications during pregnancy, labor, or delivery. The child had jaundice at birth, which delayed his discharge until 4 days of life. His peak bilirubin level was 17 mg/dl. The neonatal screen was negative, including tests for hemoglobinopathy. He has not had any other illnesses, and his growth and development are age appropriate. Examination shows an alert and playful child in no distress. The heart rate is 150 beats/min, and the temperature is 37° C. Mild scleral icterus is noted, with minimal yellowness to the skin. The spleen is palpable 4 cm below the left costal margin. No other positive physical findings are found.

A. What is the differential diagnosis for this child?
B. What additional history is useful?
C. How would you interpret the following laboratory tests?
   WBC 5000/m^3
   Hemoglobin 7.5 g/dl
   Hematocrit 24%
   MCV 79 fl
   MCH 36 g/dl
   Reticulocyte 10%
   Coombs' negative
D. What additional test would help most in determining the diagnosis?

Case 63-2

A 4-year-old girl has bruising and fever of 101.5° F. The bruising has been present for 1 week and is getting worse. The fever began today. She has been somewhat more tired than usual, with only a fair appetite for the last 2 weeks. She attends daycare. The child has complained about her legs hurting on and off for the last 2 to 3 weeks. Physical examination reveals a temperature of 101.5° F, heart rate of 150 beats/min, and respiratory rate of 24 breaths/min. She has mild pallor and lymphadenopathy in the anterior and posterior cervical areas; she has no axillary or inguinal nodes. There is a systolic flow murmur. The lungs are clear. She has no hepatosplenomegaly. Skin shows scattered petechiae and ecchymoses. The neurologic examination is unremarkable. Laboratory tests reveal the following results:

WBC 2500/mm^3
Hemoglobin 5 g/dl
Hematocrit 15%
Platelets 15,000/mm^3
Neutrophils 3%
Lymphocytes 50%

Monocytes 5%
Atypical cells 42%

A. What is the differential diagnosis?
B. What are the major concerns on the night of admission?
C. What other studies are necessary to finalize the diagnosis and to identify complications? Is any empirical treatment necessary?
D. If the bone marrow aspirate and immune markers confirm the diagnosis of acute lymphocytic leukemia, what important prognostic factors are noted in the history?

Case Answers

63-1 A. *Learning objective:* **Discuss the differential diagnosis for anemia in infancy.** Jaundice can result from many causes, including hepatitis, but this child very likely has hemolysis based on the presence of jaundice and splenomegaly. A hemoglobinopathy is unlikely because of the neonatal screen results. Hemolysis occurs because of RBC membrane defects, RBC enzyme defects, and microangiopathic processes.

63-1 B. *Learning objective:* **Use the history to evaluate a patient with anemia.** History should identify any prior episodes of jaundice. Ask about medications (prescription, over-the-counter, and "herbal") and diet. You should ask about a family history of anemia, splenectomy, or cholecystectomy.

63-1 C. *Learning objective:* **Interpret laboratory tests to identify basic causes of anemia.** The anemia is Coombs' negative and there is a brisk reticulocytosis. RBCs are not microcytic or hypochromic. This suggests an RBC membrane defect as the most likely cause.

63-1 D. *Learning objective:* **Recognize RBC abnormalities using microscopic examination of the peripheral blood smear.** Review the peripheral smear to look for spherocytes or elliptocytes.

63-2 A. *Learning objective:* **List the differential diagnosis for a child with pancytopenia.** Leukemia and aplastic anemia are the two most likely causes of this patient's clinical findings. Leukemia is much more common. The "atypical" cells on the differential are most likely blasts.

63-2 B. *Learning objective:* **Be prepared to manage the multiple complications of acute leukemia.** A child with acute leukemia usually has a severe anemia. If neutropenic, a patient is at high risk for infection. Thrombocytopenia causes bleeding, which is readily apparent in this case from petechiae and ecchymoses; in addition, the child might also have occult blood in the stool. When treatment is started, intravenous fluids are needed to ensure adequate hydration to avoid the tumor lysis syndrome.

63-2 C. *Learning objective:* **Select diagnostic tests to further characterize leukemia after the initial diagnosis.** Further diagnostic workup requires a bone marrow aspirate to characterize the disease process and to confirm the suspicion of leukemia. In addition, immune markers will need to be done to characterize the specific leukemia. Because of the fever, this patient should have a chest radiograph and a blood culture to identify possible infection. A febrile child with leukemia is at high risk for infection and should be started empirically on broad-spectrum antibiotics.

63-2 D. *Learning objective:* **Recognize the prognostic features in history, physical examination, and laboratory evaluation.** This child has a good prognosis for long-term survival because of her young age, female sex, absence of organomegaly and central nervous system disease, and low WBC count.

BIBLIOGRAPHY

Lanzkowsky P, editor: *Manual of pediatric hematology and oncology,* ed 4, New York, 2005, Elsevier.

Nathan DG et al, editors: *Nathan and Oski's hematology of infancy and childhood,* ed 6, Philadelphia, 2003, WB Saunders.

Pizzo PA, Poplack DG, editors: *Principles and practice of pediatric oncology,* ed 4, Philadelphia, 2002, Lippincott-Raven.

Ries LAG et al, editors: *Cancer incidence and survival among children and adolescents: United States SEER Program, 1975–1995* (NIH Publication No. 99-4649), Bethesda, MD, 1999, National Cancer Institute, SEER Program.

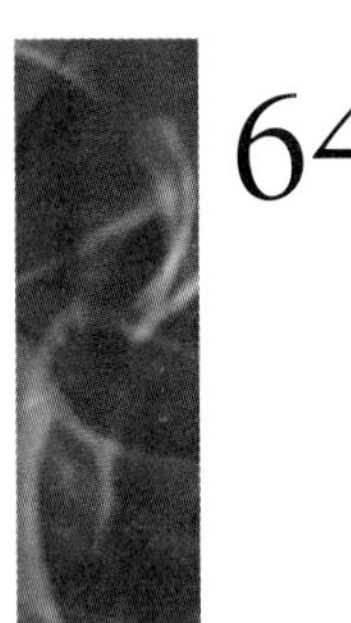

64

Infectious Diseases

WILLIAM V. RASZKA

INFECTIOUS DISEASE EMERGENCIES

ETIOLOGY

What Is an Infectious Disease Emergency?

An *infectious disease emergency* can cause rapid loss of organ function or life unless intervention is immediate. Overwhelming sepsis is the prototype infectious disease emergency. In particular, meningococcemia places a patient at high risk for organ dysfunction and death. Occasionally, even mild disease such as viral laryngotracheobronchitis or croup may lead to an emergency if the airway becomes obstructed. In many parts of the world, severe watery diarrhea causes significant morbidity and mortality. Hence, every single patient must be examined with the idea that he or she might have an infectious disease emergency. Chapter 31 describes a general approach to emergencies in children, and Chapter 59 discusses specific emergent presentations.

EVALUATION

When Should I Suspect an Infectious Disease Emergency?

Lethargy, marked irritability, and difficulty breathing are indications that a child is severely ill or "toxic." An elevated body temperature in itself is rarely a threat to long-term health. Fever is merely a sign that should be interpreted along with the heart rate, respiratory rate, and blood pressure. Lethargy or irritability implies altered central nervous system perfusion. Stridor, tachypnea, and increased work of breathing suggest serious airway problems.

TREATMENT

How Should I Treat Infectious Emergencies?

Treatment begins with the identification of the emergency situation (see Chapter 31). Hence, a high index of suspicion and a careful assessment of children whose clinical presentation suggests the possibility of an infectious emergency are mandatory if successful treatment is to be started. Treatment depends entirely on the specific infection diagnosed.

SPECIFIC INFECTIOUS DISEASE EMERGENCIES

SEPSIS

ETIOLOGY

What Is Sepsis?

Sepsis is the systemic reaction to bacteria (or other organisms). The terminology of sepsis has changed in the last decade and now reflects a progression of disease severity. The initial insult is a localized or systemic infection that provokes a systemic inflammatory response syndrome (SIRS), characterized by hyperthermia or hypothermia, tachycardia, tachypnea, and changes in the circulating white blood cell count. Once the inflammatory response is activated, the process can proceed independently of the infection. SIRS with hypotension is called ***sepsis.*** Severe sepsis is defined as sepsis with organ dysfunction, whereas ***septic shock*** is defined as sepsis with persistent hypotension despite adequate fluid resuscitation.

What Causes Sepsis?

Almost any bacterial infection can lead to sepsis, but *Streptococcus pneumoniae* and *Neisseria meningitidis* are the most common inciting organisms outside the newborn period. Both are encapsulated organisms, making them more difficult for the immune system to clear. The mortality rate of sepsis may be as high as 50% but is highly variable and dependent on the underlying condition of the patient and the initial site of infection.

EVALUATION

How Does Sepsis Present at Different Ages?

Infants and young children often present with fever, poor feeding, tachypnea, and irritability or lethargy. Adolescents may present with fever, shaking chills, confusion, and tachypnea. Additional findings in both groups include tachycardia, delayed capillary refill, hypotension or widened pulse pressure, and petechiae and purpura. The younger the infant, the more nonspecific may be the findings. Hence, particularly in children younger than 3 months, almost any child with fever and irritability is evaluated for possible sepsis (see Chapter 33).

What Laboratory Tests Help in the Diagnosis of Sepsis?

Laboratory findings include elevated prothrombin and partial thromboplastin times, reduced fibrinogen levels, neutropenia or neutrophilia, and toxic granulation of the neutrophils. Culture of blood, cerebrospinal fluid (CSF), urine, and any specific lesions often identify the infecting organism.

TREATMENT

How Is Sepsis Managed?

Management of septic patients requires immediate, aggressive fluid resuscitation, intensive care support, and prompt empirical antimicrobial therapy with a third-generation cephalosporin such as ceftriaxone with or without vancomycin. Specific antimicrobial therapy is dependent on identification of the offending agent.

Can Sepsis Be Prevented?

National immunization campaigns have made *Haemophilus influenzae* type b, once a common cause of childhood sepsis, exceedingly rare. The current 7-valent conjugate-pneumococcal vaccine given to infants has reduced the incidence of invasive *S. pneumoniae* disease in all populations. The conjugate-meningococcal vaccine, which has been highly effective in preventing meningococcal disease in English children, was approved in 2005 for universal administration to American preteens and adolescents. Close contacts of patients with meningococcal disease should be offered prophylactic treatment with rifampin, ciprofloxacin, or ceftriaxone to minimize their risk of invasive disease.

MENINGITIS

ETIOLOGY

What Causes Meningitis?

Meningitis is inflammation of the fluid and the membranes that surround the central nervous system and is caused by many different organisms. Bacterial infections are less common than viral, but can lead to serious acute and chronic complications. The most common organisms that cause bacterial meningitis outside the newborn period are *S. pneumoniae* and *N. meningitidis*. Enteroviruses are the most common viruses that cause meningitis, most often in late summer and early fall epidemics. Although children can appear quite ill, they recover very quickly and generally suffer no permanent sequelae.

EVALUATION

How Does Meningitis Present?

Younger patients with meningitis may present with fever, irritability or lethargy, poor feeding, vomiting, and a bulging fontanelle. Signs of meningismus, such as nuchal rigidity and a positive Kernig's or Brudzinski's sign, may be absent in children younger than 18 months. Older children may present with fever, decreased level of consciousness, headache, vomiting, nuchal rigidity, and positive tests for meningismus. Seizures may occur in 20% to 30% of patients.

What Tests Help with the Diagnosis?

The diagnosis of meningitis is confirmed by analysis of CSF obtained by lumbar puncture. More than 95% of patients with meningitis will have an elevated number of leukocytes in the CSF at the time of presentation. Distinguishing viral from bacterial meningitis may be difficult because of a considerable overlap in initial CSF findings. Generally, patients with bacterial disease have a low glucose and high protein level in the CSF and more than 50% of the leukocytes are polymorphonucleocytes. Blood and CSF cultures will confirm the etiology of the meningitis. Untreated patients who have signs and symptoms of meningitis and CSF pleocytosis but grow no microorganisms from CSF culture most often have viral meningitis. Some institutions will use polymerase chain reaction (PCR) technology on CSF specimens to rapidly confirm the diagnosis of enteroviral meningitis. Viral culture can also confirm the diagnosis.

TREATMENT

How Is Meningitis Treated?

Initial, empirical antimicrobial therapy is directed at the usual causative organisms, including penicillin-resistant *S. pneumoniae*. Empirical treatment of suspected pyogenic meningitis includes ceftriaxone (or cefotaxime) and vancomycin in children older than 28 days unless meningococcal disease is confirmed. Both antibiotics are continued until the microbiology laboratory verifies that the pneumococcal isolate is susceptible to penicillin or ceftriaxone, at which time vancomycin can be discontinued. Concomitant use of corticosteroids is controversial. Corticosteroid administration before systemic antibiotics may decrease the likelihood of sensorineural hearing loss. Serum sodium and intravascular volume status need to be monitored: patients with pyogenic meningitis are at risk for developing the syndrome of inappropriate antidiuretic hormone secretion, and they may also be volume depleted because of poor feeding or emesis.

What Is the Prognosis for a Patient with Meningitis?

Prognosis is dependent on the age of the child, the infecting organism, the duration of illness before initiation of appropriate care, and the sophistication of the medical support team. Pyogenic meningitis results in the death of 1% to 8% of patients. Neurologic complications such as developmental delay, seizures, and hearing loss may occur in up to one-third of patients. Of these, hearing loss is the most common complication and occurs in approximately 30% of patients with *S. pneumoniae* meningitis and in 5% to 10% of patients following *N. meningitidis* meningitis.

ENCEPHALITIS

ETIOLOGY

What Causes Encephalitis?

Encephalitis is inflammation of the cerebellar or cerebral tissue rather than just the membranes or fluid surrounding them, as occurs with meningitis. The agents that cause encephalitis are usually viral. The most important of these is herpes simplex virus (HSV). Many viruses may cause mild to moderate meningoencephalitis, but HSV is associated with severe disease that can potentially be treated.

EVALUATION

What Findings Should Make Me Suspect Encephalitis?

Patients with encephalitis commonly present with altered mental status. Patients of all ages may have fever, irritability, lethargy, myalgias, nausea, vomiting, and seizures. Some neonates may have typical HSV cutaneous vesicular eruptions. In older children, headache and depressed levels of consciousness are common symptoms.

What Are the Laboratory Tests to Order?

The diagnosis of encephalitis is usually confirmed by analysis of CSF obtained by lumbar puncture. Most patients will demonstrate a lymphocytic CSF pleocytosis and mild elevations of CSF protein. In HSV encephalitis, RBCs may become more prominent in the CSF as the disease progresses. PCR identifies the virus in the CSF of more than 90% of patients with HSV encephalitis. Viral cultures, on the other hand, identify HSV in about 50% of neonates but only 5% of older children. In HSV encephalitis, specific temporal lobe findings may be seen on computed tomography (CT) scan, magnetic resonance imaging (MRI), and electroencephalogram (EEG).

TREATMENT

Can Encephalitis Be Treated?

HSV is the only cause of encephalitis that has a specific treatment: High-dose intravenous acyclovir plus supportive care such as airway management, seizure control, and circulatory support. Although acyclovir has dramatically decreased the mortality associated with HSV encephalitis, even with therapy, many patients suffer significant neurologic sequelae.

NONEMERGENT INFECTIOUS DISEASES

SINUSITIS

ETIOLOGY

What Causes Sinusitis?

The pathophysiology, bacteriology, and treatment of acute bacterial sinusitis are similar to those of acute otitis media. Obstruction of the ostiomeatal complex or impairment of sinus mucociliary function predisposes to sinusitis. Viral illness, allergies, and exposure to smoke are frequent precipitating events. The natural history of sinusitis is not well known. Viral rhinosinusitis always accompanies viral rhinitis, and some patients develop acute bacterial infection. Some may go on to develop chronic bacterial sinusitis. The most common organisms isolated from patients with acute bacterial sinusitis include *S. pneumoniae,* nontypable *H. influenzae,* and *Moraxella catarrhalis.* In suspected chronic sinusitis, *Staphylococcus aureus* and anaerobes may play a role.

EVALUATION

How Do I Determine If a Child Has Sinusitis?

Distinguishing children with viral rhinosinusitis from those with acute bacterial sinusitis is difficult. "Classic" features of acute bacterial sinusitis, such as high fever, facial pain and tenderness, and facial edema, particularly eye swelling, are found in adults and may occur in adolescents, but they are infrequently identified in younger children. Sinusitis is usually suspected in young children because of persistent (> 10 days) upper respiratory tract symptoms such as rhinorrhea and cough. The cough is present both night and day but is often worse in the evening while the patient is supine. The diagnosis is largely clinical. Sinus x-rays and CT scans do not reliably distinguish between viral and bacterial disease.

TREATMENT

Should Sinusitis Be Treated with Antibiotics?

The treatment of sinusitis is controversial. The few randomized trials of antibiotic treatment in pediatric patients have produced conflicting results. All agree that patients with fever, facial pain and tenderness, or eye swelling should be treated with antibiotics. Patients with persistent nasal discharge and cough may also benefit from antimicrobial therapy. Antibiotic treatment should be directed at the most common organisms, including penicillin-resistant *S. pneumoniae*. Other measures that may help include nasal irrigation with normal saline, warm mist, and, in severe cases, nasal sympathomimetics. Nasal sympathomimetics such as oxymetazoline must be used very judiciously because use for more than 3 days is associated with significant complications.

EYE INFECTIONS

ETIOLOGY

What Causes Red Eyes?

Conjunctivitis is inflammation of the membrane that covers the eye and the tarsal lid surface. Allergies, foreign bodies, anatomic obstruction, systemic reactions, viruses, and bacteria all can cause conjunctivitis. Many viruses can cause conjunctivitis, including enteroviruses and adenovirus. Pharyngoconjunctival fever is an especially contagious form of adenoviral infection. The most common causes of bacterial conjunctivitis outside of the neonatal age groups are gram-positive cocci such as *S. aureus*, streptococci, and nontypable *H. influenzae*. Infants younger than 2 months may develop *Chlamydia trachomatis* conjunctivitis acquired from passage through an infected maternal cervix. Scleral injection without infection is a characteristic finding in Kawasaki disease. Distinguishing among the many causes of conjunctivitis is difficult. Eye discharge *without* conjunctival erythema is common in infants who have lacrimal duct obstruction and does not necessarily indicate the presence of conjunctivitis.

EVALUATION

How Do I Identify the Cause of Conjunctivitis?

Conjunctivitis should be diagnosed only when there is inflammation of the conjunctival tissues. An eye discharge without inflammation is not conjunctivitis. Eye inflammation exists on a spectrum ranging from mild redness with prominent conjunctival vessels, usually termed *injection,* to severe, prominent, confluent erythema, usually labeled with the term *inflammation*. Children with allergic conjunctivitis usually complain of pruritus. Examination of the tarsal conjunctivae may reveal cobblestoning. Children with a foreign body in the eye usually note the sudden onset of local irritation. Patients with systemic reactions or a systemic disease such as measles or Kawasaki disease have other symptoms and signs, including fever.

How Do I Distinguish Viral from Bacterial Conjunctivitis?

Distinguishing viral from bacterial conjunctivitis remains difficult, because considerable overlap in clinical findings exists. Viral conjunctivitis is usually associated with mild unilateral or bilateral scleral injection and clear, nonpurulent eye discharge. The discharge may lead to eyelid matting that is most noticeable on awakening. Patients with bacterial conjunctivitis may have unilateral or bilateral conjunctival injection with purulent, persistent eye discharge. Fever, prominent swelling, and erythema of the eyelids are uncommon with uncomplicated conjunctivitis. The presence of these findings should prompt an investigation for more invasive infections such as orbital cellulitis.

The occurrence of conjunctivitis along with fever, headache, and sore throat suggests the syndrome of pharyngoconjunctival fever caused by adenovirus. This is an important diagnosis to make because the infection is highly contagious and does not respond to antibiotic treatment. *C. trachomatis* infection is usually characterized by secretions that range from thin to purulent and should be suspected in infants younger than 2 months with conjunctivitis. *C. trachomatis* may be diagnosed by a rapid antigen test, Giemsa stain, or culture of conjunctival scrapings.

What if There Is a Discharge, But the Eye Is Not Red?

A discharge from the eyes without erythema of the sclera or conjunctiva should suggest nasolacrimal duct obstruction. When the duct is blocked, infants and toddlers usually have increased tearing (a "tear lake"). When the water component of the tears evaporates, the mineral and mucus components remain to cause a crusty, mucoid discharge. Nasolacrimal duct obstruction may be congenital, and it also occurs as a frequent accompaniment of upper respiratory infections. In this latter instance, mucosal edema obstructs the intranasal opening of the duct. The eye discharge does not represent conjunctival infection. Secondary infection occurs commonly, but conjunctival erythema will accompany the eye discharge.

TREATMENT

How Should Conjunctivitis Be Treated?

Both bacterial and viral conjunctivitis resolve spontaneously. Topical antibiotics, however, hasten the resolution of bacterial conjunctivitis. Infants with *C. trachomatis* infection should be treated with oral macrolide antibiotics to treat the conjunctivitis and to prevent the development of pulmonary infection. An association has been reported between oral erythromycin and the development of hypertrophic pyloric stenosis. When children younger than 6 weeks are treated with macrolides, they should be followed for this potential complication. Mothers of infants with confirmed *C. trachomatis* should be treated for *Chlamydia* cervicitis. Antibiotic treatment is not needed in nasolacrimal duct obstruction unless complicated by secondary bacterial infection; warm, moist compresses can alleviate the crusting.

ORBITAL CELLULITIS

ETIOLOGY

What Is Orbital Cellulitis?

Orbital cellulitis is vision-threatening infection of the eye and the surrounding structures, including the orbital contents, that must be distinguished from preseptal cellulitis, which is inflammation of the tissues anterior to the orbital septum. Orbital cellulitis is a bacterial infection that develops most often as a complication and extension of paranasal sinusitis. Orbital cellulitis progresses through several stages from periostitis (stage 1) to frank orbital abscess (stage 4). Progression of the disease leads to increasing amounts of edema and purulent material in the orbit. The bacteria most often implicated include *S. aureus, S. pneumoniae* and other streptococcal species, and nontypable *H. influenzae.*

EVALUATION

How Is the Diagnosis Made?

Children with orbital cellulitis have fever, eye pain, and a red, swollen eye. Physical examination shows periorbital erythema, significant eyelid edema, proptosis, ophthalmoplegia, and chemosis. The diagnosis is made clinically. CT scan of the orbits and sinuses confirms the diagnosis and the extent of the orbital involvement.

TREATMENT

What Treatment Is Necessary?

Immediate institution of parenteral antimicrobial therapy is critical. Failure to act promptly may result in loss of vision. Empirical therapy usually includes intravenous second- or third-generation cephalosporins. Some practitioners begin vancomycin as well. Surgical decompression may be necessary in those patients who do not respond to antibiotics rapidly or who have vision loss.

TUBERCULOSIS

ETIOLOGY

What Is Tuberculosis?

Tuberculosis is infection caused by *Mycobacterium tuberculosis.* The nomenclature of tuberculosis is confusing, because patients may have exposure, infection, or disease. Exposure to tuberculosis means that a patient has been exposed to an individual who has active pulmonary or laryngeal tuberculosis. Tuberculosis infection means that an individual not only has been exposed but also has become infected with *M. tuberculosis.* Infection without evidence of disease is called "latent" tuberculosis. Patients with either signs and symptoms of tuberculosis or an abnormal chest radiograph in the appropriate epidemiologic setting have "active tuberculosis." Most teens and adults with active tuberculosis have reactivated previously latent infection.

Why Is Tuberculosis a Problem in the United States?

Tuberculosis is uncommon in native-born U.S. children. Most children in the United States with tuberculosis are either immigrants from countries where tuberculosis is endemic or have had exposure to an adult from a foreign country with active tuberculosis. Immigrant children who have received bacille Calmette-Guérin (BCG) vaccine in infancy may still develop tuberculosis because the vaccine does not prevent infection with the organism. Most children with tuberculosis in the United States have latent disease, which has approximately a 10% lifetime risk of becoming reactivated to tuberculosis disease (active tuberculosis). The risk that a child with active tuberculosis will develop disseminated disease is high in children younger than 4 years, particularly infants. Morbidity and mortality are particularly high when active tuberculosis occurs in the first year of life.

EVALUATION

What Are the Clinical Findings of Tuberculosis?

Patients with latent tuberculosis infection are by definition asymptomatic. Patients with active tuberculosis may be asymptomatic or have fever, weight loss, chills, cough, and crackles on lung examination. Chest radiographs in primary tuberculosis demonstrate infiltrates (usually in the right upper lobe), hilar adenopathy, or pleural effusions. Those patients with reactivation, or adult-style disease, may have upper lobe cavities. The diagnosis of tuberculosis is suggested by a combination of epidemiologic investigation, clinical and radiographic findings, and purified protein derivative (PPD) skin testing. Culture of *M. tuberculosis* or a positive RNA hybridization test from sputum or a gastric aspirate confirms the diagnosis.

Who Should Undergo Purified Protein Derivative Testing?

A PPD is an intraepidermal injection of mycobacterial antigens that measures lymphocyte responsiveness to the antigens. The indications for PPD testing and interpretation of test results are highly dependent on the prevalence of tuberculosis in the tested population. The PPD is no longer recommended as a general screening test. "Targeted" testing relies on identification of high-risk individuals, such as those with documented exposure to an adult with active disease or immigrants from countries with a high prevalence of tuberculosis.

How Do I Interpret a Purified Protein Derivative Test?

The size of the ***induration at the PPD site,*** not the erythema, is measured 48 to 72 hours following PPD placement. Interpreting a PPD reaction is difficult and dependent on the likelihood of exposure. Positive reactions indicate infection. Negative reactions do not necessarily exclude tuberculosis infection. Induration $\geq$ 5 mm is considered positive in immunocompromised patients, in those living with an adult with active disease, or in those with clinical findings consistent with tuberculosis. Induration $\geq$ 10 mm is considered positive for children younger than 4 years, for immigrants from high-prevalence areas, for patients with chronic underlying medical conditions, and for those with repetitive exposure to a high-risk population (e.g., a child who visits an endemic country). In all other children older than 4 years, $\geq$ 15 mm of induration is considered positive.

What Tests Should I Order If the Purified Protein Derivative Test Is Positive?

A patient with a positive tuberculin skin test should have a thorough physical examination and posteroanterior and lateral chest radiographs. If both the radiographs and the physical examination are normal, the child has latent tuberculosis. The public health department should be notified because children often serve as sentinels of adult disease. The child should be treated with isoniazid for 9 months. If the child has an abnormal radiograph or a physical examination consistent with possible active tuberculosis, further evaluation will be needed. An attempt to isolate the organism from the patient or the adult index case should be made. In young children with abnormal chest radiographs, consecutive early morning gastric aspirates are collected. In older children (generally older than 10 years), sputum samples are collected. Mycobacteria can be detected by acid-fast staining techniques, nucleic acid hybridization, and culture. Recovery of the organism from the infected child or infecting adult is essential to guide therapy.

How Do I Interpret a Purified Protein Derivative Test If a Child Received Bacille Calmette-Guérin Vaccine in Infancy?

Tuberculin skin testing should be interpreted without regard to prior receipt of the BCG vaccine.

TREATMENT

How Is Tuberculosis Treated?

Patients with latent infection are treated with either daily or twice-weekly isoniazid for 9 months to decrease the patient's lifetime risk of developing active tuberculosis. Treatment of active tuberculosis depends on the susceptibility of the organism but always includes at least two antimycobacterial drugs to which the organism is susceptible.

MUSCULOSKELETAL INFECTIONS

ETIOLOGY

What Are the Causes of Musculoskeletal Infections?

Any child who presents with localized bony pain or swelling may have a musculoskeletal infection, either of a joint (septic arthritis) or of the bone itself (osteomyelitis). The principal differential diagnosis includes bone tumors or fracture. The principle etiologic agents of both septic arthritis and osteomyelitis are *S. aureus* and streptococcal species. Usually, the infection results from hematogenous seeding, although occasionally the infection is because of a penetrating injury or extension from a contiguous source.

EVALUATION

What Will I Find If a Child Has Septic Arthritis?

Children with septic arthritis have fever and pain, particularly when trying to move the joint, or may refuse to use the involved joint. Physical findings may include erythema and warmth of the affected joint and pain with motion at the joint. Plain radiographs are useful only to exclude fracture. An ultrasound or CT scan can confirm a joint effusion. ^{99}Tc radioisotope scan can show uptake at sites of inflammation or infection and is most useful in young patients who present with limp and poorly localized pain. White blood cell (WBC) count may be elevated or normal. The same is true for the erythrocyte sedimentation rate (ESR). More than 90% of children with osteoarticular infection will have elevated C-reactive protein at the time of presentation. The single best test for diagnosis is aspiration of the affected joint. Joint fluid analysis in patients with pyogenic disease usually demonstrates more than 50,000 leukocytes/ml with a polymorphonuclear predominance. Gram staining and culture can confirm the etiologic agent.

What Other Joint Problems Should I Consider?

Children with symptoms referable to a joint but whose physical examination does not demonstrate the findings consistent with bacterial infection most likely have either a viral infection or toxic synovitis, which is thought to represent a reaction to a concurrent or previous viral infection. Reactive arthritis may follow a variety of viral and bacterial diseases. A special circumstance is the arthritis of Lyme disease. Late-stage *Borrelia burgdorferi* infection can present with a migratory, monoarticular arthritis. Diagnosis of Lyme disease depends on establishing a true epidemiologic exposure to the organism, specific *B. burgdorferi* serologic tests, and a typical clinical history.

How Does Osteomyelitis Present?

Children with osteomyelitis have bone pain. Young children may have only fever and limp, refusal to walk, or irritability. The physical findings depend on the age of the patient and the extent of the disease. Osteomyelitis begins as metaphyseal abscess. At this stage, patients may only have pain with deep palpation. As the disease extends beyond the cortex and periosteum, findings become more apparent and may include erythema, warmth, and tenderness at the site. Plain films are useful to exclude fracture or tumor. Osteomyelitis does not lead to bony changes seen on plain films unless the infection has been present for more than 10 days. CT and MRI scans can show characteristic bony involvement. ^{99}Tc scans localize infection in more than 90% of patients outside the neonatal age group. The white blood cell count and the ESR may be normal or minimally elevated. The C-reactive protein is elevated in more than 95% of patients at the time of presentation, but an etiologic agent is recovered from blood or bone in only 50% to 80% of patients.

TREATMENT

What Are the Treatment Options?

Early treatment, particularly of septic arthritis, is imperative because delay can lead to destruction of the articular surfaces of the joint. Treatment consists of antibiotics directed at staphylococcal and streptococcal species initially given intravenously and then orally. Correct diagnosis is important because unrecognized or inadequately treated osteoarticular infection can lead to chronic dysfunction or infection.

KEY POINTS

- Lethargy, irritability, stridor, and increased work of breathing suggest the possibility of an infectious disease emergency.
- Sepsis is a systemic inflammatory response with hypotension.
- Bacterial meningitis causes hearing loss and other neurologic sequelae in survivors.
- Tuberculosis testing must be done for immigrants from countries with high rates of endemic disease.

Case 64-1

A 3-month-old boy is brought to the physician because of persistent fever, decreased oral intake, and decreased activity for the past 48 hours. He has not had nasal discharge, cough, diarrhea, or rashes. He received his first set of immunizations 1 month earlier. His temperature is 39.5° C, heart rate 190 beats/min, and respirations 28 breaths/min. He is irritable and difficult to console. He will not smile at either his mother or you. Aside from his irritability, his examination does not identify a focus of infection.

A. What is your initial differential diagnosis in this patient?
B. What are the findings that most concern you? Based on the history and examination, can you narrow the differential diagnosis?
C. What would be the approach to the management of this child?
D. If you were to begin antibiotics, which organisms would you be most concerned about?

Case 64-2

A previously healthy 10-year-old boy presents with 2 weeks of persistent, thick nasal discharge and a hacking cough. The cough is worse in the evening but is also present during the day. He has not had fevers but feels a little tired. He appears nontoxic. His temperature is 37.5° C, heart rate 88 beats/min, and respiratory rate 18 breaths/min. He has mild tenderness over the ethmoid and maxillary sinuses with deep, firm palpation. The rest of the examination demonstrates nasal congestion, mouth breathing, injected pharyngeal mucosa, and mucopurulent material draining down the posterior pharynx.

A. What is the differential diagnosis?
B. What is the most likely explanation for this patient's findings?
C. How would you manage this patient?
D. What possible complications can develop from untreated sinusitis?

Case 64-3

A 4-week-old girl is brought to the physician because of persistent bilateral eye discharge for the past 3 days. Otherwise, she has been feeding well and has been afebrile. She appears well. Her temperature is 37° C, heart rate is 140 beats/min, and respiratory rate is 30 breaths/min. She has very mild scleral and tarsal plate injection and a white-yellow purulent discharge from both eyes, particularly at the corners. The rest of the examination is unremarkable.

A. What is the most likely diagnosis in this patient?
B. How would you confirm a diagnosis?
C. Would antimicrobial therapy be important in this patient? Why or why not?

Case 64-4

A mother brings a 2-year-old boy to the physician for a routine health supervision visit. Both were born and raised in Zaire and arrived in the United States 2 months earlier. No records are available, but the mother recalls no tuberculosis testing for either herself or her son. The 2-year-old has been healthy and has no problems. Physical examination reveals a healthy-appearing boy. His examination is unremarkable except that he has a small scar on the left deltoid that looks like a BCG scar.

A. Should this boy be tested for tuberculosis?
B. Would the BCG immunization prevent this child from becoming infected with *M. tuberculosis*?
C. How would you interpret the PPD?
D. If the PPD is positive, what recommendations would you make for evaluation and management?

Case 64-5

A 10-year-old boy has complained of left leg pain for the past 7 days, and developed low-grade fevers 2 days ago. He fell 2 weeks ago while riding his bike but recalls no significant injury at the time. He appears tired but not toxic. His temperature is 38° C, pulse is 96 beats/min, and respiratory rate is

18 breaths/min. He has point tenderness over the distal anteromedial aspect of the left femur. He has no erythema or warmth over the site and has complete, painless range of motion of the left knee.

A. What is the differential diagnosis in this patient?
B. What are the most appropriate steps to make a correct diagnosis in this patient?

Case Answers

64-1.A. *Learning objective:* **Identify the most likely infections in a febrile, irritable infant.** A febrile, irritable infant could have any number of processes, including a viral infection such as enteroviral meningoencephalitis, but of most concern would be possible meningitis, sepsis, or urinary tract infection. Other bacterial infections that must be considered include septic arthritis and osteomyelitis.

64-1 B. *Learning objective:* **Use observation and physical examination to identify a toxic-appearing infant.** The differential diagnosis cannot be narrowed much at this point. Any infant that cannot be consoled or has a heart rate greater than 180 beats/min is seriously ill. Even though he has no evidence of meningismus, this infant is at risk for having meningitis. Sepsis and urinary tract infection are also possible. Pneumonia is possible although less likely given the absence of lung findings or tachypnea. Osteomyelitis or arthritis seem unlikely as they usually lead to extremity findings in children this age.

64-1 C. *Learning objective:* **Discuss the evaluation and initial management of the toxic-appearing infant.** Because this young infant appears toxic, the diagnostic approach should include a blood culture, a urine culture, and a lumbar puncture. A complete blood count with differential is often obtained but is not diagnostic. The child will need intravenous access for fluid resuscitation and antimicrobial therapy.

64-1 D. *Learning objective:* **Discuss treatment of the toxic-appearing infant.** Antibiotics are directed at the most likely organisms based on the presumed site of infection. The most common organisms causing sepsis or meningitis in a young infant are *S. pneumoniae* and *Neisseria meningitidis*. Exposure to *S. pneumoniae* and risk of infection are decreasing as immunization with the conjugate vaccine becomes more widespread. Group B streptococcus infections can occur in children this old but are more common in children younger than 3 months. Although he has had only one immunization against *Haemophilus influenzae* type b, herd immunity makes this infection very rare in the United States. Coliform organisms may cause urosepsis.

64-2 A. *Learning objective:* **Discuss the differential diagnosis for persistent nasal discharge.** The differential diagnosis includes bacterial sinusitis and viral rhinosinusitis. Allergic disease seems less likely without sneezing or pruritus.

64-2 B. *Learning objective:* **List the diagnostic criteria for sinusitis.** This patient meets the criteria proposed by the American Academy of Pediatrics for acute sinusitis. These include all of the findings common in adults and adolescents (fever, pain, swelling) but do not demand that they all be present. Persistent purulent nasal discharge with cough for more than 10 days are key findings in young children. The diagnosis is clinical: radiographs and computed tomography are not recommended.

64-2 C. *Learning objective:* **Discuss the management of acute bacterial sinusitis.** Antibiotics are often prescribed when acute bacterial sinusitis is suspected. Antibiotics should be directed at the most common organisms *(S. pneumoniae, H. influenzae, Moraxella catarrhalis).* Reasonable choices include amoxicillin or amoxicillin-clavulanate. Other treatment modalities could include saline washes, humidified air, and oral (or rarely topical) sympathomimetics.

64-2 D. *Learning objective:* **Identify orbital cellulitis in a febrile patient.** Orbital cellulitis can result from extension of bacterial sinusitis into the orbital space. The patient would likely be febrile, have periorbital swelling and ophthalmoplegia, and have restricted extraocular movements on the affected side.

64-3 A. *Learning objective:* **List the common causes of conjunctivitis, recognizing how the differential diagnosis is affected by the patient's age and physical findings.** This is a challenging case. A 4-week-old infant with bilateral conjunctivitis could have bacterial or viral infection, nasolacrimal duct obstruction, or, possibly, *Chlamydia trachomatis* infection. The scleral and tarsal injection suggests that some infectious or inflammatory process is occurring, which makes nasolacrimal duct obstruction less likely. Most patients with *C. trachomatis* infection present at 5 to 14 days of life, making this patient somewhat old to have this infection.

64-3 B. *Learning objective:* **Select appropriate diagnostic tests to diagnose the cause of conjunctivitis.** Confirmation of infection is not easy. Surface cultures of eyes of healthy children can grow a variety of bacterial species, although culture of a pathogen usually is interpreted as suggestive of bacterial infection. *C. trachomatis* is detected by rapid antigen testing, Giemsa staining, or culture of a conjunctival scraping.

64-3 C. *Learning objective:* **Discuss treatment options for the various causes of conjunctivitis.** Children with typical bacterial conjunctivitis who are treated with antibiotics improve more rapidly than those children not given antibiotics, but by day 7, little difference between the two groups exists. Treatment reduces the chance that the infection will be spread to caregivers and family members. Infants with *C. trachomatis* conjunctivitis become infected during birth from exposure to an infected cervix. They should be treated with systemic macrolide antibiotics, because they are at risk of developing chlamydial pneumonia. Infants given macrolides should be monitored for the development of hypertrophic pyloric stenosis.

64-4 A. *Learning objective:* **Discuss the epidemiology of tuberculosis in the United States and recognize which patients are at highest risk.** Yes, this child should be tested with a Mantoux skin test (PPD) for *Mycobacterium tuberculosis* infection because he is from a high-risk group (emigrating from a country with a high tuberculosis infection rate). The U.S. policy is to test such patients and offer "chemoprophylaxis" to those who test positive to reduce the lifetime risk of developing *M. tuberculosis* disease.

64-4 B. *Learning objective:* **Discuss the reason that BCG immunization is administered in countries with high tuberculosis infection rates.** BCG does not prevent infection with *M. tuberculosis.* Rather, it prevents disseminated tuberculosis during infancy, which has an extremely high mortality rate.

64-4 C. *Learning objective:* **Interpret the results of a Mantoux test (PPD).** Because the patient is from a high-risk population, a PPD reaction $\geq$ 10 mm of induration is considered positive. BCG vaccination does not affect the interpretation of the PPD.

64-4 D. *Learning objective:* **Develop a management plan for a patient with a positive PPD.** Any patient with a positive PPD should have a chest radiograph. If the radiograph is negative, the boy is assumed to have latent tuberculosis and should be treated with isoniazid, according to the recommendations of the state health department. If the chest radiograph is positive, the patient has active tuberculosis. The source of infection should be sought, cultures and other tests should be done to isolate the organism, and treatment with a multidrug antibiotic regimen should be started. Family members should also be tested for tuberculosis. Whether latent or active, tuberculosis must be reported to the state health department.

64-5 A. *Learning objective:* **Discuss the differential diagnosis of bony pain.** Patients with persistent bony pain usually have a fracture, malignancy, or an infection. Other processes such as bone cysts are possible. In this case, fracture seems unlikely given the absence of significant trauma. Septic arthritis is unlikely because the knee has full range of motion without pain or swelling. The leg pain, the recent development of fever, and the point tenderness raise suspicion of osteomyelitis. A malignancy such as a bone tumor or leukemia is still a possibility.

64-5 B. *Learning objective:* **Identify the cause of bone pain, including osteomyelitis, using imaging and laboratory tests.** Most physicians will start with a radiograph to help rule out a fracture or a tumor. A normal radiograph does not definitively exclude tumor but makes it less likely. A normal radiograph also does not exclude infection. A complete blood count helps exclude leukemia but, again, does not confirm or disprove infection. A positive C-reactive protein confirms inflammation but is not specific for bone infection. A normal C-reactive protein makes osteomyelitis very unlikely. A bone scan can help localize the site of rapid bone turnover and inflammation. The most important diagnostic test is culture of a specimen obtained by bone aspirate or biopsy. Only growth of bacteria from such a culture absolutely confirms osteoarticular infection.

BIBLIOGRAPHY

Meningitis

Chavez-Bueno S, McCracken GH Jr: Bacterial meningitis in children, *Pediatr Clin North Am* 52:795, 2005.

Encephalitis

Rajnik M, Ottolini MG: Serious infections of the central nervous system: encephalitis, meningitis, and brain abscess, *Adolesc Med* 11:401, 2000.

Von Rosenstiel N, von Rosenstiel I, Adam D: Management of sepsis and septic shock in infants and children, *Paediatr Drugs* 3:9, 2001.

Whitley RJ, Kimberlin DW: Herpes simplex encephalitis: children and adolescents, *Semin Pediatr Infect Dis* 16:17, 2005.

Sinusitis

American Academy of Pediatrics, Subcommittee on Management of Sinusitis and Committee on Quality Improvement: Clinical practice guideline: management of sinusitis, *Pediatrics* 108:798, 2001.

Brooks I et al: Medical management of acute bacterial sinusitis: recommendations of a clinical advisory committee on pediatric and adult sinusitis, *Ann Otol Rhinol Laryngol Suppl* 182:2, 2000.

Ramadan HH: Pediatric sinusitis: update, *J Otolaryngol* 34 (suppl 1):S14, 2005.

Eye Infections

Smith J: Bacterial conjunctivitis, *Clin Evid* 12:926, 2004.

Orbital Infection

Mawn LA, Jordan DR, Donahue SP: Preseptal and orbital cellulitis, *Ophthalmol Clin North Am* 13:633, 2000.

Wald ER: Periorbital and orbital infections, *Pediatr Rev* 25:312, 2004.

Tuberculosis

Pickering LK, editor: *2000 Red book: report of the Committee on Infectious Diseases*, ed 25, Elk Grove Village, IL, 2000, American Academy of Pediatrics, pp 593-613.

Smith KC: Tuberculosis in children, *Curr Probl Pediatr* 31:1, 2001.

Musculoskeletal Infections

Sonnen GM, Henry NK: Pediatric bone and joint infections: diagnosis and antimicrobial management, *Pediatr Clin North Am* 43:933, 1996.

Wall EJ: Childhood osteomyelitis and septic arthritis, *Curr Opin Pediatr* 10:73, 1998.

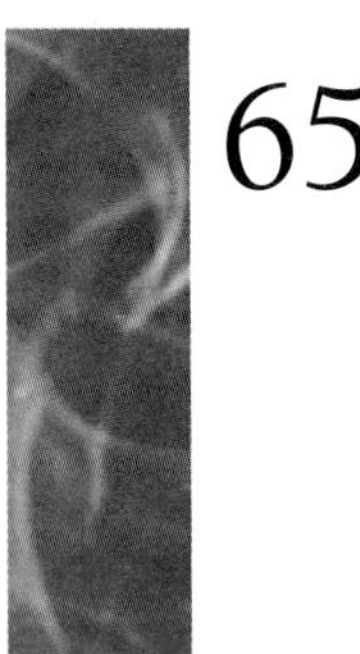

65 Nephrology

LAVJAY BUTANI and BRUCE Z. MORGENSTERN

ACUTE RENAL FAILURE

ETIOLOGY

What Is Acute Renal Failure?

Acute renal failure (ARF) refers to sudden deterioration in renal function. ARF can result from multiple anatomic problems, including acute or subacute obstruction of arteries, veins, ureters, bladder, or urethra. An alternative pathophysiologic approach categorizes ARF as caused by decreased renal perfusion, ischemic or toxic cell injury, or intrinsic renal disease. When a child has ARF with oliguria, causes can be broadly categorized:

- *Prerenal conditions* impair renal perfusion.
- *Intrinsic renal* diseases affect glomeruli, tubulointerstitium, or microvasculature.
- *Postrenal* states cause obstruction beyond the renal parenchyma.

Table 65-1 has examples of oliguric ARF in each category. Remember that not all ARF is associated with oliguria.

EVALUATION

How Can I Tell If a Patient Has Acute Renal Failure?

Renal function is decreased in ARF. Glomerular filtration rate (GFR) is the standard measure of renal function and should be 100 ± 20 ml/min/1.73 m^2 body surface area (BSA) for children older than 1 year. The most accurate measure of GFR is the clearance of inulin or iothalamate, but this technique is time-consuming, invasive, and not readily available. Serum creatinine concentration is often used as a clinical marker of renal function, but it is too insensitive to identify the early stages of renal function deterioration. The commonly used assay has a wide coefficient of variation for the values found in infants and toddlers. Also, serum creatinine concentration changes during growth from

Table 65-1

Causes of Acute Renal Failure

Prerenal	Intrinsic Renal (Most Common Category in Children)	Postrenal
TBW depletion	Glomerulonephritis	Blood clots
Gastroenteritis	Tubulointerstitial disease	Bilateral stones
IV volume depletion	Acute tubular necrosis	Intraabdominal tumors (e.g., Burkitt's lymphoma)
Septic shock	Toxic (e.g., aminoglycosides)	Posterior urethral valves
Nephrotic syndrome	Ischemic (prolonged prerenal state)	
Mechanical failure of renal perfusion	Tubulointerstitial nephritis	
Congestive heart failure	Drug-induced (e.g., NSAIDs)	
Cardiac tamponade	Infectious (e.g., EBV)	
Critical coarctation of the aorta	Microvascular disease	
Renal artery thrombosis	Hemolytic-uremic syndrome	

EBV, Epstein-Barr virus; IV, intravascular; NSAIDs, nonsteroidal antiinflammatory drugs; TBW, total body water.

infancy through adolescence as muscle mass increases and is affected to some extent by dietary protein intake.

Can Renal Function Be Estimated Easily?

The most reliable, straightforward, and simple method to estimate renal function in children uses height and serum creatinine to calculate creatinine clearance with the formula in Table 65-2. Height serves as a surrogate of muscle mass. This approach should only be used when the patient is in a steady state with respect to renal function.

Table 65-2

Formula for Estimation of Glomerular Filtration Rate (GFR) in Children*

Age of Child	Mean Value of k
Low-birth-weight infant (< 1 year)	0.33
Full-term infant (< 1 year)	0.45
2–12 years	0.55
12–17 years (female)	0.55
12–17 years (male)	0.7

*GFR (ml/min/1.73 m^2) = [k × length or height (in cm)] ÷ serum creatinine (mg/dl).
From Schwartz GJ, Brion LP, Spitzer A: The use of plasma creatinine concentration for estimating glomerular filtration rate in infants, children, and adolescents, *Pediatr Clin North Am* 34:571, 1987.

How Might a Patient with Acute Renal Failure Present?

ARF commonly presents with oliguria, edema, hypertension, and fatigue or lethargy. Absence of hypertension may indicate low circulating volume, as in dehydration. ARF can occur with either normal or elevated urine output, the latter especially with tubulointerstitial disease. A patient with ARF might have only vague symptoms, so it is important to consider renal causes in the differential diagnosis of the symptom complex, to look for hypertension and edema, and to consider blood and urine tests. Lethargy and altered mental status can result from accumulation of "uremic" toxins. ARF can occasionally occur in a completely asymptomatic patient. Table 65-3 lists causes, presenting features, and evaluation of ARF.

What Is Oliguria?

Oliguria means that urine output is below age-expected limits. For premature infants, oliguria is defined as urine output less than 2 ml/kg/hr. Full-term infants from birth up to 2 to 3 months of age are oliguric when urine output is less than 1 ml/kg/hr. For all others, oliguria is present when urine output is less than 0.5 ml/kg/hr.

What Is Anuria?

Anuria is the absence of urine output. It indicates either that the kidneys are not producing urine or that urine flow is completely obstructed. To determine the cause of anuria, insert a urinary catheter to determine whether the bladder is empty and obtain a renal ultrasound to look for dilatation of the collecting system and ureters.

How Can I Determine the Cause of Acute Renal Failure?

History, physical examination, and the initial laboratory tests used to diagnose the cause of ARF are listed in Table 65-3. The *fractional excretion of sodium* (Fe_{Na}) is particularly useful to differentiate acute tubular necrosis from prerenal causes, especially when urine output is low. This distinction is important because prompt intervention may facilitate renal recovery when ARF results from a potentially reversible cause, such as volume depletion. Even patients with intrinsic or postrenal causes for decreased GFR will benefit from appropriate fluid and electrolyte therapy if volume-depleted.

When Is a Renal Biopsy Indicated?

A renal biopsy is not routinely performed in ARF. Some indications for a biopsy include rapidly progressive renal failure of unexplained etiology and certain suspected causes of glomerulonephritis (see "Glomerulonephritis").

What Are the Risks of Acute Renal Failure?

The complications of ARF arise from severe impairment of fluid excretion (hypertension and pulmonary edema) and solute clearance (hyperkalemia,

Table 65-3

Evaluation for Causes of Acute Renal Failure (ARF)

Causes of ARF	History and Physical Findings	Urinalysis	Fe_{Na}*	Other Laboratory Tests
Prerenal				
	History of blood loss or gastroenteritis Signs of dehydration	Increased specific gravity with a normal urinary sediment	< 0.5%	Nonspecific findings that may be seen with dehydration such as acidosis and an elevated BUN that return to normal after fluid therapy
Intrinsic Renal Diseases				
Glomerulonephritis	See "Glomerulonephritis" section in text	Active urine sediment	< 0.5%	See "Glomerulonephritis" section in text
Acute tubular necrosis	Prolonged prerenal state Nephrotoxic medication use (prescription or nonprescription)	Low specific gravity Granular or tubular casts	> 2%	
Tubulointerstitial nephritis	Fever and rash Medication use or viral prodrome	Eosinophils in urine White blood cell casts	Nondiagnostic	Eosinophilia
Microvascular (HUS)	Bloody diarrhea Pallor, bruising	Active urine sediment (blood, protein, red and white blood cells)	Nondiagnostic	Microangiopathic hemolytic anemia (schistocytes on peripheral smear) and thrombocytopenia Stool positive for *Escherichia coli* O 157:H7
Postrenal				
Renal calculi	Abdominal pain (colicky) Palpable abdominal mass	No cells on urinary sediment, otherwise nonspecific Occasional crystalluria	Nondiagnostic	Renal and bladder ultrasound to look for hydronephrosis and/or hydroureter

BUN, Blood urea nitrogen; Fe_{Na}, fractional excretion of sodium; HUS, hemolytic-uremic syndrome.

***Fe_{Na} = [(urine/serum) sodium ÷ (urine/serum) creatinine] × 100%.**

hyperphosphatemia, metabolic acidosis, "uremia" causing altered mental status, and accumulation of medication metabolites).

TREATMENT

How Do I Care for a Patient with Acute Renal Failure?

Management depends on the underlying cause. General measures include the following:

- Monitor blood pressure and manage hypertension
- Limit fluid intake, *except* in prerenal ARF
- Correct hyperkalemia with intravenous calcium, insulin and glucose, beta-adrenergic agonists, or oral potassium-binding resins
- Prevent further insult to the kidneys by minimizing exposure to nephrotoxic agents and modifying drug dosages for the level of renal function
- Optimize nutritional intake to minimize the hypercatabolic state often associated with ARF
- Implement acute dialysis when needed

CHRONIC KIDNEY DISEASE

ETIOLOGY

What Is Chronic Kidney Disease?

Chronic kidney disease (CKD) refers to impaired renal function, *irrespective of the GFR*, that persists for at least 3 months. The terms chronic renal insufficiency (CRI) and chronic renal failure (CRF) refer to the degree of GFR impairment and are no longer used. There are 5 stages of CKD based on the severity of renal impairment (Table 65-4). A patient does *not* need to have reduced GFR to be categorized as

Table 65-4

Classification of Chronic Kidney Disease (CKD)

Stage of CKD	Description
Stage I	Kidney damage with normal or even higher than normal GFR (> 90 ml/min/1.73 m^2 surface area) (e.g., patients with renal scarring/reflux nephropathy, or diabetic nephropathy)
Stage II	Mild impairment of renal function (GFR 60–89 ml/min/1.73 m^2 surface area)
Stage III	Moderate impairment of renal function (GFR 30–59 ml/min/1.73 m^2 surface area)
Stage IV	Severe impairment of renal function (GFR 15–29 ml/min/1.73 m^2 surface area)
Stage V	Kidney failure (GFR < 15 ml/min/1.73 m^2 surface area or patient on dialysis)

GFR, Glomerular filtration rate.

having CKD. A patient with stage I CKD has normal GFR with reduced renal mass, either acquired or congenital, and must be monitored for possible worsening of renal function. A patient with stage V CKD has end-stage renal disease (ESRD) and may need dialysis or renal transplantation. Loss of renal function causes impairment of other organ systems. Incidence of CKD and ESRD in children is less than 15 cases per million population in North America.

What Causes Chronic Kidney Disease in Children?

Almost 50% of all children with advanced CKD/ESRD have congenital anomalies such as hypo-dysplastic kidneys or obstructive uropathies. Other causes of CKD include renal scarring/reflux nephropathy (see "Urinary Tract Infection") and chronic glomerulonephritis (see "Glomerulonephritis").

EVALUATION

How Might a Child with Chronic Kidney Disease Present?

Congenital renal anomalies are often detected on routine prenatal ultrasound. Children with obstructive uropathies may have recurrent urinary tract infections. Failure to thrive occurs commonly in infants with CKD. Children with chronic glomerulonephritis may present with gross hematuria. A relatively asymptomatic child with CKD occasionally may be identified when short stature, urinary incontinence, hypertension, or proteinuria and hematuria are discovered. Sometimes CKD is diagnosed only when a child develops complications such as uremic encephalopathy, hypertensive crisis, or pulmonary edema.

What Is the Laboratory Evaluation for Suspected Chronic Kidney Disease?

The initial laboratory approach to CKD mirrors that for ARF (Table 65-3). Laboratory tests useful in the long-term management of children with CKD include serum electrolytes, blood urea nitrogen, serum creatinine, calcium and phosphorus, parathyroid hormone level, and the complete blood count (CBC). Other tests depend on the disease that caused the CKD.

How Can I Tell If Renal Failure Is Acute or Chronic?

Clues that a patient with renal failure has CKD include the following:

- Relatively few symptoms despite acidosis or azotemia
- Short stature or failure to thrive
- Severe normocytic, normochromic anemia
- Secondary hyperparathyroidism (from chronic hyperphosphatemia)
- Renal osteodystrophy (bone deformities from hyperparathyroidism and vitamin D abnormalities)
- Small kidneys on renal ultrasound

Does a Renal Biopsy Help with Diagnosis?

Renal biopsy is not often needed because history, physical examination, and laboratory tests usually lead to the diagnosis. When biopsy is done, findings suggestive of CKD include severe glomerulosclerosis, interstitial fibrosis, and tubular atrophy, especially if all 3 are present. Some patients with advanced CKD undergo renal biopsy to establish the etiology, if possible, because some acquired renal diseases recur in transplanted kidneys.

TREATMENT

How Do I Care for a Patient with Chronic Kidney Disease?

The care of a child with CKD is best performed at a tertiary care medical center with a multidisciplinary team that includes a pediatric nephrologist, a social worker, and a dietician. Management goals include efforts to do the following:

- Prevent or slow the decline in renal function, if possible
- Treat complications of renal failure, such as
  - Anemia, by using iron and erythropoietin therapy
  - Hyperparathyroidism, by limiting dietary phosphorus intake, using dietary phosphate binders, and prescribing vitamin D
- Prevent further insults to the kidneys by avoiding nephrotoxic medications and aggressively treating hypertension and proteinuria, if present
- Provide psychosocial and emotional support to the child and family
- Optimize nutrition
- Prepare the child for transplant or dialysis, if needed

GLOMERULONEPHRITIS

ETIOLOGY

What Is Acute Glomerulonephritis?

Glomerulonephritis (GN) is a syndrome of impaired renal function (elevated serum creatinine), some degree of oliguria, volume overload (edema, hypertension, and pulmonary vascular congestion), and hematuria of glomerular origin (see Chapter 52). It is caused by glomerular inflammation. In mild cases, hematuria may be the only sign of GN. When the onset is abrupt, GN is referred to as acute GN.

What Causes Acute Glomerulonephritis?

Causes of acute GN are listed in Table 65-5. Postinfectious GN is the most common form in children and occurs after infection by *Streptococcus pyogenes* (pharyngitis, or less commonly impetigo). Signs and symptoms of GN usually appear 10 to 14 days after the infection. The infection can sometimes be entirely asymptomatic. Postinfectious GN is mediated by an incompletely understood autoimmune process. In contrast, GN caused by IgA nephropathy ("Berger's disease") is exacerbated by infections, and symptoms appear *at the same time* as the intercurrent illness.

Table 65-5

Causes of Glomerulonephritis (GN) in Children

Primary or idiopathic
- Berger's disease (IgA nephropathy)
- Idiopathic membranoproliferative GN
- Idiopathic FSGS
- Idiopathic membranous nephropathy

Secondary
- Postinfectious GN
- Henoch-Schönlein purpura nephritis
- Secondary membranoproliferative GN
  - Hepatitis B or C
  - Bacterial endocarditis/shunt nephritis
- Systemic lupus erythematosus
- Hereditary nephritis (Alport syndrome)
- Antineutrophilic cytoplasmic antibody-positive conditions (vasculitides)
  - Wegener's granulomatosus
  - Microscopic polyangiitis
- Goodpasture's disease (rare)

Note: Although disease processes that fall under the category of hemolytic-uremic syndrome technically fulfill all the criteria for acute GN, they are not truly regarded as glomerulonephritides.
FSGS, Focal segmental glomerulosclerosis.

Will Acute Glomerulonephritis Cause Long-Term Complications?

Postinfectious GN is almost always self-limited, and progression to CKD is rare. Patients with acute GN caused by other disorders may develop progressive renal damage and CKD. Although self-limited, acute postinfectious GN may have life-threatening complications related to ARF, including hyperkalemia, severe hypertension, encephalopathy, seizures, pulmonary edema, and congestive heart failure.

EVALUATION

How Do I Evaluate for Glomerulonephritis

The workup of a child with suspected GN should first establish the diagnosis, then evaluate for complications:

- History: Tea- or cola-colored urine, oliguria, and edema
- Physical examination: Hypertension, peripheral edema, pulmonary vascular congestion or pulmonary edema, and heart failure
- Laboratory tests:
  - Urinalysis for blood and protein
  - Microscopic urinalysis for red blood cell casts
  - Serum creatinine (often elevated)
  - Serum electrolytes (hyperkalemia, acidosis)

- Serum total protein and albumin (see "Nephrotic Syndrome")
- Complete blood count (dilutional anemia; thrombocytopenia in autoimmune diseases)
- Chest x-ray if you suspect pulmonary edema

What Further Tests Are Needed?

The cause of GN is identified from history, physical examination, and selected tests (Table 65-6). C3 complement and anti-neutrophil cytoplasmic antibody (ANCA) levels help differentiate amongst the various causes of GN. Renal biopsy, when indicated, can identify the underlying etiology, provide information about the severity of the GN, verify a clinical diagnosis, or determine the degree of chronicity. In some diseases, such as systemic lupus erythematosus, a biopsy can distinguish the subclasses of GN, which has therapeutic and prognostic importance.

TREATMENT

How Do I Manage a Patient with Glomerulonephritis?

Treatment of postinfectious GN is aimed at preventing complications arising from ARF. This includes the management of hypertension, fluid overload, and electrolyte abnormalities such as hyperkalemia. Most patients with acute GN require salt and fluid restriction and many benefit from the judicious use of diuretics. Patients with chronic GN may benefit from immunosuppressive therapies.

What Is the Prognosis for a Patient with Glomerulonephritis?

Children with postinfectious GN typically have complete resolution of edema and proteinuria as glomerular inflammation resolves; recurrence rate is very low. Microscopic hematuria commonly persists for years, however, and is benign in the absence of proteinuria. Progression to CKD is extremely uncommon. Other forms of GN often have recurrences and may progress to renal failure. The precise risk is dependent on the underlying disease and the response to therapy.

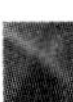

NEPHROTIC SYNDROME

ETIOLOGY

What Is Nephrotic Syndrome?

Nephrotic syndrome (NS) is characterized by the following:

- Proteinuria > 40 mg/m^2/hr (or random urine protein-to-creatinine ratio > 2.5)
- Hypoalbuminemia (serum albumin < 2.5 g/dl)
- Edema and often anasarca
- Hypercholesterolemia (in the majority of patients)

Table 65-6

Etiologic Evaluation of a Child with Glomerulonephritis

Disorder	History and Examination	Laboratory Tests
Postinfectious GN	Pharyngitis/impetigo (recent) Gross hematuria preceding edema	Transiently depressed C3 and C4 (6–8 weeks) Rapid streptococcal antigen; ASO titer
IgA nephropathy	Recurrent gross hematuria precipitated by viral infections or exercise	None
Idiopathic MPGN	Not specific: fatigue, anemia	Persistently low C3/C4
HSP	Syndrome: purpuric skin rash, periarthritis, abdominal pain, and glomerulonephritis	None: Clinical diagnosis Diagnosis confirmed by IgA deposits on skin and renal biopsy. If tested, ANA, C3/C4, and ANCA should be negative
Hepatitis B or C	Blood transfusions, sexual activity, or IV drug abuse Jaundice Maternal hepatitis SSx of chronic liver disease (+/−)	Hepatic transaminases Hepatitis B surface antigen Hepatitis C antibody C3/C4 (persistently depressed)
SLE	SSx of SLE (see Chapter 70)	C3 and C4 (depressed) ANA dsDNA/Sm antibodies
Alport's syndrome	Family history of renal failure Hearing loss or ocular abnormalities	Genetic testing possible in some families
ANCA-positive GN	Respiratory problems, sinusitis, skin rash, constitutional symptoms	ANCA (c and p)

ANA, Antinuclear antibody; ANCA, antineutrophilic cytoplasmic antibody; ASO, antistreptolysin O test; C3 and C4, third and fourth components of complement; dsDNA, double-stranded DNA; GN, glomerulonephritis; HSP, Henoch-Schönlein purpura; IgA, immunoglobulin A; IV, intravenous; MPGN, membranoproliferative glomerulonephritis; SLE, systemic lupus erythematosus; Sm, Smith; SSx, signs and symptoms +/−, variable.

What Causes Nephrotic Syndrome in Childhood?

NS is a syndrome that most often results from a primary, poorly understood, aberration in the immune system (Table 65-7). Less than 20% of NS in children is caused by an underlying systemic disorder (secondary NS). Some nephrologists feel that the only "pure" NS is "minimal change disease" (MCD) because the other forms are usually associated with hematuria and hypertension (see "Glomerulonephritis").

Table 65-7

Causes of Nephrotic Syndrome in Children

Primary or Idiopathic without Persistent Hematuria
Minimal change disease
Primary or Idiopathic with Persistent Hematuria
Focal segmental glomerulosclerosis (FSGS)
Idiopathic membranoproliferative glomerulonephritis (MPGN)
Membranous nephropathy (rare)
Secondary
Systemic lupus erythematosus
Henoch-Schönlein purpura
IgA nephropathy
Secondary MPGN associated with hepatitis B or C
Human immunodeficiency virus nephropathy
Sickle cell nephropathy

What Is Minimal Change Disease?

MCD is the commonest form of NS in children and typically occurs between 18 months and 9 years of age. The proteinuria of MCD is felt to result from cytokine-induced changes in the glomerular basement membrane and the glomerular filtration slit that allow proteins to "leak" into the urine. MCD is *not* associated with persistent hematuria. NS in patients older than 16 years is less likely to be MCD and is usually accompanied by hematuria and often by renal dysfunction. Infants younger than 3 months with NS have *congenital nephrotic syndrome,* which is rare and much more serious than usual childhood NS. Focal segmental glomerulosclerosis (FSGS) is a more ominous cause of NS that is much more common in African-American children than in Caucasian and Latino patients.

EVALUATION

How Do I Approach the Workup of Nephrotic Syndrome?

Table 65-8 lists the tests required to establish the diagnosis of NS.

Additional tests include the following:

- Serum electrolytes, to look for hyponatremia
- Serum creatinine, to evaluate renal function

Table 65-8

Tests to Establish the Diagnosis of Nephrotic Syndrome

Test	Result	Comment
Urinalysis: protein	$\geq$ 4+ ($\geq$ 300 mg/dl)	Need quantitative urine protein
Quantitative urine protein	> 40 mg/m^2/hr or urine protein to creatinine ratio > 2.5	"Nephrotic" range
Serum albumin	< 2.5 g/dl	"Nephrotic" range
Total cholesterol	> 200 (usually > 400) mg/dl	Not universally seen

- Complete blood count, to look for anemia
- Chest x-ray, to look for pleural effusions
- Purified protein derivative (PPD), to rule out exposure to tuberculosis before starting corticosteroids

How Do I Identify Secondary Nephrotic Syndrome?

Table 65-9 lists the tests to identify secondary NS. The decision to pursue further workup should be based on history, physical examination, and factors such as the regional/local prevalence of the diseases that cause NS.

Table 65-9

Etiologic Evaluation of a Child with Nephrotic Syndrome

Disease	History and Examination	Laboratory Tests
IgA nephropathy	Recurrent gross hematuria precipitated by viral infections or exercise	No reliable blood or urine tests
SLE	Signs and symptoms of SLE (see Chapter 70)	C3 and C4 (low in SLE) ANA dsDNA/Sm antibodies
HSP	Syndrome of purpuric skin rash, periarthritis, abdominal pain, and hematuria/proteinuria	Not needed because HSP is a clinical diagnosis
Hepatitis B or C	Blood transfusions, sexual activity, or IV drug abuse Jaundice Maternal hepatitis Signs and symptoms of chronic liver disease (variable)	Hepatic transaminases Hepatitis B surface antigen Hepatitis C antibody C3/C4 (persistently low)
HIV	Maternal HIV, IV drug use, cachexia, failure to thrive	Tests for HIV diagnosis
Sickle cell nephropathy	Sickle cell anemia	Tests for sickle cell diagnosis

ANA, Antinuclear antibody; C3 and C4, third and fourth components of complement; dsDNA, double-stranded DNA; HSP, Henoch-Schönlein purpura; HIV, human immunodeficiency virus; IV, intravenous; SLE, systemic lupus erythematosus; Sm, Smith.

When Is Renal Biopsy Needed?

The information provided by a biopsy may not add enough to the management plan to justify the risks of the procedure. Renal biopsy may be indicated in steroid-resistant NS (see later), and when there is high suspicion of secondary NS based on laboratory tests (e.g., low C3 level).

How Do I Treat a Patient with Nephrotic Syndrome?

The management of NS requires a combination of pharmacotherapy, dietary instructions, intensive family and patient education, and home monitoring for proteinuria. Corticosteroid treatment is the major therapy for NS. A low-salt diet is recommended to avoid worsening of edema, especially while the child is hypoalbuminemic. The family also needs instruction on the use of urine dipsticks to monitor proteinuria at home, so that relapses can be identified early and appropriate intervention instituted.

Does Nephrotic Syndrome Respond to Corticosteroid Therapy?

About 85% of children with primary NS respond completely to corticosteroids and are said to have *steroid-responsive NS*. Patients who do not respond to a standard course of corticosteroids have *steroid-resistant NS* and are more likely to have secondary NS. They usually undergo renal biopsy to establish a precise histologic diagnosis so that appropriate therapy may be offered. Treatment of secondary NS is entirely dependent on the underlying disease process.

What Is the Clinical Course of Steroid-Responsive Nephrotic Syndrome?

Children with steroid-responsive NS respond promptly to treatment but often develop relapses, often precipitated by intercurrent infections. Relapses can be diagnosed early if the family routinely monitors the child's urine for protein, noting any protein greater than 2+ on the dipstick. Each relapse usually responds to a repeat course of corticosteroids. There is a general tendency for patients to "outgrow" their disease around puberty, although this is by no means a universal phenomenon.

What Is the Clinical Course of Steroid-Resistant Nephrotic Syndrome?

Patients with steroid-resistant NS often respond to high-dose intravenous steroids, alkylating agents (cyclophosphamide), calcineurin inhibitors (cyclosporine or tacrolimus), or their combinations. A child who does not respond to these agents has a high risk of developing CKD.

What Complications of Nephrotic Syndrome Are Related to the Disease?

Complications are common in children with steroid-resistant NS, because persistent proteinuria causes urinary loss of immunoprotective and antithrombotic factors. Spontaneous bacterial peritonitis caused by encapsulated organisms such as *Streptococcus pneumoniae* is particularly dangerous. Thromboembolism may result from the patient's hypercoagulable state. Protein malnutrition may develop from chronic protein loss. CKD may also develop.

What Complications of Nephrotic Syndrome Are Related to Steroids?

Chronic treatment with corticosteroids causes osteoporosis, growth failure, hyperglycemia, hyperlipidemia, emotional lability, and cataracts. Steroids also increase risk of infections, cause or exacerbate hypertension, and result in acne, hirsutism, moon facies, and abdominal striae. These side effects justify use of alternative therapies such as alkylating agents and calcineurin inhibitors to avoid prolonged corticosteroid exposure, even for steroid-responsive patients who have frequent relapses.

URINARY TRACT INFECTION

ETIOLOGY

How Common Are Urinary Tract Infections in Children?

Urinary tract infections (UTIs) are common in infancy and are second only to upper respiratory infections as a cause of fever in children. About 5% of all febrile infants with no obvious source of fever will have a UTI. The incidence is highest in girls (7%) followed by uncircumcised male infants (3%). UTIs are less common in older children, with a reported incidence of 1% to 3%.

What Organisms Cause Urinary Tract Infections in Children?

The majority of UTIs in children are caused by *Escherichia coli*. Other organisms that cause UTIs are listed in Table 65-10.

Table 65-10

Organisms Causing Urinary Tract Infection (UTI) in Children

Organism	Comments
Escherichia coli	80%-90% of all UTIs
Klebsiella and Pseudomonas (5% each)	Immunocompromised or hospitalized patients, prior treatment with antibiotics, obstructive uropathies
Proteus (5%)	More common in male toddlers; may lead to development of "struvite" kidney stones
Staphylococcus saprophyticus/ Enterococcus	Anatomic abnormalities of the urinary tract, frequent urinary catheterization

What Factors Predispose to Urinary Tract Infection?

Host-microbial interactions are probably most important in determining which child develops a UTI. Many predisposing factors for UTIs lead to urinary stasis and bacterial overgrowth:

- Primary vesicoureteral reflux (VUR)
- Secondary VUR caused by obstructive uropathies
- Obstructive uropathies with urinary stasis such as ureteropelvic junction (UPJ) obstruction
- Obstructive uropathies with both secondary VUR and urinary stasis
  - Posterior urethral valves (PUV)—anatomic obstruction
  - Neurogenic bladder—functional obstruction
- Miscellaneous:
  - Chronic constipation
  - Poor perineal or preputial hygiene
  - Dysfunctional voiding

What Long-Term Complications Occur with Urinary Tract Infection?

Children who have a single UTI are at a high risk for recurrent infections. All UTIs in febrile children should be considered to be acute pyelonephritis. Recurrent episodes of pyelonephritis can lead to scarring of the renal parenchyma (reflux nephropathy). Reflux nephropathy is associated with a risk of developing hypertension and can progress to CKD.

EVALUATION

When Should I Suspect a Urinary Tract Infection?

Signs and symptoms of UTI include the following:

- Fever without a source (especially in a girl younger than 3 years and in uncircumcised male infants)
- Irritability, fussiness, or even diarrhea in an infant without obvious cause
- Parental report of a change in urine color, odor, or clarity
- Urgency, frequency, dysuria, or abrupt onset of secondary urinary incontinence
- Abdominal pain, flank pain, and costovertebral angle tenderness

What Laboratory Tests Help Diagnose Urinary Tract Infection?

Any patient in whom you suspect a UTI *must have a urine culture* performed because culture of a properly collected urine specimen is the only reliable way to diagnose a UTI. Urinalysis assists with the diagnosis of a UTI but is in itself insufficient. A positive nitrite or leukocyte esterase test on a urine dipstick or the presence of white blood cells or bacteria on the microscopic urinalysis should raise your suspicion for a UTI, but these tests are neither specific nor sensitive enough to be a reliable substitute for a urine culture. Table 65-11 lists the criteria for culture diagnosis of UTI, which vary with the method used to collect the urine sample.

Table 65-11

Culture Criteria for Urinary Tract Infection Diagnosis

Method of Urine Collection	Colony Count
Suprapubic (< 2 months of age)*	Any gram-negative bacteria > 1000 gram-positive bacteria
Catheterized*	> 10,000 bacteria
Clean catch	> 100,000 bacteria in females > 10,000 bacteria in males
Bag	Unreliable (very high false-positive rate)

*Gold standard method.

Can Cystitis and Acute Pyelonephritis Be Distinguished?

Because it is difficult to distinguish cystitis from acute pyelonephritis, especially in infants and young children, and because renal scarring is only seen with acute pyelonephritis, it is safest to assume that all children with a UTI have acute pyelonephritis. Early intervention to treat infection reduces the likelihood of adverse consequences. Clues that indicate acute pyelonephritis include the following:

- High fever with chills
- Nausea and vomiting
- Costovertebral angle (CVA) tenderness or flank pain
- Elevated serum creatinine without dehydration
- Elevated white blood cell (WBC) count on a CBC, or elevated C-reactive protein (CRP)
- White blood cell casts in the urine

How Do I Determine the Cause of Urinary Tract Infections?

If a child is suspected of having a UTI, the history, physical examination, and laboratory tests should aim to confirm the diagnosis and determine if an underlying factor predisposes to infection (Table 65-12). Although controversial, many healthcare professionals recommend renal and bladder ultrasound to look for obstructive uropathies and voiding cystourethrogram (VCUG) to identify possible vesicoureteral reflux (VUR) for every child with an episode of pyelonephritis and especially males (see VUR section later).

Table 65-12

Evaluation of a Child with a Urinary Tract Infection for Common Predisposing Factors

Predisposing Condition	History and Physical Examination	Laboratory Tests
VUR	History of VUR or recurrent UTIs in siblings or parents	VCUG See "Vesicoureteral Reflux" section for more details
Obstructive uropathy		
Posterior urethral valves (seen almost exclusively in males)	Weak urinary stream Difficulty urinating	VCUG Renal ultrasound
Ureteropelvic junction obstruction	Palpable renal mass (in the neonatal period) Abnormal prenatal ultrasound	Renal ultrasound Radionuclide renal scan
Bladder dysfunction		
Behavioral	Voiding pattern with infrequent urination, postponement of voiding, urinary/fecal incontinence	Serum creatinine Renal and bladder ultrasound with prevoid and postvoid images ± VCUG
Neurogenic	Urinary/fecal incontinence Bladder spasms Presence of sacral dimples, tufts of hair, lipomas Asymmetry of gluteal creases, loss of anal wink and sphincter tone Lower extremity weakness, hypotonia, and sensory loss	Consider videourodynamics Same as above, plus ultrasound or MRI of the spine (for tethering of the spinal cord)
Miscellaneous		
Constipation	History of infrequent defecation with straining; hard stools; abdominal pain; encopresis Palpable stool in rectal vault on examination	None essential; KUB may have role in confirming and documenting fecal impaction
Poor hygiene	History of improper cleaning technique after bowel movements; fecal/urinary odor to underclothes	None
Uncircumcised infant	Obvious on examination	None

KUB, Kidney-ureter-bladder x-ray; MRI, magnetic resonance imaging; UTI, urinary tract infection; VCUG, voiding cystourethrogram; VUR, vesicoureteral reflux.

TREATMENT

How Do I Manage a Patient with a Urinary Tract Infection?

The first step in acute management is to choose an appropriate antibiotic. Because *E. coli* causes most UTIs in children, empirical therapy should be based on the sensitivity pattern of the *E. coli* in your community or hospital. If the index of suspicion for a UTI is high, treatment should be started promptly while awaiting results of the urine culture. Table 65-13 lists the common antibiotic choices. Urine culture results and the sensitivity pattern of the organism will be used to modify antibiotic therapy.

Table 65-13

Antibiotic Choices for Empirical Treatment of Children with Suspected Urinary Tract Infection

Oral Antibiotics	Intravenous Antibiotics
Trimethoprim-sulfamethoxazole	Cefotaxime
Cephalexin	Ampicillin + gentamicin
Cefixime	Ceftriaxone
Amoxicillin + clavulanate	Cephalexin
Ciprofloxacin (in older adolescents and immunocompromised patients)	

When Should I Hospitalize a Child with Urinary Tract Infection?

Most children with a UTI can be safely managed at home with oral antibiotics. Hospitalization and intravenous antibiotics should be chosen if the patient is younger than 6 to 12 months, appears "toxic," has severe dehydration, cannot tolerate oral medications, or has failed a trial of oral antibiotics. A febrile patient who has a UTI usually becomes afebrile within 48 to 72 hours after the start of appropriate antibiotic treatment. Prolonged fever should prompt reevaluation, including a repeat urine culture, and may justify a renal ultrasound to search for urinary tract obstruction or for the development of a perirenal abscess.

Can Recurrent Urinary Tract Infections Be Prevented?

General measures that may prevent recurrent UTIs include increased fluid intake, frequent and "scheduled" urination, improved perineal and preputial hygiene, and treatment of underlying constipation. Prophylactic antibiotics to prevent recurrent infection should be considered for all children who have VUR, UPJ obstruction, or dysfunctional voiding. Note that large-scale randomized controlled trials of prophylaxis in children with UTI have not been reported. Additionally, some physicians also feel that all children younger than 1 year who have had an episode of pyelonephritis should be placed on prophylaxis for a short period of time (6 months), even if no predisposing factors are found, because the rate of recurrence is quite high in this age group. For detailed information on antibiotic choices and doses for prophylaxis, see the UTI section of the Bibliography. Children with neurogenic bladders may need frequent catheterization to remain infection-free. A patient who has a surgically correctable condition (such as PUV or UPJ obstruction) may also be a candidate for operative intervention.

VESICOURETERAL REFLUX

ETIOLOGY

What Is Vesicoureteral Reflux?

Vesicoureteral reflux (VUR) is a condition in which urine moves in a retrograde direction from the urinary bladder into the ureters and/or renal pelvis. About 40% to 50% of all children who develop symptomatic UTIs are found to have VUR. Figure 65-1 shows the international classification of VUR severity.

What Causes Vesicoureteral Reflux?

VUR is most commonly "primary" or idiopathic. A congenital abnormality at the ureterovesical junction (UVJ) allows urine to reflux from

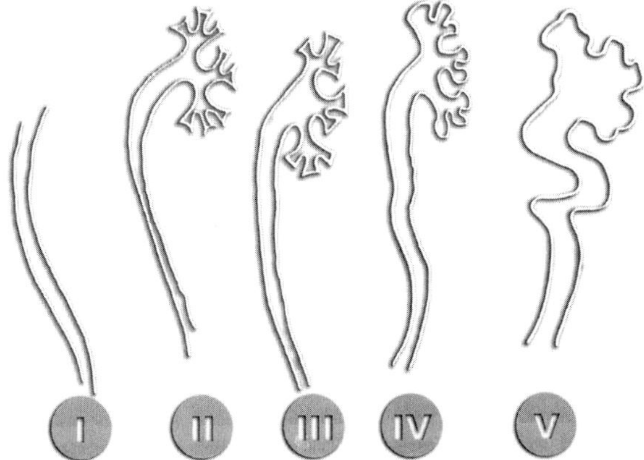

FIGURE 65-1 Vesicoureteral reflux grades (based on the international classification). Grade I: Reflux into the ureter only. Grade II: Reflux into the ureter and the renal pelvis. Grade III: Reflux up to the renal pelvis with mild dilatation of the collecting systems. Grade IV: Reflux up to the renal pelvis with moderate dilatation of the collecting systems and blunting of the calyces. Grade V: Reflux up to the renal pelvis with severe dilatation of the collecting systems, blunting of the calyces, and obliteration of the papillary impressions. (Illustrator, Christopher G. Hartung, Lazariel's Ink, Sacramento, CA.)

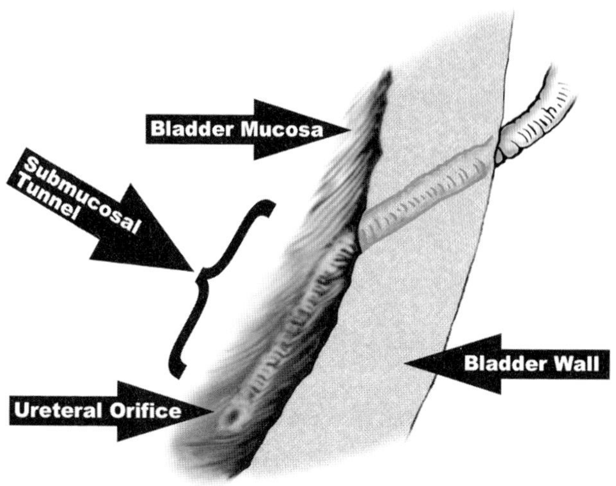

FIGURE 65-2 Anatomy of the ureterovesical junction showing the intramural and submucosal components of the ureter, both of which have an "antireflux" role. (Illustrator, Christopher G. Hartung, Lazariel's Ink, Sacramento, CA.)

the bladder into the ureter. The ureteric orifice may be abnormally large (golf-hole orifice) or more laterally directed than normal, or there may be too short a submucosal tunnel for the section of the ureter that traverses the wall of the bladder. All result in defective closure of the distal ureter or its orifice, allowing reflux of urine when the bladder fills (Figure 65-2). On occasion VUR results from bladder outlet obstruction caused by a structural abnormality such as PUV or by a neurogenic bladder or other functional bladder obstruction. VUR results from the elevated bladder pressure caused by the obstruction (secondary VUR).

When Should I Evaluate a Patient for Vesicoureteral Reflux?

There is little consensus about the specific indications for evaluation of children for the presence of VUR. Situations in which it may be reasonable to look for VUR include the following:

- Known obstructive uropathies
  - PUV
  - Neurogenic bladder
- UTI
  - Any episode of pyelonephritis
  - Any UTI in a male
  - Any UTI in a child younger than 6 years
  - More than one UTI in a girl older than 6 years
- Renal anomalies associated with VUR
  - Multicystic-dysplastic kidney

- Hypodysplastic or aplastic kidney
- Horseshoe kidney
- Family history of VUR or recurrent UTIs
  - Screening of children is controversial

How Is Vesicoureteral Reflux Detected?

VUR is most often detected with a VCUG, which detects reflux of contrast material from the bladder into the ureter or the renal pelvis. The radionuclide cystogram (RNC) uses a radioactive tracer instead of contrast. The main advantage of the RNC is its lower radiation exposure compared with the VCUG. Its disadvantages include poor anatomic resolution of the urinary tract, inability to evaluate the urethra (important in males with suspected PUV), and lack of precision in grading VUR.

When Should a Voiding Cystourethrogram Be Performed?

The timing of a VCUG after a UTI is controversial: Some physicians prefer to wait 4 to 6 weeks after a UTI, whereas others recommend immediate VCUG once the child is afebrile and the urine has been sterilized. Proponents of the first approach argue that it reduces "false-positives," which might result from edema and inflammation of the UVJ, making it incompetent. Adherents to the latter approach cite that detection of reflux, even exclusively at the time of an infection, is of importance. No consensus currently exists.

Is a Patient with Vesicoureteral Reflux at Risk of Complications?

Children who have VUR have high risk of developing recurrent UTIs, especially if the VUR was diagnosed during the evaluation of a prior UTI. Recurrent UTIs in the presence of VUR increase the risk of reflux nephropathy. Additionally, some children with VUR have associated renal dysplasia and may be at risk of developing progressive renal insufficiency. Reflux under elevated pressure, especially reflux of infected urine, poses the greatest risk for scar development. Sterile low-pressure reflux (i.e., primary VUR with no UTI) is not felt to be detrimental to renal growth, development, and function.

Does Vesicoureteral Reflux Resolve or Need Treatment?

Most children with primary VUR, especially grades I to III, have spontaneous resolution of the reflux as the UVJ matures. The likelihood of resolution is much lower with grades IV and V. To determine if VUR has resolved, you may need to repeat VCUG or RNC periodically. Once VUR has resolved, the chances of recurrence are low and further imaging studies are not needed if the patient does well.

How Should I Manage a Patient with Vesicoureteral Reflux?

Prophylactic antibiotic treatment is strongly recommended for all patients with VUR detected in the setting of a UTI. Prevention of recurrent UTIs may reduce irreversible renal scarring. Antibiotics useful for prophylaxis include trimethoprim/sulfamethoxazole, cephalexin, nitrofurantoin, and amoxicillin. The best choice is an antibiotic that is effective against the organism that caused the UTI. Once resolution of VUR has been documented by follow-up VCUG or RNC, antibiotics may be safely discontinued.

Does Surgery Correct Vesicoureteral Reflux and Prevent Renal Damage?

Surgical reimplantation of the ureter into the bladder corrects the reflux in more than 95% of cases but does not result in improved renal function. Indications for surgical correction include the following:

- Recurrent UTIs in spite of antibiotic prophylaxis
- High-grade (grade V) VUR
- Poor adherence by patient and family with prophylactic antibiotics
- Persistence of VUR into puberty (especially in females)

A potentially less invasive procedure to treat VUR is the subureteric injection of Deflux™, a material that reinforces the submucosal tunnel and eliminates the VUR.

KEY POINTS

- Renal function can be estimated using height and serum creatinine.
- Fluid and electrolyte imbalances are common in acute renal failure.
- Most childhood chronic kidney disease is caused by congenital abnormalities.
- Glomerulonephritis is most often postinfectious in children.
- Nephrotic patients have complications related to the disease and steroid treatment.
- UTI is a common cause of fever in children.
- Do not culture urine collected in "urine bags."
- VUR causes scarring in the presence of UTI, but sterile primary VUR does not.

Case 65-1

A 2-year-old boy has had a 5-day history of frequent loose watery stools and vomiting. On the day of admission he was noted to have poor urine output and lethargy. In the emergency room he was found to have dry mucous membranes and a heart rate of 150 beats/min. Weight was 11 kg and height was 88 cm. The urinalysis had specific gravity of 1.030, and no blood, protein, white blood cells, or casts. The Fe_{Na} is 0.3%. His serum creatinine is 1.0 mg/dl.

A. What evidence suggests that this patient has ARF?
B. What is the most likely cause of your patient's ARF and why?
C. What is the most important next step in the management of your patient?
D. What if the same child had a Fe_{Na} of 3%? How would his management be different?

Case 65-2

A 5-year-old boy has a 2-day history of cola-colored urine and severe headaches. His parents have noticed that he is not voiding as often as before and has now developed a cough.

A. What further information would you like to obtain from the patient?
B. What findings on physical examination should you look for?
C. How would you start the workup of this child?

Case 65-3

A 3-year-old Caucasian boy is brought to your office with a 2-week history of intermittent facial swelling, especially in the morning. He is otherwise asymptomatic. His heart rate is 80 beats/min, respiratory rate is 20 breaths/min, and blood pressure is 100/70 mm Hg (right arm). His physical examination shows periorbital and pedal edema. A urine dipstick in the office shows 4+ protein and no blood.

A. What is the child's diagnosis? Why?
B. What further information would you like from the family?
C. What further testing would you like to do?

Case 65-4

A 6-year-old girl has a 2-day history of fever and dysuria. There is no history of nausea or vomiting. She has had intermittent bedwetting and daytime enuresis for the past year, but over the last 24 hours she has been wetting herself constantly.

A. What further information do you need from the patient and parent?
B. How would you manage the patient?
C. If the urine culture is positive, what further evaluation would you do and why?

Case 65-5

A 4-year-old girl was found to have bilateral grade II VUR on a VCUG performed after an episode of acute pyelonephritis. Her renal ultrasound was normal. She has no symptoms suggestive of dysfunctional voiding.

A. What will you tell the family about the risks of VUR?
B. What treatment options, if any, would you discuss with the family?
C. Within 2 months of her first UTI, while on antibiotic prophylaxis, the child develops three more episodes of pyelonephritis, all needing hospitalization. Will you change your management approach and, if so, how?

Case Answers

65-1 A. *Learning objective:* **Use history and laboratory tests to identify ARF.** History and physical examination suggest dehydration, serum creatinine is elevated, and estimated GFR based on height and serum creatinine is 48.4 ml/min/1.73 m^2 BSA [GFR= (k $\times$ ht) $\div$ Cr]. Because reduced GFR presumably developed acutely, he has ARF. A healthy 2-year-old child should have a GFR of 100 $\pm$ 20 ml/min/1.73 m^2 BSA.

65-1 B. *Learning objective:* **Identify the cause of ARF.** This child has prerenal ARF caused by intravascular volume depletion, based on history, signs of dehydration, and low Fe_{Na}.

65-1 C. *Learning objective:* **Develop a management plan for a patient with prerenal ARF.** The Fe_{Na} of 0.3% indicates prerenal ARF, most likely from dehydration. He should be treated with aggressive intravenous fluid therapy.

65-1 D. *Learning objective:* **Use laboratory tests to distinguish different causes of ARF.** If his Fe_{Na} was 3%, one would surmise that he had developed acute tubular necrosis as a result of his prolonged dehydration and poor renal perfusion. *Initial* management would still include fluid resuscitation to treat dehydration. Once he reaches a euvolemic state, fluid and potassium should be restricted because of reduced renal function.

65-2 A. *Learning objective:* **Use the history to diagnose acute glomerulonephritis.** Cola-colored urine suggests gross hematuria, most likely from acute postinfectious GN. You should ask about a history of recent sore throat or skin infection, especially documented streptococcal infection. History of abdominal pain, rash, arthritis, and edema should also be obtained.

65-2 B. *Learning objective:* **Identify the physical findings of acute glomerulonephritis.** Key findings include elevated blood pressure, recent weight gain, and periorbital, sacral, and peripheral edema. Careful skin examination will be needed to identify rash or ecchymoses. Abdominal examination should look for pain and ascites. Examination of the joints may detect arthritis.

65-2 C. *Learning objective:* **Select diagnostic tests to evaluate a child with acute glomerulonephritis.** Test a random urine specimen for presence of protein and blood, and determine the protein-to-creatinine ratio. Obtain serum levels of creatinine, electrolytes, total protein, and albumin, and a chest radiograph to look for pulmonary vascular congestion. Base decisions about further laboratory testing on the history and examination, but at a minimum include C3 and C4 complement levels.

65-3 A. *Learning objective:* **Discuss nephrotic syndrome and how the patient's age and clinical findings affect the final diagnosis.** This child has nephrotic syndrome, identified because of edema and proteinuria. Absence of blood in the urine argues against glomerulonephritis. The most likely type would be minimal change nephrotic syndrome, based on the child's age and findings.

65-3 B. *Learning objective:* **Discuss the important history for a patient with nephrotic syndrome.** You should ask about past history of similar symptoms or of decreased urine output, puffy face, or excessive weight gain. It is also important to ask about blood transfusions in the past and whether there is a maternal history of hepatitis B or C or human immunodeficiency viral (HIV) infection.

65-3 C. *Learning objective:* **Select diagnostic tests to confirm the diagnosis of nephrotic syndrome.** Appropriate tests include random urine protein-to-creatinine ratio and serum levels of albumin, electrolytes, creatinine, and total cholesterol. If the diagnosis of nephrotic syndrome is confirmed, consider the following serologic tests: hepatitis B surface antigen, hepatitis C antibody, antinuclear antibody, C3 and C4 complement levels, and possibly an HIV screening test.

65-4 A. *Learning objective:* **Identify important information from the history to evaluate a child with suspected urinary tract infection (UTI).** The following are important in the identification of UTI: history of constipation or encopresis, voiding habits (frequency of urination and voluntary postponement of urination), and family history of recurrent UTIs or vesicoureteral reflux.

65-4 B. *Learning objective:* **Discuss initial management of suspected UTI.** Obtain a urinalysis and a urine culture, ideally with a catheterized urine specimen, and less optimally a clean-catch urine. Start empirical antibiotics: oral trimethoprim-sulfamethoxazole or cephalexin. Adjust antibiotics once urine culture and sensitivity patterns are available.

65-4 C. *Learning objective:* **Select tests to evaluate predisposing factors for and complications of UTI in children.** Consider a voiding cystourethrogram to look for VUR and a renal and bladder ultrasound (with prevoid and postvoid images) to look for obstructive uropathies and for dysfunctional voiding.

65-5 A. *Learning objective:* **Discuss the outcome of VUR in a young child.** Children with VUR may have recurrent UTI, which can lead to renal scarring/reflux nephropathy and its consequences; hypertension; and CKD, especially if treatment is delayed.

65-5 B. *Learning objective:* **Discuss the treatment of VUR.** Prophylactic antibiotics are recommended to prevent recurrent UTIs and renal scarring. General measures such as good perineal and perianal hygiene, prevention of constipation, increased fluid intake, and frequent scheduled voiding must also be discussed with the family.

65-5 C. *Learning objective:* **Discuss management of recurrent infection in a patient with VUR.** First, assess adherence of the family to the prophylactic antibiotic regimen. For this patient, either prophylaxis has failed to prevent infection or the family has not followed the treatment plan. In either case, the child is at risk for irreversible renal damage if she has more episodes of pyelonephritis. Consequently, you should strongly consider consultation with a pediatric urologist for ureteral reimplantation or subureteric injection with Deflux.

BIBLIOGRAPHY

Acute Renal Failure

Schwartz GJ, Brion LP, Spitzer A: The use of plasma creatinine concentration for estimating glomerular filtration rate in infants, children, and adolescents, *Pediatr Clin North Am* 34:571, 1987.

Urinary Tract Infection

American Academy of Pediatrics (AAP), Committee on Quality Improvement: Practice parameter: the diagnosis, treatment, and evaluation of the initial urinary tract infection in febrile infants and young children, *Pediatrics* 103:843, 1999.

Vesicoureteral Reflux

Mahant S, To T, Friedman J: Timing of voiding cystourethrogram in the investigation of urinary tract infections in children, *J Pediatr* 139:568,2001.

Wald ER: Vesicoureteral reflux: the role of antibiotic prophylaxis, *Pediatrics* 117:919, 2006.

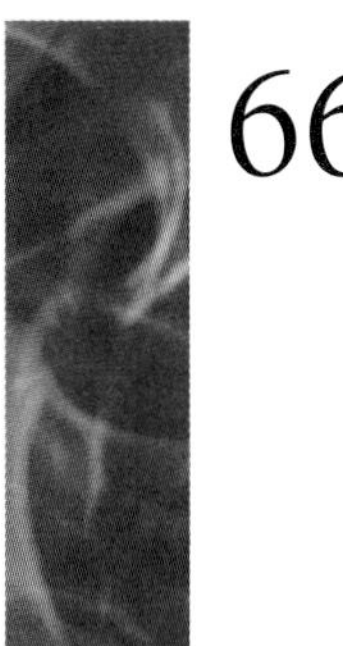

66

Neurology

ADAM HARTMAN

ACQUIRED NEUROLOGIC CONDITIONS

ETIOLOGY

What Acquired Neurologic Conditions Might I See?

Injuries to the brachial plexus occur commonly in newborn infants. Stroke occasionally occurs in childhood. Brain tumors, although relatively infrequent, cause major morbidity and mortality.

What Causes Brachial Nerve Plexus Palsies?

Erb's palsy and Klumpke's palsy are the result of brachial plexus injury. The nerve tracts are injured because the neck and arms are sometimes malpositioned in utero or during a difficult delivery. Fractures of the clavicle and ribs can be associated with either. Erb's palsy involves the upper brachial plexus (C5-C7), which affects shoulder and arm muscles. Diaphragm paralysis occurs if C3-C5 are also injured. Klumpke's palsy involves the lower brachial plexus (C8-T1), which affects the hand. Klumpke's palsies tend to be more severe because lower plexus injuries are often caused by avulsion of the spinal roots. Upper plexus injuries more commonly involve stretching injuries of the trunks.

What Causes Strokes in Children?

The incidence of strokes in children outside the neonatal period is about 2.5 to 5 events per 100,000 children per year. Stroke can present as hemiparesis, seizures, irritability, headache, fever, dystonia, vomiting, papilledema, or lethargy. Risk factors associated with strokes in neonates include hypoxic-ischemic injuries, trauma, infections, polycythemia, hypotension, congenital heart disease, clotting abnormalities, and cocaine. In older children, strokes are associated with congenital heart disease, infections (including varicella), prothrombotic and clotting disorders, sickle cell disease, trauma, vasculitis, moyamoya disease, migraines, malignancy, and sequelae of perinatal infections.

How Common Are Brain Tumors in Children?

Brain tumors occur in 2.5 to 4 per 100,000 children per year, making them the second most common form of cancer in children and the most common solid tumor of childhood. Their incidence has been increasing in recent years. Most brain tumors in children older than 1 year arise in the infratentorial compartment of the brain.

TREATMENT

How Are Brachial Plexus Injuries Treated?

Treatment is primarily supportive, including management of associated injuries such as clavicle fracture. If the palsy does not improve within the first 6 months of life, it is likely to persist.

Can Stroke Be Treated?

Treatment is aimed at the underlying disorder and also must support the child during the immediate poststroke period. Rehabilitative services may be needed and generally will involve a multidisciplinary team.

How Are Brain Tumors Treated?

Primary surgical resection and chemotherapy are the primary treatment modalities, depending on the type of tumor. Cranial radiation is used for certain tumors in older children. The long-term sequelae of treatment include learning problems, focal neurologic deficits, and endocrinologic problems, in addition to the sequelae that occur with treatment of other tumors (e.g., immunosuppression, cytopenia, and second tumors). The prognosis depends on the histology of the tumor, age at presentation, and presence of metastases.

CONGENITAL MALFORMATIONS

ETIOLOGY

What Congenital Malformations Affect the Central Nervous System?

Central nervous system (CNS) malformations most commonly occur at the distal and caudal ends of the developing neural tube. Spina bifida occulta and myelomeningocele will be encountered most often. Table 66-1 lists some abnormalities in the formation of the CNS.

What Causes Neural Tube Defects?

The neural tube closes like a zipper during the third and fourth weeks of gestation, starting in the middle and extending to the ends. Failure of distal closure leads to a condition called *spinal dysraphism*. The defect may be benign, such as a sacral dimple or spina bifida occulta, or more

Table 66-1

Selected Congenital CNS Malformations*
Anencephaly
Schizencephaly
Lissencephaly
Heterotopias
Holoprosencephaly
Encephalocele
Agenesis of the corpus callosum
Septo-optic dysplasia
Dandy-Walker cyst
Diastematomyelia
Myelomeningocele
Spina bifida occulta
Lipomeningocele
Teratoma
Tethered cord

*In order of caudal to rostral.
CNS, Central nervous system.

severe such as meningocele or myelomeningocele (MMC). Failure of caudal closure leads to encephalocele and anencephaly. *Maternal folate deficiency* causes a significant number of neural tube defects. Supplementation with folate before conception is largely responsible for the recent decreased incidence of neural tube defects.

Why Are Midline Malformations Concerning?

Malformations such as encephaloceles and midline "cysts" may indicate the presence of more complex congenital lesions. In addition, they can communicate with underlying CNS tissue. Decompression or drainage of these malformations should only be done by a neurosurgeon.

What Is a Dandy-Walker Malformation?

It is a malformation of the fourth ventricle characterized by cerebellar vermis hypoplasia or aplasia, a dilated fourth ventricle, and an upwardly displaced tentorium. It is associated commonly with hydrocephalus and other malformations of the CNS, such as cortical dysplasias or agenesis of the corpus callosum. Clinically, it can cause macrocephaly, ataxia, or signs of increased intracranial pressure.

EVALUATION

What Are Clinical Findings of Neural Tube Defects?

The level at which the defect occurs determines the impact on neurologic function and the long-term prognosis. A child with spina bifida occulta may have no visible defect and no physical findings, the diagnosis having been made incidentally with a radiograph. Occasionally, enuresis or encopresis may lead to the diagnosis of "occult" spinal dysraphism. Conversely, infants with severe MMC may have marked neurologic and structural dysfunction (Table 66-2) and may develop life-threatening infection of the nervous system.

TREATMENT

How Are Children with Neural Tube Defects Managed?

Care is best managed where multidisciplinary medical, surgical, and supportive clinical services can be obtained. A general pediatrician has a critical role to coordinate various aspects of care. Because the spinal cord level of the lesion largely dictates the severity of involvement, treatment must be based on an *individualized management plan* that focuses on the specific lesion and on the many problems that result from that lesion. Children with neural tube defects often develop allergy to latex, so latex-containing materials should be avoided. Services to address social, developmental, and physical therapy needs are crucial to successful management, as is education about the disorder for parents and older children. In addition, coordination with schools will be necessary to develop individualized educational plans for each child. Prenatal surgery is being investigated in this condition.

MOVEMENT DISORDERS

ETIOLOGY

What Movement Disorders Occur in Childhood?

During infancy and early childhood, dyskinetic movements may be appropriate for the stage of development. As the child's nervous system matures, these developmental dyskinetic movements disappear. Their persistence, or the appearance of new movement disorders, may be a sign of underlying disease. *Tics and Tourette syndrome* are the movement disorders most often seen by general pediatricians. *Sydenham's chorea* is

Table 66-2

Organ System Dysfunction in Meningomyelocele

Brain	Arnold-Chiari II malformations, hydrocephalus, seizures, learning problems
Endocrinologic	Precocious puberty, obesity, short stature
Eyes	Strabismus
Kidney/ bladder	Neurogenic bladder, urinary tract infections, vesicoureteral reflux
Orthopedic	Contractures, lower extremity malformations, scoliosis, kyphosis
Skin	Decubitus ulcers

occasionally seen, but its incidence has declined dramatically because rheumatic fever rates have decreased. *Torticollis* is a form of dystonia usually caused by a hematoma in the sternocleidomastoid muscle, although infection, tumors, and congenital malformations should be considered in the differential diagnosis. Other dystonias include opisthotonic posturing in infants caused by gastroesophageal reflux (Sandifer syndrome) and blepharospasm. Myoclonus and tremors also can be seen in children. Movement disorders may be seen in patients with Wilson disease, lupus, neuroblastoma, and toxic ingestions. Movement disorders associated with multiple neurologic signs require evaluation by an expert.

EVALUATION

How Do I Evaluate Movement Disorders?

Your major diagnostic tools are a careful history and meticulous physical neurologic examinations. Observation of the patient during routine activities will help you describe in detail the movements. Videotapes obtained from parents may allow you to compare current movements with those exhibited before the onset of the disorder. Laboratory tests and imaging will only be needed if a specific disorder is suspected as the cause of the abnormal movement. Psychological assessment can be important for many patients.

What Are Simple Tics?

Simple motor or habit tics, such as blinking and arm jerks, are common. Careful evaluation of neurologic function, behavior, and development is important. Tics not associated with other problems will eventually disappear. If tics persist or cause problems at home or school, a referral should be made to a child neurologist.

How Do I Identify Tourette Syndrome?

Tourette syndrome is a complex disorder that includes both motor and vocal tics, and often has associated behavior problems such as obsessive-compulsive disorder (OCD) and attention deficit hyperactivity disorder (ADHD). Evaluation must focus on the spectrum of presenting features. Tourette syndrome has onset before 21 years of age and a variable clinical course with a duration of at least 1 year. It is common for children to be referred for an allergy evaluation of sniffing or vocalizations before the diagnosis of Tourette syndrome is made. Many children with Tourette syndrome are first diagnosed with ADHD and receive medical therapy with stimulants, such as methylphenidate. The syndrome, not psychostimulant medication, is the cause of the tics. Coprolalia is not as common in patients with Tourette syndrome as has been portrayed on television.

How Is Sydenham's Chorea Diagnosed?

The characteristic choreoathetoid movement presents up to 6 months after the onset of rheumatic fever and is often the sole manifestation of the disease. The writhing, flowing movements of the extremities may be integrated into routine behavior such as combing hair. Handwriting may be particularly affected as the syndrome develops. Emotional outbursts are common. Symptoms recur with repeat streptococcal infections; recurrence during pregnancy is also possible. If Sydenham's chorea presents early in rheumatic fever, erythrocyte sedimentation rate will be elevated and antistreptococcal antibodies will be positive; later onset makes diagnosis difficult.

TREATMENT

What Treatment Is Effective for Tourette Syndrome?

Education about Tourette syndrome for patients, families, and teachers is the key to effective management. Pharmacotherapy for tics is guided by the severity of symptoms and their impact on the patient's daily life and includes a variety of medications, including clonidine, guanfacine, pimozide, risperidone, and many others. Comorbid conditions, such as OCD and ADHD, also may need symptomatic treatment.

How Is Sydenham's Chorea Treated?

Therapy includes penicillin to treat acute streptococcal infection and as prophylaxis to prevent recurrent infection. If necessary, immunomodulatory agents such as adrenocorticotropic hormones, steroids, or intravenous immune globulin may be useful adjuncts.

NEUROPHAKOMATOSES

ETIOLOGY

What Are the Neurophakomatoses?

These neurocutaneous disorders typically have characteristic pigmented skin lesions and neurologic abnormalities. Remember that some neural crest cells become melanocytes. The most often encountered disorders are neurofibromatosis, tuberous sclerosis, ataxia-telangiectasia, and Sturge-Weber syndrome.

How Is Neurofibromatosis Type 1 Diagnosed?

The diagnosis of neurofibromatosis type 1 (NF-1) requires presence of two or more of the criteria listed in Table 66-3. Criteria 1 to 4 are listed in the usual order of appearance. Criteria 5 and 6 are unusual but can be seen by ages 1 and 3 years, respectively. Most children meet the diagnostic criteria by the age of 8 years; all patients do so by 20 years. The gene for NF-1 is located on chromosome 17 and encodes a protein called neurofibromin.

Table 66-3

National Institutes of Health (NIH) Diagnostic Criteria for Neurofibromatosis Type 1 (NF-1)

1. Six or more café au lait macules over 5 mm in greatest diameter in prepubertal individuals and over 15 mm in greatest diameter in postpubertal individuals
2. Axillary or inguinal skin freckling
3. Two or more Lisch nodules
4. Two or more neurofibromas of any type or one plexiform neurofibroma
5. Osseous lesions, such as sphenoid dysplasia or thinning of the cortex of long bones (with or without pseudoarthrosis)
6. Optic glioma
7. A first-degree relative with NF-1

What Are the Characteristics of NF-2?

NF-2 is characterized by bilateral acoustic neuromas *or* a first-degree relative with NF-2, *and* either a unilateral eighth cranial nerve mass *or* two of the following: neurofibroma, meningioma, spinal astrocytoma, schwannoma, or posterior subcapsular cataracts. The gene is located on chromosome 22 and encodes a protein called merlin.

What Is Tuberous Sclerosis Complex?

Tuberous sclerosis complex (TSC) is a multisystem disorder. Its diagnosis is based on the clinical features and classified as definite, probable, or suspect. The genes causing TSC are on chromosomes 9 (hamartin) and 16 (tuberin). Clinical features of TSC are listed in Table 66-4.

What Is Ataxia-Telangiectasia?

Ataxia-telangiectasia is a multiorgan disease involving conjunctival or cutaneous telangiectases, ataxia, immunologic dysfunction (including T- and B-cell dysfunction and IgA, IgM, and IgE abnormalities), and

Table 66-4

Tuberous Sclerosis Complex

Common Findings	Less Common Findings
Skin: facial angiofibromas, ungual fibromas, and shagreen patches	*Kidneys*: angiomyolipomas, cysts
CNS: cortical tubers, subependymal nodules, giant cell astrocytomas	*Heart:* rhabdomyomas
Eyes: retinal astrocytomas	*Teeth:* pits
	Bone: cysts
	Lungs: lymphangiomyomatosis

CNS, Central nervous system.

malignancies (including leukemia and lymphomas). Frequent infections are common and are a leading cause of death in this patient population. The ATM protein is on chromosome 11.

What Is Sturge-Weber Syndrome?

Sturge-Weber syndrome is characterized by a facial port wine stain (classically in the first division of the trigeminal nerve) and intracranial angiomatosis. Focal seizures are seen in 80% of patients, and contralateral hemiplegia is seen in 50%. Intracranial calcifications are seen on radiographic studies. Occasionally, there is involvement of the anterior chamber of the eye resulting in glaucoma and mental retardation.

EVALUATION

How Do I Evaluate Neurocutaneous Disorders?

Careful description of the skin lesions, neurologic deficits, seizures, developmental delay, and eye problems is critical. The findings should be compared against published criteria for the specific diseases. Studies should be done to determine the extent of organ system involvement.

TREATMENT

How Do I Treat These Disorders?

Most associated abnormalities are treated symptomatically. Referral to specialists in neurology, neurosurgery, dermatology, plastic surgery, cardiology, nephrology, ophthalmology, and rehabilitative services will depend on the extent of the patient's disease. The pediatrician serves a key role to coordinate care among multiple specialists and to assist families with the stress of raising a child with a multisystem disorder.

SLEEP DISORDERS

ETIOLOGY

What Sleep Disorders Occur in Children?

Many different phenomena occur during sleep in children. Those most commonly seen by pediatricians are the parasomnias: night terrors, sleepwalking, and nightmares. Sleep-associated breathing disorders, such as obstructive sleep apnea, are observed with some frequency. Movement disorders, such as periodic limb movements of sleep or restless leg syndrome, and narcolepsy also occasionally come to the pediatrician's attention.

EVALUATION

What Symptoms May Indicate a Sleep Disorder?

Children with night terrors typically are toddlers who wake up in the middle of the night screaming. They have no recollection of the event the following day. Night terrors occur during stage III or IV of non-rapid eye movement (REM) sleep, early in the night. In contrast, nightmares tend to occur later in the night, during one of the REM cycles, and patients may recall details. Children with obstructive sleep apnea often snore and may have headaches, enuresis, and daytime sleepiness. Obese children and adolescents have increased frequency of obstructive sleep apnea.

TREATMENT

How Do I Treat a Child with a Sleep Disorder?

For most parasomnias, reassurance is all that is necessary, because children outgrow these episodes. Sometimes, safety measures must be taken for sleepwalkers. Medication is reserved for severe cases. Children with sleep-associated apnea that is not associated with snoring should be seen by a pulmonologist. Children who snore benefit from referral to an otolaryngologist. Weight management is essential for obese children. Restless leg syndrome may be associated with iron deficiency and is treated in some cases with dopaminergic agents, such as pramipexole. Children with suspected narcolepsy should be evaluated by either a neurologist or sleep expert.

NEURODEGENERATIVE DISORDERS

ETIOLOGY

What Causes Neurodegenerative Disorders?

This family of disorders has many causes. Although individual disorders are rare, they are not uncommon when considered as a group. Examples are listed in Table 66-5.

EVALUATION

What Are the Signs of Neurodegenerative Disorders?

Symptoms and signs that indicate a possible neurodegenerative disorder include loss of previously attained milestones, poor growth, behavioral

Table 66-5

Neurodegenerative Disorders

Affected System	Example
White matter	Metachromatic leukodystrophy
Gray matter	Neuronal ceroid lipofuscinosis
Inborn errors of metabolism	Wilson disease
Genetic mutation	Rett syndrome
Diseases of specific organelles	Mitochondrial cytopathies

regression, and intractable epilepsy. Organ systems outside the nervous system also may be affected (e.g., adrenal insufficiency in patients with adrenoleukodystrophy). Many congenital metabolic disorders are now detected shortly after birth by expanded neonatal screening. Certain features of the patient's presentation may suggest a specific diagnosis and guide rational testing. For example, a girl with developmental delay, wringing hand movements, static head circumference, and seizures may have Rett syndrome. Testing for the gene mutation (MECP2) is indicated.

TREATMENT

How Are Neurodegenerative Diseases Treated?

In addition to symptomatic treatment for seizures, nutritional modifications, and educational support, some neurodegenerative disorders can be managed with specific therapy. One example is dietary management in children with phenylketonuria.

KEY POINTS

- Myelomeningocele and other neural tube defects require multidisciplinary team management.
- Simple tics disappear with time. Tics that accompany ADHD may indicate Tourette syndrome.
- Neurofibromatosis and other neurocutaneous diseases have a wide range of associated neurologic disorders.
- Obtain a sleep history for any child with behavior problems, headaches, or obesity.
- The hallmark of a neurodegenerative disorder is loss of milestones.

Case 66-1

A 5-year-girl with MMC comes for a routine health supervision visit. She was diagnosed at birth and has been followed in a multidisciplinary clinic at a university hospital in another state until the family moved to your community last month. The girl has lower extremity, bladder, and bowel dysfunction but has made good developmental progress socially and cognitively. She uses a walker and a specially designed wheelchair.

A. The mother would like her child to be referred to a multidisciplinary clinic. What medical specialties should be involved in the care of a child with MMC?

B. The family is planning to have another child, and the mother would like to know if there is anything she could do to decrease the risk of having another child with MMC. What will you tell her?

C. Is there anything the family should know about finding a school for the girl?

Case 66-2

An 8-year-old boy has been impulsive and hyperactive since preschool. He has had shoulder shrugging and throat clearing at home and school for the past 6 months. The children at school are starting to make fun of him and he is very upset as a result. Aside from the obvious movement disorder, his neurologic examination identifies no generalized or focal abnormalities.

A. What is the most likely diagnosis?

B. Is there any other testing that you should do?

C. What are the management options for this patient?

Case 66-3

A family brings a newly adopted 4-year-old son for a routine health supervision visit. He was born in another country and the parents were told that he had no medical problems. The parents voice no concerns, but they are interested in his developmental progress because he uses very few words. Weight and length are at the 25th percentile; head circumference is at the 90th percentile. He is alert and shy and walks well. On examination, you count 12 café au lait spots, and he has extensive axillary freckling. You also notice white lesions on his iris. He seems to be able to see only out of his left eye. He has no other visible abnormality.

A. What is his diagnosis?

B. What other anomalies might this child have that should be investigated?

C. How would you counsel this family and manage the patient?

Case Answers

66-1 A. *Learning objective:* **Discuss the management of the multiple systems involved in patients with myelomeningocele (MMC).** The multispecialty MMC clinic will evaluate the girl to identify her specific needs and provide ongoing support. This girl most likely must see an orthopedic surgeon, a neurosurgeon, and a urologist, and must have occupational and physical therapy. Developmental specialists will also follow her to document her current development and to monitor progress. The primary-care physician should manage routine health and prevention services (including immunizations) but must be aware of the patient's special needs.

66-1 B. *Learning objective:* **Discuss the known causes of neural tube defects and outline preventive strategies.** Folate supplementation has significantly reduced the incidence of MMC when it is taken before conception. All women of childbearing age should have a daily supplement of 400 g of folate. The mother should discuss this with her obstetric provider. In addition, if she is taking any medicines herself (e.g., valproic acid), she should also discuss their use.

66-1 C. *Learning objective:* **Discuss the social and educational support needed for children with MMC.** You should investigate community resources for preschool activities for children with special needs. Once she reaches the age for formal schooling, the school system should be able to accommodate her. Schools are required to develop an individualized education plan (IEP) for each child with special needs and to provide the services necessary for continued development and activities of daily living. Specific medical needs, such as intermittent urinary catheterization or administration of medications, should be managed at school.

66-2 A. *Learning objective:* **Discuss the differential diagnosis of tics.** The patient has a movement disorder associated with hyperactivity, a combination that points to Tourette syndrome (TS). Other diagnoses, such as simple tics, are less likely because of the associated behavioral problem. The movements described are not consistent with those seen in Sydenham's chorea.

66-2 B. *Learning objective:* **Discuss the evaluation of a movement disorder such as TS.** The diagnosis of TS is made by history and observation of the tics. Laboratory testing is not needed. The patient has a history of hyperactivity at school and should have a neuropsychological evaluation. Parental and teacher observations of behavior can be of great help in the identification of attention deficit hyperactivity disorder (ADHD). Additionally, he should be evaluated for comorbidities, including learning disabilities, obsessive-compulsive disorder, and depression.

66-2 C. *Learning objective:* **Develop a management plan for a patient with a movement disorder such as TS.** Management must be based on a firm diagnosis, which may require referral to a physician with expertise in TS. The primary-care physician should coordinate diagnostic and management services and maintain ongoing contact with the patient and family. Patient education is one of the pillars of therapy for TS. Families can gain much from support organizations developed by families of children with TS. Information is available in many forms, printed and electronic. You should become familiar with reliable information sources, such as Web sites developed by reputable organizations, so that you may recommend them to families. If the patient is also diagnosed with ADHD, he will benefit from the behavioral and medical therapy for that disorder. If the tics are causing problems in school or home, consideration should be given to medical treatment with clonidine or guanfacine. After medical treatment and support systems are in place, self-esteem is significantly improved for most patients.

66-3 A. *Learning objective:* **Identify the neurocutaneous disorders associated with café au lait macules.** The numerous café au lait macules, the axillary freckling, the Lisch nodules, and the diminished vision in the left eye fulfill the diagnostic criteria for neurofibromatosis 1 (NF-1). Children with NF-1 also have large head circumference.

66-3 B. *Learning objective:* **Select diagnostic studies to identify systemic manifestations of neurocutaneous disorders.** The family history should be reviewed carefully to identify anyone with possible NF-1. Because this boy was adopted internationally, details of family history may be difficult or impossible to obtain. Decreased vision in the left eye should be investigated with a brain magnetic resonance imaging (MRI) study to search for an optic glioma, which occurs commonly in NF-1. Bone dysplasia is another abnormality commonly found with NF-1 and should be investigated with radiographs. He should have a formal developmental assessment and should be followed closely for seizure activity.

66-3 C. *Learning objective:* **Develop a management plan for a newly diagnosed patient with neurofibromatosis.** This family has undergone a tremendous amount of emotional stress as a result of the adoption. The diagnosis of NF-1 is potentially devastating for parents and they will need time to absorb the information and grieve for their loss (in this case, the loss of the "ideal" adopted child). Time for further discussion of the diagnosis and its implications should be scheduled at a future date that meets the parents' needs. Medical management will be dependent on the results of imaging studies. The pediatrician has a critical role to coordinate services, provide a "medical home," and answer questions.

BIBLIOGRAPHY

Congenital Malformations

Volpe JJ: *Neurology of the newborn*, ed 3, Philadelphia, 2001, WB Saunders.

Acquired Neurologic Conditions

Levy AS: Brain tumors in children: evaluation and management, *Curr Probl Pediatr Adolesc Health Care* 35:230, 2005.

Lynch JK, Han CJ: Pediatric stroke: what do we know and what do we need to know? *Semin Neurol* 25:410, 2005.

Movement Disorders

Schlaggar BL, Mink JW: Movement disorders in children, *Pediatr Rev* 24:39, 2003.

Singer HS Tourette's syndrome: from behaviour to biology. *Lancet Neurol* 4:149, 2005.

Neurophakomatoses

DeBella K, Szudek J, Friedman JM: Use of the National Institutes of Health criteria for diagnosis of neurofibromatosis 1 in children, *Pediatrics* 105:608, 2000.

Roach ES et al: Report of the Diagnostic Criteria Committee of the National Tuberous Sclerosis Association, *J Child Neurol* 7:221, 1992.

Sleep Disorders

Hoban TF: Sleep and its disorders in children, *Semin Neurol* 24:327, 2004.

Neurodegenerative Disorders

Crumrine PK Degenerative disorders of the central nervous system, *Pediatr Rev* 22:370, 2001.

Fong CT Principles of inborn errors of metabolism: an exercise, *Pediatr Rev* 16:390, 1995.

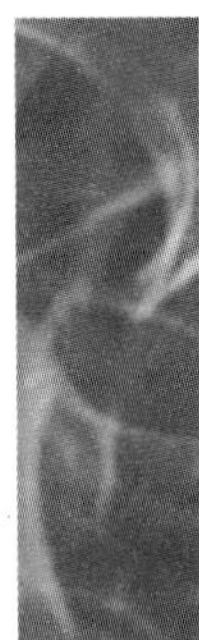

67

Newborn Issues

MICHAEL GIULIANO

THE JAUNDICED NEWBORN

ETIOLOGY

What Causes Jaundice?

Jaundice is the term used to describe the clinical appearance of a patient who has elevated indirect or direct bilirubin. Almost half of all newborns develop jaundice in the first week of life, in most cases as a physiologic process caused by elevation of indirect bilirubin. This "physiologic jaundice" develops when indirect bilirubin levels reach a peak of 8 mg/dl by the fourth day of life. Elevated direct bilirubin is uncommon, reflects a pathologic process, and usually does not become clinically apparent until several weeks of age.

What Causes Elevated Indirect Bilirubin?

Bilirubin is a breakdown product of hemoglobin. The red blood cells (RBCs) of newborns have a short life span, which means that a relatively large amount of hemoglobin is released into the circulation as the cells break down. Hemoglobin is converted first to biliverdin and then to indirect bilirubin, which is insoluble in water and must be conjugated by the liver into water-soluble direct bilirubin for excretion into the gut. Each of these steps is immature in the newborn, leading to an expected or physiologic elevation of indirect bilirubin.

What Else Causes Indirect Bilirubin to Rise?

Anything that leads to increased destruction of red blood cells, such as bruising, a cephalohematoma, or hemolysis, will result in hemoglobin breakdown and cause an abnormal elevation of bilirubin levels. Breast-feeding, dehydration, and anything that slows gastrointestinal motility can also cause elevated bilirubin levels. Rarely, infection or inborn errors of metabolism can be the cause.

What Are the Effects of Elevated Indirect Bilirubin?

Indirect bilirubin is a neurotoxin that causes central nervous system (CNS) damage when high levels cross the blood-brain barrier and produce kernicterus. The healthy full-term newborn has no risk of kernicterus at bilirubin levels *below* 25 mg/dl. A newborn infant with hemolysis, acidosis, hypoxia, or dehydration, however, has a high risk of kernicterus at much lower bilirubin levels. For example, if hemolysis is present and the bilirubin level is rising quickly, a level of 20 mg/dl appears to be the threshold at which kernicterus becomes possible. The fear of kernicterus drives almost all of the diagnostic and treatment decisions related to elevated bilirubin levels. It is important to note that premature infants may develop kernicterus at bilirubin levels much lower than for full-term newborns.

What Causes Direct Bilirubin to Become Elevated?

Direct bilirubin elevation can be seen with congenital infections, inborn errors of metabolism, liver dysfunction, and obstruction of the bile duct system. Each of these problems has a characteristic clinical presentation and associated findings that usually make the diagnosis straightforward. Direct bilirubin does not cause kernicterus, but the underlying diseases can lead to significant morbidity and mortality.

EVALUATION

How Do I Determine the Cause of Newborn Jaundice?

First, you must determine if the bilirubin is indirect or direct: Measuring total and direct bilirubin will allow calculation of the indirect fraction and immediately tell you the type of bilirubin causing the problem. The total bilirubin concentration and the age of the infant in hours can be used to predict risk for development of kernicterus using the Bhutani curve (see the Jaundice section of the Bibliography). Timing of the bilirubin elevation also helps identify the cause: If indirect bilirubin rises in the first 24 hours of life, you should suspect hemolysis caused by conditions that sensitize fetal RBCs, such as ABO incompatibility and Rh incompatibility. Elevation of indirect bilirubin after 48 hours of life is most commonly seen with physiologic jaundice, a condition that may last several days. Physical examination will often reveal bruising or a large cephalhematoma as a possible cause of jaundice. Breast-fed infants who experience difficulties with fluid intake in the first few days of life can also have elevated bilirubin, so-called breast-feeding jaundice. If indirect bilirubin rises in the second week of life, it may reflect "breast-milk jaundice," a condition thought to be caused by factors in human milk that inhibit conjugation of bilirubin. Other risk factors for elevated indirect bilirubin include prematurity, a previous sibling requiring treatment for jaundice, or East Asian race. If the cause of indirect bilirubin elevation is unclear, complete blood count (CBC), reticulocyte count, review of the peripheral blood smear, and direct Coombs' test will usually clarify the etiology. Direct bilirubin elevation is always pathologic and demands careful evaluation, although the cause is usually obvious from the history or physical examination findings.

TREATMENT

How Do I Treat a Jaundiced Baby?

Most infants with physiologic hyperbilirubinemia do not need treatment. Phototherapy is the most common treatment for elevated bilirubin. It uses light energy to change the shape of the bilirubin molecule, making indirect bilirubin water soluble so that it can be excreted into the urine. Indications for phototherapy are based on the cause of hyperbilirubinemia, the level of bilirubin, and the infant's age in hours, all of which contribute to risk of kernicterus (see the Jaundice section of the Bibliography). The uncommon infant with extremely elevated levels of indirect bilirubin must be treated aggressively to prevent kernicterus. This requires a double-volume exchange transfusion, a procedure that reduces bilirubin to nontoxic levels, but it is invasive and can have serious complications. Full-term newborns with hemolysis undergo exchange transfusion when indirect bilirubin levels are greater than 20 mg/dl, whereas those without hemolysis can tolerate 25 mg/dl before needing this procedure. Premature and ill infants may require aggressive treatment at lower levels. A new medication, tin mesoporphyrin, blocks hemoglobin breakdown, which limits bilirubin production and may decrease the need for exchange transfusion. The treatment of direct hyperbilirubinemia must address the underlying process.

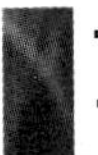

THE BLUE/CYANOTIC AND TACHYPNEIC NEWBORN

ETIOLOGY

What Causes Newborn Cyanosis and Tachypnea?

The blue or cyanotic newborn represents a medical emergency, with or without respiratory distress. First, you must decide if the infant is really blue or just bruised. Facial bruising may sometimes mimic cyanosis, but the two conditions can be distinguished by examining the mucous membranes and the rest of the body. Many problems in the newborn can cause cyanosis, but the key distinction is between cardiac and pulmonary disease. Congenital cyanotic heart disease will often present shortly after birth, although cyanosis may be delayed several days in some cases. Pulmonary disease is by far the most common cause of cyanosis and respiratory distress in the newborn.

What Are the Cardiac Causes of Cyanosis?

Lesions can range from transposition of the great vessels to hypoplasia of the right or left side of the heart. Patients with many of these lesions depend on a patent ductus arteriosus (PDA) to bring blood to the lung or body. Without a PDA these patients quickly decompensate and die, but a PDA may delay the appearance of cyanosis, making the infant look amazingly "normal."

What Pulmonary Conditions Cause Cyanosis?

Cyanosis and respiratory distress may be caused by retained fetal fluid, aspiration of meconium or blood, pneumonia, pneumothorax, surfactant deficiency, or congenital structural abnormalities of the lungs. Infants with any of these conditions will usually have tachypnea and increased work of breathing, with "grunting," intercostal space retractions, nasal flaring, and prominent abdominal breathing. Transient tachypnea of the newborn (TTN) results from retained fetal fluid and usually resolves within 24 hours, although oxygen may be needed.

EVALUATION

How Should I Evaluate a Cyanotic Infant?

Give oxygen immediately and move the baby to an environment where the temperature can be controlled and the infant can be monitored. Assess the response of the infant to the oxygen. Look for persistence or improvement of cyanosis while monitoring oxygen saturation with pulse oximetry: If administration of 100% oxygen brings the oxygen saturation to 100%, the infant probably has a pulmonary process. If oxygen saturation remains low despite 100% O_2, congenital cyanotic heart disease must be considered. The history, physical examination, and a chest radiograph will often be the only diagnostic tests that you need to determine the cause of cyanosis. The gestational age of the newborn is important: A premature infant will be at risk for surfactant deficiency, whereas an infant born after 40 weeks' gestation or who is meconium-stained will more likely have meconium aspiration syndrome. A history of resuscitation in the delivery room using positive pressure ventilation or a physical examination that demonstrates asymmetrical breath sounds would argue for a pneumothorax. Blood culture and CBC should be done routinely and antibiotics should be started while the diagnostic evaluation continues because sepsis and pneumonia can be overwhelming in the newborn. A maternal history suggestive of infection would add to this concern. The arterial blood gas (ABG) is most useful for detection of metabolic or respiratory acidosis.

TREATMENT

What Should I Do First for a Cyanotic Infant?

Provide 100% oxygen and monitor with pulse oximetry. No matter the cause of cyanosis, the overarching goal in treatment is to maintain oxygenation. If congenital cyanotic heart disease is diagnosed, intravenous administration of prostaglandin will often be needed to maintain the patency of the ductus arteriosus until corrective surgery can be done. For all pulmonary causes of cyanosis, the cornerstone of therapy is oxygen, which may require endotracheal intubation and mechanical ventilation. Close monitoring of arterial blood gas levels will be necessary in this setting. Each etiology has a specific treatment: Pneumothorax will often need to be evacuated, surfactant deficiency can be treated with surfactant replacement, pneumonia is treated with antibiotics, and the aspiration syndromes require supportive therapy. Many of the congenital structural abnormalities of the lung will require surgical treatment. Examples include diaphragmatic hernia, pulmonary sequestration, and congenital cystic adenomatoid malformation.

THE NEWBORN WITH A MURMUR

ETIOLOGY

What Causes a Heart Murmur in a Newborn Infant?

Most murmurs heard in the immediate newborn period are caused as the PDA closes in response to increasing oxygen tension and decreasing prostaglandin levels, usually in the first 3 days of life. As the PDA closes, it creates turbulent blood flow that can be heard as a murmur. A murmur may also indicate an underlying cardiac defect such as a ventricular septal defect, pulmonary stenosis, coarctation of the aorta, aortic stenosis, or tricuspid regurgitation. Newborns with congenital cyanotic heart disease can also present with a murmur, although the cyanosis is usually the first indication of heart disease.

EVALUATION

How Can I Determine the Cause of a Heart Murmur?

You should make every effort to describe the murmur that you hear. Although certain heart diseases have characteristic murmurs, both the quality and the location of murmurs in newborns may be difficult to characterize. Because most newborn murmurs result from the physiologic closing of the PDA, the initial evaluation involves a check of the oxygen saturation and four-extremity blood pressures. If the murmur persists on follow-up examinations, an electrocardiogram (ECG) will help identify the lesions of acute concern: Healthy full-term newborns have a right axis on ECG; infants with a lesion obstructing flow from the left ventricle will have a left axis on ECG. Infants with suspected aortic stenosis or coarctation of the aorta should be evaluated promptly with an echocardiogram. Careful palpation of femoral pulses will aid in detection of coarctation of the aorta. Most other infants can be followed and evaluated by echocardiogram at a later date if the murmur persists.

TREATMENT

How Is Congenital Heart Disease Treated?

Most newborns with heart murmurs do not need special treatment in the nursery. Support, monitoring, and, occasionally, oxygen usually suffice while the diagnostic evaluation is being done. An infant who has a persistently open PDA will need surgery or catheter ablation to close the PDA because of the high risk of developing bacterial endocarditis. Most infants with ventricular septal defect need no treatment unless congestive heart failure develops. Pulmonary stenosis must be followed closely to monitor the adequacy of blood flow to the pulmonary circuit. In time, this lesion may also require treatment via a catheter. Coarctation of the aorta and aortic stenosis require surgical repair. The congenital cyanotic heart lesions require complex surgical repair. Guidelines for SBE prophylaxis have been changed (see Chapter 56).

THE SMALL BABY

ETIOLOGY

How Are Small Newborns Classified?

An infant whose weight falls below the 10th percentile for gestational age is labeled "small for gestational age" (SGA). SGA babies are a heterogeneous group and are usually categorized into two patterns of growth: Infants with weight alone below the 10th percentile have *asymmetrical* growth retardation; infants who are small in all parameters (weight, head circumference, and length) have *symmetrical* growth retardation.

What Causes Asymmetrical Growth Retardation?

The etiology for asymmetrical infants usually lies with the mother's health or with the placenta. Maternal hypertension or preeclampsia commonly results in asymmetric growth retardation of a newborn infant. A small placenta caused by an abnormal uterus or a multiple-gestation pregnancy (e.g., twins) can also be the cause. Generally, the asymmetrical SGA infant has an excellent prognosis.

What Causes Symmetrical Growth Retardation?

The infant with symmetrical growth retardation is of much more concern because the underlying cause is usually fetal: Congenital infections, chromosomal abnormalities, inborn errors of metabolism, or a toxin exposure all need to be considered in the differential diagnosis. The most prominent infections include toxoplasmosis, rubella, cytomegalovirus (CMV), herpes, and syphilis. These are all included under the category of TORCHS infection (the "O" stands for "other").

EVALUATION

How Do I Evaluate the Small-for-Gestational-Age Newborn?

The physical examination should first assess the infant's gestational age. Using this information you then plot length, weight, and head circumference on a growth chart to determine whether the infant has asymmetrical or symmetrical growth retardation. *Asymmetrical growth retardation* will require mainly a review of the mother's history and the details of pregnancy, labor, and delivery. A careful physical examination will identify any anomalies. Ask the obstetrician to examine the placenta. Laboratory and imaging studies will be selected after you have considered the available information. Evaluation of *symmetrical growth retardation* is more involved.

How Do I Evaluate Symmetrical Growth Retardation?

Maternal history may disclose preeclampsia, hypertension, or chronic disease. Find out if the mother had fevers, infections, or exposure to infections during the pregnancy, especially during the first trimester. These may suggest the likelihood of TORCHS infections. Ask about family history of previous newborns with metabolic disorders and whether there any toxins in the home or work environment. Weight, length, and head circumference will already have identified the growth retardation. You should examine skin, heart, lungs, and neurologic systems. An examination of the eyes may identify cataracts. Hepatosplenomegaly will often accompany congenital infections. Dysmorphic features can be seen in the newborn with chromosomal abnormalities; look especially at the face, the ears, and the extremities.

What Tests Help in Symmetrical Growth Retardation?

The diagnostic evaluation should be guided by the findings of the history and physical examination. If no etiology is obvious in the symmetrically growth-retarded infant, a search for a congenital infection should be initiated, including IgM antibodies for specific infections, a head ultrasound, and liver function tests. Detection of metabolic acidosis would lead to a series of metabolic studies. Chromosome analysis may be needed to evaluate dysmorphic features.

TREATMENT

What Problems May Need Treatment?

Growth-retarded infants often have hypoglycemia immediately after birth, so careful attention to blood glucose level is important. Hypothermia may also develop. Babies whose birth weight is the only abnormality generally gain weight and thrive with adequate nutrition and supportive care.

Can Symmetrical Growth Retardation Be Treated?

Most conditions that cause symmetrical growth retardation do not have specific treatment, with a few exceptions: Congenital toxoplasmosis can be effectively treated with the combination of pyrimethamine, sulfadiazine, and folinic acid; some inborn errors of metabolism can be treated with dietary modification. The mainstay of treatment for most growth-retarded infants involves supportive therapy to prevent hypothermia, because SGA infants lack body fat for insulation, and hypoglycemia, because glucose stores are inadequate to maintain blood glucose levels. Close monitoring of both body temperature and blood glucose level is warranted.

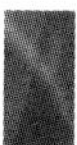

THE LARGE BABY: INFANT OF THE DIABETIC MOTHER

ETIOLOGY

Why Is the Infant of a Diabetic Mother Large?

Newborn infants whose weight is above the 90th percentile for gestational age are labeled "large for gestational age" (LGA). Poorly controlled maternal diabetes is an important cause of fetal overgrowth. Maternal hyperglycemia causes elevated glucose levels in the fetus that trigger increased fetal insulin levels. Insulin acts in the fetus as a growth hormone, leading to excessive growth and macrosomia (weight, length, and head circumference). Even infants born prematurely to diabetic mothers are LGA.

Why Does the Infant of a Diabetic Mother Develop Hypoglycemia?

Birth stops the continuous supply of glucose that was provided in utero by the placental circulation. Hyperinsulinemia caused by exposure of the fetus to chronically elevated maternal glucose persists in the newborn after the placental supply of glucose stops, placing the infant of a diabetic mother (IDM) at great risk for hypoglycemia in the hours after birth. In addition, the IDM often fails to induce the biochemical pathways for gluconeogenesis to compensate for the loss of the glucose supply. The combination of excessive insulin-induced removal of glucose from the blood and inadequate production of glucose results in significant hypoglycemia.

What Other Problems Are Common in an Infant of a Diabetic Mother?

These infants often have hypocalcemia and polycythemia and are at a higher risk for jaundice. Congenital anomalies such as cardiac defects and sacral agenesis are also more common. Respiratory distress syndrome can develop when IDMs are born prematurely.

What Are Additional Risks for the Large Infant?

The immediate risk to LGA infants occurs at the time of birth because of a much higher likelihood of birth trauma. Injuries to the brachial plexus and facial nerve occur commonly, as do cephalhematoma and caput succedaneum. An additional problem is the underdiagnosis of prematurity: An LGA infant is often assumed to be more mature than is really the case. Birth weight should not be the sole criterion used to judge a newborn's maturity. A careful assessment of gestational age with the Ballard Scale should be done for all infants. If prematurity is identified, you must make careful observations to identify complications related to prematurity.

EVALUATION

How Do I Assess Risks for an Infant of a Diabetic Mother?

A complete review of the maternal history will help estimate the risks. Has the mother had long-standing diabetes, or did it start during this pregnancy? Does the mother have any medical complications from her diabetes, especially renal or eye disease? How well was her diabetes controlled during her pregnancy? Was she on dietary control, or did she require insulin? What was the estimated size of the infant? What was the mode of delivery? The Apgar scores may give some indication of birth asphyxia. Careful assessment of gestational age with the Ballard examination is important to identify the LGA premature infant. A detailed physical examination should look for respiratory distress, congenital anomalies, and signs of birth trauma.

Are Laboratory Tests Helpful?

IDMs need to be closely monitored, using serial blood glucose determinations to detect low glucose levels. Any infant with serum glucose below 40 mg/dl needs intervention (oral or intravenous glucose) and close follow-up. A baseline CBC should be done to assess for polycythemia. The need for blood tests for calcium and bilirubin levels will depend on physical examination findings.

TREATMENT

Can Complications of Maternal Diabetes Be Prevented?

If diabetic mothers are identified early and well controlled during pregnancy, many of the problems discussed previously for the infant will never be seen. Tight control of maternal diabetes will reduce the exposure of the fetus to hyperglycemia, preventing fetal hyperinsulinemia and all of its consequences.

How Do I Manage an Infant of a Diabetic Mother?

The consequences of exposure to elevated maternal glucose should be anticipated. If the infant is expected to be LGA, a cesarean section might be planned to avoid the trauma of vaginal birth. If birth trauma occurs, it should be identified early and followed carefully. A clavicular fracture may be a tip-off that a brachial plexus injury has occurred. Most such injuries are transient and resolve with time, but surgery is sometimes required for severe brachial plexus injuries. A large cephalhematoma will likely lead to elevated bilirubin levels as the hemoglobin is reabsorbed and broken down. The jaundice is usually controlled with phototherapy. As previously noted, IDMs are at risk for polycythemia. When the hematocrit exceeds 65%, these infants should be treated with an isovolemic exchange transfusion to reduce the hematocrit. Hypocalcemia rarely is significant. After birth, LGA infants need to be fed early and often to provide adequate glucose. If blood glucose falls despite early feeding, the infant will need parenteral glucose. Most commonly, infants with hypoglycemia receive a rapid (bolus) intravenous infusion of D10W to provide 0.25 g/kg of glucose, followed by a continuous infusion of 5 to 8 mg/kg/min of glucose using D10W solution at about 100 ml/kg/day. These infants rarely need intravenous support for more than a day because their endogenous ability to generate glucose improves and their insulin levels fall.

KEY POINTS

- Most neonatal jaundice is caused by elevated levels of indirect bilirubin.
- Jaundice before 24 hours of age is most often from hemolysis.
- Administration of oxygen to a cyanotic newborn usually raises oxygen saturation if pulmonary disease is the cause of the cyanosis.
- Both SGA and LGA infants are at risk for hypoglycemia.

Case 67-1

The staff nurse notifies you that an infant in the newborn nursery is jaundiced. He was born 18 hours earlier, at full term, to a G1P1A0 healthy mother. Apgar scores were 8 at 1 minute and 9 at 5 minutes.

A. What are the most likely reasons for this jaundice?
B. What initial tests should you order?
C. What treatment(s) would be considered?
D. Your patient's bilirubin stabilized at 15 mg/dl on day 3. Do you need to do anything before he goes home?

Case 67-2

You are called to evaluate a newborn baby in the delivery room who "won't pink up." The baby was born by vaginal delivery and no problems were noted immediately. The Apgar score was 8 at 1 minute and 7 at 5 minutes.

A. What should you do first for this infant?
B. What would you look for on physical examination?
C. What would be your first diagnostic test?

Case 67-3

A 3-day-old newborn has had a murmur since birth. His oxygen saturation is 100% on pulse oximetry, and his four-extremity blood pressures are equal. His mother is eager to go home.

A. Is there any need for further diagnostic evaluation?
B. What do you tell the mother about any needed follow-up?

Case 67-4

An infant born to a mother who had no prenatal care weighs 2800 g at birth. Apgar scores were 8 at 1 minute and 9 at 5 minutes. Both the length and head circumference are below the 5th percentile for a full-term infant. Physical examination confirms that physical maturity and neurologic findings are consistent with 40 weeks' gestational age.

A. How would you classify this infant?
B. What information from the history and physical examination will assist you to evaluate this infant?
C. What immediate risk(s) does this infant face?

Case 67-5

You are called to attend a vaginal delivery at term for a diabetic mother. The estimated fetal weight was 4800 g. The delivery is complicated by shoulder dystocia. The infant is born crying and active, with Apgar scores of 8 at 1 minute and 9 at 5 minutes. You note in the delivery room that the right arm is not moving.

A. What is the most likely diagnosis? What other physical finding might you identify?
B. The parents want to know what is wrong. What do you tell them?
C. Two hours after birth the infant becomes lethargic and will not eat. What is the most likely cause for this problem?
D. How would you treat this infant?

Case Answers

67-1 A. *Learning objective:* **List the causes of newborn jaundice; recognize the importance of the age of the infant at the time jaundice is noticed.** This infant most likely has a hemolytic process caused by sensitization of fetal red blood cells by antibody from the mother, as occurs in ABO or Rh incompatibility. Intrinsic red blood cell (RBC) abnormalities such as spherocytosis can also cause early hemolysis and jaundice. Because jaundice was noted before 24 hours of age, physiologic jaundice is unlikely. Rh incompatibility is unlikely to be the cause in this case because this is the mother's first pregnancy, and she has no history of abortions that might have sensitized her. The most likely cause of hemolysis is ABO incompatibility.

67-1 B. *Learning objective:* **Select laboratory tests to evaluate newborn jaundice.** Blood should be sent to determine levels of total and direct bilirubin; the laboratory will calculate the indirect bilirubin level. Because you suspect a hemolytic process, it is also appropriate to send a sample of the infant's blood to obtain a CBC, a peripheral blood smear to determine RBC morphology, a Coombs' test, and blood type and Rh. Mother's blood should be tested to determine blood type (ABO), Rh (D), and unusual isoimmune antibodies. Further tests will depend on the results of the initial battery of studies.

67-1 C. *Learning objective:* **Explain the basic concepts that must be considered when deciding on treatment for newborn jaundice.** Treatment depends on the rate of rise of the indirect bilirubin level, the gestational age, and the health of the infant. Because hemolysis is the likely cause of jaundice, the process can be expected to continue as long as sensitized cells are in the circulation. Phototherapy may well be needed. A double-volume exchange transfusion will be needed if indirect bilirubin exceeds 20 mg/dl.

67-1 D. *Learning objective:* **Discuss management of jaundice after discharge from the nursery.** You should check the CBC to make certain that his hematocrit has not fallen too low. A reticulocyte count can be used to gauge the bone marrow response to anemia. The CBC should be followed at routine health-supervision visits. The infant should return to the clinic or office to have repeat bilirubin and hematocrit done 24 to 48 hours after discharge. In addition, because the most likely cause of this infant's jaundice is ABO incompatibility, the mother should know that hemolysis and jaundice might occur in subsequent newborn infants.

67-2 A. *Learning objective:* **Identify the cyanotic newborn infant and provide immediate management.** Cyanosis in a newborn might have a respiratory or cardiac cause. Because a respiratory problem causes the most immediate concern, you must first ensure that the airway is patent and that the infant can breathe and oxygenate the blood. The initial and 5-minute Apgar scores suggest that there is no airway obstruction, but you should check to be certain.

67-2 B. *Learning objective:* **Identify respiratory and cardiac causes of cyanosis in the newborn.** You should assess the extent of cyanosis (central vs. peripheral) and the presence of any respiratory distress (respiratory rate, nasal flaring, grunting, retractions). Listen to the heart for a murmur and to the lungs to assess breath sounds. Inspect and palpate the abdomen to identify a possible diaphragmatic hernia.

67-2 C. *Learning objective:* **Discuss the steps to evaluate a cyanotic newborn.** Measure oxygen saturation in room air with pulse oximetry, then administer 100% oxygen by face mask and reassess oxygen saturation. Subsequent tests will depend on the differential diagnosis that is developed after oxygen administration directs attention to the lungs or the heart as the cause of the cyanosis. In most cases, both a chest radiograph and an electrocardiogram will be necessary.

67-3 A. *Learning objective:* **Discuss the diagnostic evaluation of a heart murmur in a newborn infant.** If there were any concern about a left-sided obstructive lesion, an electrocardiogram and perhaps a chest radiograph would be justified. However, if the murmur is characteristic of a PDA it will disappear when the PDA closes spontaneously. No further diagnostic evaluation is needed unless the murmur persists. Another possible cause of the murmur is a small ventricular septal defect.

67-3 B. *Learning objective:* **Counsel the parents of a newborn infant about heart murmurs.** It will be important to explain that the murmur most likely represents a physiologic process, not heart disease. Routine health-supervision visits should be scheduled, at which time the heart murmur will be reevaluated. Parents should be alert to poor feeding, rapid respiratory rate, and poor weight gain.

67-4 A. *Learning objective:* **Differentiate between symmetrical and asymmetrical growth retardation in a newborn infant.** This infant has symmetrical growth retardation, because head circumference, weight, and length are all affected.

67-4 B. *Learning objective:* **List key history and physical examination findings in symmetrical growth retardation.** You should ask about general maternal health, the pregnancy, exposure to TORCHS infections, and substance abuse. Ask about the health of infants born from any previous pregnancies. Family history should attempt to identify metabolic disorders or hereditary conditions. Physical examination should search for any dysmorphic features or signs of infection.

67-4 C. *Learning objective:* **Discuss the management of the small-for-gestational-age infant.** The immediate risks include hypoglycemia and hypothermia. Later, the complications of the underlying condition must be dealt with.

67-5 A. *Learning objective:* **Identify the risks faced by the infant of a diabetic mother.** This LGA infant of a diabetic mother has most likely suffered a brachial plexus injury during vaginal birth. A clavicular fracture commonly occurs with shoulder dystocia.

67-5 B. *Learning objective:* **Explain how control of maternal diabetes reduces fetal macrosomia and hence birth trauma.** You should explain that poorly controlled maternal diabetes caused the large size of the infant, which in turn resulted in the birth trauma. It would also be important at some point to discuss control of diabetes in subsequent pregnancies to prevent such problems.

67-5 C. *Learning objective:* **Identify the metabolic complications encountered by an infant born to a poorly controlled diabetic mother.** The infant likely has hypoglycemia. Hyperinsulinemia develops in the fetus in response to chronic maternal hyperglycemia. The hyperinsulinemia persists after birth, and the newborn will rapidly develop low blood glucose and become symptomatic unless provided with an exogenous source of glucose.

67-5 D. *Learning objective:* **Discuss management of the infant of a diabetic mother.** A blood glucose test should be done immediately after birth and the infant should be fed. If he will not feed, intravenous glucose should be administered. The infant should also be monitored for other complications including polycythemia, jaundice, hypocalcemia, and congenital heart disease.

BIBLIOGRAPHY

Jaundice

American Academy of Pediatrics, Subcommittee on Hyperbilirubinemia: Management of hyperbilirubinemia in the newborn infant 35 or more weeks of gestation, *Pediatrics* 114:297, 2004. *www.pediatrics.org/cgi/content/full/114/1/297.*

The Small Baby

Stearns MR et al: Small for gestational age: a new insight? *Med Hypotheses* 53:186, 1999.

The Large Baby: Infant of The Diabetic Mother (IDM)

Carrapato MR: The infant of the diabetic mother: the critical developmental windows, *Early Pregnancy* 5:57, 2001.

Cornblath M et al: Controversies regarding definition of neonatal hypoglycemia: suggested operational thresholds, *Pediatrics* 105:1141, 2000.

Lapunzina P: Risks of congenital anomalies in large-for-gestational-age infants, *J Pediatr* 140:200, 2002.

Sperling MA, Menon RK: Infant of the diabetic mother, *Curr Ther Endocrinol Metab* 6:405, 1997.

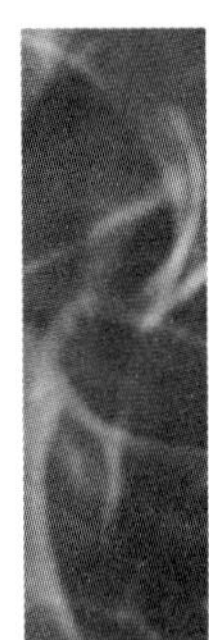

68 Orthopedics: A Practical Approach

MICHAEL R. LAWLESS

NEWBORN INFANT

ETIOLOGY

What Common Orthopedic Problems Affect Newborns?

Almost all newborns have bowing or internal curvature of the legs to some degree. Crossing one's arms and placing each hand on the opposite shoulder simulates the intrauterine position of the legs and feet of the fetus, readily explaining this transient deformity seen in the newborn. There is no force to correct this bowing until the child begins to bear weight on the legs for standing and walking. Parental reassurance may be needed.

What Is Developmental Dysplasia of the Hip?

Developmental dysplasia of the hip (DDH) is the orthopedic condition most likely to cause an adverse outcome unless diagnosed in early infancy. Identification of DDH is one of the most important goals of the newborn examination. Formerly called congenital dislocation of the hip, DDH refers to dislocation of the femoral head from the acetabulum because of incomplete formation of the acetabular roof. Predisposing factors include having a family history of DDH, being first-born, being female (9:1 female/male ratio), or being in the breech position in utero.

What Foot Problems Are Identified in the Newborn?

Metatarsus varus is a common finding, whereas talipes equinovarus (clubfoot) occurs uncommonly. Metatarsus varus, also referred to as metatarsus adductus or "C-foot," most often is a flexible positional deformity and less commonly is a rigid structural deformity. Clubfoot is a rigid deformity of the bony structures in the ankle and foot.

It can be idiopathic (75%) or may occur in association with other neuromuscular disorders.

EVALUATION

How Do I Detect Developmental Dysplasia of the Hip?

Careful examination of the hips is mandatory for all newborns. The Ortolani maneuver identifies the dislocated hip, and the Barlow maneuver identifies the dislocatable hip. Careful attention to proper technique is critical (See Chapter 5 and Figure 5-4). You must be able to distinguish DDH from a capsular or ligamentous click, which is a benign finding similar to the "popping" that might occur in your own joints. This click is very different from the gross "clunk" felt when a hip is reduced or dislocated by the Ortolani or Barlow maneuver, respectively. The examination for DDH is done on each physical examination until the age of 1 year, but after age 2 to 3 months, the dislocated hip cannot be reduced by the Ortolani maneuver, and limited abduction is the abnormal finding in DDH. Ultrasonography is the preferred imaging modality when DDH is suspected.

How Do I Distinguish the Various Foot Deformities?

All foot deformities are identified by visual inspection and by manipulation to determine whether the deformity is flexible or rigid. The lateral border of the sole of the foot should be a straight line. Metatarsus varus (Figure 68-1D) is present if the foot curves inward (like the letter C). If the curve can be easily straightened, it represents a flexible deformity. A fixed deformity cannot be easily straightened. Talipes equinovarus or clubfoot requires three features for diagnosis: hindfoot equinus (plantarflexion of the foot at the ankle), hindfoot varus (inversion deformity of the heel), and forefoot varus. This deformity cannot be straightened by simple manipulation.

TREATMENT

Does Developmental Dysplasia of the Hip Require Surgical Correction?

If DDH is diagnosed early, stabilization of the femoral head in the acetabulum by use of a harness that maintains the femurs in abduction is curative. The Pavlik harness is one example of such a treatment device. Use of "double" or "triple" diapers is not an acceptable treatment for the newborn with DDH. In more severe cases, generally meaning those in which recognition was delayed, DDH is managed by casting or surgery, and the likelihood of a good outcome is less.

Is Treatment Needed for Physiologic Deformities?

Physiologic or positional deformities of the foot and tibia do not require any treatment. Flexible metatarsus varus is often "treated" by daily stretching to straighten the lateral border of the foot, but there is little evidence that such manipulation hastens correction of the curve. Advise patience and remind parents that tibial bowing will correct when the child begins to bear weight on the legs for standing and walking.

How Are Rigid Deformities Managed?

Rigid metatarsus varus will respond to casting for 2 to 3 weeks. This is generally best left to an orthopedist familiar with pediatric problems. Talipes equinovarus is a much more serious problem that can significantly impair ankle and foot function if left untreated. Current management involves serial casting and long-term orthopedic follow-up. Surgical repair may be needed in the most severe cases.

OLDER INFANTS AND TODDLERS

ETIOLOGY

What Orthopedic Problems Affect This Age Group?

Older infants and toddlers commonly have deformities of the extremities, mainly of the legs, that provoke parental concern. Most do not cause long-lasting problems and do not require any treatment, but you must be able to identify them so that you can reassure worried parents. The deformities reflect physiologic variations of "normal" and include either angulation at a joint or rotation along a long bone (Figure 68-1). Angular deformities affect the knees (genu valgus and genu varus) and the feet (metatarsus varus—also called metatarsus adductus). Although metatarsus varus should be identified and managed in the newborn, it may be undetected until the child begins to walk and parents experience problems finding shoes that fit. Rotational deformities affect the femur (femoral anteversion or retroversion) and the tibia (tibial torsion). Femoral anteversion describes internal rotation of the femur, and femoral retroversion describes external rotation. Both cause the feet to turn away from the expected straight position and may be associated with tripping or gait patterns that concern parents. Internal tibial torsion (ITT) refers to rotation along the long axis of the bone, not bowing. The rotation of ITT is toward the midline, resulting in the feet also "turning in" toward the midline.

What Is Nursemaid's Elbow?

The term *nursemaid's elbow* refers to subluxation of the head of the radius. This common toddler injury often happens when the toddler trips while holding an adult's hand. The adult reflexively attempts to bring the falling child back to his or her feet. The child's arm is sharply pulled against resistance, which causes the annular ligament to slide over the head of the radius. The child dramatically stops using the arm and complains of pain.

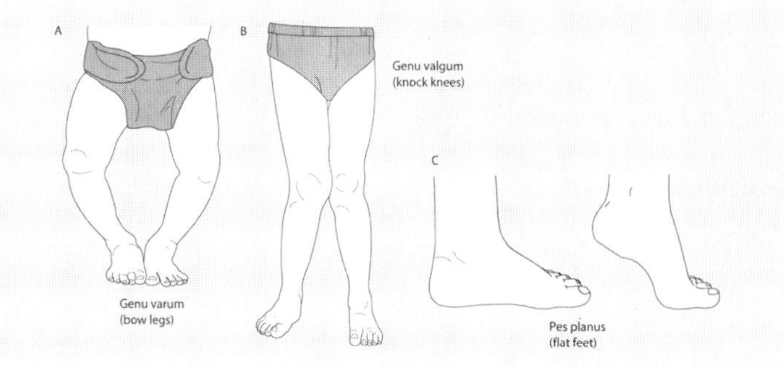

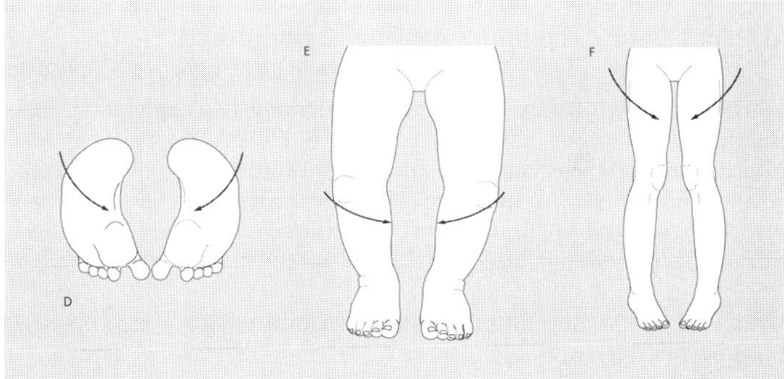

FIGURE 68-1 Physiologic variations of feet and legs. **A,** Genu varum (bow leg). **B,** Genu valgum (knock knees). **C,** Pes planus (flat feet). **D,** Metatarsus adductus. **E,** Medial tibial torsion. **F,** Femoral anteversion. (From Pang D, Newson B, editors: *Crash course paediatrics,* ed 2, London, 2005, Mosby.)

EVALUATION

How Are Positional Leg Deformities Detected?

Parents often bring these deformities to the attention of the physician by expressing concern that "toes turn in" or that "the legs are bowed." "Tripping" is another concern brought up by parents of toddlers. Whether angular or rotational, positional deformities are detected by inspection of the affected extremity and comparison with the opposite. Knowledge of the range of physiologic variation is important and is described for the specific conditions that follow. Watching the child walk helps to identify the problem.

How Do I Describe an Angular Deformity?

The first term of a condition names the anatomic location of the extremity, such as metatarsus; the second term describes the position of the extremity distal to that location in relationship to the midline. *Varus* means tilted toward the midline. *Valgus* means tilted away from the midline. Therefore, the term *metatarsus varus* indicates that the part of the foot distal to the metatarsal is tilted toward the midline. Applying this terminology scheme, does the term *genu valgus* describe knock-knee or bowleg?

How Do I Detect Internal Tibial Torsion?

ITT is most objectively assessed by palpation of the tibial tuberosity in the midline of the tibia to center the leg. Then palpate the medial and lateral malleoli. The medial malleolus should be 10 to 15 degrees anterior to the lateral malleolus in the horizontal plane. In the presence of moderate ITT, the malleoli are in the same plane. With severe internal torsion, the lateral malleolus is anterior. When affected children are viewed straight-on while standing, the knees seem to be aligned, but the feet are turned inward.

How Do I Detect Femoral Rotational Deformities?

The range of rotation of the femur is 100 to 110 degrees. With the child lying supine, grasp each lower leg, then internally and externally rotate the femurs to determine if rotation is excessive in either direction. Very few children (or adults) have equal inward and outward rotation of the femur. Most individuals have some degree of either excessive internal or external rotation. In contrast to ITT, when affected children are viewed straight on while standing, both the knees and the feet turn inward (or outward).

What Will I Find on Examination of a Child with Nursemaid's Elbow?

The child usually refuses to use the arm, holding it in a pronated and slightly flexed position, and resists any movement. The key to recognition is the history of sudden pulling or jerking of the arm. Because of lack of ossification of the radial head, no radiographic abnormality is visible, so radiologic studies are not needed.

TREATMENT

How Are Positional Deformities Treated?

Growth and weight bearing resolve almost all positional deformities without need for treatment. An important part of the pediatrician's job is to recognize physiologic variations in children and explain them to parents, thus reducing parental worry and preventing unnecessary referrals. Children are usually slightly bowlegged when they begin to walk. ITT usually improves within 3 to 6 months from the onset of walking. By age 3 to 4 years, the norm is to have some degree of genu valgus, or knock-knee. Straight alignment of the tibia and femur occurs by age 8 to 9 years, although many individuals remain slightly knock-kneed as adults. Both internal and external femoral rotation tend to self-correct toward the midline as the child grows up to 8 to 10 years of age. Some parents request prescriptions for shoes or orthotic inserts as treatment for various leg and foot "problems." As a general rule, shoes and inserts do not affect the physiologic progression that will eventually resolve the problem. Referral to a pediatric orthopedist may be needed to convince parents that such devices are not needed.

What If a Problem Is Severe or Does Not Improve?

Once you identify a serious or refractory problem, referral of the child to a pediatric orthopedist will ensure the best management. You must maintain contact with the family and include assessment of the child's orthopedic problem in regular health assessment visits. Regular communication with the orthopedist is also essential.

Can Nursemaid's Elbow Be Treated in the Office?

To reduce a nursemaid's elbow, hold the affected elbow in one hand and put pressure over the radial head. Then fully supinate the forearm while moving the arm from full flexion to full extension. This maneuver usually reduces the annular ligament, typically with a palpable click. Successful treatment of nursemaid's elbow results in immediate resolution of the pain and prompt return of full use of the arm.

How Do I Give Advice about Shoes for a Toddler?

Satisfactory development of the human foot does not depend on shoes. The main purpose of shoes, other than fashion, is protection of the feet. Shoes are not essential to support the ankle or to assist in balance of the child who is now walking. The more support or work done naturally by the child's feet and ankles, the better. Desirable features of toddler shoes include a flexible, flat sole without a heel, adequate size to accommodate rapidly growing feet, and moderate traction. These criteria are easily met by relatively inexpensive shoes. There is no need for expensive high-top leather shoes with thick, rigid soles. A child's arch develops gradually over the first 6 to 8 years of life. Having an apparent flat foot in a young child is a variation of normal that does not require special shoes.

CHILD AND ADOLESCENT

ETIOLOGY

What Orthopedic Problems Should Concern Me?

Worrisome orthopedic problems that come to the general pediatrician's attention include aseptic necrosis of the hip (Legg-Calvé-Perthes disease [LCPD]), slipped capital femoral epiphysis (SCFE), and scoliosis. Some knowledge of sports medicine is also important for pediatricians and other physicians who care for adolescents.

What Is Legg-Calvé-Perthes Disease?

This condition is one cause of limp and persistent hip pain, most commonly in preschool to early-school-age boys at a mean age of 6 to 7 years.

Although the exact pathophysiology of LCPD remains unclear, the femoral head appears to undergo avascular necrosis resulting in synovitis. Permanent disability may result if the degeneration is advanced.

What Causes Slipped Capital Femoral Epiphysis?

In SCFE, slippage occurs in the epiphysis of the femoral head, causing pain that may be felt either directly in the hip or referred to the knee. A key to identification of SCFE, especially when it presents as knee pain, is awareness that it characteristically occurs in the obese preadolescent or early adolescent in whom the epiphyses have not yet closed. It can also occur in tall, thin adolescents who are experiencing a rapid growth spurt. In the mature adolescent, SCFE is no longer a consideration because epiphyses have closed.

What Should I Know about Scoliosis?

Idiopathic scoliosis is the most common form of lateral curvature of the spine (see Figure 5-5). It occurs and progresses only in the growing spine, so it is most commonly detected during the adolescent growth spurt. Once skeletal maturity is achieved and growth is completed, there should be no further progression of mild or moderate scoliosis. Scoliosis caused by vertebral abnormalities is usually detected earlier in life and is typically more severe than the idiopathic form.

What Should I Know about Sports Medicine?

Participation in sports by school-aged children and adolescents can be a positive experience but may be associated with injuries. All school districts require that a physician provide "clearance" for sports participation in high school. Hence, athletes receive a preparticipation medical evaluation, after which the physician may authorize unlimited participation, advise limited participation, or request additional evaluation of the athlete. Few conditions completely exclude a young athlete from participation in all sports. The physician may provide guidance as to which sport is best suited for the athlete in question.

What Is Osgood-Schlatter Disease?

Osgood-Schlatter disease (OSD) is a common cause of recurrent knee pain in the young athlete. It is seen especially during the adolescent growth spurt and is an example of an overuse syndrome caused by repetitive microtrauma to affected ligaments, tendons, or bones. In this case, repetitive traction of the powerful quadriceps muscle on its insertion at the tibial tuberosity results in inflammation and painful swelling of the surrounding soft tissue. The pain progressively worsens if a high level of activity continues.

When Does Ankle Trauma Cause a Growth Plate Injury?

An ankle injury in a young adolescent is more likely to damage the epiphysis than cause a sprain. A pulling or twisting force will disrupt the integrity of the open epiphysis or growth plate of the distal tibia before the ligaments of the ankle stretch or tear. A similar force and mechanism of injury in a mature adolescent or adult will cause the ligaments to stretch or tear (a sprain), whereas the fused epiphysis and metaphysis are unyielding.

EVALUATION

How Do I Diagnose Legg-Calvé-Perthes Disease?

The history of mild or intermittent pain and limp in a 4- to 6-year-old child should prompt careful examination of the hip. Muscle spasm with limitation of abduction and internal rotation of the affected leg may be found on physical examination. Radiologic assessment is needed because the degree of degeneration and subsequent reossification of necrotic bone in the healing process determine the shape and appearance of the femoral head on plain radiograph of the hip.

What Findings Suggest Slipped Capital Femoral Epiphysis?

Physical findings seen with slippage of the femoral head epiphysis include external rotation of the affected femur when a straight-leg raise is done or limited internal rotation of the affected femur. When SCFE is suspected, radiographic confirmation should be sought immediately and weight bearing should be avoided until the condition is ruled out. The femoral head is usually displaced medially and posteriorly relative to the femoral neck.

What Is a Sports Preparticipation Evaluation?

This evaluation should identify any medical concerns that would put the young athlete at risk during sports participation. An examination should always be accompanied by a careful review of family and personal medical history, including history of previous injury. A personal history of syncope, chest pain, or palpitations with exercise or a family history of sudden death or serious cardiovascular problems would merit further evaluation before clearing the athlete for sports participation. In addition to cardiovascular assessment, a general musculoskeletal examination is done to assess joint range of motion, gross muscle strength, and muscle asymmetry (Figure 68-2). History of injury or findings suggestive of injury should prompt specific orthopedic examination.

How Is Scoliosis Identified?

The earliest manifestation of scoliosis is vertebral rotation. In the erect position, the spine may appear straight, but in the forward-bending position, early vertebral rotation is seen as asymmetrical elevation of the thoracic or lumbar spine. The forward-bending test (see Figure 5-5) allows early recognition of the condition and of the potential for progressive scoliosis. Age 8 to 10 years, just before the adolescent growth spurt, is a key time to examine for scoliosis. Incorporating the erect and

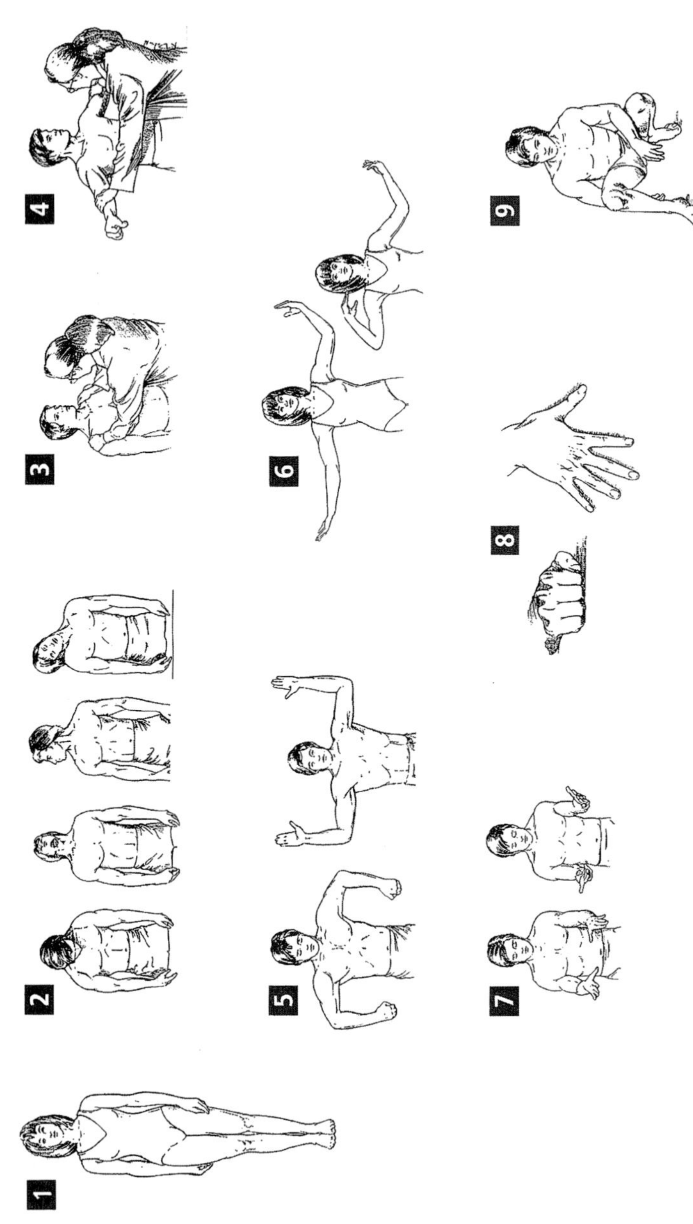
1
2
3
4
5
6
7
8
9

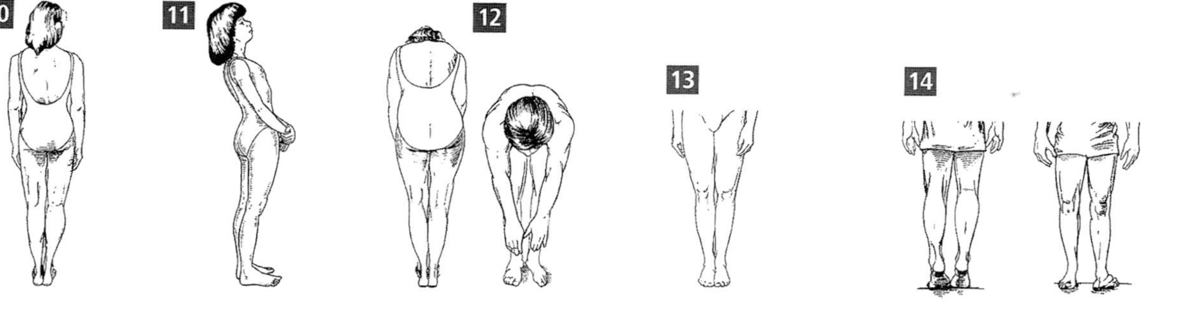

1. Inspection, athlete standing, facing toward examiner (symmetry of trunk, upper extremities);
2. Forward flexion, extension, rotation, lateral flexion of neck (range of motion, cervical spine);
3. Resisted shoulder shrug (strength, trapezius);
4. Resisted shoulder abduction (strength, deltoid);
5. Internal and external rotation of shoulder (range of motion, glenohumeral joint);
6. Extension and flexion of elbow (range of motion, elbow);
7. Pronation and supination of elbow (range of motion, elbow and wrist);
8. Clench fist, then spread fingers (range of motion, hand and fingers);
9. "Duck walk" four steps (motion of hip, knee, and ankle; strength; balance);
10. Inspection, athlete facing away from examiner (symmetry of trunk, upper extremities);
11. Back extension, knees straight (spondylolysis/ spondylolisthesis);
12. Back flexion with knees straight, facing toward and away from examiner (range of motion, thoracic and lumbosacral spine; spine curvature; hamstring flexibility);
13. Inspection of lower extremities, contraction of quadriceps muscles (alignment, symmetry);
14. Standing on toes, then on heels (symmetry, calf; strength; balance).

FIGURE 68-2 The "two-minute" musculoskeletal screening examination. (From Smith, 1997. American Academy of Family Physicians, American Academy of Pediatrics, American Medical Society for Sports Medicine, American Orthopaedic Society for Sports Medicine, and American Osteopathic Academy of Sports Medicine.)

forward-bending spinal examination routinely in the physical examination of all school-aged children will decrease the chance of omitting it in the early-adolescent child. When curvature is apparent, radiography of the spine is needed to determine the extent of the scoliosis.

Are Tests Needed to Evaluate Osgood-Schlatter Disease?

OSD is diagnosed clinically when physical examination identifies swelling and tenderness of the tibial tubercle. Radiography is not needed. If obtained, a radiograph of the tibia shows soft tissue swelling and often some degree of avulsion or fragmentation of the affected tibial tubercle; the unaffected knee may show a similar x-ray appearance of the tibial tubercle.

How Do I Recognize a Growth Plate Injury?

In the mildest form of growth plate injury, radiography of the ankle will show no abnormality. A clue that the pain and swelling are because of growth plate injury rather than a ligament sprain is the presence of point tenderness directly over the lateral malleolus at the growth plate junction. Pain of a sprained ankle is maximal in the soft tissue when the joint is stressed. In more severe growth plate injury, fracture through the growth plate or the tibial metaphysis is evident on radiograph.

TREATMENT

How Are Legg-Calvé-Perthes Disease and Slipped Capital Femoral Epiphysis Treated?

Although largely a self-healing process, containment of the femoral head in the acetabulum and maintaining good mobility of the joint are important to successful remolding and optimal outcome for LCPD. In SCFE, surgical closure of the epiphysis is usually required.

How Is Scoliosis Treated?

The finding of scoliosis in a preadolescent should result in referral to an orthopedist with follow-up at the interval recommended. In most cases of idiopathic scoliosis, no treatment will be needed. Progressive idiopathic scoliosis will require bracing, managed by a pediatric orthopedist. Scoliosis caused by vertebral anomalies may require surgical correction.

What Treatment Is Appropriate for Osgood-Schlatter Disease?

OSD, like other overuse syndromes, responds to a relative decrease in the level of activity, icing of the affected tissue following exercise, and oral antiinflammatory medication such as ibuprofen. A protective pad over the tibial tuberosity is helpful to some athletes. Quadriceps strengthening exercises may help prevent recurrence.

How Should a Growth Plate Injury Be Treated?

A growth plate injury should be immobilized by casting.

KEY POINTS

- You must assess all infants for developmental dysplasia of the hip.
- Growth and weight bearing resolve almost all positional deformities.
- Slipped capital femoral epiphysis should be suspected in an obese preadolescent with hip or knee pain.
- The sports preparticipation examination screens all major joints for range of motion and deformities.

Case 68-1

A 12-hour-old 3500-g term infant girl is seen in the newborn nursery for her admission physical examination. Pregnancy, labor, and delivery were uncomplicated, and Apgar scores were 8 and 9 at 1 and 5 minutes, respectively. Your attending physician asks you how you will assess this infant for orthopedic abnormalities.

A. What are the common orthopedic problems of the newborn infant?
B. What is the role of intrauterine position in newborn orthopedic findings?
C. Which of the newborn orthopedic problems require immediate intervention?

Case 68-2

An 18-month-old boy is seen in the office for his health-supervision visit. He has been walking since age 13 months. His mother is concerned that he is "pigeon-toed." He tripped last week while holding her hand and developed "nursemaid's elbow" that was treated in the emergency department. She wants to know if braces would correct the pigeon-toe or if special shoes would help him walk better. If not, she asks what type of regular shoe is recommended.

A. What are the common orthopedic problems seen in older infants and toddlers?
B. What should the parents know about selecting shoes for a toddler?
C. What is "nursemaid's elbow" and how does it occur?

Case 68-3

An 11-year-old boy soccer player comes to your office for a sports physical examination. He has a 2-month history of right leg pain, now accompanied by a limp. The limp is especially noticeable following soccer practice. He wants you to sign the form that will allow him to play soccer again this coming year.

A. What problems related to sports participation does a pediatrician see? What might this patient's problem be?
B. What is different about an examination for sports participation?
C. What serious orthopedic problems occur in the older child and adolescent?

Case Answers

68-1 A. *Learning objective:* **State the common orthopedic problems of the newborn infant.** The most common orthopedic problems of the newborn infant are deformities from intrauterine position, developmental dysplasia of the hip, metatarsus varus, and talipes equinovarus (clubfoot).

68-1 B. *Learning objective:* **State the role of intrauterine position in newborn orthopedic findings.** Intrauterine positioning of the feet and legs can result in bowing of the tibias and varus positioning of the foot and may predispose to developmental dysplasia of the hip.

68-1 C. *Learning objective:* **Recognize which of the newborn orthopedic problems require immediate intervention.** Rigid metatarsus varus, talipes equinovarus (clubfoot), and developmental dysplasia of the hip(s) all require intervention in the immediate newborn period.

68-2 A. *Learning objective:* **State the common orthopedic problems seen in older children and toddlers.** The common orthopedic problems seen in infants and toddlers include internal tibial torsion, internal and external femoral rotation, and nursemaid's elbow.

68-2 B. *Learning objective:* **State the recommendations to parents in selecting shoes for their child.** Shoes for the infant/toddler should be roomy and have a flat and flexible sole, a porous upper shoe, and reasonable traction. Shoes are not essential to healthy development of the child's foot.

68-2 C. *Learning objective:* **Define nursemaid's elbow and explain its occurrence.** Nursemaid's elbow is subluxation of the head of the radius. It results from sudden and forceful traction on the toddler's extended arm. This commonly occurs when a child trips while holding the hand of an adult. It causes immediate pain but is easily reduced.

68-3 A. *Learning objective:* **State some of the problems seen by the pediatrician related to sports participation.** The pediatrician may see Osgood-Schlatter disease and other overuse syndromes, as well as growth plate injuries that may resemble sprain injuries in mature athletes. The patient in this case is young for Osgood-Schlatter disease. He may well have an overuse injury, but an injury to the growth plate must be considered in the differential diagnosis.

68-3 B. *Learning objective:* **Describe the unique aspects of the examination done for sports participation.** The sports preparticipation examination must identify information from the personal and family history that might put the athlete at risk. It also includes an expanded musculoskeletal assessment.

68-3 C. *Learning objective:* **State several serious orthopedic problems that occur in the older child and adolescent.** Some of the serious orthopedic problems of the older child and adolescent are scoliosis, slipped capital femoral epiphysis, and Legg-Calvé-Perthes disease.

BIBLIOGRAPHY

Huurman WW, Ginsburg GM: Musculoskeletal injury in children, *Pediatr Rev* 18:429, 2004.

Metzel JD: Preparticipation examination of the adolescent athlete: I, *Pediatr Rev* 22:199, 2001.

Metzel JD: Preparticipation examination of the adolescent athlete: II, *Pediatr Rev* 22:227, 2001.

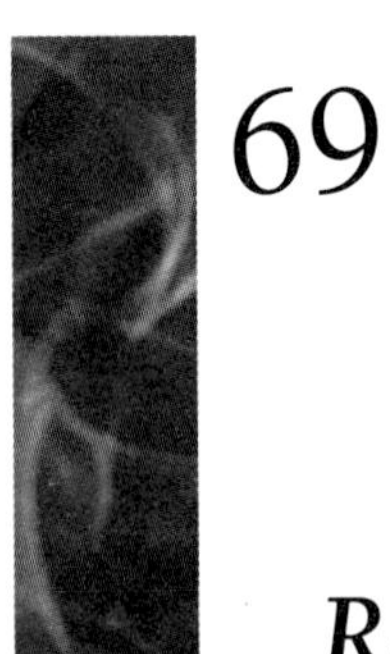

69 Respiratory Conditions

TIMOTHY D. STARNER and ROBIN R. DETERDING

ASTHMA

ETIOLOGY

What Is Asthma?

Asthma is characterized by hyperresponsiveness to a variety of stimuli that provoke reversible airway obstruction. Airway obstruction is caused by two main processes: *bronchospasm* from constriction of smooth muscles around the airway and *inflammation* with edema of the respiratory mucosa and increased mucus production. Symptomatically, airway obstruction may produce cough, chest tightness or pain, decreased air flow, and wheezing.

What Are the Common Clinical Patterns of Asthma?

Intermittent asthma is the most common pattern of asthma in children. Other patterns are *persistent asthma* and *seasonal allergic asthma* (Table 69-1). Although the National Asthma guidelines classify intermittent asthma as "mild," symptoms during an exacerbation of intermittent asthma in a child may be severe enough to warrant hospitalization. Therefore, intermittent asthma in childhood is best considered to have a range of severity from mild to severe. Young children commonly have a pattern of frequent, recurrent exacerbations of asthma, usually triggered by viral upper respiratory infections (URIs). Approximately 15% of children have 12 or more URIs a year, each of which may trigger an acute asthma exacerbation. This translates to approximately one URI-triggered asthma "attack" every 3 to 4 weeks for many young asthmatics during the fall and winter viral infection season. The frequency of URI-induced exacerbations makes the distinction between intermittent and persistent asthma difficult in infants and toddlers.

Table 69-1

Common Patterns of Asthma in Infants and Children

Classification	Onset	Symptoms	Allergic Rhinitis
Intermittent (mild/ moderate/severe)	Infancy	Mainly with URIs, none in between	Rare
Persistent (mild/ moderate/severe)	Infancy-childhood	Daily with episodic exacerbations	Common
Seasonal allergic	Childhood	Depends on specific allergy(ies)	Yes

URIs, Upper respiratory infections.

Do the National Asthma Guidelines Apply to Children?

The guidelines from the National Asthma Education and Prevention Program (NAEPP) place major emphasis on persistent asthma, the most common form in adults. The guidelines classify asthma as mild intermittent, mild persistent, moderate persistent, and severe persistent. Asthma in infancy and early childhood tends to have an intermittent pattern, although as children reach school age, the prevalence of atopic, IgE-mediated, and persistent asthma increases. Frequent recurrent viral-induced intermittent exacerbations that are commonly seen in early childhood are less well covered by the guidelines. As mentioned earlier, symptoms of intermittent asthma in children range from mild to severe.

Table 69-2

Common Triggers for Asthma

Cause	Season
Viral illness	Fall–spring
Exercise	With exercise, year-round
Irritant (smoke, perfume, etc.)	With exposure, year-round
Cold air	Winter
Allergies	
Molds	Spring and fall
Pollens	Spring–summer
Cats/dogs	Year-round
Grasses	Spring–summer
Dust mites	Year-round
Cockroaches	Year-round

What Are Common Triggers for Childhood Asthma?

Table 69-2 shows common triggers for asthma and their usual timing. All patterns of asthma can be exacerbated by viral illnesses. Up to 85% of acute exacerbations that require emergency department (ED) or hospital care are associated with viral illnesses.

EVALUATION

What History and Examination Findings Are Important?

The asthmatic child or adolescent often comes to attention because of cough (see Chapter 25). Table 69-3 shows important history and physical findings in asthma. Asthma diagnosis is primarily made from the patient's history and response to medications.

Table 69-3

Findings in Asthma

History	Physical Examination
Response to albuterol (immediate)	Increased respiratory rate
Response to oral steroids (1-3 days)	Expiratory wheezing
Symptoms between exacerbations	Decreased air movement during forced expiration
Triggers of asthma	Increased expiratory phase
Frequency and timing of exacerbations	Anxiety, fatigue, or confusion
History of intubations, ICU hospitalizations, or ED visits	Nasal flaring, retractions, and accessory muscle use
Cough at night	Inability to speak in complete sentences
Cough with exercise	Eczema
Allergic rhinitis symptoms	
Pet and tobacco exposures	
Family history of asthma	

ED, Emergency department; ICU, intensive care unit.

What Tests Are Helpful in Diagnosing Asthma?

Pulmonary function tests can document reversibility of airway obstruction. Pulse oximetry obtained during an asthma exacerbation may show decreased oxygen saturation, and any value below 92% should be viewed with concern as this is the start of the steep portion of the oxygen desaturation curve. A blood gas determination will occasionally detect increased $PaCO_2$, but this is a late finding that may indicate impending respiratory failure. If a chest radiograph is obtained, it may show hyperinflation but could also have areas of streaky atelectasis and peribronchial thickening, similar in pattern to viral bronchiolitis. Methacholine challenge or exercise testing can provoke bronchoconstriction in a patient who is not currently symptomatic. Radioallergosorbent testing (RAST) or skin testing can be useful to identify potential allergens. A symptom diary helps identify the timing, pattern and triggers of asthma.

How Does a Therapeutic Trial Help with Diagnosis?

A therapeutic trial of bronchodilators usually relieves symptoms of bronchospasm, but there may be little or no relief if bronchospasm is accompanied by airway inflammation. A therapeutic trial of oral corticosteroids (5 to 7 days, maximum 10 days) should completely reverse the inflammation and relieve all asthma symptoms. If a patient's symptoms fail to clear completely after an adequate course of steroids, then diagnoses other than asthma should be considered.

How Can Peak Flow Meters Be Used to Monitor Asthma?

Peak expiratory flow rate falls during asthma exacerbations. A child older than 5 or 6 years can usually be taught to use a peak flow meter to allow symptom monitoring, which can guide medication use. The peak flow meter is especially useful for those patients who underestimate or do not recognize the severity of their symptoms. The predicted average peak flow for a child is based on height, but peak flow should be determined individually for each child by frequent measurements when the patient is well.

TREATMENT

How Would I Treat an Acute Exacerbation of Asthma?

An inhaled bronchodilator should be the first medication prescribed. Oral bronchodilators are much less effective than inhaled forms and have increased side effects. If there is incomplete response to inhaled bronchodilators, or if treatments are needed more often than every 4 hours (or more than four times a day), then a short course of oral corticosteroids should be started. For older patients who are able to check peak flows, persistent flows in the "red zone" should also prompt treatment with oral steroids. Early intervention with oral steroids can decrease hospitalizations by 90% and clinic visits by 50%. Pediatricians often prescribe oral steroids to be kept on hand at home and teach parents how to recognize symptoms that warrant use of steroids. This decreases the time to initiation of therapy and duration of symptoms.

When Should an Asthmatic Be Hospitalized?

Most asthmatics can be treated as outpatients. Table 69-4 shows key reasons for hospitalization.

How Are Oral Steroids Prescribed for Acute Asthma?

For acute exacerbations of asthma, daily oral prednisone or prednisolone is typically prescribed at a dose of 1 to 2 mg/kg/day divided into two equal doses and continued until the patient's symptoms are entirely resolved for at least 1 day. This generally takes from 5 to 7 days. Discontinuation of treatment before complete resolution of symptoms may result in a rebound of cough and wheeze. There is usually a 1- to 3-day lag time between starting oral steroids and improvement of

Table 69-4

Criteria for Hospital Admission in Asthma

Criteria
Critically ill
Severe airway obstruction with respiratory distress
Increased $PaCO_2$
Poor response to emergency department therapies
Greater than 3 or 4 bronchodilator treatments
Oxygen saturations < 90%
Social considerations
Unreliable parents, transportation, or telephone
Home is far from nearest medical facility

symptoms, although response may be slower if the inflammation is severe or more chronic. Oral steroid treatment for asthma generally should not be continued past 10 days.

Should Steroids Be Tapered?

Tapering of steroids is not necessary for courses shorter than 14 days. Tapering increases the length of steroid therapy, subjects the patient to subtherapeutic doses that are not clinically useful, and increases the potential for side effects.

What Are the Side Effects of Steroids?

Short courses of oral steroids generally have minor, but often distressing, temporary side effects that include increased appetite, irritability, joint aches, and stomach ache. If steroids must be used frequently in short courses or for prolonged courses (> 14 days), more prominent side effects may occur, including Cushingoid features and hyperglycemia. Table 69-5 shows common corticosteroid side effects. Oral steroids also have a bitter taste, which complicates adherence to the treatment plans for young children.

Table 69-5

Corticosteroid Side Effects

Minor	Major
Behavior changes	Growth suppression
Sleep disturbances	Osteoporosis
Appetite changes (usually increase)	Hypothalamic-pituitary axis suppression
Acne or puffy red cheeks	Cushingoid appearance
Gastrointestinal upset and bowel habit changes	Skin thinning or striae
Oropharyngeal candidiasis (inhaled steroids)	Hirsutism
Joint aches	Immunosuppression
Weight gain	Hyperglycemia

How Is Persistent Asthma Treated?

Patients with persistent asthma have daily or near-daily symptoms, including difficulty with exercise and night waking with shortness of breath or cough. These patients often use albuterol daily but have inadequate relief of symptoms. Maintenance medications taken daily may reduce or prevent the symptoms of persistent asthma. Intermittent asthmatics do not benefit from maintenance asthma medications because these medications neither prevent symptoms of viral-induced intermittent asthma nor decrease the frequency of asthma exacerbations.

How Do I Choose a Medication for Persistent Asthma?

Table 69-6 lists different classes of maintenance medications for persistent asthma and shows some advantages and disadvantages of each. *Inhaled steroids* are generally the first line treatment for persistent asthma. The newer inhaled steroids—budesonide (Pulmicort), fluticasone (Flovent), or beclomethasone HFA (Qvar)—are more effective at lower doses than older preparations. Although *long-acting beta-agonists* are not as effective as inhaled steroids for monotherapy, medications such as salmeterol (Serevent) act synergistically with inhaled steroids and allow a decrease in steroid dose. They are available in combination with inhaled steroids, such as fluticasone/salmeterol

Table 69-6

Maintenance Medications for Asthma

Class	Advantages	Disadvantages
Inhaled steroid	Daily-BID dosing Long half-life	Can have growth suppression at high doses
Long-acting beta-agonists	BID dosing	Less effective as monotherapy Small but significant increase in asthma-related deaths, especially in African-Americans
Combination therapy: inhaled steroids and long-acting beta-agonists	Improved control with lower inhaled steroid doses Antiinflammatory + bronchodilator	Both inhaled steroid and long-acting beta-agonist disadvantages
Leukotriene modifiers	Oral medication Few side effects (Singulair)	Usually only effective in mild persistent asthmatics
Theophylline	Oral medication	Narrow therapeutic window Requires drug levels
Mast cell stabilizers	Minimal side effects QID dosing	Minimal therapeutic effects

BID, Twice per day; QID, four times per day.

(Advair). Recently, a small but significant increase in asthma-related deaths or life-threatening experiences was found in African-Americans older than 12 years using salmeterol in addition to their usual asthma care (Nelson et al., 2006). Montelukast (Singulair) is the preferred *leukotriene modifier* because it is a once-a-day medication with almost no side effects. Other leukotriene modifiers are either more difficult to administer or have more side effects: zileuton (Zyflo) must be given four times a day and can have hepatotoxicity, and zafirlukast (Accolate) must be given twice a day and has some drug-drug interactions. *Mast cell stabilizers*, cromolyn (Intal) and nedocromil (Tilade), have almost no effective role in the treatment of childhood asthma. Although *theophylline* (Theo-Dur, Slo-bid) is effective, it is not often prescribed because of the potential side effects and narrow therapeutic window.

What Dose of Inhaled Steroid Should I Prescribe?

The preferred approach to inhaled steroid dosing is to start at a mid- to-high-level dose (400 or 800 mg/day) to establish good control of the asthma. The dose should then be decreased every few months until the minimum dose is reached that maintains good control (usually 100 to 200 mg/day). Growth delay can occur with inhaled steroids when total daily dose is above 500 mg/day; doses less than 500 mg/day are generally believed to be safe in children older than 5 years. For younger children and infants, safety is not well studied, and lower doses should be used if possible.

When Should I Make a Referral to a Pulmonologist?

The decision to make a referral to a pulmonary specialist depends on the severity of the asthma, the experience and comfort of the physician, and the comfort level of the family. In general, patients are referred to a specialist when asthma is not well controlled on one maintenance medication, when they have severe or frequent exacerbations, or when the history is complicated or confusing.

BRONCHIOLITIS

ETIOLOGY

What Is Bronchiolitis?

Bronchiolitis is an acute viral infection that occurs most commonly in the winter months, usually affects children younger than 2 years, and is most problematic in young infants. Prematurity, congenital heart disease, and chronic lung disease greatly increase the risk of adverse outcomes. Bronchiolitis causes inflammation and edema of the bronchioles and is characterized by wheezing and respiratory distress. Respiratory syncytial virus (RSV) accounts for about one-third of cases. Other less common causes include parainfluenza virus, adenovirus, rhinovirus, enterovirus, influenza A and B, and *Mycoplasma pneumoniae*.

EVALUATION

What History and Examination Findings Are Important?

History and examination findings for bronchiolitis are shown in Table 69-7.

What Tests Are Helpful in Diagnosing Bronchiolitis?

RSV can be identified rapidly by a direct fluorescent antibody test or by antigen detection with enzyme immunoassay [EIA]. Other respiratory viruses are detected by direct or indirect fluorescent antibodies. Viral cultures can be obtained but take 2 to 4 days to grow. All patients with suspected bronchiolitis should have pulse oximetry to guide use of supplemental oxygen. An infant whose respiratory rate is more than 60 breaths/min is likely to be hypoxic. A chest radiograph should be obtained in severe cases.

TREATMENT

When Should I Hospitalize an Infant with Bronchiolitis?

An infant with bronchiolitis should be hospitalized for severe respiratory distress, hypoxia, dehydration, poor feeding, or complicating social reasons. Most hospitalizations last 2 to 5 days, but the length of the hospital stay depends on the severity of respiratory distress, the requirement for supplemental oxygen, and the ability of the patient to take adequate oral fluids. Patients who have mild respiratory distress, who are able to take adequate fluids, and whose oxygen saturation by pulse oximetry is above 94% can be managed on an outpatient basis with close follow-up. Symptoms usually resolve by 2 weeks but can last for 4 weeks in about 10% of patients.

Do Steroids or Bronchodilators Help in Bronchiolitis?

The use of oral corticosteroids in bronchiolitis is controversial. Most studies have failed to show benefit from steroid administration in terms of length of hospital stay or improvement of symptoms.

Table 69-7

Findings in Bronchiolitis

History	Physical Examination
Viral prodrome	Expiratory wheezing and/or crackles
Copious rhinorrhea	Tachypnea (> 60 breaths/min)
Poor feeding	Respiratory distress (grunting, nasal flaring, retractions, etc.)
Apneic episodes (> 20 sec)	Lethargy and fatigue
Cyanosis	Signs of dehydration

Guidelines (2006) recommend that oral steroids should *not* be used routinely for bronchiolitis. Either nebulized albuterol or epinephrine can reduce wheezing in some patients. Oral albuterol should not be used.

What Other Medications Are Used for Bronchiolitis?

RSV immune globulin (RSV-IGIV) or paluvizamide (Synagis) can be given during the RSV outbreak season to prevent serious complications of infection in premature infants and those with congenital heart disease or chronic lung disease. A combination of RSV-IGIV and ribavirin has been used to treat patients with compromised immune systems. Antibiotics should be used only if secondary bacterial pneumonia complicates bronchiolitis.

What Is the Prognosis of Bronchiolitis?

Patients with RSV or other viral bronchiolitis that is severe enough to warrant hospitalization have up to a 50% chance of having episodes of recurrent wheezing with subsequent URIs. The parents or caretakers should be counseled to monitor closely future viral illnesses for increased or prolonged respiratory difficulties. It is not necessary to perform repeat chest radiographs if the clinical picture is consistent with bronchiolitis as long as the patient has complete clinical recovery.

PNEUMONIA

ETIOLOGY

What Is Pneumonia?

Pneumonia is an infection of the lung parenchyma that causes fever, cough, and respiratory distress. Most pneumonias are viral. Patients with bacterial pneumonia almost always appear toxic and have significant respiratory distress. Exceptions to this are pneumonias caused by *M. pneumoniae* ("walking pneumonia") and *Bordetella pertussis* ("whooping cough").

What Causes Bacterial Pneumonia at Different Ages?

The bacterial and bacteria-like pathogens that cause pneumonia vary at different ages, as shown in Table 69-8. Neonatally acquired *Chlamydia trachomatis* is often associated with a history of conjunctivitis. If pulmonary abscesses are present, *Staphylococcus aureus* is the most likely organism. Anaerobic organisms need to be considered in aspiration pneumonias. Recurrent pneumonias are often associated with underlying chronic diseases such as cystic fibrosis, ciliary dyskinesia syndrome, or immunodeficiencies. These diseases can lead to less common bacterial infections, such as *Pseudomonas aeruginosa* in cystic fibrosis and *Pneumocystis carinii* in immunocompromised patients.

Table 69-8

Common Causes of Bacterial Pneumonia at Different Ages

Age	Pathogen
Newborn	Group B streptococci, *Listeria monocytogenes*, gram-negative rods
1-3 months	*Chlamydia trachomatis, Bordetella pertussis*
Childhood and adolescence	*Streptococcus pneumoniae, Haemophilus influenzae, Staphylococcus aureus, Mycoplasma pneumoniae, Chlamydia pneumoniae*, group A streptococci

What Complications Occur with Pneumonia?

Bacterial pneumonias can cause respiratory failure, abscess, empyema, pleural effusion, pneumatocele, pneumothorax, and pyopneumothorax. Viral pneumonias occasionally can be severe and cause respiratory failure but generally have far fewer complications than bacterial disease. One exception is adenoviral pneumonia, which can cause bronchiolitis obliterans.

EVALUATION

What History and Examination Findings Are Important?

Important history and examination considerations are listed in Table 69-9. Some physical findings may be less prominent in infants. For example, decreased breath sounds or dullness to percussion may not be apparent. Tachypnea is almost always present.

Table 69-9

Findings in Pneumonia

Common Findings	Findings More Common with Bacterial Pneumonia
Cough	Toxic appearance
Crackles	Focal areas of decreased breath sounds
Dyspnea	Dullness to percussion
Tachypnea	Pleuritic chest pain
Fever	Underlying chronic disease
Lethargy	Persistent high fevers unresponsive to antipyretics

What Tests Help to Diagnose and Manage Pneumonia?

All patients with pneumonia should have pulse oximetry. Patients with suspected bacterial infection should have a chest radiograph, to look for lobar and lobular infiltrates. Complete blood count (CBC) may show an increased white blood cell (WBC) count (> 10,000/mm^3) but has poor sensitivity and specificity for differentiating between viral and bacterial pneumonias. Rapid diagnostic testing can be used to identify viral pathogens from samples obtained with nasopharyngeal washings. Sputum or blood culture can be useful to identify bacterial pathogens. Bacterial cultures are optimally obtained before antibiotics are started.

What Are the Goals of Therapy?

Therapy must first manage respiratory distress and maintain adequate ventilation and oxygenation. Subsequent goals include management of complications, treatment of any underlying illness (e.g., cystic fibrosis), and maintenance of hydration and nutrition. Antibiotic therapy should be used when appropriate.

When Should Antibiotics Be Used?

The decision to treat pneumonia with antibiotics depends on the ability to distinguish bacterial from viral pneumonia, which can be difficult. A patient with bacterial pneumonia who receives an antibiotic to which the organism is susceptible generally improves significantly within 1 day of beginning therapy. When the cause of pneumonia is not certain at the time of diagnosis, treatment is usually started with broad-spectrum antibiotics and coverage is later narrowed, either based on culture results or on clinical improvement if no culture results are available. Mild-to-moderate pneumonia is usually treated on an outpatient basis, often with macrolide antibiotics (erythromycin, azithromycin) because these drugs cover *Mycoplasma* and *Chlamydia* species. This benefit must be weighed against the increasing resistance of *Streptococcus pneumoniae* to macrolides. Semisynthetic beta-lactamase–resistant antibiotics, such as amoxicillin-clavulanate (Augmentin), are also widely used, although they have no effect against *Mycoplasma* species.

CROUP

ETIOLOGY

What Is Croup?

Croup is a viral syndrome that causes swelling of the laryngeal and subglottic areas and is also known as laryngotracheobronchitis. It is characterized by a barking cough, hoarseness, inspiratory stridor, and respiratory distress. It most commonly affects infants and toddlers.

What Are the Common Causes of Croup?

The common causes of croup are shown in Table 69-10. Other rare causes include adenovirus, enterovirus, and rhinovirus.

Table 69-10

Common Causes of Croup

Cause	Percentage
Parainfluenza (1–3)	75
RSV	10
Influenza (A and B)	7
Mycoplasma	4

RSV, Respiratory syncytial virus.

EVALUATION

What History and Examination Findings Are Important?

Important elements in the history of stridor are listed in Table 38-2. The most important physical signs to consider are the amount of respiratory distress and the degree of inspiratory stridor. Signs of "toxicity" must also be looked for. *Epiglottitis* is rare because of immunization against *Haemophilus influenzae* type b (Hib); however, this disease should still be carefully considered in toxic patients with severe croup. Patients with epiglottitis are usually 2 to 7 years of age (older than typical patients with croup), have a more acute and toxic presentation, and often present with the 4 D's: dysphagia, dysphonia, drooling, and distress. *Bacterial tracheitis* occurs more commonly today than epiglottitis and can also be life-threatening if not recognized. Patients have more toxic symptoms than patients with viral croup and have stridor that is less responsive to treatment. A subset of younger patients with bacterial tracheitis may appear less severely ill initially but may still need aggressive management of the tracheal membranes (Salamone et al., 2004). *Foreign-body aspiration* and *retropharyngeal abscess* should also be considered in the differential diagnosis of croup.

What Tests Help Diagnose and Manage Croup?

Patients with viral croup usually have a CBC that shows a "viral" pattern, although leukocytosis of greater than 15,000/mm^3 occurs in 20% of patients. Hypoxia by pulse oximetry or elevated pCO_2 on blood gas are late findings and indicate advanced disease. Neck radiographs classically show a narrowed subglottic area (steeple sign), but this sign is not reliably present. *Never send a child with suspected epiglottitis or bacterial tracheitis for a neck radiograph!* Such patients will need careful airway management and usually require intubation. Direct laryngoscopy in the operating room can verify the diagnosis of epiglottitis, but this is now rarely needed except in cases of bacterial tracheitis.

TREATMENT

What Medications Reduce Croup Symptoms?

Nebulized racemic epinephrine and oral or intramuscular dexamethasone are the two medications used most often to treat croup (Table 69-11). A patient who requires nebulized racemic epinephrine in the ED should also receive dexamethasone. High-dose nebulized budesonide has shown some benefit in croup but is less effective and more expensive than intramuscular or oral dexamethasone. There is evidence that dexamethasone can effectively control croup at even the low dose of 0.15 mg/kg (Geelhoed et al., 1996). Intramuscular dexamethasone should be administered to patients with severe respiratory distress and those unable to tolerate oral dosing.

Table 69-11

Medications for Croup

Medication	Route	Dose	Onset	Duration
Racemic epinephrine	Nebulized	0.5 ml of 2.25% solution or 5 ml of 1:1000	Immediate	< 1 hr
Dexamethasone	PO or IM	0.6 mg/kg	2-6 hr	36+ hr

IM, Intramuscularly; PO, per os (by mouth).

When Can a Patient with Croup Safely Return Home?

A child with croup may be discharged to home from the ED if pulse oximetry is greater than 95% *and* if stridor at rest and intercostal retractions have been absent for 2 to 3 hours after treatment with nebulized epinephrine and dexamethasone. The family must have access to a functioning telephone and also have transportation in case return to the ED is needed.

LARYNGOMALACIA

ETIOLOGY

What Is Laryngomalacia?

Laryngomalacia is a congenital disorder that causes upper airway obstruction because of collapse of the supraglottic laryngeal structures. Stridor (Chapter 38) is produced when "floppy" structures such as the aryepiglottic folds or the epiglottis are drawn into and obstruct the airway during inspiration. Laryngomalacia is associated with other airway abnormalities in some patients, but most of these are not significant. Gastroesophageal reflux is hypothesized to aggravate laryngomalacia by causing inflammation and edema of the supralaryngeal structures, leading to increased edema and obstruction.

EVALUATION

What History and Examination Findings Are Important?

Common history and physical findings in laryngomalacia are shown in Table 69-12. Laryngomalacia will classically have its onset at 2 weeks to 2 months of age, have an increase in symptoms until around age 6 to 10 months, and then resolve spontaneously by 2 years of age.

Table 69-12

Findings in Laryngomalacia

History	Physical Examination
Stridor begins shortly after birth	Stridor
Worse when breathing harder (URI, crying)	Retractions
Worse in supine position with neck flexed	Thoracic deformities
Better in prone position with neck extended	Poor growth
Poor feeding	

URI, Upper respiratory infection.

When Should the Patient Be Evaluated by Bronchoscopy?

A presumptive diagnosis of laryngomalacia can be made from the history and by observation of the child, but the definitive diagnosis is made during bronchoscopy by direct visualization of the invaginating supralaryngeal structures during inspiration. Any infant with significant persistent stridor and respiratory distress should be evaluated by bronchoscopy. Bronchoscopy can also identify other causes for stridor including vocal cord anomalies, laryngeal webs, hemangiomas, lymphangiomas, vascular abnormalities, and mucus retention or brachial cleft cysts.

TREATMENT

What Are the Treatment Options for Laryngomalacia?

Because laryngomalacia typically resolves spontaneously, observation or conservative treatment is generally the best approach and will allow the infant to "outgrow" the laryngomalacia. Changing feeding positions or feeding the infant slowly can sometimes be helpful. Severe laryngomalacia can cause life-threatening airway obstruction or cor pulmonale. Generally, surgical correction with laryngoplasty is reserved for infants who demonstrate poor growth or have recurrent episodes of severe respiratory distress. Laryngoplasty is highly successful in most patients, and tracheostomy is rarely needed.

Does a Trial of Antireflux Medications Help?

A trial of antireflux medications is relatively benign and should be tried for patients who are candidates for surgery. A therapeutic trial can also be tried for patients with less severe symptoms, especially if there is significant parental concern over the infant's symptoms. The medication trial should last at least 1 month to document any improvement. Medications include proton pump inhibitors (omeprazole, lansoprazole) or H_2-receptor antagonists (ranitidine, cimetidine) with or without the addition of a motility agent (metoclopramide).

HYPOXIA

ETIOLOGY

What Are the Common Causes of Hypoxia?

The most common cause of hypoxia is ventilation-perfusion (V/Q) mismatch. Cardiac diseases cause hypoxia only when there is shunting of unoxygenated blood from the right to left side of the heart. Table 69-13 shows the four main causes of hypoxia. A fifth and less common cause would be decreased PaO_2, which is seen mainly at high altitude.

What Tests Help Determine the Cause of Hypoxia?

Hypoxia from cardiac lesions can be distinguished from hypoxia caused by respiratory problems because it does not improve with supplemental oxygen, as exemplified by the infant with complete transposition of the great arteries. If hypoventilation is severe enough to cause hypoxia, a blood gas test will have an elevated $PaCO_2$ even when the PaO_2 is increased with supplemental oxygen. Pulmonary function testing can detect a decreased adjusted diffusion capacity of the lung for carbon monoxide (DLCO) that indicates diffusion impairment. A V/Q scan can reveal areas of V/Q mismatch; however, a plain chest radiograph can usually locate these same areas of infiltrate or atelectasis.

Table 69-13

Hypoxia

Cause of Hypoxia	Common Mechanisms	Changes in O_2 Saturations with Supplemental O_2
V/Q mismatch	Asthma, pneumonia, atelectasis	Increased
Hypoventilation	Obstructive sleep apnea, muscular weakness, neurologic impairment	Increased
Shunting	Cardiac abnormalities (e.g., ASD, VSD) Intrapulmonary arteriovenous malformation	No change
Diffusion impairment	Interstitial lung disease	Increased

ASD, Atrial septal defect; V/Q, ventilation-perfusion ratio; VSD, ventricular septal defect.

TREATMENT

How Is Hypoxia Treated?

In general, oxygen is administered while the underlying disorder is identified. See Chapter 59 for a discussion of the emergency management of a child with respiratory distress and hypoxia.

When Can Oxygen Be Harmful to a Hypoxic Patient?

Giving oxygen to a hypoxic patient can be harmful in several situations. Oxygen acts as a pulmonary vasodilator and can cause pulmonary edema in a patient with a left-to-right cardiac shunt. Oxygen dilates the pulmonary arteries and can decrease pulmonary vascular resistance, which results in more shunting, increased pulmonary blood volume, and eventual congestive heart failure. Chronic treatment with higher than 40% oxygen can cause oxygen toxicity to growing organs. Premature infants and neonates are particularly vulnerable to oxygen toxicity because their organs are undergoing substantial growth. In particular, they develop retinopathy of prematurity and bronchopulmonary dysplasia as a result of oxygen toxicity.

KEY POINTS

- Effective treatment of asthma must include antiinflammatory drugs (corticosteroids) if symptoms persist despite bronchodilator therapy.
- Respiratory rate greater than 60 breaths/min in infants with bronchiolitis is correlated with hypoxia.
- Community-acquired pneumonia is most often caused by a virus, *Mycoplasma pneumoniae,* or *Streptococcus pneumoniae.*
- Never send a child with suspected epiglottitis for a lateral neck x-ray.
- V/Q mismatch results in hypoxia.

Case 69-1

A 2-year-old child presents to clinic with a 5-week history of cough. He originally caught a cold in January from his 5-year-old brother. Nasal congestion resolved, but the cough has persisted and is present all the time. He coughs during the night, waking occasionally, and he sometimes coughs so hard that he "throws up." He had two other bad coughing episodes associated with colds last winter and again in the fall; both cleared up slowly. He has not had fever. His weight is following the curve at the 10th percentile. Otherwise he has been healthy, has age-appropriate development, and is fully immunized. On physical examination the lung fields are clear.

A. What is the likely explanation for his cough?
B. Can asthma be present if wheezing is not detected on lung examination?
C. What are the options for treatment?

Case 69-2

An 8-month-old child is seen in the clinic in mid-January with first-time wheezing, cough, low-grade fever, and rhinorrhea. An albuterol treatment in the clinic did not change the symptoms.

A. What additional information from the history and physical examination will assist you to make a diagnosis?
B. What is the most likely organism responsible for this child's problem?
C. How will you treat this particular child? Was albuterol treatment appropriate?

Case 69-3

A 3-year-old child is seen in the clinic for fever and cough that have worsened over the past 24 hours. He had an abrupt onset of fever 2 days ago, and the cough developed yesterday. His mother says that he looks more ill than she has ever seen him. On examination his temperature is 39.2° C, respiratory rate is 30 breaths/min, and he has intercostal retractions. Crackles are heard in the right lung.

A. What additional history should you obtain to assist development of a differential diagnosis?
B. Are diagnostic studies needed?
C. How will you treat this child now, before you have confirmation of the specific organism that causes his illness?

Case 69-4

A previously healthy 24-month-old child is seen in the emergency department in the early morning hours for marked shortness of breath, stridor, rhinorrhea, low-grade fever, and a brassy/harsh cough.

A. What criteria should you use to determine initial management?
B. What is the most likely cause of this clinical picture?
C. How should this child be treated?

Case 69-5

A 4-month-old infant has had a hoarse cry and noisy breathing since shortly after birth. In addition, she "snores" when she sleeps. Her parents are concerned that she might have allergies or enlarged tonsils and request a referral to an otolaryngologist.

A. What information will help you identify the cause of the problem?
B. What is the most likely explanation for this infant's symptoms?
C. Does she need a tonsillectomy?

Case 69-6

A 7-year-old boy with severe asthma is seen in the emergency department (ED) in moderate distress with diffuse wheezing. He has been ill for the past week and has used his inhaler four to six times each day. Today he had difficulty climbing the stairs at school. When he arrived in the ED, his respiratory rate was 28 breaths/min and his oxygen saturation was 90% on room air. His chest radiograph demonstrates scattered atelectasis. After his third treatment with nebulized albuterol, his oxygen requirement increases from 1 to 3 L, even though his wheezing seems to have decreased.

A. Because his wheezing is less apparent than on arrival in the ED, why is he not improved?
B. What is the most likely mechanism for his worsening oxygen requirement?
C. What additional treatment will benefit this boy?

Case Answers

69-1 A. *Learning objective:* **Discuss the causes of wheezing and recognize the history that suggests asthma.** This boy most likely has viral-induced asthma. Symptoms are triggered by viral infections. Between infections, he is asymptomatic.

69-1 B. *Learning objective:* **Identify asthma from the history and physical examination.** Asthma most commonly presents with wheezing, but not all asthmatic patients wheeze. Some have only a chronic cough. Others, with intermittent asthma, will cough and wheeze only when asthma is active; between asthma flareups the patients do not cough or wheeze. An asthmatic with severe bronchospasm and airway inflammation may have such poor air exchange that wheezing is not apparent. This latter situation is a predictor of respiratory failure.

69-1 C. *Learning objective:* **Select the appropriate treatment for a child with asthma.** This child will need inhaled bronchodilators, such as albuterol, whenever a viral infection is accompanied by a cough.

If the cough persists for more than a few days or if it worsens, then an antiinflammatory medication such as prednisone or prednisolone should be prescribed. A symptom diary is an important adjunct to treatment because it helps the family and the physician detect patterns of illness.

69-2 A. *Learning objective:* **Use the history and physical examination to identify the likely cause of respiratory illness.** You must ask about details of the illness, including exposures, time course, and severity of symptoms. Review the immunization history. Ask about family history of acute and chronic respiratory illness, especially asthma. In addition, you should be aware of the respiratory illnesses in your community and must factor in the season and the child's age.

69-2 B. *Learning objective:* **Identify the causative organism for common respiratory infections.** This child most likely has bronchiolitis, which is caused by respiratory syncytial virus.

69-2 C. *Learning objective:* **Select the appropriate treatment for common respiratory illnesses.** The trial of albuterol was reasonable given the prominent wheezing. Failure to respond to albuterol, the patient's age, and the season, all make bronchospasm unlikely as a cause and instead points to bronchiolitis. In most cases, bronchiolitis resolves spontaneously and does not require treatment. When respiratory distress is severe, the infant may need supportive care, including oxygen. When respiratory rate is above 60 breaths/min, hypoxia is common. Some studies suggest that antiinflammatory medications such as dexamethasone hasten the resolution of the disease and reduce the severity of symptoms. Antiviral agents have benefit only for premature infants and those with congenital heart disease or chronic lung disease. Antibiotics should be used only if a frank pneumonia complicates bronchiolitis.

69-3 A. *Learning objective:* **Use the history to aid in development of differential diagnosis for a child with a febrile respiratory illness.** In addition to more details about the acute illness, you should ask about daycare attendance and other exposures. History of immunization is important, especially the 7-valent conjugate pneumococcal vaccine (PCV-7). Past medical history should focus on growth, infections, and respiratory diseases.

69-3 B. *Learning objective:* **Select diagnostic studies for a child with findings on lung examination.** Because you suspect pneumonia in this ill child, you should obtain a chest radiograph. The severity of symptoms and the rapidity of the onset of illness suggest a bacterial infection, so you should also order a complete blood count with differential, and a blood culture.

69-3 C. *Learning objective:* **Develop a treatment plan for a child with a febrile respiratory illness.** This child has fever, increased work of breathing, and signs of pneumonia on physical examination.

You should assume that he has a bacterial infection and treat accordingly. The time course of the illness and the severity of symptoms suggest infection with *Streptococcus pneumoniae,* so antibiotic treatment must cover that organism. If he attends daycare, he is at increased risk of infection with an organism that is resistant to many commonly used antibiotics. Empirical treatment can be started with intramuscular ceftriaxone. This may be administered once daily until blood culture results are available (sputum cultures are not reliable in children). If blood culture is negative, continued treatment will be based on symptomatic response, and an oral antibiotic such as amoxicillin-clavulanate may be substituted.

69-4 A. *Learning objective:* **Identify the patient who has stridor and provide initial management based on clinical findings.** You must immediately assess his airway, breathing, and circulation, taking into account any signs of systemic disease. This child has respiratory distress and should have oxygen saturation monitored by pulse oximetry. He may benefit from oxygen administration. The fact that he has a harsh cough and a low-grade fever makes epiglottitis unlikely, but you should find out whether he has received the immunization against *Haemophilus influenzae* type b (Hib vaccine). You should also ask about the possibility that he aspirated something. Listen carefully to his lungs.

69-4 B. *Learning objective:* **Discuss the common causes of stridor.** This child has the clinical features of croup, which is usually caused by a viral infection that results in inflammation and swelling of the subglottic region of the airway.

69-4 C. *Learning objective:* **Select the appropriate treatment for a child with stridor.** This child may benefit from oxygen, nebulized racemic epinephrine, and oral or intramuscular steroids. Because of the degree of respiratory distress, he may also need observation overnight in the hospital. The average child with croup has less respiratory distress and usually needs only supportive care. In fact, many such children improve on the way to the emergency department because the cool, moist night air reduces the airway inflammation and edema.

69-5 A. *Learning objective:* **Identify the cause of chronic stridor using the history and physical examination.** You should ask about the onset of symptoms and their progress. Do symptoms worsen when the infant is agitated, lying supine, or ill with an upper respiratory infection? Does she "spit up" often after feedings? Does she have a chronic cough, or does she cough during feedings? Has she any facial, oral, or chest wall deformities? Does she have stridor or retractions at rest on physical examination? Does she have any evidence of growth retardation?

69-5 B. *Learning objective:* **Describe the causes of chronic stridor. This infant most likely has laryngomalacia.** A previous history of intubation could suggest subglottic stenosis and history of thoracic surgery for heart disease such as patent ductus arteriosis ligation would suggest recurrent laryngeal nerve damage with vocal cord paralysis. Other less likely causes include vocal cord anomalies, laryngeal webs, hemangiomas, lymphangiomas, vascular abnormalities, and mucus retention or brachial cleft cysts.

69-5 C. *Learning objective:* **Discuss the evaluation and treatment of laryngomalacia.** Tonsillectomy is not indicated in laryngomalacia. This infant probably must be evaluated with bronchoscopy. Treatment will depend on the findings of the study, but most infants outgrow symptoms before the first birthday and need no specific treatment. Supportive management includes modification of feeding position and occasionally treatment with medication to reduce gastroesophageal reflux. Infants with severe stridor may need surgical repair of the airway.

69-6 A. *Learning objective:* **Recognize the signs of worsening hypoxia.** This asthmatic patient is bronchodilator resistant because he has used his inhaler excessively over the past week. He has less wheezing because air exchange is decreasing as airway inflammation and obstruction worsen.

69-6, B. *Learning objective:* **Discuss the causes of airway obstruction in asthma that lead to hypoxia.** In this case, the airway obstruction is caused by inflammation and mucus plugging not bronchospasm. Albuterol dilates both airways and vasculature (although the airway action is generally greater). Continued use of albuterol dilates the vasculature, without affecting the airway obstruction. The end result is a worsening ventilation-perfusion ratio.

69-6 C. *Learning objective:* **Discuss treatment for a hypoxic patient.** Because this asthmatic patient has not responded to bronchodilators, he likely has significant airway inflammation and obstruction. He will need antiinflammatory medication such as prednisone or dexamethasone. Continued administration of oxygen will be needed. In addition, he is at risk for respiratory failure, so he should be hospitalized in an intensive care unit where ventilation can be managed and supported.

BIBLIOGRAPHY

Asthma

The National Asthma Education and Prevention Program (NAEPP) guidelines: *www.nhlbi.nih.gov/guidelines/asthma/asthgdln.htm.*

Nelson H et al: The Salmeterol Multicenter Asthma Research Trial. A comparison of usual pharmacotherapy for Asthma of Usual Pharmacotherapy Plus Salmeterol, *Chest* 129:15, 2006.

Bronchiolitis

American Academy of Pediatrics Clinical Practice Guideline: Diagnosis and management of bronchiditis, *Pediatrics* 118:1774, 2006.

Croup
Geelhoed GC, Turner J, Macdonald WB: Efficacy of a small single dose of oral dexamethasone for outpatient croup: a double blind placebo controlled clinical trial, *BMJ* 313:140, 1996.
Salamone FN et al: Bacterial tracheitis reexamined: is there a less severe manifestation? *Otolaryngol Head Neck Surg* 131: 871, 2004.

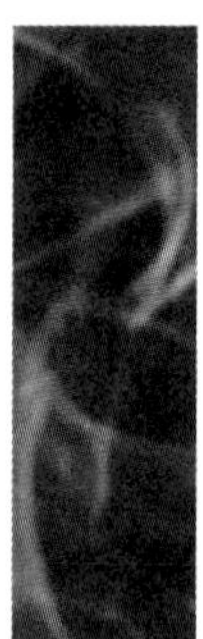

70 Rheumatologic Diseases

MARY C. OTTOLINI

JUVENILE RHEUMATOID ARTHRITIS

ETIOLOGY

What Causes Juvenile Rheumatoid Arthritis?

Although a specific trigger has not been identified, T lymphocytes of genetically predisposed children are chronically activated to recruit other inflammatory cells, leading to synovitis. The prevalence of juvenile rheumatoid arthritis (JRA) is about 1.3 in 1000 children in the general population.

EVALUATION

What Is the Typical Clinical Presentation of Juvenile Rheumatoid Arthritis?

All cases of JRA are characterized by chronic arthritis (joint pain, limitation of range of motion, joint swelling, and/or warmth) for at least 6 weeks without another etiology such as Lyme disease. Morning stiffness is common, but severe pain, especially at night, should raise concerns about another diagnosis such as leukemia. There are three general presentations for JRA based on clinical findings during the first 6 months of disease.

1. *Pauciarticular*: Involves *fewer than 5 joints*, with large joints such as the knee usually the most affected. Rarely, the hip is the presenting joint. Young girls are most commonly affected. Ophthalmologic examination is necessary to identify uveitis, which occurs commonly but may be clinically silent until irreversible damage occurs. Frequent follow-up is needed to prevent permanent vision loss.
2. *Polyarticular*: Involves *more than 5 joints*, most often in the wrists and hands. This form is more common in older girls. Rheumatoid nodules and erosive joint damage develop often.

3. *Systemic onset:* This form of JRA usually presents with high fever (> 39° C) for several weeks in children who appear systemically ill. Anemia, hepatosplenomegaly, pericarditis or pleural effusions (serositis), and a salmon-colored rash commonly accompany the fever. The rash may come and go with fever. Arthritis may be either pauciarticular or polyarticular; it may not be present initially but becomes the prominent finding as the systemic symptoms resolve.

What Laboratory Tests Should I Order?

Complete blood count (CBC) may reveal anemia of chronic disease or iron-deficiency anemia from gastrointestinal blood loss caused by nonsteroidal antiinflammatory drugs (NSAIDs). The erythrocyte sedimentation rate (ESR) is often elevated. Antinuclear antibody (ANA) and the rheumatoid factor (RF) may be variably positive, as indicated in Table 70-1. Patients on NSAIDs are monitored for liver toxicity by checking liver enzymes and for renal dysfunction by periodically checking a urinalysis.

Do Laboratory Test Results Predict Disease and Prognosis?

In general, patients with positive ANA have a better prognosis than those with positive RF. Overall, however, clinical signs and symptoms are the best indicators of prognosis and disease control rather than lab tests. Joint destruction and unremitting disease progressing into adulthood are most common in patients who are positive for RF.

Table 70-1

Findings and Prognosis in Rheumatoid Arthritis

Type	ANA	Rheumatoid Factors	Clinical Findings	Prognosis for Remission
Pauciarticular	Frequently positive	Usually negative	Young girls Knee swelling common Uveitis	Good if uveitis is controlled, except in 25% who develop polyarthritis
Polyarticular	Frequently negative	Frequently positive	Older girls Hand and wrist Nodules develop frequently	Poor if RF positive Good if RF negative
Systemic onset	Negative	Negative	Fever, lymphadenopathy, rash, and arthritis	Good except in 25% who develop polyarticular disease

ANA, Antinuclear antibody; RF, rheumatoid factor.

Modified from Cassidy JT, Petty RE: *Textbook of pediatric rheumatology,* ed 3, Philadelphia, 1995, WB Saunders.

TREATMENT

How Is Rheumatoid Arthritis Treated?

The mainstays of treatment are the NSAIDs. Disease-modifying drugs such as methotrexate and biologic therapies are reserved for those with persistent symptoms and radiologic evidence of erosions. Etanercept, a recombinant anti-TNF, has proven efficacy for patients with moderate to severe polyarticular JRA unresponsive to NSAIDs or methotrexate but is associated with an increased risk of infection. Sulfasalazine is also being used to treat patients with unresponsive JRA but has been associated with a risk of severe hypersensitivity reactions, such as Stevens-Johnson syndrome. Corticosteroids may be used systemically to quiet the inflammation seen in systemic-onset JRA. Chronic use of steroids should be minimized to avoid side effects. Steroids are also used in joint injections or topically as ophthalmic drops to treat uveitis. One of the primary concerns with long-term steroid use is poor bone mineralization during treatment. Various agents such as alendronate are being studying to help ameliorate osteopenia resulting from long-term steroid use, but their role in management of JRA is not yet clear.

SYSTEMIC LUPUS ERYTHEMATOSUS

ETIOLOGY

What Is the Cause of Systemic Lupus Erythematosus?

A single etiologic agent cannot explain systemic lupus erythematosus (SLE), a complex autoimmune disorder involving autoantibodies to a variety of tissues throughout the body. It is thought that a combination of hormones and environmental stimuli activate B lymphocytes in genetically predisposed individuals, triggering production of autoantibodies. Disease prevalence varies between 4 and 250 cases per 100,000 children, depending on gender and ethnicity. SLE is more common among Native American, Asian, Latino, and African-American children than in white patients. Girls are four times more likely to develop SLE than are boys before puberty and eight times more likely afterward.

EVALUATION

How Do Patients with Systemic Lupus Erythematosus Present?

Most of the physical findings in SLE result from vasculitis. SLE can present at any age from the newborn period into adult life. The typical patient with SLE is an African-American adolescent girl with weight loss, fatigue, arthralgias, and rash, all of which often are induced by sun exposure. Over the course of the illness, 80% develop glomerulonephritis. Neonatal lupus manifests as rash and heart block in a newborn infant, resulting from placental transfer of autoantibodies from a mother with the disease. Outside of the neonatal period, SLE is uncommon in males and in children younger than 10 years. SLE should be considered in the differential diagnosis when children or adolescents present acutely with unusual findings, such as thrombosis, psychosis, or pericardial or pleural effusions (serositis). Table 70-2 depicts the most common multiorgan system findings in SLE. Diagnosis is based on the combination of clinical findings plus laboratory test results.

Table 70-2

1982 Revised Criteria for Diagnosis of Systemic Lupus Erythematosus

1982 Revised Criteria for Diagnosis of Systemic Lupus Erythematosus
Skin/mucous membrane
Malar rash: Red, "butterfly" flat or raised rash over malar eminences, tending to spare the nasolabial folds
Discoid rash: Red plaques with scales potentially leading to atrophic scarring
Photosensitivity: Appearance or worsening of a rash with sun exposure
Oral: Painless oral or nasopharyngeal ulcers
Arthritis
Nonerosive arthritis involving two or more peripheral joints, with tenderness and swelling
Serositis
Pleuritis—evidence of a pleural effusion, or
Pericarditis—documented exam, ECG, or echocardiogram findings of pericardial effusion
Renal disorder
Persistent proteinuria > 0.5 g/day, or
Cellular casts—may be RBC, granular, tubular, or mixed
Neurologic disorder
Seizures—in the absence of offending drugs or metabolic abnormalities, or
Psychosis—in the absence of offending drugs or known metabolic abnormalities
Hematologic disorder
Hemolytic anemia (frequently Coombs' positive)
WBC: Leukopenia ($< 4000/mm^3 \times 2$)
Lymphopenia ($< 1500/mm^3 \times 2$)
Platelets: Thrombocytopenia ($< 100,000/mm^3$)
Immunologic disorder
Positive LE cell preparation, or
Anti-DNA antibody to native DNA in abnormal titer, or
Anti-Sm—presence of antibody to Sm nuclear antigen, or
False-positive serologic test result for syphilis for at least 6 months
Antinuclear antibody (ANA)
Abnormal ANA titer in absence of drugs known to cause false-positive results

ANA, Antinuclear antibody; ECG, electrocardiogram; LE, lupus erythematosus; RBC, red blood cell; Sm, Smith antigen; WBC, white blood cell.

From Tan EM et al: The 1982 revised criteria for the diagnosis of systemic lupus erythematosus, *Arthritis Rheum* 25:1271, 1982, with permission.

To categorize patients as having SLE for clinical research studies, 4 of the 11 findings in Table 70-2 must be present. In clinical practice, the diagnosis is often made with fewer than four findings.

What Laboratory Tests Help to Diagnose and Monitor Systemic Lupus Erythematosus?

No single laboratory test can be used to diagnose SLE. In addition to nonspecific findings of inflammation, such as an elevated ESR, several *autoantibodies* may be found. The ANA has high sensitivity but low specificity for SLE. Anti-SSA and anti-SSB antibodies occur more often with Sjögren's syndrome than with SLE. Anti-Smith antibody is specific for SLE but is not an indicator of disease activity. Anti–double-stranded DNA is specific for SLE and reflects disease activity, although decreased levels of complement (CH50, C3, C4) are better markers of disease activity. Autoantibodies can cause a range of laboratory and clinical abnormalities, depending on the organ system affected. All of the cell lines on the CBC can be depressed because of antibodies produced against white blood cells (ANA), red blood cells (Coombs'), or platelets. Other autoantibodies can be associated with hypothyroidism (antithyroid antibodies), cerebritis (antiribosomal P antibody), and coagulopathy or thrombosis (lupus anticoagulant/antiphospholipid antibodies). Elevations in transaminases reflect autoimmune hepatitis. Hematuria and proteinuria as seen on urinalysis reflect renal disease.

TREATMENT

How Is Systemic Lupus Erythematosus Treated?

Specific treatment may vary, depending on the organ system involved. NSAIDs can be used to treat arthritis, but creatinine and liver transaminases should be monitored closely because patients with SLE are more susceptible to NSAID-related renal and hepatic damage. Hydroxychloroquine may also be used to treat arthritis, arthralgia, skin rash, and fatigue. Patients should be advised to use sunscreen liberally because SLE is exacerbated by exposure to ultraviolet (UV) light. Patients presenting with signs of vasculitis such as thrombosis from antiphospholipid antibody should be treated with anticoagulant medications until the disease is under control. Systemic corticosteroids are often used both in low doses to control disease and in high doses to treat renal, central nervous system, or pulmonary complications. Cytotoxic agents, such as cyclophosphamide and azathioprine, are standard treatment for the patient with renal disease.

Does Treatment Affect the Long-Term Prognosis?

Lupus is a lifelong illness that requires meticulous clinical and laboratory follow-up. Signs of increasing disease activity may be identified from clinical findings such as fatigue, rash, and weight loss, and from laboratory tests including proteinuria and decreased complement. Any increase in disease activity affecting organ function must be treated promptly with appropriate immunosuppressive medications. Clinicians must have a low threshold for suspecting and treating potential infectious complications such as pneumonia or sepsis. Signs of infection such as fever, elevated white blood cell (WBC) count, and elevated ESR will be unreliable indicators of bacterial infection because of the ongoing immunosuppression caused by both the disease and treatment.

JUVENILE DERMATOMYOSITIS

ETIOLOGY

What Causes Juvenile Dermatomyositis?

The factors that trigger autoimmune activation in this disease are unknown, but some epidemiologic studies point to infectious triggers such as enteroviruses. Disease prevalence is about 3 per 1 million children. It is twice as common in girls as in boys. The mean age of onset is 6 years, with two peaks between preschool and 9 years and between 10 and 14 years. Younger children generally have a better prognosis than adolescents.

EVALUATION

What Is the Clinical Presentation of Juvenile Dermatomyositis?

As the name implies, the two primary features of the disease are skin and muscle inflammation. Fatigue, weight loss, fever, and weakness may precede the rash. A few patients have only the skin manifestations and little to no myositis.

What Is the Characteristic Rash?

The characteristic "heliotrope" rash is purplish in color and noted over the eyelids, often with facial edema. The purple rash may also occur on the trunk, the extensor surfaces of the arms and legs, the ankles, and the buttocks. Sun exposure can be a trigger, so the rash may initially appear during the summer.

Are There Other Skin Findings?

Other skin findings include Gottron's papules, which are violaceous papules over the metacarpal and proximal interphalangeal joints. Patients with long-standing disease may also develop nail-bed telangiectases, infarction of areas of the oral epithelium, and calcinosis and ulceration involving the extensor surfaces of the hands and extremities, resulting in areas of hyperpigmentation or vitiligo.

Besides Rash, What Other Findings Are Likely?

Skeletal muscle weakness is the most common finding other than rash. Weakness is greatest in the proximal muscles and is noted with activities such as climbing stairs but may be insidious until severe. The involved muscles are often painful to palpation. Smooth muscle weakness of the pharynx and the gastrointestinal tract may cause hoarseness, dysphagia, and constipation. Cardiomyopathy and/or conduction defects can also occur. Central nervous system, liver, and kidney can be involved. Retinitis or iritis may also occur.

What Laboratory Tests Are Useful for Diagnosis and Management?

Elevations in muscle enzymes such as creatine phosphokinase, aldolase, serum glutamic-oxaloacetic transaminase, and lactic acid dehydrogenase reflect myositis. The ANA is positive and has a speckled pattern in most patients at the time of diagnosis. In primary dermatomyositis without other associated connective tissue disease, antibodies to rheumatoid factor, SSA, SSB, Sm, RNP, and DNA are negative. ESR may be increased. CBC may reveal anemia of chronic disease. Myositis is confirmed as the etiology for weakness by electromyography, magnetic resonance imaging (MRI), and muscle biopsy. MRI can be used to guide muscle biopsy to confirm the diagnosis. Electrocardiography may reveal conduction defects and often shows myocardial contraction dysfunction.

TREATMENT

What Treatment Is Recommended for Dermatomyositis?

A child with dermatomyositis must use sunscreen assiduously to prevent sun exposure–induced flare-ups of disease. If skin manifestations are the only disease manifestation, a patient may be managed with hydroxychloroquine and relatively low doses of oral prednisone. Those with myositis require higher doses of systemic steroids to control disease. Intravenous steroids are required if there is dysphagia or other evidence of gastrointestinal smooth muscle involvement. Steroid doses are titrated to alleviate symptoms and to normalize muscle enzymes. Methotrexate may also be added if muscle enzymes fail to decline to acceptable levels with steroids or if the steroid dose cannot be tapered to acceptable levels. Occasionally, other immunosuppressive drugs, intravenous immunoglobulin (IVIG), and biologic therapies are required to control disease.

What Is the Prognosis?

With aggressive management, the period of active inflammation can be reduced substantially and repair of muscle damage may occur. Meticulous follow-up will allow prompt treatment when laboratory or clinical evidence demonstrates disease exacerbation. Complete recovery is possible, but prognosis is poor with active severe muscle disease, calcinosis, and lipodystrophy. Careful assessment of swallowing ability is important, because aspiration pneumonia can be a complication of dysphagia. Calcinosis can lead to draining skin lesions, which may become secondarily infected. A high index of suspicion should be maintained for secondary bacterial infection because treatment renders patients immunocompromised. Lipodystrophy, or loss of subcutaneous fat, can occur in a few patients and persist into adulthood.

KEY POINTS

- Uveitis is a severe, preventable complication of juvenile rheumatoid arthritis.
- Sun exposure causes flare-up of systemic lupus erythematosus and juvenile dermatomyositis.
- More than three-quarters of patients with systemic lupus erythematosus develop glomerulonephritis.

Case 70-1

A 4-year-old girl has been limping for the past several months and recently developed knee swelling. Her mother says that her daughter limps for several hours every morning, after she gets out of bed, and for a shorter time each afternoon, after her nap. She does not limp at any other time and has not complained of pain. She has not had any major trauma and has not had fever. Her temperature today is 36.7° C. Your physical examination identifies a warm, swollen left knee, without ecchymoses. The left knee has limited extension and flexion. In addition, you note left quadriceps atrophy, and the left leg is 1.5 cm longer than the right leg. There are no other involved joints.

A. Does this child have arthralgia or arthritis? What clinical features demonstrate this?
B. What feature in the case points to an inflammatory cause rather than a mechanical cause?
C. What diseases would you include in your differential diagnosis?
D. What are the different forms of JRA in childhood? Explain the differences.
E. If this child has pauciarticular JRA, what other organ system is most likely to be involved? How would you identify the involvement?

Case 70-2

A 14-year-old African-American girl comes to your office complaining of fever, pain in her hands and feet, and sunburn on her face. Physical examination shows her temperature to be 101° F, pulse 90 beats/min, and respiratory rate 20 breaths/min. She has a red rash on her cheeks and swollen, tender knuckles and toes. In addition, you note that she has alopecia.

A. Which clinical findings point to the most likely cause of this patient's illness? What is the likely diagnosis?
B. What laboratory tests would you order to evaluate this patient? Which results are likely to be abnormal?
C. What organ system(s) would you expect to be involved for this patient? Which predicts the worst prognosis?

D. What clinical signs and laboratory tests should be used to follow the course of SLE?
E. Why does a physician need to have a low threshold for treating SLE patients with antibiotics?

Case 70-3

An 8-year-old girl has difficulty running. Recently, her mother noted she could not get up off the floor. Lately, she has choked on several occasions while eating and has complained of difficulty swallowing. Your examination reveals a pale girl who cannot sit up on her own or rise out of a chair without pulling herself up with her hands. She has swollen eyes and full range of motion of her hips.

A. What are the major systems involved in this child and what is the likely diagnosis?
B. What are the emergencies for which you need to watch?
C. What is the mainstay of therapy for this illness and what are the major side effects of that therapy?

Case Answers

70-1 A. *Learning objective:* **Distinguish between arthritis and arthralgia.** This patient has arthritis, because there is objective evidence of inflammation: joint swelling accompanied by decreased range of motion and warmth. Although pain and erythema are not noted in this patient, arthritis often causes both. Arthralgia is the subjective complaint of joint pain, without any objective evidence of inflammation.

70-1 B. *Learning objective:* **Differentiate inflammatory arthritis from arthritis caused by trauma or other mechanical causes.** The child has no history of trauma. Overuse injuries of the knee (patellar-femoral syndromes) do not occur in prepubertal children. Without significant trauma, the knee swelling and the decreased range of motion indicate an inflammatory rather than a mechanical problem. Infection usually has a more acute onset, with high fever and obvious redness, swelling, and pain. The chronicity of this patient's problem is evident from the history and from the quadriceps atrophy and leg-length discrepancy. Chronic noninfectious joint inflammation causes overgrowth of the affected limb in children younger than 9 years and physeal arrest with limb shortening after age 9 years.

70-1 C. *Learning objective:* **List causes of arthritis in childhood.** Because this child has no evidence of trauma and nothing to suggest an acute bacterial infection, you should consider JRA and reactive arthritis, such as Lyme disease, in your differential diagnosis.

70-1 D. *Learning objective:* **Differentiate among the various types of JRA.** Pauciarticular JRA affects young children, has few joints involved (usually the knee), and is associated with uveitis. Systemic-onset JRA is also rheumatoid factor negative but has high fever and other systemic involvement, including carditis, hepatitis, lymphadenopathy, and rash. Polyarticular JRA may be either rheumatoid factor positive or negative. If positive, the patient has a high risk for a chronic, relapsing course.

70-1 E. *Learning objective:* **Discuss the systemic effects of JRA.** Pauciarticular JRA has a strong association with uveitis, which is often asymptomatic. An ophthalmologic examination must be done at the time of diagnosis, and yearly thereafter.

70-2 A. *Learning objective:* **Identify systemic lupus erythematosus using the history and physical examination.** The combination of fever, arthritis, and malar rash should make you consider SLE. SLE is more common among African-American adolescents. Although other rheumatologic disorders may also have some of the same clinical findings, the specific constellation in this patient points to SLE.

70-2 B. *Learning objective:* **Select laboratory tests to identify SLE.** You should order the tests and would expect the results shown in the following table.

Laboratory Study Results in Systemic Lupus Erythematosus

Test	Expected Results
CBC	Normochromic, normocytic, Coombs' positive anemia, low total WBC and lymphocyte count, thrombocytopenia
Urinalysis	Proteinuria, hematuria, leukocyte esterase positive, WBCs, and granular casts on microscopic evaluation
ESR	Elevated
ANA	Positive > 1:80

70-2 C. *Learning objective:* **Discuss the organ system involvement and the progression of the disease process in a patient with SLE.** Multiple organ systems are involved by SLE. Renal disease is most common and often progresses to end-stage renal disease. Central nervous system involvement occurs less commonly but has the worst prognosis.

70-2 D. *Learning objective:* **Discuss how monitoring of physical findings and laboratory test results aids in long-term management of SLE.** Clinical symptoms may reflect increasing activity of SLE: weight loss, decreased activity level, declining school performance, and mental status changes. Similarly, evidence of new rash, arthritis, signs of peripheral vascular insufficiency, and serositis (cardiomyopathy, pleural effusion, and hepatomegaly) should be sought on physical examination. Laboratory tests used to follow disease include complete blood count, erythrocyte sedimentation rate, complement levels, urinalysis, serum creatinine, liver enzymes, and anti–double-stranded DNA.

70-2 E. *Learning objective:* **Recognize the infectious risks of the immunosuppression caused by SLE.** Serious bacterial illnesses are one of the major risks because SLE is a severe autoimmune disease. Patients with SLE have decreased ability to mount an appropriate immune response to infection. In addition, treatment with immune modulators, such as corticosteroids, further impedes the patient's ability to mount an appropriate immune response, which makes the usual signs of infection unreliable and impairs a patient's ability to localize infection.

70-3 A. *Learning objective:* **Identify dermatomyositis using history and physical examination.** The history suggests extensive muscle involvement, including weakness of skeletal muscles and smooth muscle of the gastrointestinal tract. Physical examination confirms the skeletal muscle involvement and demonstrates that this child also has involvement of skin. The most likely diagnosis is dermatomyositis. You should examine the heart carefully, because cardiac involvement is common.

70-3 B. *Learning objective:* **Discuss the life-threatening complications of dermatomyositis.** Cardiomyopathy or arrhythmias may lead to cardiac failure; weakness of the diaphragm and pharyngeal muscles can cause respiratory failure. Smooth muscle involvement of the gastrointestinal tract can cause perforation.

70-3 C. *Learning objective:* **List the options for treatment of dermatomyositis and understand the complications of therapy.** Steroids are the main therapy for dermatomyositis and can cause growth failure, diabetes, cataracts, Cushing's syndrome, and pathologic fractures.

BIBLIOGRAPHY

Juvenile Rheumatoid Arthritis

Ilowite NT: Current treatment of juvenile rheumatoid arthritis, *Pediatrics* 109:109, 2002.

Lovell DJ et al: Etanercept in children with polyarticular juvenile rheumatoid arthritis, *N Engl J Med* 342:763, 2002.

Systemic Lupus Erythematosus

Lang BA, Silverman ED: A clinical overview of systemic lupus erythematosus in childhood, *Pediatr Rev* 14:194, 1993.

Rheumatologic Diseases

Lehman TJ: A practical guide to systemic lupus erythematosus, *Pediatr Clin North Am* 42:1223, 1995.

Juvenile Dermatomyositis

Pachman LM et al: Juvenile dermatomyositis at diagnosis: clinical characteristics of 79 children, *J Rheumatol* 25:1198–1204, 1998.

Practice Examination

1. A 15-month-old boy is brought for routine evaluation. He was last seen at 12 months of age. Development is age-appropriate. He prefers whole milk to all other foods, and drinks 32 to 40 ounces of cow's milk daily from a bottle. He is pale and has a heart rate of 150 beats/min, respiratory rate of 20 breaths/min, and blood pressure of 95/64 mm Hg. Weight is at 90th percentile and height is 50th percentile. He has a grade 2/6 systolic ejection murmur that decreases when he sits up; there is no diastolic murmur. The remainder of the examination is unremarkable. Which laboratory test will you order to evaluate this child?

   A. ECG
   B. Hematocrit
   C. Lead level
   D. Serum creatinine
   E. Thyroid studies

2. A 4-year-old child has developed bruises over the past 2 days. Four days ago he had diarrhea that had some streaks of blood, which has resolved. His face has been "puffy" for the last day, and urine frequency has decreased. Examination shows heart rate of 150 beats/min, respiratory rate of 20 breaths/min, and blood pressure of 148/90 mm Hg. Diffuse petechiae and ecchymoses are seen over the face, trunk, and extremities. The sclerae are mildly icteric, and the face is slightly puffy. CBC shows WBC 8000/μl, hematocrit 15%, hemoglobin 5g/dl, and platelets 20,000/μl. Which of the following additional laboratory test results would you expect for this patient?

   A. Bone marrow aspirate shows all cell lines reduced
   B. Bilirubin 0.5 mg/dl
   C. Creatinine 3.0 mg/dl
   D. Hemoglobin electrophoresis = SS
   E. Osmotic fragility test positive

3. A 3-year-old boy has had bruising and fever to 101.5° F for the past 4 days and has seemed more tired than usual for the past week. He has not had blood in the stool or urine, and there is no history of trauma. Examination shows an alert child with diffuse ecchymoses and petechiae on the face, trunk, and extremities. He has cervical lymphadenopathy and a palpable spleen. The liver is not palpable. Laboratory data show WBC 1500/μl, hemoglobin 8.5 g/dl, hematocrit 26%, platelets 10,000/μl, and reticulocytes 0.5%. WBC differential shows

neutrophils 5% and lymphocytes 80%. Prothrombin time is 12.5 seconds and partial thromboplastin time is 29 seconds. Which of the following is the most appropriate next step in diagnosis?

A. Bone marrow aspiration
B. Contact child protection services
C. Epstein-Barr virus antibody
D. Factor VIII level assay
E. Platelet antibodies

4. An 18-month-old girl is brought to the clinic for a health-supervision visit. The family has just moved from another city. The toddler was diagnosed with sickle cell disease at birth. She currently takes no medications. Her mother says that the last immunizations were given at 12 months, but she does not have a record. She will let you give only one immunization today. Which of the following organisms is the most important to immunize this child against?

A. *Bordetella pertussis*
B. *Salmonella typhi*
C. *Staphylococcus aureus*
D. *Streptococcus pneumoniae*
E. Varicella

5. A 4-year-old child is brought to the physician because the mother noted a swelling in the abdomen when she bathed him last night. The child has been well and has had no pain, fever, night sweats, or weight loss. Examination shows a well-appearing child with a firm, nontender mass in the left flank. The child has no lymphadenopathy, no pain with palpation of the extremities or movement of any joints, and no bruising. Which of the following is the next step in management?

A. Abdominal ultrasound
B. Aortic angiography
C. Inferior venacavogram
D. Surgical exploration of the abdomen
E. Voiding cystourethrogram

6. A 2-year-old child has had watery diarrhea for the last 3 months. She is at the 50th percentile on the weight and height growth charts and her physical examination is unremarkable. Which of the following laboratory test results is most likely?

A. Elevated endomysial antibody titer
B. Fecal osmotic gap of 10
C. Hemoglobin of 12 g/dl
D. Positive fecal assay for *Clostridium difficile* toxin
E. Stool pH 6.5

7. A 2-year-old child has had diarrhea for 3 months and has lost weight. The parents note that his abdomen is more prominent than in the past. His height is at the 50th percentile and weight at the 3rd percentile. The physical examination identifies an irritable child with minimal body fat. Which of the following would you most likely find on stool analysis?

   A. Fat droplets
   B. Occult blood
   C. Pinworm ova
   D. *Shigella flexneri*
   E. Stool pH < 5.5

8. You are asked to evaluate a 12-year-old girl with a 9-month history of abdominal pain. Which of the following would make you concerned about a serious underlying illness?

   A. Cramping, intermittent abdominal pain
   B. History of marked pallor during attacks of pain
   C. Pain that awakens child from sleep at 2 a.m.
   D. Periumbilical location of pain
   E. Unable to attend school for the past 2 months

9. You are asked to evaluate a 3-week-old infant with jaundice. The infant is breast-fed and has been gaining weight well. Which of the following laboratory test results would make you most concerned about congenital liver disease?

   A. Total bilirubin 19 mg/dl, direct bilirubin 0.2 mg/dl
   B. Total bilirubin 4.2 mg/dl, direct bilirubin 3.2 mg/dl
   C. Total bilirubin 11.1 mg/dl, direct bilirubin 1.0 mg/dl
   D. Total bilirubin 4.2 mg/dl, decreased from 6.4 mg/dl 1 week ago
   E. Total bilirubin 4.2 mg/dl, increased from 2.9 mg/dl 1 week ago

10. A 3-year-old child is rushed to your office after vomiting bright red material. He has red stains on his shirt when you examine him. What is the first thing that you should do?

    A. Administer 0.5 ml/kg of liquid antacid.
    B. Insert 2 large-bore intravenous lines for fluid resuscitation.
    C. Perform Hemoccult or Gastroccult test on stains.
    D. Schedule urgent upper endoscopy.
    E. Send blood for type and cross match.

11. A 2-day-old infant in the nursery has passed a dark red stool that has a positive test for occult blood. He was born after an uncomplicated pregnancy and has had a benign course in the newborn nursery. Which of the following is the most likely cause of the bloody stool?

    A. α_1-Antitrypsin deficiency
    B. Anal fissure

C. Bleeding ulcer
D. Esophageal varices from biliary atresia
E. Swallowed maternal blood

12. Before delivery, a pregnant woman requests that her newborn not have any blood tests done, including glucose tests and neonatal screening. She is concerned that the pain will cause behavioral changes. Pregnancy has been uncomplicated, and there is no personal or family history of infections, metabolic diseases, or diabetes mellitus. Which of the following will you emphasize when you talk to the mother?

    A. Federal law requires that all newborns be screened.
    B. Hypothyroidism has characteristic clinical findings identifiable at birth.
    C. Low blood glucose can be detected just as well by symptoms as by blood test.
    D. Neonatal screen detects problems before they become clinically apparent.
    E. Only African-American babies need to be screened for hemoglobinopathies.

13. A 12-year-old boy was found to have 2+ protein on his urine dipstick analysis 2 weeks ago at the time of a sports physical. In your office today his height and weight are at the 90th percentile for age, BMI is > 95th percentile, and blood pressure is 110/65 mm Hg. Repeat urinalysis shows specific gravity 1.015, pH 7.5, 2+ protein, and no blood, white blood cells, or casts. He is asymptomatic, and his physical examination is unremarkable except for overweight. Which of the following tests would be the next step in the evaluation?

    A. First morning urine protein
    B. Renal biopsy
    C. Serum albumin level
    D. Serum complement levels
    E. Serum creatinine level

14. A 3-year-old girl has a 4-day history of "puffy eyes." She is otherwise feeling well. On examination, her height, weight, and BMI are at the 50th percentile for age, and her blood pressure is 100/60 mm Hg. She has mild periorbital edema and mild pretibial pitting edema. Urinalysis in the office demonstrates specific gravity 1.020, pH 7.0, 4+ protein, and no blood. How would you start to manage this patient?

    A. Admit her to hospital for a diagnostic workup.
    B. Begin corticosteroid treatment.
    C. Determine serum albumin, cholesterol, and creatinine.
    D. Obtain a urine protein electrophoresis.
    E. Repeat dipstick urinalysis in 1 week.

15. At a routine health-supervision visit, the mother of a 7-year-old girl mentions to you that the girl is wetting the bed at night and has always done so. She has no abdominal pain, fever, voiding discomfort, constipation, or other health problems. Physical examination reveals a healthy-appearing girl at the 75th percentile for height and weight. BP is 102/64 mm Hg. Examination of her abdomen, spine, and genitourinary and neurologic systems identifies no abnormalities. Urinalysis in the office laboratory reveals specific gravity 1.015, protein negative, blood negative, glucose negative, and leukocyte esterase negative. Which of the following clinical problems will you discuss with the girl and her mother?

A. Poor renal concentration

B. Primary enuresis

C. Secondary enuresis

D. Type 2 diabetes

E. Urinary tract infection

16. A 5-year-old girl has microscopic hematuria detected at a routine urinalysis at the county health clinic. Urine has specific gravity of 1.020, no white cells, protein, or casts. The girl has been entirely asymptomatic. Blood pressure is 92/56 mm Hg, height and weight are at the 75th percentile, and physical examination is unremarkable. Repeat urinalysis 1 week later confirms microscopic hematuria, and urine culture shows no growth. What is the next test in your evaluation?

A. C3 and C4 complement levels

B. Calcium-to-creatinine ratio in urine

C. Renal ultrasound

D. Serum creatinine

E. Timed urine for total protein

17. A 2-year-old girl is brought to you with recent onset of painful urination, urinary incontinence and fever of 102° F for the past 3 days. She started to vomit this morning. On examination, she appears ill. Her temperature is 102.5° F, heart rate is 110 beats/min, respiratory rate is 26 breaths/min, and blood pressure is 100/65 mm Hg. On examination she is exquisitely tender to palpation in the right flank. What should you do next?

A. Apply a urine bag to obtain urine for urinalysis.

B. Empirically start oral antibiotics as an outpatient.

C. Request a renal ultrasound.

D. Send a catheterized urine specimen for urinalysis and culture.

E. Schedule an urgent voiding cystourethrogram.

18. Hispanic parents bring an 8-month-old boy to the community free medical clinic for a health-supervision examination. Through an interpreter you determine that the family moved to your community

1 month ago. The baby was born in California and has never been in Mexico. He is exclusively breast-fed, but the mother is worried that he is not gaining enough weight. He has received some immunizations, but parents do not remember which ones because the record was left at home. Both weight and length are at the 25th percentile for age. The infant is sociable, alert, and in no respiratory distress. He sits unaided, crawls, and pulls to stand on furniture. Which of the following will you tell the parents?

A. Developmental assessment should be requested.
B. He should be tested for tuberculosis.
C. Immunizations must be restarted from scratch.
D. Mother should switch from breast to formula.
E. Weight and length are age-appropriate.

19. A 17-year-old male comes to the office for a sports physical examination. The parents ask you in private to do a drug screen on their son without his knowledge because they found drug paraphernalia in his bedroom 2 weeks ago. The adolescent told his parents that he was holding the paraphernalia for a friend, but they do not believe him. You inform the parents that you will interview the adolescent alone and then develop a management plan. During the interview, he admits to trying marijuana on one occasion but denies other drugs. Which of the following is the most appropriate management plan?

A. Inconspicuously obtain a hair sample and perform a drug screen on the hair.
B. Inform the adolescent that he must comply with his parents' request for a urine drug screen.
C. Obtain urine for routine urinalysis and do a drug screen without informing the adolescent.
D. Perform the urine drug screen only if the adolescent consents.
E. Tell the adolescent that federal law mandates a urine drug screen.

20. A 13-year-old boy has had a tender "lump" in his left breast for the past month. He is worried that he has cancer. He does not take prescription or street drugs and he takes no nutritional supplements. His height, weight, and BMI have been at the 50th percentile for the past 3 years and he has had no growth spurt. Vital signs are age-appropriate. Physical examination identifies a 1 cm diameter, slightly tender disk of tissue in the left breast. He is at Tanner stage III for pubic hair and genitalia. The remainder of the physical examination is unremarkable. Which of the following is the most likely diagnosis?

A. Adrenergic steroid use
B. Benign gynecomastia
C. Breast cancer
D. Marijuana-induced gynecomastia
E. Pseudogynecomastia

21. A 15-year-old girl is concerned that she has not yet started menstruating. She reports that her breasts started enlarging at age 11 years. Her height, weight, and BMI are at the 25th percentile and the physical examination is unremarkable. Breasts and pubic hair are Tanner stage IV. Which of the following is the most appropriate approach for evaluation?

A. Bone age radiograph
B. Chromosome evaluation
C. Gonadal steroid levels
D. Pelvic examination
E. Reassurance that development is age-appropriate

22. A 16-year-old boy presents with a 6-week history of fatigue. His appetite is decreased and he has lost weight. He has not had fever, vomiting, diarrhea, or other localizing symptoms. He dropped out of basketball and is having difficulty sleeping. His grades have dropped from primarily A's and B's to C's and D's. Complete blood count, urinalysis, and blood urea nitrogen show no abnormalities. Which of the following is the most likely diagnosis?

A. Chronic fatigue syndrome
B. Depression
C. Diabetes mellitus
D. Eating disorder
E. Mononucleosis

23. A 13½-year-old girl complains of cramping pain in her lower abdomen, lower back, and the posterior aspect of her thighs at the time of her menstrual period. Menarche was 9 months ago. The cramping has been present for only the last 3 months. Her menstrual periods occur every 4 to 6 weeks. She is not sexually active. She denies any vaginal discharge or dysuria. Which of the following is the most appropriate initial approach to this patient?

A. Ibuprofen treatment at the time of menses
B. Perform a pelvic examination
C. Therapeutic trial of oral contraceptives
D. Ultrasound examination of the abdomen and pelvis
E. Urinalysis and urine culture just before her next period

24. A 15-year-old boy is concerned that he is not as well developed as his peers. He has always been healthy. Height has been tracking at the 5th percentile for age, weight is at the 10th percentile for age, and BMI is 20.3 (50th percentile). The general physical examination is unremarkable. He is at Tanner stage I for all development. Which of the following findings is the best indicator that his pubertal development is delayed?

A. Body mass index below 25
B. Height at the 5th percentile

C. Lack of axillary hair
D. No pubic hair
E. Testicular length < 2.5 cm

25. A 17-year-old male had had dysuria without frequency or urgency for 10 days. He has noticed a stain on his underwear for the past 3 days. He is sexually active with several partners and does not regularly use condoms. Physical examination reveals Tanner stage V pubic hair. There is no pain to palpation of the testicles or epididymis. A milky white discharge is expressed from the urethra. Which of the following is the most appropriate initial step in your approach to diagnosis and treatment?
   - **A.** Antibiotic treatment for *Escherichia coli* infection
   - **B.** Empirical treatment for *Gardnerella* infection
   - **C.** Identification of sexual contacts
   - **D.** Routine urinalysis
   - **E.** Urethral swab to test for *Chlamydia* and gonorrhea

26. A 12-year-old girl comes to clinic for a routine health-maintenance visit. She tells you that she noted tender "bumps" in her breasts about 2 weeks ago and would like to know what this means. After a physical examination, you explain that the "bumps" are breast buds that signal the onset of puberty. Which of the following information will you provide about the events that occur during puberty in girls?
   - **A.** A thick, malodorous vaginal discharge commonly occurs in the first 6 months of puberty.
   - **B.** Axillary hair most commonly appears after menarche.
   - **C.** Menarche occurs only after a girl has stopped growing.
   - **D.** Rapid growth begins immediately following the appearance of breast buds.
   - **E.** The first period occurs within 6 months of the appearance of breast buds.

27. A 4-month-old baby is brought by her parents to the emergency department at 10 p.m. Parents tell you that the baby rolled off the couch that morning and has been crying all day. Physical examination reveals an alert infant with tenderness and swelling of the left thigh. X-ray of the left leg shows an acute fracture of the femur. What is the most appropriate next step in the child's management?
   - **A.** Head CT scan
   - **B.** Serum calcium level
   - **C.** Skeletal survey
   - **D.** Skin biopsy for osteogenesis imperfecta testing
   - **E.** Technetium 99 bone scan

28. A 7-year-old girl is brought to your office after disclosing to her mother that an adult male cousin had been" touching her" for the past several months, most recently 1 week ago. She tells you that her cousin "put his private in my butt." The mother wants to know how she can find out whether her daughter has been sexually abused. Which of the following is the appropriate information to tell the mother about the expected findings from the evaluation process?

   A. A large hymenal orifice must be identified to confirm the child's history.
   B. Gonorrhea testing is important, regardless of the child's symptoms.
   C. History from a young child is generally regarded as unreliable.
   D. Physical examination in sexual abuse often shows no trauma.
   E. Semen is likely to be found in the girl's vagina.

29. A 2-month-old baby is brought to the emergency department by ambulance after her parents called 911 to say that the infant "won't wake up." They state that she was perfectly fine when put to bed several hours ago. On physical examination, the infant is afebrile and does not respond to voice. She has a bulging anterior fontanelle and a small facial bruise. No other bruises, rashes, or bleeding are identified. How will you interpret the injuries to plan further evaluation?

   A. Absence of extensive trauma makes skeletal survey unnecessary.
   B. Bruises are common in young infants and do not raise suspicion of abuse.
   C. Bulging fontanelle indicates the need for lumbar puncture to detect meningitis.
   D. Lethargy should be investigated with a drug screen.
   E. Subdural effusion caused by violent shaking should be sought with head CT.

30. Parents of an 8-year-old boy bring him to the office for evaluation of behavior. They have a note from the teacher and a list of his concerning behaviors. Which of the following behaviors is most likely to be noted by the teachers and parents if the child has attention deficit hyperactivity disorder (ADHD)?

   A. Failure to gain pleasure from playing with other children
   B. Frequent fighting and bullying of other children at recess
   C. Impulsive behavior that results in frequent injuries
   D. Low scores on achievement tests
   E. Shyness and reluctance to participate in class discussion

31. Parents request advice from you about their son who is struggling with reading in second grade. The teacher suspects ADHD because the boy is "not working up to his potential" and becomes distracted during reading time. Parents note no behavioral problems at home

or play groups. You suspect that he may have a learning disability. Which of the following will help manage the boy's problem?

A. Cognitive testing to compare ability with school performance
B. Eye exercises to strengthen extraocular muscles
C. Neurologic examination to identify fine motor deficits
D. Observation in the classroom to identify the behaviors specific for learning disability
E. Treatment with methylphenidate

32. A 5-year-old African-American child has a patch of alopecia of 2 weeks' duration. Within the patch are black dot hairs and scale. Which of the following is the most appropriate treatment?

A. Cephalexin orally
B. Griseofulvin orally
C. Hydrocortisone 1% topically
D. Miconazole nitrate topically
E. Nystatin topically

33. A 6-year-old child has had a rash for 2 days. On physical examination you find a well-appearing, afebrile child with red cheeks and lacy, reticulated erythema of the extremities. Which of the following is the most likely diagnosis?

A. Atopic dermatitis
B. Erythema infectiosum
C. Lyme disease
D. Rubella
E. Scarlet fever

34. A 15-year-old girl has had a rash on the trunk for several months. During her physical examination, you observe small, scaling hypopigmented macules on the chest and back. On the central back, the macules have coalesced into a large patch. Which of the following is the most appropriate therapy?

A. Ketoconazole orally
B. Miconazole nitrate topically
C. Mupirocin topically
D. Triamcinolone 0.1% topically
E. Selenium sulfide 2.5% topically

35. A 7-month-old infant has a recurring eruption composed of erythematous, chapped-appearing patches on the face and erythematous, slightly scaling patches on the trunk and extremities. The family history is remarkable for asthma in an older sibling. Which of the following is the most appropriate initial treatment for this infant's rash?

A. Cephalexin orally
B. Griseofulvin orally

C. Hydrocortisone 1% topically
D. Miconazole nitrate topically
E. Prednisone orally

36. A 6-year-old adopted child arrived from Thailand last week. Fever and rash developed 2 days ago and the rash has progressed. Physical examination reveals an unhappy child with a temperature of 38.4° C (101.1° F). There are numerous vesicles on the trunk and extremities. Each vesicle is on an erythematous base, and some of the vesicles have ruptured forming crusts. Which of the following is most likely to occur over the next 3 days?

A. Cough, conjunctivitis and worsening fever
B. "Crops" of skin lesions with progressive crusting
C. Fever resolution at the time the rash abruptly disappears
D. Inflammation of oral mucosa accompanied by shock
E. Swelling of hands and feet with desquamation of fingertips

37. A 2-year-old boy has generalized weakness, leg calf hypertrophy, and a positive Gowers' sign. During the clinic visit, his parents ask about the risk of having another child with this disease. Which mode of inheritance will you explain to the family to answer their question?

A. Autosomal dominant
B. Autosomal recessive
C. Chromosome trisomy
D. Multifactorial transmission
E. X-linked

38. A 2-year-old girl had an episode of generalized arm and leg "jerking" that lasted about 5 minutes. After the episode was over her temperature was 103.5° F. Her mother gave a dose of acetaminophen, then brought the girl to the office. She has met all developmental milestones on time. In your office she is alert and talkative. Her temperature is 101.6° F. She has an inflamed, bulging right tympanic membrane and nasal congestion. The remainder of the physical examination is unremarkable. In addition to treating her ear infection, what is your next step in management?

A. Admit to hospital for intravenous phenytoin therapy.
B. Begin oral phenobarbital 3 mg/kg/24 hours.
C. Discuss the benign nature of the seizure.
D. Perform lumbar puncture with cultures and chemistries.
E. Refer the child to a neurologist for an EEG.

39. A 7-year-old girl has had a headache about twice a month for the past 3 months. She describes a throbbing sensation all over her head. She had nausea, photophobia, and phonophobia with each episode. The mother is concerned that her child has a brain tumor.

The physical examination, including ocular funduscopic and neurologic examinations, is unremarkable. Which of the following evaluations will most likely provide information that will help you answer the mother's concerns and also be useful in long-term management of this child's headaches?

A. Computed tomographic study of the head
B. Headache diary
C. Lumbar puncture
D. Magnetic resonance imaging study of the head
E. Psychiatric consultation

40. The parents of an 8-year-old boy bring him to your office to discuss the recent onset of "strange behavior." He shrugs his left shoulder, blinks his left eye, and clears his throat often while he is awake. There are no serious illnesses or injuries in his past medical history, and his physical examination is unremarkable except for the repeated tics. Which of the following comorbid problems will you need to investigate?

A. Attention deficit hyperactivity disorder
B. Conduct disorder
C. Oppositional defiant disorder
D. Schizophrenia
E. Suicidal ideation

41. A previously healthy 5-year-old boy has had low-grade fever, malaise, upper respiratory congestion, and conjunctivitis for 5 days. When he awoke this morning he could not walk to the bathroom. On examination, he has a wide-based unsteady gait and slightly slurred speech. What additional finding on physical examination is most consistent with the likely diagnosis?

A. Bilateral gastrocnemius muscle hypertrophy
B. Conjunctival and cutaneous telangiectases
C. Muscle strength 5/5 symmetrically in upper and lower extremities
D. Patellar reflexes 1+/4+ bilaterally
E. Scoliosis visible on forward-bending test

42. A 16-month-old girl is not yet walking. She is beginning to pull herself up on furniture but can stand only for a few seconds. She has a pincer grasp and transfers objects. She says "ma-ma" and "da-da" specifically for her parents but has no other words. The child was born at 27 weeks' gestation weighing 900 g, after a pregnancy complicated by toxemia in the third trimester. Her neonatal course was complicated by mild respiratory distress, jaundice, and feeding problems. She has been well since hospital discharge. Physical examination demonstrates an alert, socially responsive child with symmetrical movement, strength, and muscle bulk. She has

symmetrical reflexes and demonstrates no primitive reflexes or fasciculations. Which of the following will you discuss with the mother?

A. Delayed independent walking suggests muscle weakness.
B. Development is appropriate for adjusted gestational age.
C. Inability to stand independently suggests cerebral palsy.
D. Language delay indicates high likelihood of mental retardation.
E. Premature infants rarely walk before 2 years of age.

43. A 15-month-old child has not yet begun to walk. He was born at full term, after an uncomplicated pregnancy. He met all of the developmental milestones up to the 12-month assessment. On examination you find an alert, socially aware toddler who crawls rapidly, plays with toys, responds to parental requests, and cries when you approach him to perform the examination. During his tantrum you observe that he has symmetrical muscle strength. Which of the following is the most appropriate plan for evaluation and management?

A. Consult a pediatric neurologist.
B. Prescribe twice weekly physical therapy.
C. Reassure the mother that she should not worry about her child.
D. Refer for developmental evaluation at a tertiary care center.
E. Review developmental progress at the 18-month visit.

44. Parents new to your practice bring their 10-month-old girl for evaluation because she cannot sit unsupported. She first rolled over at 8 months, and she just started to reach for objects with a raking grasp. On the examination table, the infant lies supine with hips abducted and flexed in the "frog-leg" position and arms hanging at her sides. Spontaneous movement is minimal. When you pick her up under the arms her legs dangle below her and she feels as if she is slipping through your hands. She has no persistent primitive reflexes. Which of the following best characterizes the physical examination findings?

A. Cerebral palsy
B. Hypotonia
C. Myoclonus
D. Paraplegia
E. Spasticity

45. A 3-year-old boy has just started to combine words into 2-word phrases but mostly communicates with pointing and gestures. He is affectionate and playful and loves the company of other children. He can walk and run well and can throw and kick a ball. He is able to dress and to brush his teeth with help. Parents have noted no regression of development. Physical examination shows no middle ear effusion, ear infection, or palatal clefting. The remainder of the examination is unremarkable. Which of the following additional information is most relevant to the evaluation of this child?

A. Audiometry results
B. Head circumference
C. Family history of autism
D. Genetic testing
E. Temper tantrum frequency

46. A 3-year-old boy immigrated to the United States with his family from Somalia several months ago. He is brought to the free medical clinic for an evaluation. His height, weight, and head circumference are below the 5th percentile for age. He is essentially nonverbal, although he can babble. He can sit if propped but cannot walk. He holds his left arm close to his body, with the elbow flexed and the hand fisted. He uses his right arm to bat at toys and makes no hand-to-hand transfers. When you pick him up he arches away from you and scissors his legs. Bending his arms and legs is extremely difficult. Which of the following is the best way to discuss this boy's condition with his family?

A. He has a degenerative disorder caused by a progressive neurologic disease.
B. His condition will steadily improve with intensive physical therapy.
C. Malaria at age 12 months caused these findings.
D. Neuromuscular findings reflect a non-progressive brain injury.
E. The multiple findings suggest a genetic syndrome.

47. A 5-year-old boy began limping with his left leg about 4 days ago. The limp has become much more noticeable in the past 2 days. According to his mother, he has not appeared ill nor has he had any obvious trauma. His development and past medical history are entirely unremarkable. Which of the following findings on physical examination best supports the most likely diagnosis?

A. Diameter of the left thigh is 2 cm smaller than the right thigh.
B. Left knee is tender, swollen, and warm.
C. Passive internal and external rotation of the left leg causes pain in the knee and hip.
D. Temperature is 39.6° C.
E. Weight is above the 97th percentile.

48. A 3-year-old child has a limp, morning stiffness, a swollen, red right knee, and a diffuse maculopapular rash. Which of the following test results would be most likely?

A. Antinuclear antibody 1:120
B. Erythrocyte sedimentation rate 42 mm/hr

C. Hemoglobin 9.9 g/dl, mean corpuscular volume 70 fl
D. Urinalysis with 3+ blood and 2+ protein
E. WBC 15,000/mm^3 with 50% neutrophils and 20% bands

49. You have recently diagnosed systemic lupus erythematosus (SLE) in a 15-year-old girl who has joint pains, fever, and a rash. After starting treatment with prednisone, you counsel her about her disease. Which of the following should you recommend for your patient?

A. Daily antibiotic prophylaxis to prevent infection
B. Electrocardiogram every 6 months to detect heart block
C. Regular urinalysis to detect signs of nephritis
D. Sun block to prevent flare-up of SLE myositis
E. Yearly ophthalmologic evaluation to detect uveitis

50. An 8-year-old boy has had "allergies" since age 2 years. Symptoms include runny nose, congestion, and cough. Which of the following is the best indicator that this symptom complex is caused by an allergy?

A. He has dry, itchy skin each winter.
B. Family history is positive for seasonal allergies.
C. Skin test shows a 3+ wheal and flare to both dog hair and histamine.
D. His symptoms worsen around grandmother's cat.
E. Tobacco smoke causes increase in symptoms.

51. A 12-year-old comes to the office in late May with complaint of headache, nasal congestion, decreased hearing, and lack of appetite. She has not had fever. Her past history shows that she has "hay fever" for 2 months every spring. Symptoms abate in early July every year. She demonstrates an "allergic salute," has a stuffy ("denasal") voice, and has thickened, poorly mobile tympanic membranes without inflammation. Her nasal and conjunctival mucosae are pale and edematous. Nasal discharge is thin and watery. Which of the following medication combinations would be most appropriate for management?

A. Amoxicillin for 10 days plus pseudoephedrine daily while symptomatic
B. Beclomethasone nasal spray, hydroxyzine, and pseudoephedrine daily
C. Cromolyn sodium nasal spray
D. Oxymetazoline nasal spray and hydroxyzine daily for the duration of symptoms
E. Prednisone daily for the duration of symptoms

52. A 12-month-old infant is scheduled to undergo elective palatal surgery as part of the staged repair of cleft lip and palate. He will be NPO for 12 hours before surgery and for an unpredictable period after surgery. Which of the following is most important to take into consideration when planning his perioperative management?

A. Core body temperature
B. Daily maintenance fluid requirements
C. Fluid losses from surgical drains
D. Stool quantity
E. Urine output

53. A 2-month-old infant has had progressively worsening nonbilious vomiting for 4 days. He vomits after each feeding and is fussy and hungry. He has dry mucous membranes, sunken fontanelle, tachycardia, and capillary refill > 4 seconds. Which of the following laboratory test results is most likely?

A. Bicarbonate level 18 mEq/L
B. Blood glucose 100 mg/dl
C. Serum chloride 88 mEq/L
D. Serum creatinine 0.3 mg/dl
E. Urine pH 5

54. An infant with chronic mild eczema develops gastroenteritis, fever, and poor feeding. You are concerned that the infant will become dehydrated because he has several problems that increase total fluid needs. Which of the following is most likely to increase the insensible water loss?

A. Decreased fluid intake
B. Diarrhea
C. Eczema
D. Fever
E. Vomiting

55. A 15-month-old infant has had severe watery diarrhea for 3 days and has had no urine output for 18 hours. He weighs 10 kg and has a heart rate of 180 beats/min, capillary refill > 4 seconds, and parched mucous membranes. Serum sodium is 134 mEq/L, bicarbonate is 12 mEq/L, and serum creatinine is 0.9 mg/dl. What is the first fluid to administer to this patient?

A. 3% NaCl solution
B. D5W plus {1/2} normal saline with 20 mEq/L KCl
C. Isotonic saline
D. Packed red blood cells
E. Plasmanate

56. After evaluating a 2-year-old child who has had diarrhea for 3 days, you determine that the child is only minimally dehydrated. You

decide to manage him at home and instruct parents in the use of oral fluids. Which of the following physical findings led to your conclusion and recommendation for therapy?

A. Absent tears

B. Capillary refill < 2 seconds

C. Diminished social responsiveness

D. Dry, sticky oral mucous membranes

E. Pulse 150 beats/min

57. You are assigned to a clinic for migrant workers and are asked to evaluate a 33-month-old Hispanic boy. He was born in Mexico and lives there except during the harvest season, when his family travels to the United States. He received Bacille Calmette-Guérin (BCG) vaccine at birth and PPD was nonreactive last month. He has been healthy except for minor illnesses. Weight is at the 90th percentile and length at the 10th percentile. He speaks Spanish and is developmentally on track. His physical examination is unremarkable. Which of the following screening tests should be done at this visit?

A. Audiogram

B. Blood lead level

C. Chest x-ray

D. Stool for ova and parasites

E. Urinalysis

58. A 13-month-old girl has had fever for the past 24 hours. She vomited once this morning after a dose of acetaminophen. She has had two loose stools since last night. She has received all of her immunizations, including PCV-7 and Hib. Her urine output is decreased, based on diaper count, and her mother thinks that the urine "smells bad." In the office she has a temperature of 39.8° C and appears toxic with rapid, labored respirations and mottled skin. After a workup identifies the most likely cause for her findings, what is the most appropriate management plan?

A. Admit to hospital for intravenous fluids and antibiotics.

B. Give a dose of oral ibuprofen and observe in clinic until all test results are available.

C. Inject ceftriaxone intramuscularly and send her home.

D. Request a consultation with pediatric urology.

E. Schedule voiding cystourethrogram.

59. Parents of a 3-month-old boy who was just diagnosed with cystic fibrosis request that the 3-year-old brother and 7-year-old sister have sweat testing to determine whether they have the disease. In addition, they want to know the chance that either child might be a carrier. Which of the following will you recommend to the family?

A. Both sweat test and DNA testing must be done now to detect the carrier state.

B. DNA testing of siblings is not needed because cystic fibrosis is not present in either parent.
C. Genetic testing should be done when the siblings reach reproductive age.
D. Sweat test is not necessary if the other children are healthy.
E. Testing will be needed for the other children only if they have asthma.

60. A newborn infant is diagnosed with a VSD. He was born at full term after an uncomplicated pregnancy, weighing 7 pounds 8 ounces (3.4 kg) and has no other congenital anomalies. Which of the following information will you discuss with the parents?

A. Asymptomatic maternal diabetes during pregnancy caused the VSD.
B. DNA testing to detect cardiac disease is available for future pregnancies.
C. Family members should undergo cardiac ultrasound.
D. Single malformations, such as VSD, occur in 2% to 3% of all newborns.
E. Structural cardiac defects are most often caused by chromosomal abnormalities.

61. A 14-year-old girl is concerned because she is much shorter than her classmates. She also notes that unlike her friends, she has not yet started to have breast development. Her growth in height has always been below the 5th percentile. Today her height is below the 5th percentile for age, and she is at stage I pubertal development. Which of the following additional physical findings would you expect?

A. Cataracts
B. Elevated blood pressure
C. Pectus excavatum
D. Thin, fragile hair
E. Webbing of the toes

62. A 3-year-old girl has a 4-day history of cough, congestion and low-grade fever but has been able to eat, play, and interact normally with her brother. The cough is mild and occurs both day and night. On examination she has nasal congestion, pharyngeal injection, gray tympanic membranes with visible landmarks and light reflexes, and vesicular breath sounds with equal aeration. Which of the following is the most likely cause of this cough?

A. Asthma
B. Bacterial pneumonia
C. Foreign-body aspiration
D. Pertussis
E. Viral URI

63. A 2-year-old child has been coughing for 2 weeks, day and night. He has never had a significant cough before. He was entirely well when the cough started suddenly one day at home. Since then, his mother thinks that he has been short of breath. On physical examination, breath sounds are decreased in the right base, and a faint expiratory wheeze is audible on the right. What further information from the history is most likely to identify the cause of the cough?

A. A cousin has cystic fibrosis.
B. Father and brother both have asthma.
C. Parents refused DTaP immunizations over concern about side effects.
D. The 5-year-old brother says that one of his Lego blocks is missing.
E. Two children at daycare have fever and cough.

64. A 4-year-old child has had a daily cough for as long as her mother can remember. The girl does not seem to be able to gain weight despite the fact that she eats more than her 6-year-old brother. In addition, she has less "stamina" than her brother did at the same age. She has not had recurrent fever. On physical examination, weight is below the 5th percentile. Respiratory rate is 24 breaths/min. She has faint crackles in both lung bases and an occasional wheeze. She has minimal body fat, but otherwise has no concerning findings. Which of the following diagnostic tests would most likely confirm the diagnosis?

A. Chest radiograph
B. Ova and parasite test of stool
C. Pulmonary function testing
D. Sweat chloride test
E. Tuberculosis skin test

65. An 8-month-old child is seen in clinic in mid-January with first-time wheezing, a tight cough, low-grade fever, and rhinorrhea. Respiratory rate is 60 breaths/minute, and oxygen saturation is 92% in room air. She has prominent intercostal space retractions and abdominal breathing. A treatment with nebulized albuterol did not change the respiratory findings. Which of the following is the next step in management?

A. Acyclovir, orally
B. Ceftriaxone injection
C. Nebulized prednisolone
D. Oxygen by nasal prongs
E. Repeat albuterol treatment

66. A 6-week-old female infant is seen in clinic during the month of March for cough and breathing problems that the mother says have been getting worse over the past 2 weeks. On examination, the child

is afebrile and in mild respiratory distress, with respiratory rate of 50 breaths/min and intercostal space retractions. Oxygen saturation is 96% in room air. Diffuse crackles are heard on auscultation of the lungs. A chest radiograph shows interstitial infiltrates. Complete blood count shows an increase in the absolute number of eosinophils without other abnormalities. What organism is the most likely cause of this infant's findings?

A. *Bordetella pertussis*
B. *Chlamydia trachomatis*
C. Group B streptococcus
D. Respiratory syncytial virus
E. *Streptococcus pneumoniae*

67. A 3-year-old child with cystic fibrosis has developed fever and worsening respiratory problems. His immunizations are complete for age. His weight has fallen below the 5th percentile over the past 6 months. On examination, his temperature is 38.2° C and his respiratory rate is 28 breaths/min. Auscultation reveals crackles in both lung bases. A chest radiograph shows scattered infiltrates. What is the most likely organism causing this patient's problem?

A. *Bordetella pertussis*
B. *Mycoplasma pneumoniae*
C. *Pseudomonas aeruginosa*
D. Respiratory syncytial virus
E. *Streptococcus pneumoniae*

68. A 1-month-old healthy girl is brought to clinic by her mother who just heard that a friend's baby died of sudden infant death syndrome. She wants to do everything possible to prevent this from happening to her child. The infant was born at full term, had no postnatal problems, and is formula fed. The baby is a restless sleeper and "spits up" after almost every feeding. The mother smoked cigarettes throughout pregnancy and continues to do so. The physical examination is completely unremarkable. What would you recommend to this mother?

A. Add a tablespoon of rice cereal to each bottle of formula to prevent reflux.
B. Have the infant tested with a sleep study.
C. Limit cigarette smoking to the living room and kitchen, never in the bedrooms.
D. Obtain an apnea monitor from the local medical supply store.
E. Place the infant to sleep on her back.

69. The parents of a 6-month-old inform you that they discontinued formula last week and started cow's milk. Parents tell you that it is more convenient and less expensive to buy cow's milk for the baby and her 18-month-old brother. The infant has grown well on formula, and she is currently at the 50th percentile for weight and length. What information should you give to the family to encourage use of formula?

A. Cow's milk is not a suitable food because it is low in folic acid.
B. Eczema develops in 25% to 30% of infants fed cow's milk in the first year.
C. Lactose intolerance is much more likely to develop if an infant drinks cow's milk.
D. Malabsorption of protein from cow's milk often causes poor growth.
E. Use of cow's milk before 12 months causes iron deficiency.

70. The mother of a 24-hour-old newborn asks about switching from breast-feeding to formula. She has noticed that her breast milk is pale bluish in color and appears "thin." She says that her own mother has recommended that she switch to formula so her infant will receive "better" nutrition. In addition to explaining that the color and consistency of her breast milk is typical for colostrum, which of the following should you emphasize in an attempt to encourage her to continue with breast-feeding?

A. Calories in colostrum help combat cold stress.
B. High iron content of colostrum prevents iron deficiency.
C. Large fluid volume of colostrum prevents dehydration.
D. Immunoglobulins in colostrum protect against infection.
E. Proteins that are present only in colostrum provide important nutrients.

71. A 3.2-kg newborn male infant develops respiratory distress 30 minutes after delivery. He was born to a 26-year-old, obese mother who had no prenatal care. You suspect that this may be an infant of a diabetic mother and that the infant's respiratory problems reflect prematurity. Which of the following physical examination findings suggests that this is a large for gestational age premature infant?

A. Absent lanugo
B. Breast buds > 1 cm
C. Flexed position when undisturbed
D. Prominent creases on the soles of the feet
E. Undescended testicles

72. On the second day of life a newborn infant is noted to be lethargic and a poor feeder. Her temperature is 34.9° C, skin is mottled, and capillary refill is prolonged. She also has jaundice that was first noted this morning. Total bilirubin is 8 mg/dl and direct bilirubin is 2.4 mg/dl. Which of the following should be the next step in this infant's management?

A. Blood and CSF cultures

B. Examination of the peripheral blood smear for evidence of hemolysis
C. Liver function testing
D. Phototherapy
E. Workup for TORCHS infections

73. A 2.6-kg female infant was born at 42 weeks' gestational age to a G2P2 mother. Maternal history includes ½ pack-per-day cigarette smoking and regular consumption of beer throughout the pregnancy. Which of the following represents the most immediate concern for this infant?

A. Fetal alcohol syndrome
B. Hyperbilirubinemia
C. Hypoglycemia
D. Sudden infant death
E. TORCHS infection

74. At the time of discharge of a healthy full-term boy from the newborn nursery, parents ask what they should watch for over the next several weeks. You review common problems, safety, and nutrition for the newborn. Which of the following will you include in your discharge discussion with the parents?

A. A strict 4-hour feeding schedule will help establish regular habits.
B. "Back to sleep" only applies for the first 4 weeks.
C. Either front or back seat is OK for the automobile safety seat.
D. Jaundice commonly develops during the second or third week.
E. Parents will be notified if neonatal screening detects any abnormalities.

75. A male infant is born at term to a G1P1 mother. The parents had visited your office 1 month before birth for a prenatal discussion about nutrition, immunizations, and general care of a newborn. After you examine the infant in the newborn nursery, you speak with the mother to remind her of important issues regarding breast-feeding. Which of the following advice will you give?

A. An infant must nurse for 20 to 25 minutes at each breast, at every feeding, to obtain enough milk.
B. Breast milk is deficient in vitamins A and C, so a vitamin supplement is needed.
C. Breast-fed infants usually have < 6 wet diapers per day to conserve body water.
D. Healthy newborn infants may nurse as often as every 90 minutes.
E. The mother should not breast-feed if she has an upper respiratory infection.

76. A 2-year-old boy has had a "cold" with fever for 5 days and has refused to walk today. He appears irritable. His temperature is 38.9° C, pulse is 140 beats/min, and respirations are 30 breaths/min. He refuses to stand and will not bear weight on his left foot. On the examination table he holds his left hip flexed and slightly adducted. He cries whenever the hip is moved. What is the most likely diagnosis?

A. Bacterial arthritis
B. Legg-Calvé disease
C. Lyme disease
D. Rheumatoid arthritis
E. Toxic synovitis

77. A previously healthy 6-month-old girl has been ill for 2 days with vomiting, irritability, and decreased activity. The emesis is not yellow or blood stained. No other family members are ill. Her mother cannot console her in the examination room. She has not received any immunizations. Temperature is 38.6° C, heart rate is 178 beats/min, and respirations are 58 breaths/min. She is unresponsive to your attempts to interact with her. Her fontanel is bulging and oral mucous membranes are somewhat dry. No other focus of infection can be identified on physical examination. Which of the following is the next most appropriate step in the management of this child?

A. Administer D-5-W.
B. Begin oral amoxicillin.
C. Obtain a urinalysis.
D. Order a CT scan of the head.
E. Perform a lumbar puncture.

78. A 10-year-old boy is brought to the physician's office for the first time. He was born in Burlington, Vermont, and recently moved to your city when his parents accepted teaching positions at the local university. His family plans to spend 1 month traveling through India, and the boy needs travel immunizations. The boy and all family members are healthy. His immunizations are complete for age and his physical examination is age-appropriate. You immunize him against hepatitis A and provide advice for malaria prophylaxis. His mother wants to know if he should be tested for tuberculosis before departing for India. Which of the following is the most appropriate response to the mother's question?

A. Explain that the boy does not need testing for tuberculosis.
B. Obtain a baseline chest radiograph before the family leaves on the trip.
C. Place an intradermal Mantoux test (PPD) on the boy.
D. Treat him prophylactically with isoniazid for the duration of the trip to India.
E. Vaccinate the boy with bacille Calmette-Guérin (BCG).

79. A 12-year-old girl has had fever, sore throat, and malaise for 3 days. Her temperature is 38.9° C, heart rate is 106 beats/min, and respirations are 22 breaths/min. Her pharynx is red and tonsils are enlarged. She has several mildly tender 1-cm lymph nodes in both the anterior and posterior cervical chains. Her spleen can be palpated 2 cm below the left costal margin. Hemogram shows WBC = 12,500, HCT = 37%, and platelets = 300,000. Differential is pending. What is the most likely diagnosis in this child?

A. Acute lymphocytic leukemia
B. Cat scratch disease
C. Coxsackie virus infection
D. Epstein-Barr virus infection
E. Streptococcal pharyngitis

80. A 3-year-old boy presents with 5 days of fever and irritability. His temperature is 39° C, heart rate is 130 beats/min, and respirations are 26 breaths/min. He has a red throat and tongue, cracked lips, and a diffuse, erythematous macular rash on his trunk. His hands appear swollen and he has a 2-cm moderately tender lymph node in the left anterior cervical chain. Both sclerae are intensely red without any purulent discharge noted. Which of the following is the most likely explanation for the patient's findings?

A. Adenovirus pharyngoconjunctival fever
B. Bacterial conjunctivitis
C. *Chlamydia trachomatis* infection
D. Kawasaki disease
E. Viral conjunctivitis

81. A 7-year-old child comes to the emergency department by ambulance after a fall from a bicycle. He was not wearing a helmet. The emergency medical technician team provided urgent management at the scene before transport to the emergency department. He has been comatose since the fall. By report from the EMT the boy had oxygen saturation of 95% in the ambulance. In the emergency department, he is wearing a cervical spine collar and his blood pressure is 76/48 mm Hg. He has a thready pulse, perioral cyanosis, and oxygen saturation of 90% in room air. He also has a compound fracture of his right humerus. Which of the following should be done first?

A. Administer ½ normal saline via a large-bore intravenous line.
B. Create a splint for the arm.
C. Determine the Glasgow Coma Scale score.
D. Give oxygen by face mask.
E. Order an immediate head CT scan.

82. A 3-year-old child is brought to the emergency department because he has been actively seizing for about 10 minutes. According to the rescue personnel, he was cyanotic when the team arrived 5 minutes after the seizure began, but has had oxygen saturation in the mid-90s since 100% oxygen was administered by face mask. The boy has a peripheral intravenous line in place. He continues with generalized tonic-clonic seizure activity during your primary assessment. Oxygen saturation is 97% on 100% oxygen. What is the next step in management?

A. Administer intravenous phenobarbital.
B. Draw blood for glucose and electrolytes.
C. Give diazepam rectally.
D. Obtain an emergency head CT.
E. Perform a lumbar puncture.

83. A 15-year-old girl is brought to the emergency department by her parents because she has been combative and irrational for the past hour. She has had type 1 diabetes mellitus for 6 years. Her parents do not know anything about her use of insulin. She recently broke up with her boyfriend and has been moody and tearful for the past week. While waiting to be seen by the triage nurse, the girl suddenly begins to seize and falls to the floor. You are the first one to reach her. She has stopped seizing but is unresponsive. What should you do?

A. Assess oxygenation with a pulse oximeter.
B. Begin immediate ventilation with a bag-valve-mask.
C. Initiate cardiopulmonary resuscitation.
D. Insert an intravenous line.
E. Use a jaw-thrust maneuver to open the airway.

84. The mother of an 11-year-old boy expresses concern about the family history of diabetes at her son's health-supervision visit. Two maternal aunts and the maternal grandmother have diabetes. Both parents and a sibling are overweight. The boy drinks four cans of soda each day and "eats more than his father." His height and weight are both at the 95th percentile. What physical examination finding would suggest that this boy is at risk for complications of type 2 diabetes?

A. Blood pressure = 121/78 mm Hg (90th percentile for age and height)
B. Body mass index = 21.2 (90th percentile)
C. Moon facies
D. Short stature
E. Waist circumference–to–height ratio = 0.58

85. A 12-year-old girl wishes to play basketball in seventh grade next autumn. She gives you the sports participation form, and you note several positive responses to questions in the medical history. The physical examination is entirely unremarkable. When you discuss the history and physical examination with the girl and her mother, you tell them that you cannot authorize participation in sports because of a positive answer to one question. The girl will need further evaluation. Which of the following questions led to this decision?

A. Are you susceptible to recurrent injury?
B. Did you ever pass out during strenuous exercise?
C. Do you have asthma?
D. Have you ever had head trauma with loss of consciousness?
E. Is there a family history of early heart attacks?

86. An unimmunized 4-year-old child cut his foot while playing in the city park and was taken by his mother to the emergency department to have the laceration sutured. The wound was carefully cleansed and the child was examined. Which of the following is the most appropriate next step in management?

A. Administer tetanus toxoid (DTaP).
B. Give ceftriaxone intramuscularly.
C. Inject tetanus immune globulin.
D. Obtain a radiograph of the foot.
E. Suture the laceration.

87. A 9-month-old boy was noted to have a heart murmur at the WIC clinic last week. His mother was told to have the child evaluated. Your colleague follows this child and has noted a "functional murmur" at past visits. The boy's mother says that she did not know that her son had a murmur. Today you hear a grade 2/6 systolic murmur, best heard at the left upper sternal border while the infant is supine. The murmur decreases in intensity when the infant sits up. Which of the following additional physical findings is most likely to accompany this murmur?

A. Bounding pulses
B. Diastolic rumble
C. Physiologically split S_2
D. Systolic click
E. Systolic murmur heard in the back

88. A 9-year-old Native-American boy has blood pressure of 120/76 mm Hg. Both systolic and diastolic pressures are at 90th to 95th percentile for age and stature. His weight is at the 90th percentile, height is at the 75th percentile, and BMI is > 95th percentile. He has acanthosis nigricans in his axillae and on his neck. Physical examination including ocular fundus examination is otherwise unremarkable. Family history is positive for hypertension in the father and his family and for type 2 diabetes in the mother's family. After discussing a program to increase physical activity and reduce food consumption, which of the following is the next step in management?

A. BP checks weekly at school

B. Oral glucose tolerance test

C. Renal ultrasound with Doppler study

D. TSH and free T_4 levels

E. Urinary cortisol levels

89. Parents of a 7½-year-old boy are concerned because he has "large tonsils" and has become "skinny" over the past year. They request tonsillectomy so that he will gain weight "and not catch so many colds." On physical examination his weight is 25th percentile, height is 75th percentile, and BMI is 25th percentile. His tonsils are moderately enlarged without inflammation. He has a few small, nontender anterior cervical lymph nodes and no nasal airway obstruction. Which of the following treatment plans will you recommend?

A. Antibiotics

B. Antihistamines

C. Nonsteroidal antiinflammatory drugs

D. Reevaluation at the 8-year checkup

E. Tonsillectomy

90. A 15-month-old girl developed fever of 103.5° F 24 hours ago. Fever responds to 100 mg of ibuprofen but returns about 6 hours after each dose. Fluid intake is reduced, and she has had a decrease in the number of wet diapers. Immunizations are completely up to date for age. Vital signs recorded by the office nurse while the girl was crying include temperature 38.3° C, respiratory rate 28 breaths/min, and pulse rate 150 beats/min. When you enter the room, the child watches you carefully. As long as you speak with the parents, she sits quietly on her mother's lap, but when you approach, she cries. Physical examination does not identify a specific source for fever. Which finding should make you consider a bacterial infection?

A. Elevated heart rate

B. Gender

C. Lack of response to ibuprofen

D. Negative reaction to examination

E. Tachypnea

91. At a health-supervision visit for a 2-year-old child, you reach the conclusion that motor development is somewhat behind expectations. You have regularly assessed development since age 15 months, when he first began to walk. Which of the following findings on physical examination today made you concerned about delayed gross motor development?

A. Attempts to balance on one foot cause him to fall.

B. He cannot hop on two feet.

C. He is unable to stoop to pick up an object.

D. Walking up steps can be done only while holding his parent's hand.

E. When he walks backward, he sometimes stumbles.

92. During the physical examination of a full-term newborn girl, you identify physical findings that suggest congenital adrenal hyperplasia. Which of the following is likely to be present if your patient has this disorder?

A. Epicanthal folds

B. Fusion of the labia

C. Low-set ears

D. Short arms and legs

E. Umbilical hernia

93. A 12-month-old infant is found to have a blood lead level of 14 µg/dl at a routine screening. The family lives in a home built in 1936 and has been renovating the house for the past 6 months. Which of the following physical examination findings is most likely for this infant?

A. Bulging fontanelle

B. Delayed motor development

C. Pallor

D. Periorbital and pretibial edema

E. Unremarkable physical examination

94. A child has had upper respiratory symptoms for the past 3 days and now has right ear pain and fever. The physical examination is consistent with the diagnosis of acute otitis media. Which of the following patient characteristics would allow you to select the option to observe the child with pain control rather than to immediately prescribe antibiotic treatment?

A. 30-month-old child

B. Fever = 103.5° F

C. Inconsolable crying

D. Parents have no telephone

E. Purulent discharge is found in the ear canal

95. A 2-year-old boy has had fever for the past 3 days. Temperature has responded to ibuprofen 100 mg every 6 hours, but when temperature increased again this afternoon to 104° F the boy's father brought him to the office for evaluation. He appears ill. Which of the following would prompt you to perform a sepsis workup on this boy?

A. A school-age child in your community has pertussis.

B. He has crackles in the right posterior lung fields.

C. Left ear canal is filled with a purulent discharge.

D. Parents refused immunizations during infancy.

E. Pharynx is inflamed with multiple vesicles.

96. A newborn infant is found to be hypotonic during the physical examination immediately after birth. In addition, multiple findings suggest to you that the infant has Down syndrome. Which of the following findings led to this diagnosis?

A. Cleft lip and palate

B. Extra digits on hands and feet

C. Long, narrow skull

D. Midfacial hypoplasia

E. Short arms and legs

97. A 13-year-old boy was diagnosed with type 1 diabetes mellitus 5 years ago and has had intermittently poor control of blood glucose levels. He currently uses a combination of short- and long-acting insulin to manage his diabetes. He has had behavioral problems this year at home and school and was recently picked up by the police with a small amount of marijuana. After recommending counseling for the boy and his family, the physician discusses a plan for long-term management. Which of the following should his physician monitor closely over the next several years?

A. Blood levels of cannabinol

B. Elevated body mass index

C. Pulmonary function tests

D. Urine protein

E. Visual acuity

98. Parents of a 2-month-old infant do not want you to administer any vaccine that contains live organisms because they read on a Web site that these vaccines can cause disease. Which of the following vaccines that are currently recommended for administration between birth and 12 months will be affected by the parental decision?

A. *Haemophilus influenzae* (Hib)

B. Hepatitis B

C. Trivalent polio

D. *Streptococcus pneumoniae* (PCV-7)

E. Varicella (Varivax)

99. An adolescent collapsed during a choir concert and was taken by ambulance to the emergency department. Eyewitnesses report that she suddenly fell to the floor but had no unusual movements. She was awake when her classmates came to her assistance. In the emergency department her pulse was 82 beats/min, respirations were 18 breaths/min, BP was 116/76 mm Hg, and oxygen saturation was 99% in room air. She had an unremarkable physical examination. Which of the following diagnoses is most consistent with this event?

A. Absence seizure
B. Basilar artery migraine
C. Cardiac arrhythmia
D. Hypoglycemia
E. Neurally mediated syncope

100. A 14-year-old with trisomy 21 (Down syndrome) comes to the office for a health-supervision visit. He is accompanied by his mother. He lives at home with both parents and a younger sister. He attends the local junior high school, where he has an individual education plan and resource teachers. Review of his chart shows that last year he was at Tanner stage 2 in his pubertal development. How will you structure today's visit so that you can address pubertal issues with this patient?

A. Ask him and his mother about sexual activity, alcohol, tobacco, and drugs.
B. Avoid sensitive issues such as tobacco, alcohol, sexual activity, and drugs.
C. Interview the boy without involving his mother.
D. Speak with the patient and his mother together to determine their wishes for the session.
E. Talk with the mother about puberty but do not bring this topic up with the boy.

Answers and Explanations

1. **The answer is B: Hematocrit.** The history of excessive milk consumption, pallor, tachycardia, and relatively limited dietary iron point to iron deficiency anemia caused by an imbalanced diet.

2. **The answer is C: Creatinine 3.0 mg/dl.** Bruising after a diarrheal illness with edema and elevated BP, plus low Hct, Hb, and platelet count point to hemolytic-uremic syndrome; hence, elevated creatine would be expected.

3. **The answer is A: Bone marrow aspiration.** Bruising and bleeding are accompanied by a CBC that shows depression of all cell lines, most consistent with leukemia. Bone marrow is needed.

4. **The answer is D: *Streptococcus pneumoniae*.** Because immunization status is unclear, this child with sickle cell anemia needs immunization against *S. pneumoniae*. Functional asplenia puts the child at risk for infection with encapsulated organisms.

5. **The answer is A: Abdominal ultrasound.** The most common origin of an abdominal mass in an infant or young child is the kidney. It is best evaluated with ultrasound.

6. **The answer is C: Hemoglobin of 12 g/dl.** This clinical pattern most likely reflects "toddler's diarrhea" from excessive consumption of sweetened drinks. It does not cause weight loss or abnormal lab test results. This is an osmotic diarrhea, so fecal osmotic gap would be > 50. Weight loss would accompany celiac disease, and 3 months of *C. difficile* toxin diarrhea is very unlikely. Lactase deficiency would produce GI symptoms and acid stool. The age-appropriate Hb of 12 g/dl is the best answer.

7. **The answer is A: Fat droplets.** This child's diarrhea is accompanied by weight loss and wasting, most likely the result of fat malabsorption that would be detected by presence of fat droplets in the stool.

8. **The answer is C: Pain that awakens a child from sleep at 2 a.m.** Pain that awakens a child during the night is a "red flag" for serious underlying disease.

9. **The answer is B: Total bilirubin 4.2 mg/dl, direct bilirubin 3.2 mg/dl.** Persistence of jaundice at 3 weeks of age plus an elevated direct bilirubin level point to cholestasis.

10. **The answer is C: Perform Hemoccult or Gastroccult test on stains.** The first step in evaluation of vomited "blood" is to ensure that it is indeed blood with Hemoccult or Gastroccult. This child most likely vomited a red beverage.

11. **The answer is E: Swallowed maternal blood.** This well newborn has passed a dark red stool that is positive for occult blood. The infant most likely swallowed maternal blood during delivery. An anal fissure would cause streaks of bright red blood. Ulcer and varices are far less likely. α_1-Antitrypsin deficiency does not cause GI bleeding.

12. **The answer is D: Neonatal screen detects problems before they become clinically apparent.** Neonatal screening is done because the conditions tested for are unlikely to be identified clinically before they cause harm to the newborn. Universal screening is *not* mandatory but is needed to ensure that these serious disorders are all detected, especially hypothyroidism. Hypoglycemia may be asymptomatic yet cause irreparable damage. Hemoglobinopathies may occur in children of any race or family background.

13. **The answer is A: First morning urine protein.** The only abnormality detected is 2+ proteinuria. Because it has persisted, the next step is to check a first-voided morning urine for protein. A negative test would support the diagnosis of orthostatic proteinuria. Serum albumin is not necessary because he has no edema. Renal disease is unlikely because of the absence of hematuria.

14. **The answer is C: Determine serum albumin, cholesterol, and creatinine.** This child most likely has nephrotic syndrome. She has no hematuria or hypertension to suggest nephritis. Serum albumin is likely to be low, cholesterol elevated, and creatinine age-appropriate.

15. **The answer is B: Primary enuresis.** Approximately 7% of 7-year-old children have enuresis. This otherwise totally healthy child has an unremarkable urinalysis. Because she has never been dry at night, she has primary enuresis.

16. **The answer is B: Calcium-to-creatinine ration in urine.** The best test is the calcium-to-creatinine ratio in urine, because this child has no evidence for infection or glomerulonephritis. A renal stone is unlikely because of the absence of pain.

17. **The answer is D: Send a catheterized urine specimen for urinalysis and culture.** This clinical picture is most likely caused by pyelonephritis. Urine culture is important, and the specimen must be obtained by catheter, not a urine bag. Ultrasound and VCUG may be necessary at a later date, but not now. It is inappropriate to treat with antibiotics without cultures.

18. **The answer is E: Weight and length are age-appropriate.** This is a healthy child, thriving on breast feeding. Development is age-appropriate. He does not need TB testing because he was born in California. Immunization records can be obtained from the previous physician.

19. **The answer is D: Perform the urine drug screen only if the adolescent consents.** Drug testing must only be done with the assent/consent of the adolescent. The physician risks losing the patient's confidence if specimens are taken surreptitiously. There is no federal mandate for drug testing. Encouraging communication between the adolescent and his parents is a good idea.

20. **The answer is B: Benign gynecomastia.** Benign pubertal gynecomastia is common at this boy's stage of puberty. He is not obese, so he does not have pseudogynecomastia. Prolonged adrenergic steroid use would be associated with increased muscle bulk and early growth spurt. He has no drug history that would explain the mass. Cancer is rare.

21. **The answer is D: Pelvic examination.** A pelvic examination is the proper evaluation to assess the structural integrity of the genital tract. This girl had onset of puberty at age 11 years and is now at stage IV puberty. Menarche should have occurred by age 13 or 14 years. Hormonal and radiologic tests are unneeded because pubertal development is age-appropriate.

22. **The answer is B: Depression.** Fatigue, poor appetite, weight loss, and poor school performance all point to depression.

23. **The answer is A: Ibuprofen treatment at the time of menses.** Menstrual cramps occur only with ovulatory periods, which begin within the first year after menarche. It is appropriate to use nonsteroidal antiinflammatory agents. More evaluation is not needed for this otherwise-healthy adolescent unless she does not respond to the initial management or other signs and symptoms develop.

24. **The answer is E: Testicular length < 2.5 cm.** This boy is still prepubertal at age 15 years. He is short and is most likely to have stage I testicular development (< 2.5 cm). Axillary and pubic hair only appears after testicular enlargement occurs. Short stature could be genetic. BMI is age- and stature-appropriate.

25. **The answer is E: Urethral swab to test for *Chlamydia* and gonorrhea.** This adolescent's history, symptoms, and examination findings are consistent with a sexually transmitted infection. A urethral swab test will most likely identify *Chlamydia* or gonorrhea. His symptoms are not consistent with *E. coli* UTI, and treatment would only be started if a urine culture identified the organism. *Gardnerella* can colonize the urethra in males but is asymptomatic. Identification of sexual contacts will be appropriate after STI has been confirmed.

26. **The answer is D: Rapid growth begins immediately following the appearance of breast buds.** Rapid growth begins once breast buds appear at stage II puberty in girls. A thin, odor-free discharge commonly occurs around the time of puberty onset. Menarche occurs approximately 2 years after onset of puberty, just after the peak of the growth spurt at stage IV puberty.

27. **The answer is C: Skeletal survey.** The history of injury is not consistent with the severity of the fracture. In addition, the delay in seeking medical attention is a "red flag." Skeletal survey is the most appropriate next step in evaluation. Head CT may be needed as the investigation proceeds, but it is not the first study for this alert infant. Other studies listed are not appropriate.

28. **The answer is D: Physical examination in sexual abuse often shows no trauma.** This child's history must be considered seriously. Physical examination is most likely to be unremarkable. Physical findings such as genital trauma or a large hymenal orifice are not necessary to make the diagnosis of sexual abuse. She is unlikely to have positive culture for gonorrhea or the presence of semen in the vagina.

29. **The answer is E: Subdural effusion caused by violent shaking should be sought with head CT.** An infant with altered level of consciousness, a bulging fontanel, and a history that is inconsistent with the findings must be considered to be a possible victim of abuse. Head CT is the most appropriate evaluation.

30. **The answer is C: Impulsive behavior that results in frequent injuries.** Of the behaviors listed, impulsivity is most consistent with ADHD.

31. **The answer is A: Cognitive testing to compare ability with school performance.** A child with a learning disability may be labeled with a behavior problem such as ADHD. This boy manifests his concerning behavior only at school. Children with ADHD have problem behavior in more than one environment. Cognitive and other neuropsychological testing will assist with the diagnosis of learning disorder. There are no neurologic findings or behaviors

specific for learning disability. Medications have no place in management of learning disabilities nor do eye exercises.

32. **The answer is B: Griseofulvin orally.** The "black dot" alopecia is characteristic of tinea capitis and must be treated with systemic griseofulvin. Antibiotics, hydrocortisone, and topical antifungal agents will have no effect.

33. **The answer is B: Erythema infectiosum.** The rash described is most consistent with erythema infectiosum (fifth disease), caused by parvovirus B19.

34. **The answer is E: Selenium sulfide 2.5% topically.** The rash described is tinea versicolor and is best treated with selenium sulfide lotion 2.5%.

35. **The answer is C: Hydrocortisone 1% topically.** The rash has lesions and distribution characteristic of atopic dermatitis. The patient's age and the family history of asthma (atopy) are also consistent with the diagnosis. The best treatment among those listed is hydrocortisone 1% topically.

36. **The answer is B: "Crops" of skin lesions with progressive crusting.** This adopted child has varicella. It is likely that he did not receive the varicella vaccine at age 1 year. The characteristic rash of varicella is crops of vesicles that appear daily for 5 to 7 days with progressive crusting.

37. **The answer is E: X-linked.** Duchenne muscular dystrophy is transmitted as an X-linked trait.

38. **The answer is C: Discuss the benign nature of the seizure.** This child has had a simple febrile seizure, a benign condition. She needs no further workup or treatment.

39. **The answer is B: Headache diary.** This girl has recurrent, acute headaches that have characteristics of migraine. A headache diary is the best approach to obtain more information. She has no findings that suggest the need for an extensive workup at this time.

40. **The answer is A: Attention deficit hyperactivity disorder.** Tics are associated with ADHD and may reflect Tourette syndrome.

41. **The answer is C: Muscle strength 5/5 symmetrically in upper and lower extremities.** Appearance of acute ataxia following a viral upper respiratory infection is consistent with acute cerebellar ataxia. Aside from the unsteadiness and slurred speech, he should have no other abnormal findings. Strength and reflexes will be equal and age-appropriate in all extremities. There would be no findings of a progressive disease.

42. **The answer is B: Development is appropriate for adjusted gestational age.** This girl has appropriate development for her corrected gestational age of approximately 12 to 13 months.

43. **The answer is E: Review developmental progress at the 18-month visit.** Most 15-month-old children born at term will be walking. Everything else in this boy's history and physical examination point to appropriate development, so the most reasonable approach is to reassess him at the 18-month visit. No other testing is needed now, nor are referrals to a neurologist, physical therapist, or developmental specialist. "Reassurance" will not help the mother stop worrying.

44. **The answer is B: Hypotonia.** This 10-month-old is hypotonic.

45. **The answer is A: Audiometry results.** Delayed language development often occurs when children have impaired hearing. Audiometry is the best first test for this boy. He has no clinical findings for autism, and the other options have little relevance.

46. **The answer is D: Neuromuscular findings reflect a static brain injury.** This child has "cerebral palsy" with spasticity, microcephaly, hemiplegia, and delayed development, all of which reflect a static brain injury. He is not weak or hypotonic. Malaria is not a likely cause. He is not likely to progress, nor will he improve with the treatments listed.

47. **The answer is C: Passive internal and external rotation of the left leg causes pain in the knee.** Knee pain with rotation of the left leg points to a problem in the hip. Symmetrical muscle bulk plus *absence* of swelling, fever, and obesity make transient synovitis most likely. A child with atrophy of the left thigh muscles might have a chronic problem. High fever would suggest osteomyelitis or arthritis (with appropriate additional findings).

48. **The answer is B: Erythrocyte sedimentation rate 42 mm/hr.** The characteristic features of juvenile rheumatoid arthritis will be associated with an elevated ESR. He would be unlikely to have renal disease, microcytic anemia, or a positive ANA.

49. **The answer is C: Regular urinalysis to detect signs of nephritis.** Patients with SLE have high likelihood of developing nephritis and should be monitored for the appearance of proteinuria and hematuria. Antibiotics, ECG, and eye examinations are not needed routinely. SLE typically does not cause myositis.

50. **The answer is D: His symptoms worsen around grandmother's cat.** A reaction that flares on exposure to an antigen (cat dander) is likely to be allergic. Family history is helpful but not specific. "Winter dry skin" is not the same as atopic dermatitis. Tobacco smoke is a nonspecific irritant that should be avoided by all children. The skin test reaction to dog hair is the same as to histamine, thus it is nonspecific.

51. **The answer is B: Beclomethasone nasal spray, hydroxyzine, and pseudoephedrine daily.** The best combination includes an antihistamine (hydroxyzine), a decongestant (pseudoephedrine), and an antiinflammatory nasal spray (beclomethasone). She does not need antibiotics. Cromolyn is ineffective. Oxymetazoline is an effective

decongestant but should not be used for more than 3 days. Systemic prednisone is likely to cause major side effects if used for 2 months.

52. **The answer is B: Daily maintenance fluid requirements.** He *must* have maintenance fluids before and after operation: IV before and by mouth as soon as tolerated after surgery. He will not likely have surgical drains, has no diarrhea, and should have no reason for diminished urine output. Temperature will be monitored but will not likely affect management, unless it becomes elevated.

53. **The answer is C: Serum chloride 88 mEq/dl.** The characteristic clinical picture of pyloric stenosis and the duration of vomiting place this infant at risk for hypochloremic metabolic alkalosis and dehydration. Creatinine may well be elevated.

54. **The answer is D: Fever.** Fever causes increased insensible water loss. Eczema should not affect insensible loss. Diarrhea and vomiting are components of pathologic fluid loss.

55. **The answer is C: Isotonic saline.** This infant is severely dehydrated, has signs of vascular insufficiency (shock), and has reduced renal function manifested by an elevated serum creatinine. He needs a rapid infusion (bolus) of isotonic saline ("normal saline"). Using his current weight of 10 kg, he will be given 200 ml of isotonic saline (20 ml/kg) over a 30-minute period. The other fluids are inappropriate (3% NaCl) or not needed. The ½ NS is hypotonic and will not be effective to reverse the hypovolemia. Potassium is dangerous in a dehydrated child with reduced renal function! Packed RBCs or Plasmanate may be needed if he does not respond to two treatments with the isotonic saline.

56. **The answer is B: Capillary refill < 2 seconds.** Brisk capillary refill shows that this child has only mild dehydration. Oral rehydration is recommended. All other findings listed suggest more severe dehydration.

57. **The answer is B: Blood lead level.** He needs a blood lead level test because of the high likelihood of exposure in Mexico. PPD is negative, so CXR is not needed. The other tests are not indicated.

58. **The answer is A: Admit to hospital for intravenous fluids and antibiotics.** This toddler is dehydrated and toxic with a UTI. Catheterized urine will demonstrate protein, blood, leukocytes, and motile bacteria. A culture will eventually be positive, but the diagnosis of UTI is clinically apparent. Because she is toxic appearing, she should be treated in hospital. She needs IV fluids and antibiotic therapy in hospital until she is afebrile and clinically improved. Consult may or may not be needed. VCUG will be part of the workup at a later date.

59. **The answer is C: Genetic testing should be done when the siblings reach reproductive age.** Genetic testing to detect the carrier state for cystic fibrosis is best delayed until the siblings reach reproductive age and can make informed decisions.

60. The answer is D: Single malformations, such as VSD, occur in 2% to 3% of all newborns. A single congenital malformation may be found in 2% to 3% of all newborns. VSD is the most common congenital heart defect, but it is not caused by a chromosomal abnormality and DNA testing is not indicated. Cardiac defects do occur in infants born to poorly controlled diabetic mothers, but this infant's mother had no signs of diabetes during pregnancy and the infant had none of the findings of an infant of a diabetic mother. Study of family members is not indicated.

61. The answer is B: Elevated blood pressure. A short, prepubertal adolescent may have Turner syndrome. Hypertension as a result of coarctation of the aorta must be looked for. Shield chest, low hairline, and webbed neck are additional findings.

62. The answer is E: Viral URI. This child has a URI.

63. The answer is D: The 5-year-old brother says that one of his Lego blocks is missing. The disappearance of the Lego block (small enough to be aspirated) combined with the sudden onset of coughing, persistence of cough for 2 weeks, asymmetrical wheezing, and diminished right-sided breath sounds suggest a foreign body aspiration. The cough of pertussis starts after a prodrome of runny nose. Asthma would have more diffuse wheeze. Viral illness may persist for 2 weeks, but other findings point away from this diagnosis.

64. The answer is D: Sweat chloride test. Failure to gain weight and a voracious appetite suggests malabsorption, which is likely to be caused by cystic fibrosis. The chronic cough adds additional support for this diagnosis. Diagnosis is confirmed by the sweat chloride test. Neonatal screen for CF was likely not available.

65. The answer is D: Oxygen by nasal prongs. An infant with hypoxia, tachypnea, and wheeze in the winter likely has RSV bronchiolitis. Because of the respiratory distress and low oxygen saturation, she needs oxygen and supportive treatment. Further albuterol is unlikely to help. If a corticosteroid is administered, it should be dexamethasone orally or IM. Antibiotics and antiviral agents are not indicated.

66. The answer is B: *Chlamydia trachomatis*. This infant's clinical course is most consistent with pneumonia caused by *Chlamydia trachomatis*, transmitted during the birth process. She would be much more ill if she had infection with *S. pneumoniae* or Group B streptococcus. RSV would likely cause more hypoxemia.

67. The answer is C: *Pseudomonas aeruginosa*. When children with cystic fibrosis have chronic respiratory disease, they commonly have infection with *Pseudomonas aeruginosa*. *S. pneumoniae* would likely cause much higher fever, and the immunization with PCV-7 vaccine would reduce likelihood of infection. The pattern of illness is not consistent with RSV or *B. pertussis* infection.

68. **The answer is E: Place the infant to sleep on her back.** This infant has many risk factors for sudden infant death syndrome. The most immediately effective intervention would be "back to sleep." Smoking anywhere inside the home exposes the infant to the dangers of secondhand smoke. Cessation of cigarette smoking by the mother would definitely benefit the infant, as would smoking outside of the home. Apnea monitors and sleep studies have no proven benefit. The "spitting up" is not a risk factor for SIDS.

69. **The answer is E: Use of cow's milk before 12 months causes iron deficiency.** Occult GI bleeding caused by cow's milk fed to infants in the first year of life is a common cause of iron deficiency. Milk ingestion does not trigger development of lactose deficiency, nor is cow's milk protein malabsorbed. Although eczema may develop in infants fed cow's milk, it is not specifically associated with milk intake. Cow's milk is rich in folic acid.

70. **The answer is D: Immunoglobulins in colostrum protect against infection.** Colostrum is low in volume and nutrients, but rich in immunoglobulins, cells, and many other nonnutritive substances that protect the newborn against infection.

71. **The answer is E: Undescended testicles.** He is LGA and premature. Premature boys commonly have undescended testicles. The rest of the findings listed are those found in full-term newborns.

72. **The answer is A: Blood and CSF cultures.** The major concerning findings are lethargy, poor feeding, inability to maintain temperature, evidence of shock, and the elevated direct bilirubin. This combination suggests sepsis and requires blood and CSF cultures plus empirical antibiotic treatment.

73. **The answer is C: Hypoglycemia.** This SGA post-term infant is at risk for hypoglycemia in the immediate postnatal period and blood glucose must be monitored closely. She is at increased risk of fetal alcohol syndrome and also has an increased risk of SIDS. Workup for TORCHS infections may also be needed later if specific findings are identified.

74. **The answer is E: Parents will be notified if neonatal screening detects any abnormalities.** The neonatal screening results will be provided if abnormalities are identified. Feeding schedules are not recommended. "Back to sleep" is recommended until the infant rolls spontaneously. Safety seats belong in the back seat. Physiologic jaundice occurs at about 2 days of life; late onset jaundice may reflect liver disease.

75. **The answer is D: Healthy newborn infants may nurse as often as every 90 minutes.** A breast-fed newborn may feed as often as every 90 minutes and should have 6 or more wet diapers per day if the mother's milk supply is adequate. An infant who nurses ~10 minutes at each breast will obtain most of the milk from the breasts.

The only nutrients in human milk that are inadequate are iron and vitamins D and K. Maternal URI should not preclude nursing.

76. **The answer is A: Bacterial arthritis.** This toxic-appearing, febrile boy is holding his leg in the position that minimizes pain in the hip, a position seen with septic (bacterial) arthritis. Toxic synovitis is a postviral syndrome and is not accompanied by such serious findings. Legg-Calvé disease is not an infectious process and would not present with toxicity. Lyme disease and rheumatoid arthritis are also not likely given the clinical findings.

77. **The answer is E: Perform a lumbar puncture.** An unimmunized, febrile, lethargic, toxic-appearing infant with a bulging fontanel likely has meningitis. Lumbar puncture is the appropriate procedure. She also needs a blood culture and IV antibiotics. She is dehydrated and needs a rapid infusion of isotonic fluid (normal saline), NOT hypotonic fluid (D5W). Other tests may be needed later.

78. **The answer is A: Explain that the boy does not need testing for tuberculosis.** This boy has no need for a PPD, CXR, INH therapy, or BCG immunization.

79. **The answer is D: Epstein-Barr virus infection.** The clinical picture described is most consistent with Epstein-Barr virus infection. Streptococcal pharyngitis does not cause splenomegaly. Generalized lymphadenopathy and splenomegaly occur with leukemia, but the CBC would usually show anemia and thrombocytopenia. Cat scratch disease is usually localized to the nodes in the drainage pattern of the scratch. Coxsackie virus commonly causes a vesicular rash.

80. **The answer is D: Kawasaki disease.** The clinical picture fits Kawasaki disease. Bacterial conjunctivitis usually has a purulent discharge. Viral conjunctivitis does not have the other findings demonstrated by the child. Adenovirus can cause fever and intense conjunctival erythema, but not the rash and swollen extremities. Chlamydial conjunctivitis also does not fit the clinical picture.

81. **The answer is D: Give oxygen by face mask.** *First* he needs oxygen, because oxygen saturation has fallen and he has perioral cyanosis. He will *next* need isotonic IV fluids (NOT ½ NS) to restore circulating volume and combat shock. The other options will be deferred until the boy is stable.

82. **The answer is B: Draw blood for glucose and electrolytes.** Check blood glucose and electrolytes first, then manage the seizure. IV glucose may be beneficial, as may rectal diazepam.

83. **The answer is E: Use a jaw-thrust maneuver to open the airway.** Use a jaw-thrust maneuver to open her airway and call for assistance as you do so. Maintain the airway until help arrives.

84. **The answer is E: Waist circumference-to-height ratio = 0.58.** Waist-circumference-to-height ratio > 0.5 is associated with adverse outcomes of type 2 DM. BP and BMI at 90th percentile are concerning

but not as closely linked to adverse outcomes of DM type 2. Moon facies and short stature result from excess corticosteroid (either exogenous or endogenous).

85. **The answer is B: Did you ever pass out during strenuous exercise.** Loss of consciousness during exercise may be caused by cardiac outflow obstruction, such as hypertrophic cardiomyopathy. This is a contraindication to physical activity and must be evaluated promptly. Asthma can be managed medically. Concussion may or may not have sequelae that interfere with activity.

86. **The answer is C: Inject tetanus immune globulin.** This unimmunized boy needs immediate passive (preformed) immunity in the form of immune globulin. He will also need the tetanus toxoid, but it should be given after the immune globulin. Antibiotic use, x-ray, and suturing will be determined clinically.

87. **The answer is C: Physiologically split S_2.** Physiologically split S_2 accompanies a flow or "functional" murmur. The murmur changes with position. The other findings point to cardiac pathology.

88. **The answer is A: BP checks weekly at school.** Follow BP on a regular basis to establish its pattern and to see if it is consistently at or above 90th percentile. Oral GTT is not indicated, but it would be appropriate to order a fasting blood glucose and lipid panel at a later date. The boy's growth pattern is not consistent with hypothyroidism or Cushing's syndrome. Renal ultrasound is not needed.

89. **The answer is D: Reevaluation at the 8-year checkup.** Reevaluation at his next scheduled visit is the best answer. The tonsils and lymph nodes respond to recurrent viral infections and may remain persistently prominent. Tonsils are not "large" and the boy's weight and BMI are within the expected range. Tonsillectomy will not prevent viral infections. Allergy does not cause tonsils to enlarge.

90. **The answer is B: Gender.** This child's biggest risk factor is her gender, because febrile girls have a high rate of urinary tract infections. She is alert, wary about your presence, and cries when you approach. She is not lethargic or irritable. Tachycardia reflects the elevated temperature and crying during vital signs. Respiratory rate is age-appropriate. Fever response is non-specific.

91. **The answer is C: He is unable to stoop to pick up an object.** A 2-year-old child routinely stoops and recovers objects from the floor. Because this child cannot do this, you should assess motor skills. The other motor skills listed are age-appropriate.

92. **The answer is B: Fusion of the labia.** A girl with congenital adrenal hyperplasia will be virilized and have fused labia. The other findings listed are not associated with CAH, although epicanthal folds may occur in healthy children, in addition to many different syndromes.

93. **The answer is E: Unremarkable physical examination.** This child has elevated blood lead at a level that would not be expected to cause

any physical findings. The examination would be unremarkable. Although chronic lead exposure can cause developmental delay, the findings usually appear later in life as behavioral problems or cognitive deficiencies.

94. **The answer is A: 30-month-old child.** Observation with pain control is a management option for children older than 24 months who have acute otitis media with mild symptoms, low-grade fever, and the ability to contact the physician if the symptoms worsen. A purulent discharge in the canal is likely the result of a TM perforation and generally is treated with antibiotics.

95. **The answer is D: Parents refused immunizations during infancy.** This boy did not receive immunization against *S. pneumoniae* and *H. influenzae* type b. A sepsis workup is indicated because he has high risk for bacteremia, meningitis, and other invasive infections caused by these organisms. Pneumonia, otitis media, and viral pharyngitis can cause fever but usually do not require sepsis workup. Pertussis is a risk for this boy, but his illness currently has no features of this disease.

96. **The answer is D: Midfacial hypoplasia.** Midfacial hypoplasia is characteristic of Down syndrome (trisomy 21). Extra digits can be found on otherwise healthy children and also with many different syndromes. The other findings are not characteristic of Down syndrome.

97. **The answer is D: Urine protein.** The boy is at risk for the vascular complications of DM, especially renal. Proteinuria will be an early sign of renal involvement. Regular evaluations by an ophthalmologist are recommended, but decreased visual acuity will not be one of the likely abnormalities caused by DM complications. Obesity with elevated BMI is most often a precursor of Type 2 DM. Social dysfunction as manifested by marijuana use will need management but not with blood levels of cannabinol.

98. **The answer is E: Varicella (Varivax).** Varivax is the only vaccine on the list that has live, attenuated organisms. The vaccine occasionally causes a localized vesicular rash at the site of injection, but this is not a contraindication to its use.

99. **The answer is E: Neurally medicated syncope.** The events surrounding the episode fit best with neurally mediated syncope, which causes transient loss of consciousness or "fainting" without findings that point to a more serious cause. The prompt return to lucidity does not fit with a seizure, arrhythmia, migraine, or hypoglycemia.

100. **The answer is D: Speak with the patient and his mother together to determine their wishes for the session.** The best approach is to observe how the boy and his mother interact and to ask them both how they wish the session to be handled. This boy's level of maturity will influence the extent to which you ask him about personal habits. It is not appropriate to *assume* that he can or cannot discuss pubertal topics or that his mother will make all decisions.

Index

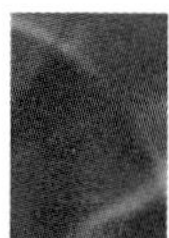

Page numbers followed by an *f*, *t*, or *b* indicate figures, tables and boxed material, respectively; **bold** refers to case answers.

B

C

E

F

G

H

I

M

N

O

R

T

U

W

X

Y